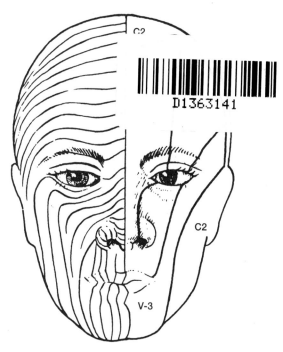

Left side: Relaxed skin tension lines. *Right side*: Dermatome chart—sensory root fields.

Note: The illustrations on the inside covers and facing front cover, dermatome charts and relaxed skin tension lines, represent approximations, since there is much overlap and individual variation. Denervation of one posterior root will not produce complete anesthesia within the corresponding dermatome. The direction of the relaxed skin tension lines (RSTL) should always be assessed before making an ellipsoidal incision parallel to, or a punch biopsy with skin stretched perpendicular to, these lines (see Fig. 37-1, p. 256). In areas of flexion creases, flex and note the direction of the majority of "wrinkle" lines, that is, the direction of the RSTL. In nonflexion areas, the RSTL is determined by picking up skin folds between thumb and index finger and pinching, proceeding in a clockwise direction, until it is clear in which direction wrinkle lines are most numerous, straight, and parallel to one another. In certain areas it is difficult or impossible to find the RSTL. In that situation, make a small circular incision or "punch" to see in which direction the ellipse forms.

MANUAL OF DERMATOLOGIC THERAPEUTICS

ition

t, MD

sicians

husetts

itology

ecticut

tology)

School

ipshire

neritus

School

husetts

I, MD

sicians

husetts

tology)

School

ipshire

kins

Acquisitions Editor: Susan Rhyner
Managing Editor: Lauren Aquino
Project Manager: Alicia Jackson
Senior Manufacturing Manager: Benjamin Rivera
Marketing Manager: Kimberley Schonberger
Designer: Terry Mallon
Cover Designer: Becky Baxendell
Production Services: Laserwords Private Limited, Chennai, India
Printer: RR Donnelley-Crawfordsville

© 2007 by LIPPINCOTT WILLIAMS & WILKINS, a Wolters Kluwer business

530 Walnut Street
Philadelphia, PA 19106 USA
LWW.com

6th edition, © 2002 Lippincott Williams & Wilkins

Printed in the USA

Library of Congress Cataloging-in-Publication Data

Arndt, Kenneth A., 1936-
  Manual of dermatologic therapeutics / Kenneth A. Arndt, Jeffrey T.S. Hsu.—7th ed.
    p. ; cm.
  Includes bibliographical references and index.
  ISBN-13: 978-0-7817-6058-4
  ISBN-10: 0-7817-6058-5
  1. Dermatology—Handbooks, manuals, etc. 2. Skin—Diseases —Treatment—Handbooks, manuals, etc.   I. Hsu, Jeffrey T. S. II. Title.
  [DNLM: 1. Skin Diseases—therapy—Handbooks. 2. Skin Diseases —diagnosis—Handbooks. 3. Skin Diseases—physiopathology—Hand-books.   WR 39 A747m 2007]
  RL74.A75 2007
  616.5—dc22
                                    2006031492

10 9 8 7 6 5 4 3 2 1

To my family, with love: Anne, David, Jennifer, Pablo, Alexander, and Benjamin.

Kenneth A. Arndt

To my father, my mother, my wife Anita, and my mentors for their encouragement and inspiration.

Jeffrey T.S. Hsu

CONTENTS

II: PROCEDURES AND TECHNIQUES

III: TREATMENT PRINCIPLES AND FORMULARY

$\mathcal{T}$he first six editions of the *Manual of Dermatologic Therapeutics* have been greeted with considerable enthusiasm. It is gratifying that such an approach to rational therapeutics has found such widespread use throughout the world, and that this information has been disseminated through several editions in Spanish, Portuguese, French, Italian, Indonesian, Japanese and Taiwanese editions.

The seventh edition has been totally revised and rewritten in collaboration with many talented colleagues. Each chapter and section has undergone close scrutiny, and has been updated, revised significantly, or totally rewritten. New textual reference and tabular material has been added.

The *Manual* presents up-to-date information on the pathophysiology, diagnosis, and therapy of common cutaneous disorders. Diagnostic procedures and surgical and photobiologic techniques are explained in both theoretical and practical terms. The pharmacology and optimal use of dermatologic medication are discussed in detail.

The first portion of the *Manual* is organized so that a disease is defined initially and its pathophysiology is discussed according to the problem-oriented record system. Each disease is then subdivided into subjective data (symptoms), objective data (clinical findings), assessment, and therapy sections. A sequence of therapeutic interventions and alternative approaches to treatment is emphasized. The remainder of the text is concerned with procedures, techniques, treatment principles, and discussion of the pharmacodynamics, and usage of specific medications employed in treating cutaneous disease.

We hope that the seventh edition of the *Manual* is as helpful an educational and practical guide to therapeutics and disease management as the previous six have been.

Kenneth A. Arndt, MD
Jeffrey T.S. Hsu, MD

R. Sonia Batra, MD, MSc, MPH
Clinical Assistant Professor
Department of Dermatology
University of Southern California;
Keck School of Medicine
Los Angeles, California;
Section Head
Dermatology and Dermatologic Surgery
City of Hope National Medical Center
Duarte, California

Ashish C. Bhatia, MD
Assistant Professor of Clinical Dermatology
Department of Dermatology
Northwestern University
Feinberg School of Medicine
Chicago, Illinois;
Director
Department of Dermatology
and Dermatologic Surgery
River North Dermatology and
Dermatologic Surgery
DuPage Medical Group
Naperville, Illinois

Melissa A. Bogle, MD
Director
The Laser and Cosmetic Surgery
Center of Houston;
Clinical Assistant Professor
Department of Dermatology
The University of Texas
MD Anderson Cancer Center
Houston, Texas

Karen Chen, MD
Clinical Assistant Professor
Department of Dermatology
University of Minnesota;
Dermatologist
Department of Dermatology
Minneapolis VA Medical Center
Minneapolis, Minnesota

Jennifer Nam Choi, MD
Chief Resident
Department of Dermatology
Yale University School of Medicine
Yale-New Haven Hospital
New Haven, Connecticut

Sola Choi, MD
Adult and Pediatric Dermatology
Concord, Massachusetts

Danielle M. DeHoratius, MD
Resident
Department of Dermatology
Yale-New Haven Hospital
New Haven, Connecticut

Adrienne M. Feasel, MD
Clinical Dermatology
Ladera Park Dermatology
Austin, Texas

David E. Geist, MD
Resident
Department of Dermatology
Tufts-New England Medical Center
Boston, Massachusetts

Elaine S. Gilmore, MD, PhD
Research Fellow;
Dermatology Resident
Department of Dermatology
Yale University School of Medicine
New Haven, Connecticut

Kira R. Giovanielli, MD
Affiliate
Department of Dermatology
Medical Center of Aurora, South
Aurora, Colorado

John G. Hancox, MD
Mohs Surgeon
Department of Dermatology
Mountain State Medical Specialities
Clarksburg, West Virginia

Shih-Ping Hsu, Pharm D
Pharmacist
Department of Pharmacy
Swedish Medical Center
Seattle, Washington

Jennifer Hunter-Yates, MD
Fellow in Laser and Cosmetic Dermatology
Boston Dermatology and Laser Center;
Massachusetts General Hospital
Boston, Massachusetts

Joseph L. Jorizzo, MD
Professor and Former "Founding Chair"
Department of Dermatology
Wake Forest University School of Medicine
Winston Salem, North Carolina

Wanla Kulwichit, MD
Assistant Professor
Division of Infectious Diseases
Department of Medicine
Faculty of Medicine
Chulalongkorn University;
Assistant Professor
Department of Medicine
King Chulalongkorn Memorial Hospital
Bangkok, Thailand

Ken K. Lee, MD
Associate Professor
Departments of Dermatology, Surgery,
Otolaryngology-Head and Neck Surgery;
Director of Dermatologic
and Laser Surgery
Oregon Health and Science University
Portland, Oregon

Khosrow M. Mehrany, MD
Assistant Clinical Professor
Department of Dermatology
University of California
San Francisco, California

Janine D'Amelio Miller, MD
Clinical Fellow
Department of Dermatology
Case Western Reserve University,
University Hospitals of Cleveland
Cleveland, Ohio;

Maryam Moinfar, MD
Los Angeles, California

Julie A. Neville, MD
Clinical Instructor
Department of Dermatologic Surgery
Yale University School of Medicine
New Haven, Connecticut

Manisha J. Patel, MD
Senior Resident
Department of Dermatology
Wake Forest University
Winston Salem, North Carolina

Brian Poligone, MD, PhD
Research Fellow;
Dermatology Resident
Department of Dermatology
Yale University School of Medicine
New Haven, Connecticut

Peter C. Schalock, MD
Instructor of Dermatology
Department of Dermatology
Harvard Medical School;
Assistant in Dermatology
Department of Dermatology
Massachusetts General Hospital
Boston, Massachusetts

Jeffrey M. Sobell, MD
Assistant Professor
Department of Dermatology
Tufts University School of Medicine
Boston, Massachusetts
SkinCare Physicians
Chestnut Hill, Massachusetts

Steven Q. Wang, MD
Assistant Attending Physician
Department of Medicine, Dermatology
Service
Memorial Sloan Kettering Cancer Center
New York, New York

Penpun Wattanakrai, MD
Assistant Professor
Division of Dermatology
Department of Medicine
Ramathibodi Hospital, Mahidol University
Bangkok, Thailand

Christopher B. Yelverton, MD, MBA
Research Fellow
Department of Dermatology
Wake Forest University Health Sciences
Winston Salem, North Carolina

Ethel Ying, MD, FRCP(C)
Assistant Professor
Department of Pediatrics
University of Toronto;
Director of Nurseries
Department of Pediatrics
St. Michael's Hospital
Ontario, Canada

Gil Yosipovitch, MD
Professor
Department of Dermatology
Wake Forest University School of Medicine
Winston-Salem, North Carolina

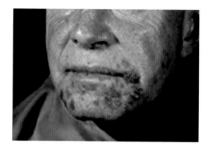

Color Plate 1. Impetigo.

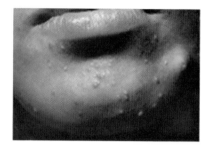

Color Plate 2. Molluscum contagiosum.

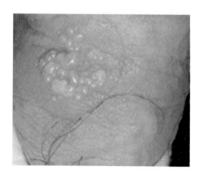

Color Plate 3. Herpes simplex.

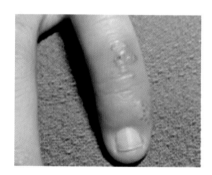

Color Plate 4. Herpetic whitlow.

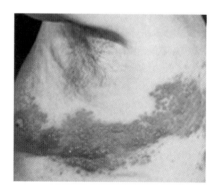

Color Plate 5. Herpes zoster.

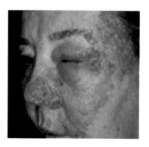

Color Plate 6. Herpes zoster—Ramsay Hunt syndrome.

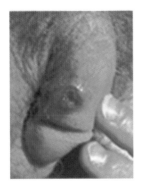

Color Plate 7. Primary syphilis.

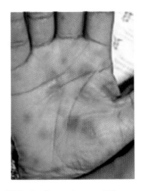

Color Plate 8. Secondary syphilis.

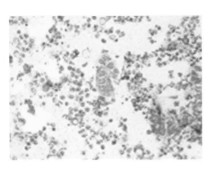

Color Plate 9. Tzanck preparation.

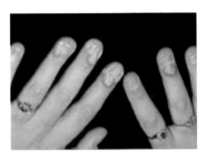

Color Plate 10. Periungual warts.

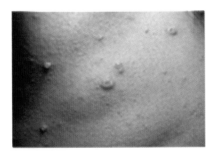

Color Plate 11. Varicella.

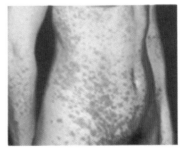

Color Plate 12. Pityriasis rosea.

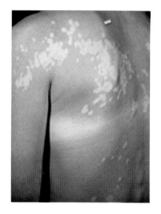

Color Plate 13. Tinea versicolor.

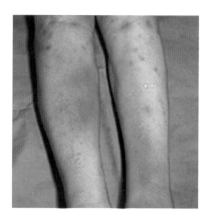

Color Plate 14. Erythema nodosum.

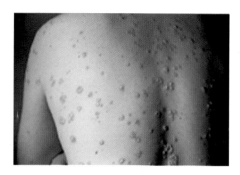

Color Plate 15. Guttate psoriasis.

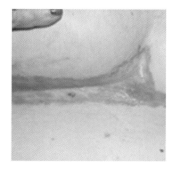

Color Plate 16. Intertrigo.

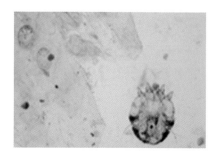

Color Plate 17. Scabies.

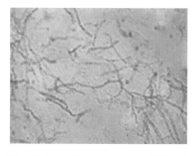

Color Plate 18. Fungal scrapings: KOH with Schwartz-Lamkin stain.

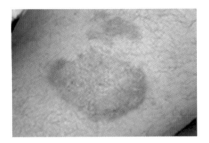

Color Plate 19. Tinea corporis.

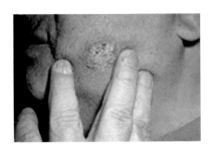

Color Plate 20. Tinea barbae with onychomycosis.

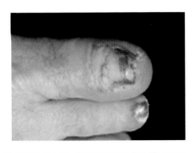

Color Plate 21. Onychomycosis with acute paronychia.

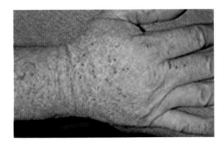

Color Plate 22. Acute contact dermatitis.

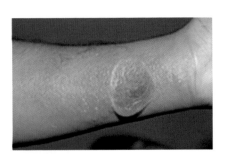

Color Plate 23. Burn with cellulitis.

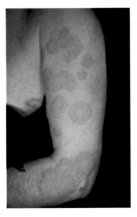

Color Plate 24. Urticaria.

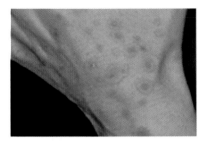

Color Plate 25. Erythema multiforme.

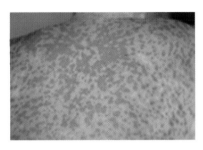

Color Plate 26. Stevens-Johnson syndrome.

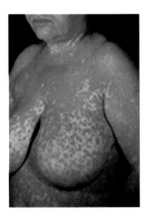

Color Plate 27. Drug eruption.

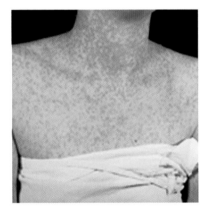

Color Plate 28. Viral exanthem.

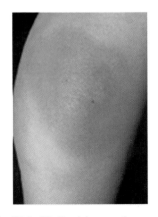

Color Plate 29. Fixed drug eruption.

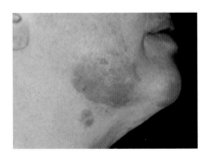

Color Plate 30. Insect bite hypersensitivity.

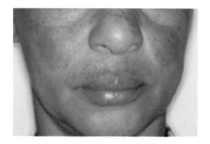

Color Plate 31. Melasma.

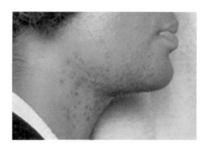

Color Plate 32. Pseudofolliculitis.

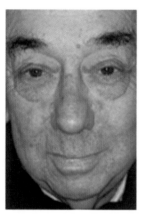

Color Plate 33. Rosacea.

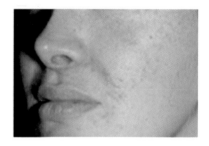

Color Plate 34. Perioral dermatitis.

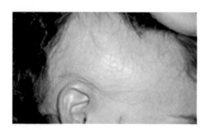

Color Plate 35. Alopecia areata.

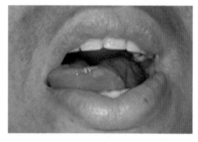

Color Plate 36. Aphthous ulcer.

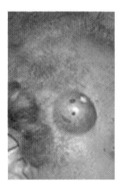

Color Plate 37. Epidermal inclusion cyst.

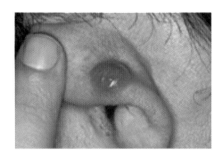

Color Plate 38. Kaposi's sarcoma.

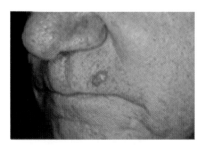

Color Plate 39. Nodular basal cell carcinoma.

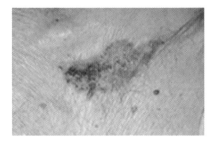

Color Plate 40. Superficial basal cell carcinoma.

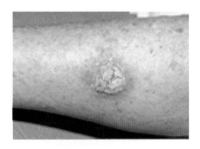

Color Plate 41. Squamous cell carcinoma.

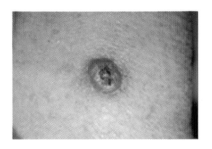

Color Plate 42. Keratoacanthoma.

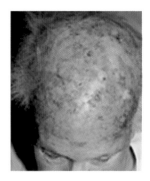

Color Plate 43. Actinic keratoses (treatment with Efudex).

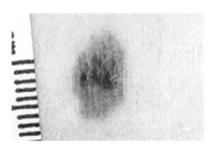

Color Plate 44. Dysplastic nevus.

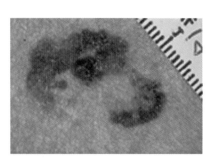

Color Plate 45. Superficial spreading melanoma.

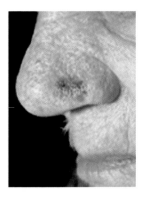

Color Plate 46. Lentigo maligna melanoma.

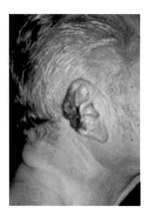

Color Plate 47. Nodular melanoma.

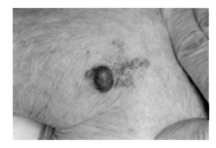

Color Plate 48. Melanoma (in transit metastasis).

Common Dermatologic Diseases: Diagnosis and Therapy

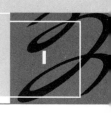

I

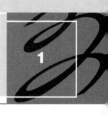

I. DEFINITION AND PATHOPHYSIOLOGY. Acne vulgaris is a very common, chronic disorder, involving inflammation of the pilosebaceous units that can be varied in presentation and difficult to treat. Acne lesions include comedones, inflamed papules, pustules, and nodules. Acne typically involves areas with the largest number of pilosebaceous glands: the face, chest, and back (1). Most adolescents (80%) experience some acne; however, it may linger into adulthood, particularly in women with hormonal acne flares during the menstrual cycle. Lesions may begin as early as ages 8 to 10 at adrenarche, when androgens of adrenal origin begin to stimulate pilosebaceous units on the face (2). In girls, this may precede menarche by more than a year. Prevalence increases steadily throughout adolescence and then decreases in adulthood. Although girls often develop acne at a younger age than boys, severe disease affects boys 10 times more frequently (up to 15% are involved). Patients with severe cystic acne often have a family history of the same (3).

Neonatal acne or cephalic pustulosis is self-limited with an onset around 2 to 3 weeks of age. Almost one in five newborns is affected by at least mild neonatal acne characterized by erythematous nonscarring papules on the face and neck, most commonly on the cheeks and nasal bridge. This disorder spontaneously resolves within 1 to 3 months. Recent data implicates *Malassezia* spp. in its pathogenesis (4). Topical 2% ketoconazole cream as well as benzoyl peroxide have been shown to be effective treatments, although parental reassurance alone is often sufficient, given the transient and benign nature of the eruption. Infantile acne (usually at age 3 to 6 months) includes persistent comedones and inflammatory lesions with an increased risk of scarring. Immature infantile adrenal glands lead to elevated dehydroepiandrosterone (DHEAS) levels until the age of 12 months. Boys are more often affected than girls because of additional high testosterone levels between the ages of 6 to 12 months. Infantile acne usually resolves within 1 to 2 years; however, individuals with infantile acne may have more severe teenage acne than their peers. Some of these infants may eventually require systemic isotretinoin. Acne in midchildhood may be a marker for adrenal or gonadal tumors.

A significant increase in adult acne has been observed over the last several decades. A study by Goulden found the prevalence of acne in a group aged 25 to 58 years to be 3% of men and 12% of women. Eighty-two percent of the affected individuals had experienced acne since teenage years and most did not see a decrease until after age 45 (5). In another study by Goulden, 50% of patients with adult acne had a first-degree relative with postadolescent acne; one third of the women had at least one symptom of hyperandrogenism and 37% of the entire group had failed a course of Accutane (6).

The principal factors involved in the pathogenesis of acne are androgen-mediated stimulation of sebaceous glands, abnormal keratinization of the follicular epithelium leading to follicular plugging, proliferation and activity of *Propionibacterium acnes* within the follicle, and inflammation (7). Severity of involvement often corresponds to the amount of sebum secreted; patients with severe acne will usually have large and active sebaceous glands with prominent follicular openings ("pores") and oily skin ("seborrhea"). Altered follicular growth and differentiation fosters an environment in which *P. acnes* proliferates, and the resultant host-immune response to the bacterium with proinflammatory cytokines results in inflamed lesions.

Early-onset acne may be the first sign of an underlying hormonal abnormality, especially if there is an associated advanced bone age and early pubic hair development. Early comedonal acne development is predictive of later, more severe disease. At puberty, hormonal stimuli lead to increased growth and development of sebaceous follicles. Female patients with severe acne or evidence of virilization often have abnormally high levels of circulating androgens. Several studies have demonstrated that many female patients with milder forms of acne and no evidence of virilization may still have ovarian and/or adrenal overproduction of androgens. In those patients with normal circulating levels of androgens, there is some evidence that suggests a heightened end-organ responsiveness of the sebaceous glands to androgenic stimulation. This heightened end-organ response may result in increased conversion of testosterone to dihydrotestosterone (DHT) and other 5-α-reduced metabolites or suppressed follicular testosterone metabolism. Male acne patients tend to have higher levels of androstenedione, testosterone, free androgen index, and 11-deoxycortisol (8).

The enlarged gland secretes sebum into a dilated follicle that contains an elevated number of normal cutaneous bacteria. Sebum contains free and esterified fatty acids as well as unsaponifiable lipid components. The anaerobic diphtheroid *P. acnes* enzymatically produces free fatty acid (FFA) from sebum in the follicle. These FFAs are the primary irritating substances in inflammatory acne. As triglyceride levels rise, so does the population of *P. acnes*. The bacterium also produces low-molecular-weight peptides, which act as chemoattractants for polymorphonuclear leukocytes. Patients with severe acne demonstrate cell-mediated immunity directed toward *P. acnes*, and the severity of inflammation is proportional to the anti-*P. acnes* immunity. In addition, toll-like receptor 2 (TLR-2) has been implicated in acne pathogenesis. TLR-2 is a pattern recognition receptor activated by *P. acnes*. TLR-2 activates a transcription factor to upregulate the production and release of proinflammatory cytokines including interleukin-12 (IL-12) and IL-8 from monocytes. TLR-2 is expressed on inflammatory cells around the pilosebaceous unit in patients with acne, and its expression increases as the acne lesion becomes older and more inflamed (9). Attraction and killing of leukocytes by comedonal components, the resultant inflammatory cascade, and specific immunologic events probably contribute to the final appearance of an inflammatory acne lesion.

Disordered shedding of the cells that line sebaceous follicles is another factor in the pathogenesis of acne lesions. Sticky desquamating horny cells are retained in the follicular orifice, and the dilated opening becomes plugged by entrapped sebum forming a closed comedo ("whitehead"). If this comedonal mass protrudes from the follicle, it is recognized as an open comedo ("blackhead"). The dark color is due to oxidized lipid, melanin, or densely packed keratinocytes and bacteria, and *not* dirt. As hydrolytic enzymes released from polymorphonuclear leukocytes induce follicle walls to leak or rupture, sebum (with its irritant and chemoattractant factors), keratin, bacteria, and hair are released into the dermis and result in an inflammatory mass (papule, "pimple," pustule, nodule, cyst, and/or abscess). Activation of the classic and alternative pathways of complement by *P. acnes* enhances the inflammation. Experimentally, follicular hyperkeratosis is induced by IL-1 α and epidermal growth factors; isotretinoin inhibits this process.

Most acne papules or pustules result from the rupture of an intrafollicular microcomedo rather than a visible one. Patients with large numbers of comedones usually have only small numbers of inflammatory lesions, whereas patients with severe cystic acne usually have few comedones. In adult life, the cells lining the follicle presumably become less susceptible to comedogenic materials. Spontaneous resolution of acne may also be related to a decreased dermal reactivity to irritant substances.

As many as one third of adult women are affected by a low-grade acneiform eruption that may start *de novo* or merge imperceptibly with preexisting adolescent acne. The eruption may be induced by chronic exposure to comedogenic substances such as isopropyl myristate, cocoa butter, and fatty acids present in some creams and moisturizers, by androgenic stimuli from progestins present in some oral contraceptives, by recent cessation of oral contraceptives, or by unknown causes.

Inflammatory acne may yield both scarring and pigmentary changes. Early treatment is essential to prevent and minimize the cosmetic disfigurement associated with acne scarring. Adequate therapy will, in all cases, decrease its severity and may entirely suppress this disease. However, if left alone, most inflammatory acne tends to disappear slowly in the early twenties in men and somewhat later in women. Permanent pitted or nodular hypertrophic scars may result.

II. SUBJECTIVE DATA

A. Acne has a significant impact on the patient's self-image and quality of life, and the psychological toll of acne may be comparable to that of asthma or epilepsy (10). Even clinically mild acne may cause considerable social embarrassment to the patient. As with all medical and psychological conditions, the patient's perception of the severity of the problem is an important factor in choosing treatment. Decisions by the physician about the severity of objective disease and therapeutic plans must be evaluated in this context.

A quality of life scale has been developed specifically for the patient with acne (11). Respondents answer on a grade of 0 to 3 to what extent they have experienced each item. The scale may be used to help the clinician evaluate the relationship between acne severity and psychosocial impact and morbidity, especially among mild to moderately affected patients for whom quality of life issues are often a major consideration in deciding whether to institute therapy.

1. Feeling self-conscious in the presence of others.
2. Decrease in your socialization with others.
3. Difficulties in your relationships with your spouse or partner.
4. Difficulties in your relationships with your close friends.
5. Difficulties in your relationships with your immediate family.
6. Feeling like an "outcast" most of the time because of the effect of acne upon your appearance.
7. People making fun of your appearance.
8. Feeling rejected in a romantic relationship because of the effect of acne upon your appearance.
9. Feeling rejected by your friends because of the effect of acne upon your appearance.

B. Inflammatory lesions of acne may itch as they erupt and may be very painful or tender.

III. OBJECTIVE DATA (See color insert.)

A. **Noninflammatory lesions.** The initial lesion is the closed comedo; visible as a 1- to 2-mm white bump (whitehead) most easily seen when the skin is stretched. If follicle contents extrude, a 2- to 5-mm, dark-topped, open comedo (blackhead) results.

B. **Inflammatory lesions.** Erythematous papules, pustules, cysts, and abscesses may be seen. Patients with cystic acne also tend to show "double," or polyporous comedones, which result from prior inflammation during which epithelial scarring caused fistulous links between neighboring sebaceous units. Acne lesions are seen primarily on the face, but the neck, chest, shoulders, and back may be involved. One or more anatomic areas may be involved in any given patient, and the pattern of involvement, once present, tends to remain constant.

C. The skin, scalp, and hair are frequently oily.

D. Pustules and cysts often rupture spontaneously and drain a purulent and/or a bloody but odorless discharge.

IV. ASSESSMENT. Several points regarding etiology or therapy should be considered with each patient:

A. Are endocrine factors important in this patient? Sudden onset of acne, treatment-resistant acne, and acne associated with signs of androgenism should lead one to suspect an endocrine abnormality.

1. Is the acne accompanied by irregular menstrual periods or concomitant hirsutism? Stein–Leventhal syndrome, Cushing's syndrome, 21-hydroxylase deficiency, and other endocrinopathies are frequently accompanied by acne. Polycystic ovarian syndrome is defined by menstrual irregularities, acne, pelvic ultrasound imaging of subcapsular ovarian cysts, and an elevated luteinizing hormone (LH) to follicle-stimulating hormone (FSH) ratio (a level greater than 2 to 3 is suggestive). The testosterone elevations are modest in the range of 80 to 150 ng/dL.

Men and women with mild to severe cystic acne, especially those who do not respond to conventional therapy, may have elevated plasma-free testosterone and/or DHEAS levels. Hyperandrogenism is associated with acne, hirsutism, alopecia, and menstrual irregularities; other possible findings include infertility, deepening of the voice, increased libido, acanthosis nigricans, insulin resistance, type 2 diabetes mellitus and dyslipidemia. DHEAS elevations above 8,000 ng/mL suggest the presence of an adrenal tumor; a range of 4,000 to 8,000 ng/mL is indicative of congenital adrenal hyperplasia. Testosterone elevations point to an ovarian dysfunction, with levels of 150 to 200 ng/dL suggesting an ovarian tumor. Oral contraceptives can mask an underlying endocrine disorder, so testing should be done 1 month after the discontinuation of exogenous hormones. Women may have high normal levels of DHEAS and testosterone and may benefit from hormonal therapy. Postmenopausal acne occurs in dark-complexioned women with previously oily skin, with the development of small closed comedones at the periphery of the face; unopposed adrenal androgens are the presumed cause.

2. Is there a premenstrual flare-up? Premenstrual flares of acne are associated with a narrowing of the sebaceous duct orifice between days 15 and 20 of the menstrual cycle. This can lead to duct obstruction and resistance to the flow of sebum. Many women tend to do well on anovulatory drugs.

3. Is the patient on oral contraceptives, or has she stopped taking these pills within the past few months? When were the pills started? Which ones? Acne may be associated with oral contraceptive pills if recently started or discontinued and if composed of an androgenic progesterone. During the first two or three cycles on oral contraceptives, acne may worsen. Post-pill acne may continue for as long as a year after birth control pills are stopped. Although anovulatory drugs may provide excellent therapy for acne, the various pills differ enormously in their effect on the sebaceous gland (see sec. V.C.2). Oral contraceptives that contain the androgenic and antiestrogenic progestogens norgestrel and norethindrone acetate may actually provoke an acneiform eruption.

B. What is the effect of seasonal changes? Is sunlight beneficial? Has the patient recently been in a hot and humid environment? Most patients find that summer sunlight will diminish the activity of their acne. However, very humid environments or heavy sweating will lead to keratin hydration, swelling, decrease in the size of the sebaceous follicle orifice, and partial or total duct obstruction. Therefore, it is not always good advice to "get out into the sun," except in a dry climate. A small number of people with excessive sunlight exposure will develop an acneiform papular eruption related to abnormal follicular keratinization ("Mallorca," miliary, actinic acne). In addition, many sunscreens are comedogenic; facial formula and gel-based sunscreens are recommended.

C. Does the patient have occupational or other exposure to chemicals? Exposure to heavy oils, greases, polyvinyl chloride, chlorinated aromatic hydrocarbons, and tars can cause acne. These occlusive comedogenic agents will initiate lesions, as can some greasy substances used for hair care (pomade acne). Certain oily or greasy cosmetics and creams can also exacerbate acne.

D. Does the patient wear occlusive or tight clothing or have any habits that will initiate or aggravate the disease? Mechanical trauma (pressure, friction, rubbing, squeezing) from clothing or athletic wear or from behavioral habits will also cause lesions. For example, an individual with the habit of cradling the chin in his or her hand may develop unilateral lesions at that site.

E. Has the patient been on any medications known to cause acne? The most prominent among these are corticosteroids, adrenocorticotropic hormone (ACTH), phenytoin, androgens, anabolic steroids (danazol and testosterone), iodides, and bromides. Other possible stimuli include trimethadione, isoniazid, lithium, halothane, vitamin B_{12}, cobalt irradiation, and hyperalimentation therapy. Drug-induced acne often presents as an abrupt, monomorphous eruption of inflammatory papules (12).

F. Is the acne of rapid onset and associated with fever and leukocytosis (acne fulminans)? Is a destructive arthropathy present, resembling rheumatoid arthritis (acne arthropathy)? SAPHO syndrome consists of synovitis, acne, pustulosis (palmarplantar, pustular psoriasis), hyperostoses, and osteitis; this is considered one of the spondylarthropathies and has been reported with inflammatory bowel disease and pyoderma gangrenosum. The PAPA syndrome, an autosomal dominant disorder, consists of pyogenic sterile arthritis, pyoderma gangrenosum, and acne (13).

G. How has the patient's acne been treated in the past? Have antibiotics been used? If so, what were the instructions, dosage, duration, and effect of these therapies? Was tetracycline inadvertently taken with meals instead of on an empty stomach? Was the dosage adequate? (see sec. V.C.1.)

There is an increased incidence of bacterial resistance of both *P. acnes* and coagulase-negative *Staphylococcus aureus* noted after long-term antibiotic use. These resistant bacteria are found in both the patients and their close contacts. *P. acnes* resistance to antibiotics should be considered in treatment failures. This is seen particularly with erythromycin; but cross-resistance can occur with clindamycin. Multiple antibiotics should not be used at the same time and benzoyl peroxides should be added as a second agent to help minimize this possibility. The highest possible dose of an oral antibiotic should be started for as short a course as possible. Oral minocycline has the lowest risk for bacterial resistance over time. Oral isotretinoin reduces the total number of resistant *P. acnes*.

An unusual complication of chronic broad-spectrum antibiotic therapy is the development of a **gram-negative folliculitis**. Such patients will notice a sudden change in their acne, with the appearance of pustules or large inflammatory cysts that, on culture, usually grow *Proteus, Pseudomonas,* or *Klebsiella* species. Because acne cysts are sterile on routine bacteriologic culture, a sudden change in morphology warrants Gram's stain and culture of cyst/abscess contents (see Chap. 4). This condition is treated with the appropriate antibiotic or systemic isotretinoin. Gram-negative folliculitis can develop in individuals who have not been on oral antibiotics and may be associated with impaired immune function.

H. Is there any effect from stress or emotional upsets on acne activity? An acutely stressful situation may cause acne to flare (14). Are there shallow erosions covered by a serous crust? Excoriated acne (acne excoriee), especially in young women, may be confused with impetigo.

I. The number and type of lesions should be roughly quantified to assess further therapeutic responses.

V. THERAPY

A. Mild involvement (few to many comedones)

1. Bacteriostatics are thought to improve acne by decreasing the formation of harmful by-products, but not necessarily the actual number, of *P. acnes* bacteria. These agents can be applied twice daily to the point of mild dryness and erythema but not discomfort.

a. Benzoyl peroxide (see also Chap. 40, Acne Preparations, sec. II.F) has a potent bacteriostatic effect with a reduction of *P. acnes* within 2 days and a reduction in lesion count after 4 days of application. Benzoyl peroxides decrease the likelihood of bacterial resistance and should be a mainstay of every acne program, if tolerated. It is hypothesized that this agent is decomposed by the cysteine present in skin, after which free-radical oxygen is capable of oxidizing proteins in its vicinity. These proteins include the bacterial proteins of the sebaceous follicles, thereby decreasing the number of *P. acnes* and consequently the amount of FFAs. Topical 5% benzoyl peroxide lowers FFAs 50% to 60% after daily application for 14 days and decreases aerobic bacteria by 84% and anaerobic bacteria (primarily *P. acnes*) by 98%. Benzoyl peroxide will also reduce the size and number of comedones present and may inhibit sebum secretion. Contact sensitivity is observed in 1% to 3% of patients. Benzoyl peroxides can bleach the color out of clothing.

i. Benzoyl peroxide products include preparations such as clear aqueous gel (Desquam-X Desquam-E); clear alcohol gel (Benzagel, PanOxyl); clear oil-based lotion (Benoxyl); Brevoxyl in a regular and creamy base; and a glycerin and glycolic acid containing product (Triaz). Numerous other prescriptions and over-the-counter benzoyl peroxide products, ranging in strength from 2.5% to 10.0%, are also available. The 2.5% formulation is therapeutically equivalent to the 5% and 10% concentrations and induces less irritation. Patients with lesions of the chest and back may find the use of a benzoyl peroxide wash easier (Desquam-X, 5% and 10%; Benzac A-C, 5% and 10%; Brevoxyl, 4% and 8%; Triax, 3%, 6%, and 9%).

b. Topical antibiotics (see also Chap. 40, Acne Preparations, sec. II.G) may affect acne lesions by their bacteriostatic action or because of suppressive effects on the inflammatory response. Papular and pustular lesions respond best; the activity of comedonal or cystic acne may not be altered. Resistant organisms may emerge after continued therapy; combination therapy with benzoyl peroxide minimizes this risk. All topical antibiotics are applied twice daily.

   i. Clindamycin phosphate is available in 1% concentration in a hydroalcoholic vehicle (30 or 60 mL) as a gel or lotion. Although the drug has not been detected in the blood after topical use, its detection in the urine suggests that 4% to 5% of topically applied clindamycin is absorbed. There have been two reports of pseudomembranous colitis after topical use of clindamycin hydrochloride. Patients with inflammatory bowel disease should avoid topical clindamycin use, and all patients should be warned to discontinue therapy if intestinal symptoms occur. Products that combine clindamycin with benzoyl peroxide include Benzaclin and Duac.

   ii. Erythromycin base applied topically is effective and nonsensitizing. It is available as 1.5% solution (Staticin, 60 mL); 2.0% solution (EryDerm, 60 mL, A/T/S, 60 mL, Emgel, 60 mL); 2% pledgets (Erycette, T-Stat pads); 2% ointment (Akne-Mycin); or a combination 3% erythromycin and 5% benzoyl peroxide gel (Benzamycin).

   iii. Sulfacet R and Novacet have a combination of sodium sulfacetamide (an antibacterial agent) and sulfur (a comedolytic agent). These products can help decrease the redness of skin lesions, and Sulfacet comes with a skin tint to help cosmetically cover lesions.

   iv. Klaron lotion contains sodium sulfacetamide without sulfur. The solution is a water-based gel, and it is a good choice for sensitive skin. All sulfur-based products are contraindicated in patients with a sulfonamide allergy.

c. Salicylic acid is a β-hydroxy acid that penetrates into the sebaceous gland and has comedolytic and anti-inflammatory properties. It can be used as an adjunctive therapy and is found in cleansers, toners, masks, and peels. Its side effects include erythema and scaling.

d. Aluminum chloride hexahydrate (6.25% Xerac A-C) is an effective antiperspirant that has also an antibacterial effect. It may be useful in cases of acne in which sweating is prominent or appears to be aggravating the disease, but its effects have not been well studied.

e. Azelaic acid is a dicarboxylic acid that has antimicrobial, anti-inflammatory, and comedolytic activity, and it is relatively nonirritating. It is available as a cream (Azelex) or gel (Finacea) formulation. Azelaic acid may help lighten postinflammatory hyperpigmentation and is a good choice for ethnic or pigmented skin. It is not a photosensitizer and so far shows minimal tendency for bacterial resistance. This drug works best when combined with other topical preparations, for example, benzoyl peroxides or retinoids.

f. Clinac OC, indicated for oily skin, is an over-the-counter copolymer that absorbs 20 times its volume of sebum. It is applied one to three times per day, depending on the degree of oiliness. Clinac is also available in combination with benzoyl peroxide, Clinac-BPO.

g. Although the administration of systemic antibiotics will reduce comedo formation in experimental animal systems, these drugs play no role in the therapy of the usual patient with comedonal acne.

2. Exfoliants. These agents, such as elemental sulfur, resorcinol, and abrasives, produce irritation and consequent peeling and exfoliation. Not all topical irritants have the property of decreasing the presence or formation of new comedones. Most of these are a source of additional injury to already inflamed skin and may be ineffective in removing deeply rooted comedones.

a. Topical exfoliants and irritants. Clear gels or lotions (Novacet); tinted creams (Sulforcin); tinted lotions (Liquimat).

B. Mild or moderate involvement (few to many comedones, some papules and/or pustules)

1. Benzoyl peroxide gel.

2. Retinoids are one of the most effective groups of drugs for acne that help in correcting the abnormal desquamation of the follicles that leads to the formation of microcomedones. There are now three topical retinoids available in the United States. A small percentage of patients may experience a pustular flare of their acne in the first few weeks of topical retinoid therapy, a transient effect that is indicative of the effectiveness of therapy. The risk of teratogenicity with topical retinoid application is minimal. Tazarotene is labeled as Category X, on the basis of its indication for psoriasis when larger areas with an altered skin barrier are treated. Tretinoin and adapalene are Category C. All the three drugs recommend minimizing exposure to sunlight and sunlamps because of an increased susceptibility to burning, likely secondary to the thinning of the stratum corneum.

   a. **Tretinoin** (*trans*-retinoic acid; vitamin A acid) first became available 25 years ago. The irritant effects of tretinoin sometimes limit its usefulness, but these can be minimized by the correct method of application. Tretinoin, which does not function as a vitamin in its therapeutic applications, increases epidermal cell turnover and decreases the cohesiveness ("stickiness") of horny cells, thereby inhibiting the formation of comedones while helping existing comedones to loosen and be expelled. Tretinoin not only changes follicular keratinization but also decreases the number of normal cell layers of the stratum corneum from 14 to 5. This decrease in the thickness of the barrier layer may potentiate the penetration of other topical agents.

      i. **Tretinoin products.** Retin-A cream, 0.1%, 0.05%, or 0.025%; Retin-A liquid, 0.05%; Retin-A gel, 0.01% or 0.025%; Retin-A micro gel, 0.1% or 0.04%; Avita, 0.025% cream or gel. Retin-A micro, a viscous yellow gel, contains porous microspheres that release tretinoin more slowly over time, thereby making it less irritating while having the same efficacy. Patients may notice a fine white residue if they overapply this product.

      Avita uses a large polymer compound, polyolprepolymer-2 (PP-2), to create a reservoir of the drug in the upper layers of the skin and the sebaceous glands delivering the drug over 12 to 24 hours.

   b. **Adapalene** (Differin 0.1% cream, gel, solution, and pledgets) is a derivative of naphthoic acid and a selective retinoic acid analog. This product is not degraded by sunlight, is not phototoxic, and is compatible with benzoyl peroxide application at the same time. When compared with topical tretinoin 0.025% gel, there is a lower incidence of cutaneous irritation and it compares favorably in the reduction of both inflammatory and noninflammatory lesions. This effect may be secondary to its more selective binding, increased lipophilic properties, and follicular penetration. This is a good first-line therapy in colder climates or in patients with sensitive skin.

   c. **Tazarotene** (Tazorac gel/cream, 0.05%, 0.1%, Avage Cream, 0.1%) is a potent selective retinoid that binds to the retinoic acid receptors, RAR-β and RAR-γ. This drug is converted in the epidermis to its active metabolite tazarotenic acid and was originally developed for the treatment of psoriasis. Tazorac is a category X drug and must be avoided in pregnancy. This drug can be irritating and should be avoided in patients with sensitive skin or seborrheic dermatitis. The 0.1% gel is more effective than the 0.05% concentration; however, starting with the 0.05% concentration may decrease the irritation. Some investigators advocate short-contact therapy, such as 1- to 5-minute exposures every other night, especially for patients with resistant comedones. Treatment time can be gradually increased to overnight. Twice-daily short-contact therapy can be tolerated in the individual with an oilier complexion. This product is not degraded by sunlight.

3. **Instructions for use — Retinoids.** The cream base is preferred for dry skin and the gels are preferred for oily skin. Easily irritated skin should be started with adapalene (Differin) cream 0.1%, tretinoin 0.025% cream or 0.01% gel, Retin-A

Micro 0.04% gel or Avita; others may start at higher strengths. The strength of the product may be gradually increased once the patient has become tolerant of the weaker formulation.

a. Apply sparingly every other night to the entire face except around the eyes, lips, and neck. After 2 to 3 weeks, if no excess irritation, erythema, dryness or scaling is noted, increase to every night. For tretinoin, apply before bedtime on thoroughly dry skin—wait for at least 45 minutes after the face has been washed. Tazarotene is best applied over or several minutes after the application of a moisturizer at bedtime.

b. Use mild, gentle soaps not more than twice daily.

c. Avoid excessive exposure to sun. Use sunscreens.

d. Use water-based cosmetics if necessary.

e. Expect mild redness and peeling within a week, lasting 3 to 4 weeks, and a flare-up in the acne during the first 2 to 4 weeks. This is explained as the surfacing of lesions onto the skin.

f. Clearing requires approximately 3 months. Inflammatory lesions improve more rapidly, but comedones take longer. Effectiveness cannot be judged before 8 weeks and is best assessed at 12 weeks.

g. Continue retinoid application after the lesions clear.

h. Apply less frequently if the daily use of the retinoid cannot be tolerated—for example, every other night or skipping every third night.

i. Although there is negligible systemic absorption of topical retinoids, this agent should be discontinued if pregnancy is suspected. Cases of neurologic toxicity and ear malformation have been reported.

4. Combined retinoid-bacteriostatic therapy. With this mode of therapy, the retinoid prevents or removes comedones, whereas benzoyl peroxide or topical antibiotic eradicates *P. acnes*. The retinoid also enhances absorption of the other product. Irritation reactions limit the use of this combination therapy.

a. Instructions for use.

i. Apply retinoid cream or solution in the evening/bedtime, as with retinoid alone.

ii. Apply benzoyl peroxide gel or topical antibiotic in the morning.

iii. After clearing, decrease frequency of therapy and concentration of medication.

iv. If using tretinoin, apply the agents at different times, **not** simultaneously. Mixing the highly unsaturated tretinoin with reactive oxidants such as benzoyl peroxide destroys both chemicals.

C. Moderate or severe involvement (inflammatory papules, pustules, cysts, abscesses, and/or scarring). Use topical therapy as discussed previously, plus antibiotics.

1. Antibiotics. Some systemic antimicrobials suppress the growth of normal cutaneous flora (primarily *P. acnes*). As bacteria are decreased and the FFA level slowly diminishes, inflammatory lesions decrease and new lesions stop appearing within 2 to 6 weeks. The beneficial effects of antibiotics may be multifold. Not only are the number of bacteria and FFA levels decreased but antibiotics useful in acne therapy also directly interfere with local chemical and cellular inflammatory mechanisms. Tetracycline, erythromycin, and clindamycin have been shown to inhibit leukocyte chemotaxis and other neutrophil inflammatory functions and may also directly inhibit extracellular lipases responsible for the generation of inflammatory compounds. Antibiotic therapy cannot be truly evaluated until 6 to 8 weeks after starting. Antibiotic levels in sebum are not detectable until approximately 7 days after treatment has started, and, in addition, lipid formed in basal cells of sebaceous follicles may require 1 month to reach the skin surface. Although sebum composition changes, the rate of secretion remains constant; therefore, skin may remain oily. Therapy may need to be continued for several months. The overall incidence of bacterial resistance has increased from 20% noted 20 years ago, to 62% in 1996 (15). The full antibiotic dose should be utilized, and it is controversial whether to taper the oral antibiotics or to stop with no taper. Tapering may allow resistant organisms to grow more readily. Long-term use of antibiotics likely contributes to the pool of resistant organisms.

Female patients should be counseled that oral antibiotics might decrease the effectiveness of oral contraceptives, although one study showed a failure rate of only 1% to 3% with the combination of oral antibiotics and oral contraceptives (16). In addition, a recent report found that increasing cumulative days of antibiotic use may be associated with an increased risk of breast cancer in women (17). The risk was highest in women on macrolide, tetracycline, and cephalosporin classes of antibiotics, and for durations >500 days. Although the data is limited, this finding indicates that reliance on systemic antibiotics should be limited and long-term maintenance therapy should focus on topical regimens or other medications.

a. Tetracycline is often the first antibiotic prescribed. It is the least expensive, has few side effects, and is well tolerated for longer periods of time. Tetracycline is effective in low doses because high concentrations are achieved within sebaceous follicles, especially when inflammation is present.

Apart from minor gastrointestinal tract irritation, *Candida* vaginitis is a common complication. Although tetracycline can cause enamel hyperplasia and hence tooth discoloration, by age 12, growth of teeth is essentially complete. Tetracycline should neither be used in younger children nor be administered during pregnancy. There is drug interaction with the metallic ions Al^{3+}, Mg^{2+}, and Ca^{2+} present in antacid preparations and dairy products; these products should never be taken at the same time as tetracycline. Pseudotumor cerebri is an uncommon adverse reaction from tetracycline. The duration of treatment can be from 2 weeks to 10 months. The presenting symptoms are usually headache, nausea, vomiting, and double vision. With a timely diagnosis, the increased intracranial pressure will resolve.

Initiate therapy at 250 mg q.i.d. (or 500 mg b.i.d.) taken on an empty stomach (half hour before meals or 2 hours after) until there is clear improvement; then, decrease the dosage to a maintenance level (250 to 500 mg/day) or eliminate it. If inflammatory lesions have not subsided after 4 to 6 weeks, increase the dose to 1.5 g/day for 2 weeks, and if necessary to 2 g/day for several weeks to induce remission in otherwise unresponsive patients. Once remission is achieved, it is almost always possible to decrease the dosage to a lower level.

b. Erythromycin, 1 g/day, is also effective in the treatment of acne. The same dose and time responses noted for tetracycline also apply for this drug. Forty percent of *P. acnes* organisms are resistant to erythromycin. Combination with topical benzoyl peroxide helps decrease the bacterial resistance. Elevated liver function tests (LFTs) and reversible hepatotoxicity have infrequently been reported.

c. Minocycline (Minocin, Dynacin, Vectrin) is a useful but expensive antibiotic in patients unresponsive to other antibiotics. It is overall the most effective antibiotic available to treat acne, but it can have serious side effects. This antibiotic is very lipid soluble and penetrates the sebaceous follicle more effectively; it is well absorbed, even with meals. Owing to its highly lipophilic nature, it crosses the blood–brain barrier and can precipitate pseudotumor cerebri syndrome. The duration of therapy can be a week to a year, with the most common presenting symptoms being headache, visual disturbances, diplopia, pulsatile tinnitus, nausea, and vomiting.

Because minimal amounts of minocycline remain in the gut, the frequency of *Candida* vaginitis is less than in those taking tetracycline. Most tetracycline-resistant bacteria are sensitive to minocycline at a dose of 100 mg b.i.d. Dizziness, nausea, and vomiting may be a problem if full doses are administered initially. Start at 50 mg/day and slowly increase to as much as 100 mg b.i.d. Some patients may eventually achieve complete control on 50 mg/day.

Minocycline may cause a blue discoloration of acne cysts or sites of trauma; this discoloration usually does not appear until 8 months of therapy with a total cumulative dose of 70 g and is usually reversible after discontinuation of the drug. Once a cumulative dose of 100 g is reached, alternative therapies should be considered. Cases of autoimmune hepatitis, serum sickness-like reactions, pulmonary infiltrates with eosinophilia, and a syndrome similar to drug-induced lupus (DIL) have been reported secondary to minocycline. For DIL, the duration of time ranged from 6 weeks to 2 years after starting antibiotics; patients had a positive antinuclear antibody (ANA) but negative antibodies to DNA. All symptoms resolve with discontinuation of the drug. The estimated risk is an 8.5-fold increase from controls, an absolute risk of 52.8 cases/100,000 prescriptions (18). If long-term minocycline is taken (i.e., >2 years) periodic LFTs and ANA levels may be warranted. A personal or family history of systemic lupus erythematosus (SLE) or underlying liver and/or kidney disease may be relative contraindications to the use of this drug.

d. **Doxycycline** (Vibramycin, Monodox) has similar absorption and duration-of-activity characteristics. Its effectiveness in acne approaches that of minocycline, when used in the same fashion with similar dosages. Early data suggests that subantimicrobial doses of doxycycline, 20 mg (Periostat), may play a therapeutic role in acne by reducing inflammation through anticollagenolytic, antimatrix-degrading metalloproteinase, and cytokine downregulating properties (19). Patients taking doxycycline must be warned to avoid excessive exposure to sunlight because of the photosensitivity that accompanies the use of this drug.

e. **Clindamycin** (Cleocin), 300 to 450 mg/day, is an extremely effective agent for acne. However, the risk of pseudomembranous colitis limits its systemic use to only very severe cases that are unresponsive to all other modes of therapy.

f. **Trimethoprim-sulfamethoxazole** (Bactrim, Septra) has also been shown to decrease FFA levels and inhibit inflammatory acne. Trimethoprim is very lipophilic, which enhances follicle penetration. Start with one double-strength tablet at bedtime; up to two tablets/day may be used. A high rate of allergic reactions limit its use. Neutropenia may occur on long-term therapy, and a baseline complete blood count (CBC) with intermittent monitoring is recommended. Toxic epidermal necrolysis (TEN) is unlikely to occur after the first month of therapy. Cases of hepatic necrosis and aplastic anemia have also been associated with this drug.

g. **Trimethoprim** (Proloprim, Trimpex), 300 mg b.i.d., used alone, is an effective alternative therapy.

h. **Cephalosporins** may be useful in patients resistant to other antibiotics.

i. **Ampicillin** may also be helpful in certain patients, particularly pregnant women with acne, for whom the use of tetracycline, erythromycin, and minocycline should be avoided. In resistant acne patients, culture may reveal a gram-negative bacteria responsive to ampicillin.

j. **Azithromycin** in a 500-mg dose three times a week has been shown to yield a 60% reduction in inflammatory papules in 83% of patients enrolled in a 12-week study (20). There is no associated pseudotumor cerebri and, therefore, it can be used for an acne flare during early Accutane therapy.

k. Some reports suggest that nonsteroidal anti-inflammatory agents such as indomethacin or ibuprofen may exert an additive beneficial effect when given with oral antibiotics.

2. **Sebaceous gland suppression**

a. **Oral contraceptives** (estrogen given as an anovulatory agent) may be of use in unresponsive cases in young women after more conventional regimens have failed. If a patient with acne is already taking anovulatory agents for contraception, an effort should be made to use a formulation known to alleviate, rather than exacerbate, acne. Most or all the estrogen effect is the result of adrenal and androgen inhibition rather than local suppression at the gland site; small doses of androgen can overcome the sebum-suppressive effects of large doses of estrogen in women as well as in men. There is a direct correlation between the degree of sebaceous gland inhibition and acne improvement. The gland, however, responds variably to estrogen suppression. On average, there will be a decrease of 25% in sebum production on administration of 0.1 mg ethinyl estradiol. This drug and its 3-methyl ether, mestranol (which has two thirds the potency of ethinyl estradiol), are the estrogens present in oral contraceptives. All combination birth control pills are antiandrogenic because they reduce free testosterone, testosterone conversion to 5-α-androstanediol, and sex hormone–binding globulin. With combination therapy, it is important to use a pill with adequate estrogenic effect linked with nonandrogenic progesterones such as drospirenone, desogestrel, norgestimate, northindrone, and ethynodiol diacetate. Drospirenone is a new progestogen with antimineralocorticoid, progestogenic, and antiandrogenic activity. Patients may exhibit a difference in the tolerability of side effects between the various progestational agents. If a patient has been taking an oral contraceptive with minimal side effects, the clinician does not need to change the pill unless there appears to be a correlation with worsening of acne.

i. The preferable pills are Yasmin (3 mg drospirenone, 0.03 mg ethinyl estradiol), Desogen and OrthoCept (0.15 mg desogestrel, 0.03 mg ethinyl estradiol), Orthocyclen, or Ortho Tri-cyclen (0.25 mg norgestimate, 0.035 mg ethinyl estradiol), Alesse (0.1 mg levonorgestrel, 0.02 mg ethinyl estradiol), Ovcon 35 (0.4 mg norethindrone, 0.035 mg ethinyl estradiol), Brevicon (0.5 mg norethindrone, 0.35 mg ethinyl estradiol), Modicon (0.5 mg northindrone, 0.035 mg ethinyl estradiol), or Demulen (0.05 mg ethinyl estradiol, 1.0 mg ethynodiol diacetate), in decreasing order of effectiveness.

Decrease in acne should be noted within 3 months and marked improvement should be noted within 4 months of administration. The progestational agent norgestrel and norethindrone acetate should be avoided (Ovral, Ovrette, Lo-ovral, Loestrin). Estrogen therapy is rarely needed before age 16, after which time there will be no problem with growth retardation.

ii. Prednisone 2.5 to 7.5 mg, administered at night or dexamethasone 0.25 to 0.75 mg are useful in female patients, with severe acne unresponsive to conventional therapy, who suffer from adrenal gland overproduction of androgens such as congenital adrenal hyperplasia. Dexamethasone has a higher risk of causing adrenal suppression. For individuals with an acute acne flare, Prednisone can also be used in a dose of 20 mg/day for 1 week before an important occasion such as a wedding.

iii. Concomitant administration of estrogen and prednisone may act synergistically in suppressing sebum production by inhibiting both adrenal and ovarian androgen production.

iv. Spironolactone (Aldactone), used for many years as a diuretic, is also an antiandrogen that blocks the binding of androgens to androgen receptors. It is useful in treating recalcitrant acne in women with adult acne. Menstrual irregularities and breast tenderness are common side effects, and the drug may be easier to use in women taking birth control pills. The drug should not be used during pregnancy, because it may block the normal development of male genitalia. Most clinicians recommend combined use of this drug with oral contraceptives. Spironolactone alters potassium excretion (usually only at higher doses and in only 10% of patients). Serum electrolytes should be monitored during initial institution of therapy. Nausea, vomiting, and anorexia are also common (21).

Spironolactone has been shown to promote breast tumors in rats fed with doses 25 to 100 times higher than human doses. There have been no data to support this association in women on long-term therapy, although caution should be used if there is a strong family history of breast cancer.

Good candidates for this drug are individuals with a premenstrual flare-up of their acne, acne onset after the age of 25, oily skin, coexistent hirsutism, and acne that has a predilection for the lower face, especially the chin and mandible. Start patients on 50 to 100 mg/day taken with meals. If no clinical response is seen in 1 to 3 months, adjust the dose up to 200 mg/day if necessary. Once maintenance has been achieved, try to lower the dose to the lowest effective daily dose. Keep in mind that hirsutism requires higher doses and longer treatment schedules. A topical 5% gel may be developed in the future.

v. Oral cyproterone acetate is available in Europe and Canada usually in combination with ethinyl estradiol for treatment of hirsutism and acne. Topical cyproterone acetate (a sexual steroid, antiandrogen) in combination with liposomes has been shown to improve acne.

vi. Flutamide, an androgen receptor blocker, has been shown to have benefit in doses of 250 mg b.i.d. However, the risks of fatal hepatitis and lipid abnormalities make this an expensive and high-risk choice of therapy.

vii. Gonadotropin-releasing hormone agonists (GnRHas) block ovarian androgen production and are widely used in the treatment of infertility disorders. This category of drugs includes buserelin, leuprolide, and nafarelin and, theoretically, they may be used to treat acne. They are very expensive, decrease the levels of estrogen, and, therefore, increase the risk of bone loss. Endocrinologists or reproductive endocrinologists are usually involved in the care of patients with these drugs.

viii. Sebaceous glands have type 1 5-α reductase activity. Inhibitors that block this enzyme and, therefore, the conversion of testosterone to DHT may have a place in acne therapy.

b. Patients with severe recalcitrant cystic acne should be considered for treatment with **isotretinoin** (13-*cis*-retinoic acid, Accutane, Amnesteem, Claravis, Sotret). The emergence of increased bacterial resistance of *P. acnes* has resulted in an increase in the number of cases of treatment-resistant acne. Criteria for treatment with isotretinoin include less than 50% improvement after 6 months of oral and topical therapy, scarring, associated psychological distress, or acne that relapses quickly once conventional therapy is discontinued.

The beneficial effects of this synthetic retinoid are indisputable, although its mode of action remains unclear. Isotretinoin is sebostatic, inducing a decrease in sebum production rates to as low as 10% of pretreatment values. However, given that sebum production approaches pretreatment rates after therapy is completed *without* a concomitant return of acne, other mechanisms, such as an anti-inflammatory effect or correction of altered keratinization, may be equally important. Isotretinoin therapy causes a 2.6-fold decrease in androgen site–binding capacity (22).

The initial dose of isotretinoin is 0.5 to 1.0 mg/kg of the patient's body weight. Many of the problems with this drug come from starting at too high a dose. For the first month, a patient may be started at 20 mg daily. This allows for monitoring of any adverse effects and allows the patient to become accustomed to or more comfortable with the drug. The daily dose may be increased each month by an additional 20 mg (e.g., 20 mg first month, 40 mg second month, 60 mg third month, etc.) to a dose of approximately 1 mg/kg. Most physicians plan a course of therapy that reaches a total dose of 100 to 120 mg/kg, which may take up to 6 months to achieve. Some practitioners administer the drug until 2 months after complete healing, with an average treatment of 7 months. Although lower doses may achieve the same initial response rates, they are associated with a much higher recurrence rate on discontinuation of the drug.

There appears to be no advantage to single versus divided dose, but isotretinoin absorption is enhanced by taking it with meals. Because the skin will often continue to clear after drug administration has been stopped, at least a 2-month waiting period and preferably a 6-month period is advised before one commits a patient to a second course of therapy. Any woman who fails to respond to isotretinoin should be evaluated for hyperandrogenism. The response rate may be as high as 90% with one to two courses of treatment, and with adequate dosing, most patients experience prolonged remissions from their disease. In a 10-year follow-up study, 61% of patients were free from acne. Of those who relapsed, 23% required a second course of Accutane. Ninety-six percent had relapsed within 3 years of therapy; truncal acne had a higher relapse rate. Patients given a cumulative dose of 120 mg/kg overall were less likely to relapse (22).

Intermittent isotretinoin at lower doses may benefit some patients with adult acne or stubborn isotretinoin treatment failures. In one study, with isotretinoin 0.5 mg/kg/day for 1 week every 4 weeks for a total of 6 months, the acne resolved in 88% of patients, and at 1 year, 39% had a relapse of their acne (73% relapse with truncal acne) (6).

Isotretinoin is teratogenic in humans. A pregnancy prevention program was initiated in 1988. Since that time, 0.3% of treated female patients have become pregnant; 38% of live born infants had retinoid embryopathic defects. Women of childbearing age must have a negative pretreatment pregnancy test and continue adequate contraception for the duration of therapy. Because of the short half-life of isotretinoin, the current recommendation is that conception may be attempted 1 month after the cessation of treatment. Men may take isotretinoin without concern for its teratogenic effects.

The U.S. Food and Drug Administration (FDA) had received 20 spontaneous reports, over a 15-year period, of depression associated with isotretinoin use, leading to a change in the Accutane package insert in early 1998 warning of the association with psychiatric disorders including suicide. More than 50% of these reported patients had a significant personal or family history of depression. These cases may reflect an idiosyncratic response to the medication because larger, controlled studies have failed to find a causal association (23,24). Acne by itself can be associated with depression, but an increased awareness of this potential side effect of isotretinoin should be kept in mind before prescribing this drug and during follow-up.

Xerosis, cheilitis, alopecia, dry eyes, muscle and bone aches, and hypertriglyceridemia are frequent side effects, but all are reversible on discontinuation of therapy. Although patients may experience a temporary flare-up of their acne when treatment is started, this does not affect their ultimate response to isotretinoin. Excessive granulation tissue, giving a pyogenic granuloma-like picture, is a less common problem. Because of delayed or poor wound healing, incisional surgery including attempts at cosmetic scar revision should be delayed for 12 months after the completion of isotretinoin therapy.

Another concerning side effect of isotretinoin therapy is the development of vertebral hyperostoses. This finding was recognized initially in patients being treated for various disorders of keratinization who had received isotretinoin at higher dosages and for longer periods than is recommended for acne. Diffuse interstitial skeletal hyperostoses (DISH) would commonly affect the spine and is often asymptomatic. However, asymptomatic vertebral hyperostoses have since been found in patients with acne who had been treated according to the current recommendations. Only long-term follow-up will determine whether these vertebral changes will cause symptomatic disease or become a contraindication to therapy. A single course of isotretinoin may slightly decrease bone density and bone mineralization, but it is not known whether these changes are reversible or increase a patient's risk for osteoporosis and fractures when older. Baseline vertebral x-rays and bone density studies may be considered in individuals who receive three or more courses of isotretinoin.

c. Vitamin A (Aquasol A), in doses ranging from 50,000 to 500,000 units/day in divided doses, has been advocated for the treatment of severe nodulocystic acne that does not respond to other modalities. This treatment has yet to be evaluated in an adequately controlled, prospective clinical trial and is not an approved indication for the drug. However, vitamin A is available without prescription, and patients may take it on the advice of friends or the lay press. The toxic dose for adults is usually at least 50,000 IU/day over a period of a year or longer. Normal diets contain approximately 7,500 to 10,000 IU/day. Physicians should be aware of the signs and symptoms of chronic hypervitaminosis A, because patients may take an excess of the vitamin without their knowledge or approval. Signs and symptoms include dry, coarse, scaly skin, hair loss, fissures of the lips, pruritus, sore tongue or mouth, and low-grade fever. Normal serum vitamin A levels do not rule out a diagnosis of hypervitaminosis A.

D. Adjunctive therapy

1. Intralesional corticosteroids. The therapy of choice for cystic lesions and acne abscesses is the intralesional injection of small amounts of corticosteroid preparations (triamcinolone acetonide or diacetate, 0.63 to 2.5 mg/mL). The high local concentration of corticosteroid injected leads to rapid involution of these nonpyogenic, sterile, inflammatory lesions.

The stock 10-, 25-, or 40-mg/mL steroid suspension should be diluted with lidocaine or bacteriostatic normal saline and only enough injected through a 1-mL syringe with a 27- or 30-gauge needle to distend the cyst slightly (usually 0.025 to 0.1 mL). Use of undiluted solutions or injections of too large an amount may lead to temporary atrophic depressions in the skin (see Chap. 40, Anti-inflammatory Agents, sec. I). Most lesions, particularly early ones, will flatten and disappear within 48 hours of injection.

2. Acne surgery

a. Comedo expression. Gentle removal of comedones by pressing over the lesion with a comedo extractor or the opening of an eyedropper not only relieves the patient of unsightly lesions but may also prevent progression to more inflammatory lesions. Occasionally, it may be necessary to incise the follicular opening carefully with a No. 11 scalpel blade or a 25-, 27-, or 30-gauge needle. Over-rigorous attempts to express comedones may result in an increased inflammatory response. Retinoid-resistant comedones can be treated with 30% to 50% trichloroacetic acid on the wooden end of a Q-tip.

Recurrence of comedones after removal is common. Open comedones have been shown to recur within 24 to 40 days and closed comedones, within 30 to 50 days. Fewer than 10% of comedo extractions are a complete success. Nevertheless, this mode of therapy, carefully done, is useful in the appropriate case.

b. Draining of cysts. Careful and judicious incision and drainage of cysts and/or abscesses may initiate healing and shorten the duration of lesions.

c. Microdermabrasion, with aluminum oxide crystals or other abrasive substances is a newly developed technique that is advocated for treatment of acne and acne scars. Early data indicate that this modality may be a useful adjunct to other topical therapies (25).

3. Laser and light therapies

a. Blue light or photodynamic therapy (420 nm). These light sources cause an overproduction of porphyrins that are toxic to *P. acnes*. Pulsed green light (532 nm) is also approved for the treatment of acne and presumably works in the same way. Light treatments can be performed alone or with prior application of aminolevulinic acid 20% for 10 minutes to 2 hours. Protocols vary, but one standard treatment is every 3 weeks in a 3-month course. This may be performed in conjunction with other acne therapies.

b. Nonablative lasers in the infrared range rely on selective photothermolysis to target the follicle. Through transient thermal effects, *P. acnes* is reduced and sebaceous glands are heated and decreased in size. The 1320-nm Nd:YAG, 1450-nm diode, and 1540-nm Er:glass lasers show promise in the treatment of inflammatory acne and clinical improvement in acne scars (26). Treatments are typically performed monthly for 4 to 6 months. Other therapies may be continued concomitantly. The limiting factors are patient discomfort and expense.

   c. **Pulsed dye lasers** in the visible light range (585 to 595 nm) can be used to minimize erythema of active acne lesions and acne scars (27). However, data is inconsistent as to whether this laser decreases acne lesion counts (28,29).
   d. **Ultraviolet light (UVL).** Exposure to sunlight or UVB sunlamps may be moderately effective in some patients. Patients using tretinoin may show a heightened sensitivity to UVL. However, this method carries the potential for photodamage and carcinogenesis in the long term.
   4. α-**Hydroxy acids** (glycolic, lactic, pyruvic, and citric acids) and β-hydroxy acids (salicylic acid) are available in topical cream formulations or as peeling agents. These acids reduce corneocyte cohesion.
E. **Acne scars**
   1. **Laser skin resurfacing.** Ablative CO_2/Er:YAG laser skin resurfacing can improve the appearance of acne scars of all types but requires significant postoperative wound care and recovery time. A newer fractional resurfacing device, Fraxel, shows promise for remodeling acne scars through a series of treatments with less downtime. Nonablative lasers (see preceding text) are thought to stimulate collagen production and, thereby, gradually improve the appearance of pitted acne scars.
   2. **Dermabrasion** using high-speed diamond buffing drills can remove small and superficial scars and sometimes deep scars. However, this method is highly dependent on practitioner technique and can result in scarring in untrained hands.
   3. **Fillers.** Fat transfer and injection of filler substances can be used to elevate acne scars.
   4. **Surgical techniques.** Punch excision, punch elevation, and elliptical excision can be used to remove isolated ice-pick or deep boxcar scars.
F. **Patient education about long-standing misconceptions.** A number of myths circulate with regard to the relationship between habits, diet, hygiene, and acne. Patients should be counseled that if certain exposures aggravate their individual case of acne, these should be avoided. However, strict or fad diets and regimens are unlikely to affect sebaceous gland function or acne activity. Detailed information and instructions should be emphasized. Moreover, shared, realistic expectations between the physician and patient of any acne treatment regimen or therapeutic approach are essential to achieve the desired improvement.

References

1. Marcus LS. Treating acne in 2004: a review. *Cosmetic Dermatol* 2004;17:484–488.
2. Bergfeld WF. The pathophysiology of acne vulgaris in children and adolescents. Part 1. *Cutis* 2004;74:92–97.
3. Lucky AW, Biro FM, Simbartl LA, et al. Predictors of severity of acne vulgaris in young adolescent girls: results of a five-year longitudinal study. *J Pediatr* 1997;130:30–39.
4. Bernier V, Weill FX, Hirigoyen V, et al. Skin colonization by Malassezia species in neonates: a prospective study and relationship with neonatal cephalic pustulosis. *Arch Dermatol* 2002;138:215–218.
5. Goulden V, Stables GI, Cunliffe WJ. Prevalence of facial acne in adults. *J Am Acad Dermatol* 1999;41:577–580.
6. Goulden V, Clark SM, McGeown C, et al. Treatment of acne with intermittent isotretinoin. *Br J Dermatol* 1997;137:106–108.
7. Gollnick H, Cunliffe W, Berson D, et al. Global alliance to improve outcomes in acne. Management of acne: a report from a global alliance to improve outcomes in acne. *J Am Acad Dermatol* 2003;49:S1–S37.
8. Ramsay B, Alaghband-Zadeh J, Carter G, et al. Raised serum androgens and increased responsiveness to luteinizing hormone in men with acne vulgaris. *Acta Derm Venereol* 1995;75:293–296.
9. Kim J, Ochoa MT, Krutzik SR, et al. Activation of toll-like receptor 2 in acne trigger inflammatory cytokine responses. *J Immunol* 2002;169:1535–1541.
10. Thomas DR. Psychosocial effects of acne. *J Cutan Med Surg* 2004;8(suppl 4):3–5.

11. Gupta MA, Johnson AM, Gupta AK. The development of an acne quality of life scale: reliability, validity, and relation to subjective acne severity in mild to moderate acne vulgaris. *Acta Derm Venereol* 1998;78:451–456.
12. Zaengelin AL, Thiboutot DM. Acne Vulgaris. In: Bolognia JL, et al. ed. *Dermatology*. London: Mosby, 2003;531–544.
13. Lindor NM, Arsenault TM, Solomon H, et al. A new autosomal dominant disorder of pyogenic sterile arthritis, pyoderma gangrenosum, and acne: PAPA syndrome. *Mayo Clin Proc* 1997;72:611–615.
14. Chiu A, Chon SY, Kimball AB. The response of skin disease to stress: changes in the severity of acne vulgaris as affected by examination stress. *Arch Dermatol* 2003;139:897–900.
15. Cooper AJ. Systematic review of propionibacterium acnes resistance to systemic antibiotics. *Med J Aust* 1998;169:259–261.
16. Helms SE, Bredle DL, Zajic J, et al. Oral contraceptive failure rates and oral antibiotics. *J Am Acad Dermatol* 1997;36:705–710.
17. Velicer CM. Antibiotic use in relation to the risk of breast cancer. *JAMA* 2004;291:827–835.
18. Gough A, Chapman S, Wagstaff K, et al. Minocycline-induced autoimmune hepatitis and systemic lupus erythematosus-like syndrome. *BMJ* 1996;312:369–372.
19. Skidmore R, Kovach R, Walker C, et al. Effects of subantimicrobial-dose doxycycline in the treatment of moderate acne. *Arch Dermatol* 2003;139:459–464.
20. Kapadia N, Talib A. Acne treated successfully with azithromycin. *Int J Dermatol* 2004;43:766–767.
21. Yemisci A, Gorgulu A, Piskin S. Effects and side-effects of spironolactone therapy in women with acne. *J Eur Acad Dermatol Venereol* 2005;19:163–166.
22. Layton AM, Knaggs H, Taylor J, et al. Isotretinoin for acne vulgaris—10 years later: a safe and successful treatment. *Br J Dermatol* 1993;129:292–296.
23. Chia CY, Lane W, Chibnall J, et al. Isotretinoin therapy and mood changes in adolescents with moderate to severe acne: a cohort study. *Arch Dermatol* 2005;141:557–560.
24. Hersom K, Jick SS, Kremers HM, et al. Isotretinoin use and risk of depression, psychotic symptoms, suicide, and attempted suicide. *Arch Dermatol* 2000;136:1231–1236.
25. Lloyd JR. The use of microdermabrasion for acne: a pilot study. *Dermatol Surg* 2001;27:329–331.
26. Patton T. Light therapy in the treatment of acne vulgaris. *Cosmet Dermatol* 2004;17: 373–378.
27. Alster TS, McMeekin TO. Improvement of facial acne scars by the 585 nm flashlamp-pumped pulsed dye laser. *J Am Acad Dermatol* 1996;35:79–81.
28. Orringer JS, Kang S, Hamilton T, et al. Treatment of acne vulgaris with a pulsed dye laser. A randomized controlled trial. *JAMA* 2004;291:2834–2839.
29. Seaton ED, Charakida A, Mouser PE, et al. Pulsed-dye laser treatment for inflammatory acne vulgaris: a randomized controlled trial. *Lancet* 2003;362:1347–1352.

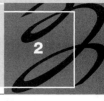
I. **DEFINITION AND PATHOPHYSIOLOGY.** Alopecia areata (AA) is a unique disorder characterized by patches of nonscarring patterned alopecia that is postulated to be an organ-specific autoimmune disease.

A. **Epidemiology.** Children and young adults are most frequently affected, and there is a positive family history in 10% to 30% of cases. Sixty percent of patients with AA are less than 20 years old. The average lifetime risk of developing AA is estimated to be 1.7% with a prevalence estimated at 0.1% to 0.2%. A case of a patient with congenital AA has been reported.

Significant human leukocyte antigen (HLA) associations with AA have been reported. HLA-DQB1*03 (DQ3) appears to be a susceptibility marker for all forms of AA, whereas HLA-DRB1*0401 (DR4) and HLA-DQB1*0303 (DQ7) are markers for severe long-standing alopecia totalis (AT)/universalis (1,2). Researchers have identified a homolog of the hairless mouse gene in a large Pakistani family with alopecia universalis (AU); this "hairless" gene is located on chromosome 8 and the implications for AA are not yet clear (3).

B. **Pathogenesis.** An aberrant interaction between T lymphocytes and HLA-DR antigens expressed by hair follicle keratinocytes has been implicated in the pathogenesis of AA. Gilhar et al. showed that 2-mm sections of scalp skin from patients with AA would grow hair when engrafted onto congenitally athymic nude mice highlighting the role of immune cells, specifically T cells. This work was expanded to show that regrowth of hair occurred when AA scalp grafts were engrafted onto nude mice. In the severe combined immunodeficiency (SCID) mouse model, T lymphocytes from patients with AA, when activated by follicular antigens, were able to induce the disease in autologous scalp transplants (4).

The inflammatory infiltrate consists of T cells, monocytes, and Langerhans cells; T helper cells predominate. Adhesion molecule receptors, specifically, intercellular adhesion molecule 2 [ICAM-2] and endothelial leucocyte adhesion molecule-1 (ELAM-1) are expressed at the beginning of the disease and mediate the trafficking of leukocytes into the dermis. Interferon-γ (IFN-γ) and interleukin-2 (IL-2) are significantly elevated in patients with more extensive AA.

C. **Etiology.** The cause is unknown; however, it is postulated to be an organ-specific autoimmune disease with the target antigens being melanocyte peptides. Genetic factors are also known to mitigate disease susceptibility and severity. A concordance rate of 55% seen in studies of identical twins suggests that environmental factors are also important.

D. **Disease associations.** Atopy, including allergic rhinitis, asthma, and atopic dermatitis, is the most common disease associated with AA. Many patients experience a seasonal flare of AA with increased atopic symptoms. Some of the most recalcitrant patients with AA have a history of atopy.

Emotional stress does not appear to play a significant role in this disorder. The disease itself is significantly stressful, and major depression, social phobias, and anxiety may develop.

Other autoimmune diseases are thought to occur in association with AA, including thyroid disease, vitiligo, and inflammatory bowel disease, specifically Crohn's disease. Autoimmune gonadal disease in male patients with AA has also been reported. Thirty percent of patients with APECED syndrome (autoimmune polyendocrinopathy mucocutaneous candidiasis-ectodermal insufficiency) type 1 were recently found to exhibit AA. Lastly, as mentioned in the preceding text, AA occurs in approximately 0.1% of the general population, but this is increased to 9% in Down's syndrome.

E. Prognosis. The course of AA is erratic and impossible to predict. In general, the younger the age of the patient at onset and the more widespread the disease, the poorer is the prognosis. Cases developing before puberty have a particularly dismal regrowth rate. One patient out of ten has hair loss only in sites other than the scalp—eyelashes, eyebrows, beard, and general body hair—and approximately 10% of patients progress to loss of all scalp hair AT. Regrowth of hair during the first attack takes place within 6 months in 30% of cases, within 1 year in 50%, and within 5 years in 75%; complete recovery occurs in approximately 30%; in up to 33%, the hair never regrows. New lesions reappear within months to years in up to 50% of cases. A prolonged and difficult course with poor outlook is associated with total loss of hair from scalp and body AU; with an ophiasis pattern; with rapid progression of disease; with eyebrow, eyelash, or beard involvement; and with severe associated nail changes.

II. **SUBJECTIVE DATA.** The hair loss is usually without discomfort; rarely, there may be itching, burning, tingling, or paresthesias in affected areas, which may precede hair shedding by 1 to 2 weeks. Patients with AU may occasionally report significant pruritus.

III. **OBJECTIVE DATA**

A. **Clinical findings.** Lesions are well defined, single or multiple, round to oval areas of nonscarring hair loss in which the skin seems very smooth and soft. There may be some slight erythema and overlying fine scale. Any hair-bearing area can be affected.

    1. In active lesions, "exclamation point hair" may be seen around the margins. These loose hairs protrude approximately 3 to 10 mm above the scalp surface and have a dark, rough, brush-like tip, a narrower, less pigmented shaft, and an atrophic root (distal end broader than proximal end). These hairs reflect the disturbed keratinization seen after injury to the growing hair follicle and with transition to a resting follicle; they are pathognomonic of expanding AA.

    2. Various patterns have been described. The more common patterns include alopecia totalis—loss of all scalp hair, alopecia universalis—loss of all scalp and body hair, and ophiasis—band-like pattern of hair loss along the periphery of the temporal and occipital scalp. Less commonly, patients may present with a diffuse pattern or reticular variant, which is characterized by recurrent patchy disease with active areas of loss and spontaneous regrowth in different areas occurring at the same time.

B. Regrowing hairs appear first as fine, downy, vellus strands that are gradually replaced by normal terminal hair. These new hairs are often lusterless, may break easily, and may be white.

C. Nail changes, present in 10% to 20% of cases, consist primarily of discrete pits in the nail surface usually arranged in horizontal or vertical rows. There is clinical overlap with psoriatic nail pitting. Other changes noted include longitudinal ridging, onycholysis, koilonychia, and rarely onychomadesis.

IV. **ASSESSMENT**

A. Patients with AA are generally healthy and do not routinely require investigative laboratory studies. Thyroid function testing should be considered, particularly in children, because the incidence of abnormalities may be as high as 24%.

B. Careful scalp examination will show no evidence of scarring alopecia. During periods of active disease, the pull test will be positive often several centimeters away from a patch of alopecia. One should examine for exclamation point hairs.

C. **Differential diagnosis.** Other patterned, nonscarring alopecias should be considered when evaluating patients. Tinea capitis, traumatic (traction alopecia) and pressure-related alopecia, self-induced hair loss (trichotillomania), androgenetic alopecia, loose anagen syndrome and secondary syphilis need to be considered. In younger patients, aplasia cutis should be suspected before biopsy.

D. Histopathology. Findings have been described as a "swarm of bees" highlighting the peribulbar lymphocytic infiltrate seen classically in active AA. The inflammatory cells, primarily Langerhans' cells and $CD4^+$ lymphocytes, can be seen in the peribulbar/perivascular areas in addition to invading the external root sheath. Apoptosis is a prominent feature during periods of active disease, as are miniaturized catagen phase follicles.

V. THERAPY

A. Reassurance about the likelihood of spontaneous regrowth and a simple explanation covering the nature and course of the disease, as well as a discussion about the poor clinical impact of most treatments, are imperative at the onset of diagnosis. Existing treatments are not a cure, and they must be continued until remission is achieved. Different portions of the scalp may respond to different treatment modalities. Spontaneous regrowth of hair may be confused with the presumed beneficial effects of therapy, especially in patients with patchy AA. When hair loss is extensive or when there is total or universal alopecia, an honest discussion of the chronic nature of AA is necessary. Despite the smooth bald appearance of the scalp, the potential for full hair regrowth exists. A wig is useful and will not affect active treatment negatively.

B. Intralesional therapy. Although they are widely used for the treatment of AA, few studies have been done evaluating their efficacy. Intralesional corticosteroid injections can be considered for patchy localized disease which is cosmetically disfiguring and persistent, particularly on the scalp or, occasionally, on the eyebrows. Regrowth may be evident 4 to 6 weeks after injections. Up to 33% of patients will not regrow hair; failures occur primarily in new and rapidly expanding plaques or in areas of long-standing hair loss.

   1. Intradermal injections around and within the plaques at 1- to 2-cm intervals with a 3-mL syringe and a 30-gauge needle.

   2. Recommendations for the dilution of triamcinolone acetonide suspension ranges from 2.5 to 10 mg/mL; approximately 0.05 to 0.10 mL should be placed with each injection for a maximum volume of 2 to 3 mL.

   3. Re-injection at 4- to 6-week intervals. If no growth is present at 3 months, it is generally not worth continuing the procedure.

   4. Areas of corticosteroid-related regrowth may begin to thin after 3 to 6 months and can be injected again if necessary. Spontaneous regrowth frequently occurs during this interval.

C. Topical corticosteroids. Again, few studies have been done to assess the efficacy of topical corticosteroid therapy. Fluocinolone acetonide cream 0.2% b.i.d., desoximetasone cream b.i.d. for 12 weeks, and betamethasone dipropionate cream 0.05% have been reported in case series with equivocal results, and many researchers believe that topical corticosteroids alone are not very effective. If tried, high or super-high potency topical corticosteroids should be used for at least 3 months, and maintenance therapy is often necessary. Many advocate weekly pulse therapy after 2 weeks of topical corticosteroids. Anecdotal reports of topical corticosteroids under occlusion have recently been stated by some authors to improve outcomes. For children, topical corticosteroids may be the most practical alternative. Their side effects include folliculitis, telangiectases, and local cutaneous atrophy.

D. Systemic corticosteroids. Treatment with systemic corticosteroids will often stimulate hair regrowth but may, infrequently, alter the basic disease course and is therefore rarely, if ever, warranted. In one small, uncontrolled study using pulse corticosteroids in children with new onset AA, 71% of the patients had complete regrowth, sustained at 12-month follow-up (5). Another prospective study showed some benefit of pulse methylprednisolone therapy in adults with early AA (6). The rate of regrowth varies greatly and is difficult to compare because different dosage regimens are used in different studies. Price et al. recommend the following regimen for adults weighing greater than 60 kg: 40 mg for 3 days, reducing the dose by 5 mg every 3 days until the patient is tapered off the drug completely—24-day regimen (7).

E. Topical immunotherapy involves the induction of an allergic contact dermatitis by the topical application of potent contact sensitizers. These therapies are generally reserved for patients older than 10 years of age and for those with greater than 50% of the scalp involved. Repeated applications of topical sensitizers such as dinitrochlorobenzene (DNCB), squaric acid dibutylester (SADBE), and diphencyprone (DPCP) have been found to induce regrowth of scalp hair in 50% to 90% of those treated. DNCB is a potential mutagen and is no longer used in most centers. The U.S. Food and Drug Administration (FDA) does not approve the use of DPCP, and but approves SADBE with the stipulation that it be administered in a physician's office. There is a paucity of double-blind, randomized studies with these agents. The mechanism of action has not been completely elucidated; however, it is thought that allergic contact sensitization changes the peribulbar T_4/T_8 ratio from 4:1 to 1:1, reduces the abnormal expression of some HLAs in the epithelium of lower hair follicles or, according to one hypothesis, may induce "antigenic competition" that inhibits autoimmune reactions. Therapy with allergic contactants must be prolonged (months), and the side effects include constant mild rash, pruritus, adenopathy and rarely erythema multiforme, vitiligo, and the possibility of an autosensitization reaction.

F. Anthralin has been used as both short-contact and overnight treatments in both children and adults with limited patchy AA. The mechanism of action is unknown. However, it is thought to create inflammation by generating free radicals, which have immunosuppressive actions. Only uncontrolled studies have been conducted to assess its efficacy with response rates ranging from 25% to 75%. Lower concentrations (0.1% to 0.4%) are used for overnight treatments, whereas concentrations of 1% to 3% are used for short contact. Anthralin is initially applied once or twice a week. The dose and frequency are both increased as tolerated to a maximum of 1.0% with overnight application. This treatment must be continued for at least 6 months before evaluating therapy; short contact therapy may be easier for young children. Combination therapy of 0.5% anthralin and 5% minoxidil has been shown to enhance the response rate. Its side effects include pruritus, erythema, scaling, folliculitis, and lymphadenopathy. Staining of skin and clothes can also be an issue.

G. Minoxidil was originally used orally to treat recalcitrant hypertension. Because its systemic use produced hypertrichosis in a significant number of patients, its efficacy as a topical therapy for AA and for androgenic alopecia has been examined. The results in patients with AA have been conflicting, with reported response rates ranging from 8% to 45%. Nonresponders are more likely to have the most extensive hair loss. Occlusion of the treatment sites maximizes the results. Despite measurable percutaneous absorption, systemic side effects have not been a clinical problem. However, allergic contact dermatitis has occasionally been seen. Minoxidil most likely has a direct mitogenic effect on epidermal cells and prolongs the survival time of keratinocytes (8). The regimen involves the application of topical 5% Minoxidil, not more than 25 drops two times a day, for 12 weeks for initial regrowth to be seen and with continued application to achieve cosmetically acceptable regrowth. Minoxidil is now available in both 2% and 5% over-the-counter solutions. However, the 5% solution appears to be more effective. The solution is well tolerated with common side effects of hypertrichosis and irritation.

H. Prolonged photochemotherapy (PUVA) may induce regrowth of scalp and body hair in 70% of those treated. PUVA therapy involves a combination of psoralen and UVA light. Hair regrowth is related to total energy delivered. Initial response is seen after 85 to 120 J/cm^2; satisfactory results may require 350 J/cm^2 for AA and 730 J/cm^2 for AT. PUVA decreases a subset of T lymphocytes and may affect AA by altering immune mechanisms. One recent study, reviewing 10 years' experience, reported an initial response rate of 43.8% for partial AA and 50% for AT and AU. After excluding patients with only vellus hair regrowth and those who relapsed within 4 months, their success rate was at best 6.3% for partial AA and 12.5% for AT and AU (9). Their side effects include increased risk of skin cancers and burning. Once the hair has regrown, the UVA light may have difficulty in reaching the scalp, and loss of efficacy (i.e., repeat hair loss) has been reported.

I. Cyclosporine inhibits the activation of T helper cells, which may be pathogenic in AA. No beneficial response has been reported using topical cyclosporine, perhaps related to the relatively large size of the molecule preventing penetration through the stratum corneum. A trial of oral cyclosporine (6 mg/kg/day) has led to cosmetically acceptable scalp hair regrowth in 50% of the patients. However, all patients relapsed within 3 months of discontinuation of therapy (10). Although systemic cyclosporine appears to be effective in AA, the high recurrence rate after discontinuation and the side effect profile make it a poor long-term choice. A paradox also exists with this drug as AA developed in patients who take the medication during transplant therapy.

J. Topical immunomodulators. Topical FK 506 (tacrolimus) has shown promise in hair regrowth in Dundee experimental bald rat (DEBR) rats with alopecia. However, they subsequently lost their hair after discontinuation of therapy as with cyclosporine. Human studies are yet to be published, and a large randomized, prospective study would be required (11). Tacrolimus and pimecrolimus are smaller molecules than cyclosporine and they do penetrate the stratum corneum, but their molecular size may limit their reaching the site of the pathology (i.e., deep dermis) in sufficient concentration to have efficacy. Combination regimens with corticosteroids and/or keratolytics and/or occlusion are being investigated.

K. Many other modalities have been studied including IFN, specifically the topical interferon inducer imiquimod, dapsone, nitrogen mustard, massage and relaxation, and acupuncture and aromatherapy, to name a few. The efficacy of these treatments needs to be further assessed in controlled studies.

References

1. Duvic M, Hordinsky MK, Fiedler VC, et al. HLA-D locus associations in alopecia areata. *Arch Dermatol* 1991;127:64–68.
2. Colombe BW, Lou CD, Price V. The genetic basis of alopecia areata: HLA associations with patchy alopecia areata versus alopecia universalis. *J Investig Dermatol Symp Proc* 1999;4:216–219.
3. Ahmad W, Faiyaz ul Haque M, Brancolini V, et al. Alopecia universalis associated with a mutation in the human hairless gene. *Science* 1998;279:720–724.
4. Gilhar A, Ullmann Y, Berkutzki T, et al. Autoimmune hair loss (alopecia areata) transferred by T-lymphocytes to human scalp explants on SCID mice with T-lymphocyte injections. *J Clin Invest* 1998;101:62–67.
5. Kiesch N, Stene JJ, Goens J, et al. Pulse steroid therapy for children's severe alopecia areata? *Dermatology* 1997;194:395–397.
6. Friedli A, Labarthe MP, Engelhardt E, et al. Pulse methylprednisolone therapy for severe alopecia areata: an open prospective study of 45 patients. *J Am Acad Dermatol* 1998;39:597–602.
7. Price VH. Treatment of hair loss. *N Engl J Med* 1999;341:964–973.
8. Baden HP, Kublius J. Effect of minoxidil on cultured keratinocytes. *J Invest Dermatol* 1983;81:558–560.
9. Taylor CR, Hawk JL. PUVA treatment of alopecia areata partialis, totalis and universalis: audit of 10 years' experience at S. John's Institute of Dermatology. *Br J Dermatol* 1995;133:914–918.
10. Gupta AK, Ellis CN, Cooper KD, et al. Oral cyclosporine for the treatment of alopecia areata: a clinical and immunohistochemical analysis. *J Am Acad Dermatol* 1990;22:242–250.
11. McElwee KJ, Rushton DH, Trachy R, et al. Topical FK506: a potent immunotherapy for alopecia areata? Studies using the Dundee experimental bald rat model. *Br J Dermatol* 1997;137:491–497.

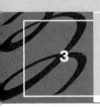

3 APHTHOUS STOMATITIS (CANKER SORES)
Jennifer Nam Choi

I. **DEFINITION AND PATHOPHYSIOLOGY.** Canker sores are recurrent, painful mucosal erosions that appear on the inner cheeks, lips, gums, ventral tongue, palate, and pharynx (nonkeratinized tissues). The prevalence of aphthous ulcerations in the general population is approximately 20%, although rates from 31% to 66% have been reported in select patient groups (1,2). It is estimated that over 1 in 5 individuals have had at least one episode of aphthous ulcers in their lifetime. Lesions may be found at any age, but the onset of disease is usually in adolescence or young adulthood, whereas disease prevalence peaks in the third to fourth decades. Although any ethnicity or socioeconomic group may be affected, being white and of a higher socioeconomic group have been found to be positive predictors of recurrent aphthous stomatitis (RAS) (3). Most published reports show a slightly higher prevalence for females than males (4,5). Multiple local and systemic triggering factors have been implicated in the pathogenesis, including stress, hormonal changes, trauma, microorganisms, food hypersensitivity, immune dysregulation, recurrent herpes labialis, family history, and deficiencies of certain vitamins, calcium, iron, and ferritin. Despite the associations, the data are conflicting, and the etiology of this syndrome remains unclear. Nicotine, on the other hand, may be a protective factor; several studies have shown a significant reduction in aphthous ulcers with the use of nicotine, in the form of tobacco smoking, nicotine patches, and nicotine-containing tablets (6–13). Premenstrual flare-ups and remissions during the third trimester of pregnancy are common.

Three types of RAS exist:

A. **Minor aphthae**, by far the most common form, account for 80% of the cases. They usually measure between 1 and 5 mm, but may be as large as 1 cm, lasting for 7 to 14 days. One to five ulcers may be present at any time. Pain is minimal to moderate and healing is spontaneous with no scarring.

B. **Herpetiform aphthae** occur in approximately 10% of patients, usually measure 1 to 3 mm in diameter and are similar to minor aphthae with the exception of being far more numerous (from 2 to 10, but as many as 100) and grouped together in a herpetiform pattern occurring on any area of the oral mucosa. Despite the name, these are not associated with herpesvirus infection.

C. **Major aphthae or Sutton's disease**, formerly known as periadenitis mucosa necrotica recurrens, are large (>1.0 cm, up to several centimeters in size), slow healing, few in number, and very painful. They frequently involve the soft palate and oropharynx. The healing may take weeks to months, often with scarring.

Recurrent lesions of aphthous stomatitis may be divided into four stages. The premonitory stage lasts up to 24 hours and is characterized by tingling, burning, painful or hyperesthetic sensations in the absence of any clinical changes. The preulcerative stage may last 18 hours to 3 days with variable but often moderately severe pain. Flat or raised indurated areas surrounded by a red halo are present and are gradually covered by a gray or yellow fibrinous membrane in the ulcerative stage. This third phase usually lasts 1 to 16 days, and lesions are severely painful until 2 to 3 days after the ulcer has formed. The healing stage lasts from 4 to 35 days with the natural history of eventual remission. Two of three patients with recurrent lesions will go into remission within 15 years, whereas one of these will continue to have lesions for up to 40 years. Patients with superficial (minor) lesions remit earlier than those with deeper, more destructive (major) lesions.

RAS can be further classified on the basis of the clinical disease severity (14). Simple aphthosis consists of recurrent attacks of any type of aphthae with distinct ulcer-free periods, most being in otherwise well, young patients. Complex aphthosis is defined as the almost constant presence of ≥ 3 oral aphthae or recurrent oral and genital aphthae in the absence of Behçet's disease. Forms of complex aphthosis include primary, idiopathic, and secondary, related to inflammatory bowel disease, human immunodeficiency virus (HIV), cyclic neutropenia, PFAPA (periodic fever, aphthous stomatitis, pharyngitis, adenitis), hematinic deficiency (iron, zinc, folate, vitamins B_1, B_2, B_6, B_{12}), gluten-sensitive enteropathy, and ulcus vulvae acutum.

Behçet's disease can present with multiple oral and genital aphthous ulcers that may occur for many years before the diagnosis (average 7 to 8 years). Criteria for establishing the diagnosis have been published by the International Study Group for Behçet's disease, as well as by O'Duffy and Goldstein (14,15). These criteria include the presence of minor, major, or herpetiform aphthae observed by physicians or reported reliably by the patient, recurrent at least three times in one 12-month period, plus two of the following: (i) recurrent genital aphthae or scarring, (ii) anterior uveitis, posterior uveitis, cells in vitreous on slit-lamp examination, or retinal vasculitis, (iii) erythema nodosum-like lesions or papulopustular lesions consistent with Behçet's disease, or (iv) positive pathergy test (neutrophilic vascular reaction or leukocytoclastic vasculitis) read by a physician at 24 or 48 hours, performed with oblique insertion of a 20-gauge or smaller needle under sterile conditions. There is no diagnostic test to predict which patients with oral aphthae will progress to Behçet's disease; close clinical follow-up is suggested (16,17).

The PFAPA syndrome has been recently described in the pediatric population. There are no known disease associations with this syndrome. The average duration of each recurrent attack is 4 to 5 days. Episodes may be aborted by a single dose of prednisone (2 mg/kg) at the beginning of the symptoms. Tonsillectomy has been curative in some patients (18–20).

Bednar's aphthae are large oral palatine ulcers in infants. Non-orthodontic nipples and pacifiers and its contact with the mucosa cause these ulcerations. Alteration of the nipple is curative, although scarring may occur (21).

Evidence for an immunopathogenesis of aphthous stomatitis related to lymphocyte-epithelial cell interaction is based on the pathologic features of early lesions, positive lymphocyte transformation, lymphocytotoxicity, and leukocyte migration tests. The presence of antimucosal antibodies indicates an immunologic reaction to damaged epithelial tissue. There is a depressed or reversed CD4:CD8 ratio, increased T cell receptor γ-δ T cells, and an increase in tumor necrosis factor-α (TNF-α) levels (findings also seen in HIV-positive patients), suggesting the imbalance of the Th1/Th2 immune pathways. An abnormal cytokine cascade is established with enhanced cell-mediated immune response directed against the normal mucosa. Elevated levels of interferon-γ, TNF-α, and IL 2,4, and 5 are present (22). A recent study compared the mean serum cytokine levels of IL-2, IL-4, granulocyte-macrophage colony-stimulating factor (GM-CSF), sFas, and FasL by ELISA for 67 patients with RAS and 72 normal controls, showing the mean serum cytokine level for patients to be significantly greater than that for controls. Additionally, the mean serum cytokine concentrations for the patient group demonstrated a diffuse pattern covering a wide range of serum concentrations, as compared with the compact range and lower mean serum cytokine concentrations of the control group (23). A recent microarray study comparing the cDNA from 29 samples of aphthae mucosa and that from 11 samples of normal mucosa has confirmed a higher expression level of the Th1 gene cluster (24). Salivary prostaglandin E2 and epidermal growth factor are decreased during the active stage of RAS (25). Significantly greater expression of both vascular cell adhesion molecule (VCAM-1) and E-selectin has been detected in the vasculature of RAS; increased keratinocyte adhesion molecules (ICAM-1) may facilitate the invasion of lymphocytes into the epithelium (26). Mast cells and factor XIII-a positive dermal dendritic cells are also increased in the infiltrate.

Human leukocyte antigens (HLA) types A_2 and B_{12} are more common in patients with RAS. HIV-positive patients have an increased incidence of RAS. The most common type is minor aphthae; patients with major aphthae tend to be more immunosuppressed. HIV infection can present as a glandular fever-like illness with shallow ulcers in the mouth or on the genitals and/or anus. Women with HIV disease may develop oral and genital aphthae.

Chemical insult, disease, and/or infection are among the potential environmental factors precipitating oral ulceration. Some reported oral ulcer–inducing chemicals include tacrolimus, alendronate, nicorandil, hydroxyurea, ferrous sulfate, cholinsalicylate gel, and piroxicam. Aphthous ulcers have also been associated with imiquimod treatment of actinic cheilitis (27). One regular finding is the isolation of a pleomorphic α-hemolytic streptococcus, *Streptococcus sanguis*, from aphthous lesions. These organisms or their cell wall material can produce lesions in animals that are histologically similar to those found in sections of human lesions, and they may produce a hypersensitivity reaction of a delayed type in animals and humans with recurrent aphthae. Streptococcal cell wall material may be pathogenic in aphthous stomatitis, with the cell wall–lacking L-form present during remissions. Whether cross-reactions between streptococcal antigens and oral mucosal antigens occur and are central to the pathogenesis of aphthous stomatitis still remains to be seen.

Other bacteria suspected to be causative of aphthous stomatitis include *Helicobacter pylori* (28), *Treponema pallidum* (29), and members of the actinomyces family (30).

Suspected viruses associated with oral ulceration include the human papilloma virus (HPV), herpes simplex virus (HSV), Epstein–Barr virus (EBV), cytomegalovirus (CMV), human herpesvirus-8 (HHV-8), HIV, and reactivation of human herpesvirus-6 (HHV-6). Recently, oral mucosal samples from 60 patients suffering from RAS were investigated by polymerase chain reaction (PCR) and southern hybridization for the presence of six different viruses (23). Among the 32 (53.3%) virus-positive results, the frequency of prevalence revealed the overall association between viruses and RAS to be HHV-8>CMV>EBV>HPV>HSV-1. No HSV-2-positive samples were found.

II. SUBJECTIVE DATA. Tingling or burning may antedate the appearance of the lesions by 24 hours. During the first 2 to 3 days, the lesions are extremely painful and may interfere with eating and speaking.

III. OBJECTIVE DATA. Aphthae appear as single or multiple, small (1- to 10-mm diameter), shallow erosions with clearly defined borders covered by a gray membrane and surrounded by an intense erythematous halo. Rarely, extremely large or exceedingly numerous lesions appear.

IV. ASSESSMENT. Morphologically similar lesions can be seen with (i) acute herpes simplex gingivostomatitis, (ii) candidiasis, (iii) Vincent's angina, (iv) traumatic ulcers, (v) ulcers in patients with agranulocytosis or cyclic neutropenia, (vi) vitamin B_{12}- or folate-deficient macrocytic anemia, (vii) iron deficiency, and (viii) celiac or Crohn's disease. Distinguishing RAS from a differential diagnosis of erythema multiforme, erosive lichen planus, pemphigus, pemphigoid, and herpangina should not be difficult. Rarely, a squamous cell carcinoma of the oral mucosa can present as a non-healing oral ulceration. Aphthae may be associated with chronic ulcerative colitis, Crohn's disease, gluten-sensitive enteropathy, lupus erythematosus, and HIV infection. The erosions of Behçet's syndrome (oral and genital ulceration associated with iritis) may be identical, and it is possible that this syndrome is a severe form of the same entity as aphthous stomatitis. A minority of patients with RAS having normal hemoglobin and red blood cell indices has been found to have deficiencies of iron (low ferritin), folate, or vitamin B_{12}. Vitamins B_1, B_2, and B_6 (thiamine, riboflavin, and pyridoxine) deficiency should be considered as a precipitating factor in RAS. Suggested evaluation for patients with complex aphthosis includes complete dermatologic examination with biopsy of ulcers or other coexisting cutaneous lesions as appropriate, complete blood count (CBC) with differential and platelet count, serum iron, folate, zinc, and vitamin B_{12} levels, and culture or PCR of ulcers to exclude HSV infection (14). Consideration of HIV, HLA-B27, antiendomysial or antigliadin antibody testing, as well as referral for gastroenterologic, rheumatologic, ophthalmologic, or neurologic evaluation should be made if appropriate.

V. THERAPY. Therapy of aphthous stomatitis is aimed at (i) controlling the pain, (ii) shortening the duration of lesions already present, and (iii) aborting new lesions. These objectives may often be attained. Prevention of further attacks is much more elusive.

A. Controlling pain

1. **Topical anesthetics.** Apply dyclonine HCl solution (Dyclone) to ulcers as often as needed. Onset of anesthesia is rapid, and duration of numbing is up to 1 hour. Lidocaine (Xylocaine, ointment 5%, or viscous) or diphenhydramine HCl (Benadryl elixir) alone or mixed with Kaopectate may be used in the same way. If local anesthetics are used over too wide an area, a disturbing "cottonmouth" feeling and total loss of taste result; frequently, these symptoms are worse than those of the original problem. A common soothing home remedy is to apply hydrogen peroxide with a cotton swab on the canker sore (one part hydrogen peroxide and one part water). Subsequently, a small amount of milk of magnesia is applied onto the canker sore three to four times a day.

   a. Benzodent is an anesthetic in a denture adhesive–like base. This product contains 20% benzocaine, 0.4% eugenol, and 0.1% hydroxyquinoline sulfate. It is applied directly to aphthous ulcers. Ora-Jel is a similar product. Kank-A contains 5% benzocaine and benzoin in a liquid vehicle.

   b. A new mucoadhesive tablet (Canker Cover), which releases natural active agents for pain reduction and rapid healing of aphthous ulcers, has been prepared and characterized. Adhesive tablets prepared by compression molding of mixed powders of cross-linked polyacrylic acid and hydroxypropyl cellulose, absorbed with citrus oil and magnesium salt, have been shown to reduce pain and decrease healing time without adverse side effects in a clinical trial on 248 patients with canker sores (31).

2. Superficial destructive therapies such as carbon dioxide laser ablation or silver nitrate stick application destroys nerve endings and may provide relief from pain for the duration of the eruption, but the ulcers may enlarge slightly and heal more slowly.

B. Aborting lesions and shortening course

1. Suppression of oral streptococci by topical antibiotics is a logical approach to therapy and is often successful.

   a. The application of tetracycline compresses is one method of choice. Gauze pledgets must be saturated with 250 to 1000 mg tetracycline dissolved in 30 mL of water or elixir of Benadryl and applied for 10 to 20 minutes four to six times a day. Nothing should be taken by mouth for the following 30 minutes. Therapy should be continued for 5 to 7 days. In many patients, this treatment effectively shortens the duration of lesions, decreases pain, and aborts early lesions, although, unfortunately, some lesions do not respond to this regimen. Patients with recurrent lesions should be instructed to initiate therapy as early as possible.

   b. Some patients acquire resistance to tetracycline. In those instances, a 1% cephalexin monohydrate compress must be used by dissolving a 250-mg capsule of cephalexin (Keflex) in 30 mL of water and applied for 10 to 20 minutes four to six times a day.

   c. Penicillin G potassium troches (Cankercillin) in 50 mg doses has been shown to be efficacious for the treatment of minor recurrent aphthous ulcers of <48 hours duration in a phase 2 double-blind, randomized placebo-controlled trial with a no-treatment arm consisting of 100 patients (32). The mouth should first be rinsed with water, then the troche placed directly over the ulcer. The troche must be directly maintained at the site of the ulcer to dissolve slowly over 5 to 10 minutes. For 1 hour after troche application, chewing, eating and drinking, and talking should be avoided. Troches should be applied over the ulcer four times daily, after meals and before bedtime. The study demonstrated a significant reduction in the time of healing and pain relief of minor aphthous ulcers with treatment for 1 week. Larger phase 3 studies are necessary to confirm these findings.

  d. Other topical treatments of some benefit include Sucralfate after meals and at bedtime; regular use of a triclosan-containing mouth rinse; use of an ultrasonic toothbrush; and avoidance of toothpaste containing the detergents sodium lauryl sulfate (SLS). Zilactin is a hydroxypropyl cellulose film that is placed over the ulcer and helps reduce the pain, without any effect on the healing time.

  e. Five percent amlexanox (Aphthasol) is a unique topical oral paste that can shorten the pain and duration of aphthous ulcers. The paste is applied to each ulcer four times a day.

2. Topical steroids can also be useful, especially if applied during the prodromal stages. Triamcinolone acetonide 0.1% or clobetasol 0.05% in a base that adheres to mucous membrane (Orabase) or other corticosteroid agents should be applied at least q.i.d. Others advocate use of 2.5-mg tablets of hydrocortisone sodium succinate or 0.1-mg tablets of betamethasone 17-valerate, allowed to dissolve slowly near the lesion, three to four times a day. Dexamethasone suspension (Decadron, 0.5 mL/5 mL) swished and spit q.i.d. can decrease the frequency and intensity of RAS with some systemic absorption. Corticosteroid inhalers have also been used and are helpful for hard-to-reach ulcers such as those in the soft palate or posterior vestibule. Oral candidiasis is a frequent side effect of long-term topical steroids on the oral mucosa.

3. Administration of systemic corticosteroids can abort attacks if taken for 4 days during the prodromal period, and it will usually induce healing of lesions in patients with severe erosive lesions. A sample regimen of oral prednisone is an initial dose of 25 mg daily for 1 day, followed by 20 mg daily for 2 days, 15 mg daily for 2 days, 10 mg daily for 2 days, and 5 mg daily for 1 day.

4. Colchicine, an alkaloid that interferes with microtubule function, has been reported to promote healing and prevent recurrences in patients with aphthous ulcers. Its beneficial effect on the cutaneous lesions of Behçet's syndrome has been known for some time. Response to a daily oral dose of 0.6 to 1.8 mg can be expected within 4 to 6 weeks; otherwise, the drug should be discontinued. The toxicity of colchicine, particularly gastrointestinal complaints, often limits its use. For long-term therapy, the physician should be particularly aware of the potential for bone marrow suppression, myopathy, and alopecia.

5. Dapsone may also be helpful for severe recurrent oral aphthae. Dosing can range from 25 to 100 mg daily and should be started after G6PD screening with concomitant hematologic monitoring. The combination of colchicine and dapsone at the full, tolerated doses has been shown to have excellent results in some patients (14).

6. Pentoxifylline at a dose of 400 mg three times a day after meals was reported to alleviate the symptoms in a small open trial.

7. Sulfapyridine at a dose of 1 g daily in combination with colchicine has been reported to be effective (14).

8. Topical 5% 5-aminosalicylic acid (5-ASA) has been shown to shorten the healing time and decrease the pain of RAS (33).

9. Thalidomide, available through Celgene Corporation as part of the STEPS (System for Thalidomide Education and Prescribing Safety) program or research protocols associated with the U.S. Food and Drug Administration (FDA), is one of the most effective drugs for severe aphthous stomatitis. In addition to being a teratogen, thalidomide may also cause or aggravate peripheral neuropathy. Dry mouth, drowsiness, and constipation are other less serious side effects. Fifty-five percent of patients had complete healing after 4 weeks of therapy (34). Unfortunately, many patients relapse after discontinuation of therapy; the goal is to establish the lowest effective drug level to control symptoms, doses usually ranging from 50 to 150 mg nightly.

10. Cyclosporine, in a topical solution, may induce remission while on therapy. Relapse is common, and administration as an oral suspension to swish and spit is very expensive.

11. Low-dose interferon-α, given orally, has shown promise in inducing significant remissions of RAS.

12. GM-CSF has been used in patients with either cyclic neutropenia or HIV disease with difficult-to-treat aphthae.

References

1. Rogers RS III. Recurrent aphthous stomatitis in the diagnosis of Behçet's disease. *Yonsei Med J* 1997;38:370–379.
2. Ship JA. Recurrent aphthous stomatitis. An update. *Oral Surg Oral Med Oral Pathol Oral Radiol Endod* 1996;81:141–147.
3. Shulman JD. An exploration of point, annual, and lifetime prevalence in characterizing recurrent aphthous stomatitis in USA children and youths. *J Oral Pathol Med* 2004;33:558–566.
4. Reichart PA. Oral mucosal lesions in a representative cross-sectional study of aging Germans. *Community Dent Oral Epidemiol* 2000;28:390–398.
5. Garcia-Pola MJ, Garcia-Martin JM, Gonzalez-Garcia M. Prevalence of oral lesions in the 6-year-old pediatric population of Oveido (Spain). *Med Oral* 2002;7:184–191.
6. Bittoun R. Recurrent aphthous ulcers and nicotine. *Med J Aust* 1991;154:471–472.
7. Espinoza I, Rojas R, Aranda W, et al. Prevalence of oral mucosal lesions in elderly people in Santiago, Chile. *J Oral Pathol Med* 2003;32(10):571–575.
8. Ussher M, West R, Steptoe A, et al. Increase in common cold symptoms and mouth ulcers following smoking cessation. *Tob Control* 2003;12(1):86–88.
9. Rizvi SW, McGrath H Jr. The therapeutic effect of cigarette smoking on oral/genital aphthosis and other manifestations of Behçet's disease. *Clin Exp Rheumatol* 2001;19(5 Suppl 24):S77–S78.
10. Scheid P, Bohadana A, Martinet Y. Nicotine patches for aphthous ulcers due to Behçet's syndrome. *N Engl J Med* 2000;343(24):1816–1817.
11. Grady D, Ernster VL, Stillman L, et al. Smokeless tobacco use prevents aphthous stomatitis. *Oral Surg Oral Med Oral Pathol* 1992;74(4):463–465.
12. Bittoun R. Recurrent aphthous ulcers and nicotine. *Med J Aust* 1991;154(7):471–472.
13. Rivera-Hidalgo F, Shulman JD, Beach MM. The association of tobacco and other factors with recurrent aphthous stomatitis in an US adult population. *Oral Dis* 2004;10:335–345.
14. Letsinger JA, McCarty MA, Jorizzo JL. Complex aphthosis: a large case series with evaluation algorithm and therapeutic ladder from topicals to thalidomide. *J Am Acad Dermatol* 2005;52:500–508.
15. O'Duffy JD, Goldstein NP. Neurologic involvement in seven patients with Behçet's disease. *Am J Med* 1976;61:170–178.
16. Al-Otaibi LM, Porter SR, Poate TW. Behçet's disease: a review. *J Dent Res* 2005;84(3):209–222.
17. Suzuki Kurokawa M, Suzuki N. Behçet's disease. *Clin Exp Med* 2004;4(1):10–20.
18. Thomas KT, Feder HM Jr, Lawton AR, et al. Periodic fever syndrome in children. *J Pediatr* 1999;135:15–21.
19. Kurtaran H, Karadag A, Catal F, et al. PFAPA syndrome: a rare cause of periodic fever. *Turk J Pediatr* 2004;46(4):354–356.
20. Galanakis E, Papadakis CE, Giannoussi E, et al. PFAPA syndrome in children evaluated for tonsillectomy. *Arch Dis Child* 2002;86(6):434–435.
21. Pedra C, Terra CM, Ejzenberg B, et al. Oral palatine ulcers of a traumatic nature in infants: Bednar's aphthae. *Int J Pediatr Otorhinolaryngol* 1996;35:39–49.
22. Buno IJ, Huff JC, Weston WL, et al. Elevated levels of interferon gamma, tumor necrosis factor alpha, interleukins 2, 4, and 5, but not interleukin 10, are present in recurrent aphthous stomatitis. *Arch Dermatol* 1998;134:827–831.
23. Lin S-S, Chou MY, Ho CC, et al. Study of the viral infections and cytokines associated with recurrent aphthous ulceration. *Microbes Infect* 2005;7(4):635–44. Epub 2005 March 28.
24. Borra RC, Andrade PM, Silva Id, et al. The Th1/Th2 immune-type response of the recurrent aphthous ulceration analyzed by cDNA microarray. *J Oral Pathol Med* 2004;33:140–146.

25. Wu-Wang CY, Patel M, Feng J, et al. Decreased levels of salivary prostaglandin E2 and epidermal growth factor in recurrent aphthous stomatitis. *Arch Oral Biol* 1995;40:1093–1098.
26. Healy CM, Thornhill MH. Induction of adhesions molecule expression on blood vessels and keratinocytes in recurrent oral ulceration. *J Oral Pathol Med* 1999;28:5–11.
27. Chakrabarty AK, Mraz S, Geisse JK, et al. Aphthous ulcers associated with imiquimod and the treatment of actinic cheilitis. *J Am Acad Dermatol* 2005;52:S35–S37.
28. Shimoyama T, Horie N, Kato T, et al. Helicobacter pylori in oral ulcerations. *J Oral Sci* 2000;42:225–229.
29. Alam F, Argiriadou AS, Hodgson TA, et al. Primary syphilis remains a cause of oral ulceration. *Br Dent J* 2000;189:352–354.
30. Alamillos-Granados FJ, Dean-Ferrer A, Garcia-Lopez A, et al. Actinomycotic ulcer of the oral mucosa: an unusual presentation of oral actinomycosis. *Br J Oral Maxillofac Surg* 2000;38:121–123.
31. Mizrahi B, Golenser J, Wolnerman JS, et al. Adhesive tablet effective for treating canker sores in humans. *J Pharm Sci* 2004;93(12):2927–2935.
32. Ross Kerr A, Drexel CA, Spielman AI. The efficacy and safety of 50 mg penicillin G potassium troches for recurrent aphthous ulcers. *Oral Surg Oral Med Oral Pathol Oral Radiol Endod* 2003;96:685–694.
33. Collier PM, Neill SM, Copeman PW. Topical 5-aminosalicylic acid: a treatment for aphthous ulcers. *Br J Dermatol* 1992;126:185–188.
34. Jacobson JM, Greenspan JS, Spritzler J, et al. Thalidomide for the treatment of oral aphthous ulcers in patients with human immunodeficiency virus infection. National Institute of Allergy and Infectious Diseases AIDS Clinical Trials Group. *N Engl J Med* 1997;336:1487–1493.

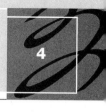

BACTERIAL SKIN INFECTIONS
Sola Choi

4

I. DEFINITION AND PATHOPHYSIOLOGY

A. Pyodermas

1. A pyoderma is a purulent infection of the skin, most commonly caused by staphylococci or streptococci. The most common forms are impetigo and folliculitis. Adults and up to 10% of children in the southeastern United States and 80% of children in endemic areas are affected. Risk factors include antecedent cutaneous lesions, obesity, treatment with steroids and chemotherapeutic agents, dysglobulinemia, acquired or inherited immune dysfunction, hematologic and immunologic disease, malnutrition, and diabetes.

   a. Impetigo contagiosa, the most superficial bacterial infection, is caused primarily by *Staphylococcus aureus* in the United States. The next most common isolate is a mixture of *S. aureus* and group A *Streptococcus*, followed by group A *Streptococcus* alone. Impetigo is usually located on the face and other exposed areas. It is very contagious among infants and young children through person-to-person contact, with a latency period of 10 to 20 days. Predisposing factors include poor health and hygiene, malnutrition, and a warm climate, as well as antecedent scabies, chickenpox, contact and atopic dermatitis, and other eruptions causing skin breakdown. Japanese researchers have noted an increase in streptococci among isolates from impetigo in patients with atopic dermatitis. There was a higher recurrence rate in those treated with topical compared with those treated with oral therapy (1).

   Impetigo can be a polymicrobial infection with both aerobes and anaerobes. Pathogens may vary depending on the body location; for example, in one study, coliforms were isolated from impetigo of the buttocks, whereas oral anaerobes were isolated from head and neck disease. However, *S. aureus* dominated in all areas, 80% of which produced the β-lactamase enzyme (2).

   Group A streptococci are unable to survive on intact skin and require at least superficial damage to the stratum corneum to establish infection. Skin surface lipids, especially free fatty acids, inhibit the growth of this organism. The primary lesion is a fragile subcorneal pustule. In patients who develop impetigo, streptococci may be cultured first from normal skin, then from lesions, and much later from the respiratory tract. In contrast, staphylococci are initially found in the respiratory tract, then on normal skin, and finally in skin lesions. *S. aureus* commonly colonizes the anterior nares; less common sites are the axillae, perineum, and toe web spaces. Untreated, nonbullous impetigo usually resolves spontaneously without scarring in 10 to 14 days.

   Postpyodermal acute glomerulonephritis is quite rare in the United States, but may occur in an epidemic setting. In tropical climates, nephritogenic strains of streptococci (M-T serotypes 2, 49, 55, 57, 60) commonly cause impetigo. An outbreak of acute poststreptococcal glomerulonephritis was reported in the southern United States in which 9 of 10 children had preceding impetigo, although 5 also had a history of pharyngitis (3). Bacteremia, cellulitis, septic arthritis, and osteomyelitis are very rare complications.

   b. Bullous staphylococcal impetigo is seen primarily in children and is caused by group II phage types 70 and 71 staphylococci and rarely by group A *Streptococcus*. These organisms elaborate an exfoliative toxin that induces an intraepidermal, subgranular cleavage plane, resulting in blister formation.

They may also cause an exfoliative dermatitis (Ritter's disease, staphylococcal scalded-skin syndrome) in infants and children.

c. Ecthyma is a deeper bacterial infection than impetigo, with ulceration beneath the crust. Unlike impetigo, ecthyma is accompanied by abrupt onset of fever and malaise, and resolves with scarring. Children, debilitated elderly, and immunocompromised hosts are at risk. Differentiation from ecthyma gangrenosum, caused by *Pseudomonas aeruginosa*, is possible by tissue culture of a punch biopsy taken from the ulcer.

d. Folliculitis is a staphylococcal infection starting around hair follicles. Superficial folliculitis usually does not represent a serious problem, but deep and/or recurrent lesions of the scalp, nose, and eyelid cilia (sties) are far more distressing. Pseudofolliculitis, otherwise known as "razor bumps" or "ingrown hairs," results from beard or body hairs that become ingrown and is seen in individuals with highly curved and tough hairs. This is a papular, pustular, follicular-based disorder that is not primarily an infection but rather a foreign body inflammatory reaction (4).

e. A furuncle involves a follicle and surrounding tissue and may develop from a superficial staphylococcal folliculitis. Furuncles are common in areas of hair-bearing skin subject to friction and maceration, especially the face, scalp, buttocks, and axillae. A group of furuncles constitutes a carbuncle. These drain at multiple points and are commonly located on the back of the neck, back, and thighs. Recurrent furunculosis inexplicably develops in an unfortunate few who do not demonstrate a specific immune deficiency or harbor particular staphylococcal strains.

f. Abscesses are walled-off collections of pus, often larger and deeper than furuncles. They may develop on hair-bearing or non-hair-bearing sites and have the same predisposing conditions as furuncles. *S. aureus* is the most common organism; recently, community-acquired methicillin-resistant *Staphylococcus aureus* (CA-MRSA) strains have been isolated from as many as 75% of abscesses in patients presenting to urban emergency rooms (5). CA-MRSA carries two characteristic markers: SCCmec type IVa, a gene complex carrying methicillin resistance and Pauton-Valentine leukocidin (6).

g. Erysipelas is a superficial dermal form of bacterial cellulitis. The most common organism is Group A β-hemolytic *Streptococcus*. Clinically, a tender, red, well-demarcated, expanding plaque is seen on the face or the leg. Cellulitis is a deep dermal and subcutaneous infection with lymphangitis and adenopathy. The most common organisms are *S. aureus* and *Streptococcus pyogenes*. Risk factors for developing cellulitis include edema, abrasions, chronic ulcers, and chronic tinea pedis with web space maceration. Fever and other systemic symptoms are seen in both.

h. There are two uncommon but distinctive forms of folliculitis in which the pathogenic organism is a gram-negative bacterium.

    i. Gram-negative folliculitis occurs in the setting of long-term antibiotic treatment of acne vulgaris. There is a male predominance. Antibiotic therapy is felt to alter the ecology of the anterior nares, allowing colonization by gram-negative organisms, mainly *Proteus, Enterobacter, Escherichia*, and *Klebsiella* species. In a small percentage of patients, dissemination to the skin will occur with the development of facial lesions. In a series of 46 patients, immunologic abnormalities such as low concentrations of immunoglobulin M were identified, with possible implications in the development of gram-negative folliculitis (7).

    ii. *Pseudomonas* folliculitis has been associated with the use of hot tubs, swimming pools, and whirlpools. Given its ability to withstand relatively high temperatures and chlorine levels, *P. aeruginosa* is well adapted to survive in such facilities. Hydration of the skin, sweating, occlusion, and abrasions further predispose to cutaneous infection. Although most commonly described in epidemiologic reports of outbreaks occurring in public facilities, private bathers may also be affected.

B. Erythrasma a mild, chronic, localized, superficial infection involving intertriginous areas of skin, is caused by *Corynebacterium minutissimum*. This organism is often part of the normal flora, and some change in the host–parasite relationship, such as increased heat or humidity, results in the development of the clinical disorder.

II. SUBJECTIVE DATA

A. Impetigo is either asymptomatic or pruritic. Perinasal or perioral lesions may follow an upper respiratory infection.

B. Deep forms of folliculitis such as sties, furuncles, carbuncles, and abscesses may be exquisitely painful.

C. Patients with *Pseudomonas* folliculitis often have pruritus. They may also have malaise, fever, headache, nausea, otitis, and sore throat and eyes.

D. Erythrasma is usually asymptomatic.

III. OBJECTIVE DATA (See color insert.)

A. Impetigo begins as a small erythematous macule that rapidly develops into a fragile vesicle with an erythematous areola. The vesicopustule breaks and leaves a red, oozing erosion capped with a thick, golden yellow crust that appears "stuck on." Satellite lesions are often seen. The presenting lesions of bullous staphylococcal impetigo are flaccid bullae that are first filled with clear, then cloudy, fluid which are replaced after rupture by a thin, varnish-like crust. Lesions may be up to 1 cm or more in diameter and may lack surrounding erythema. Regional lymphadenopathy may be present, and 50% of patients may have an increased white blood cell count. Extensive impetigo may be seen in immunocompromised patients. Infants have a predilection for impetigo in the inguinal folds and diaper area, which may later generalize.

B. Folliculitis appears as superficial or deep pustules or follicular nodules. The superficial lesions have a central hair piercing the pustule and sometimes a red rim around the pustule. The face is a common site for deep folliculitis.

C. Sties are erythematous swellings around eyelid cilia.

D. Furuncles start as firm, red, tender nodules that become fluctuant, point, and rupture, discharging a core of necrotic tissue.

E. Carbuncles appear similar to furuncles but drain at multiple points.

F. Gram-negative folliculitis most often presents as superficial pustules, without comedones, on the cheeks and chin. Occasionally, there are deeper nodules and cysts.

G. *Pseudomonas* folliculitis is polymorphous. Papular, vesicular, and pustular lesions have been described. The rash usually develops within 2 days of exposure and has a predilection for the lateral trunk, axillae, buttocks, and proximal extremities. The palms and soles are spared. Axillary lymphadenopathy is not uncommon. Cases have been reported secondary to contaminated diving suits, bath sponges, and bath toys (8–10).

H. Viral folliculitis may be secondary to atypical presentations of herpes simplex, herpes zoster, and molluscum contagiosum. It should be considered in the differential diagnosis of superficial folliculitis, especially when it does not respond to standard therapies (11).

I. Erythrasma may be seen as dry, smooth to slightly creased or scaly, sharply marginated, red-brown plaques in the inguinal, axillary, or inframammary folds; as mild scaling or fissuring between the third to fourth or fourth to fifth toe webs; or as generalized scaly patches. Lesions may be easily mistaken for those of superficial fungal infection.

IV. ASSESSMENT

A. Factors predisposing to infection should be identified, evaluated, and treated or eliminated. Low serum iron has been reported in recurrent furunculosis; improvement was noted after 3 to 4 weeks of iron supplementation (12).

B. Most cases of impetigo or folliculitis need not be routinely cultured; recalcitrant or unusual cases deserve a Gram's stain and culture of the exudate. In suspected cases of gram-negative folliculitis, culture of the nares and skin lesions is recommended.

C. Ninety percent of patients with acute glomerulonephritis secondary to pyoderma will have an elevated serum titer of anti-DNase B; only 50% of similar patients will have elevated levels of antistreptolysin O.

D. Cultures and even skin biopsies frequently fail to demonstrate any organisms in *Pseudomonas* folliculitis. A high index of suspicion, careful history taking, and, occasionally, epidemiologic investigation are necessary to establish the diagnosis.

E. Erythrasma is diagnosed by the characteristic coral red fluorescence of lesions when viewed under the Wood's light. Fluorescence is caused by a water-soluble porphyrin and may be lacking if the patient has bathed recently. The organisms appear as gram-positive rod-like filamentous and coccoid forms and are best viewed under $45\times$ magnification or oil immersion after Gram's or Giemsa's stain of affected scales. Culture is rarely required and needs special media.

V. THERAPY

A. Impetigo caused by both streptococci and staphylococci may be treated with either topical or systemic antibiotics. Systemic treatment may be justified because (i) impetigo may have a protracted course and may become widespread and (ii) antibiotics can shorten the healing time and decrease the number of recurrences. Unfortunately, there is no convincing evidence that treating pyodermas prevents subsequent glomerulonephritis (3). Penicillin resistance of *S. aureus* is so common that penicillin is considered ineffective. Oral semisynthetic penicillinase-resistant penicillins, such as dicloxacillin, are effective, but the oral suspensions are poorly tolerated by children because of the taste. Cephalexin and cefdinir are roughly equivalent in efficacy and are well-tolerated (13). Erythromycin is less costly, but resistance is common. In recalcitrant cases, combination therapy with cephalexin and rifampin has been efficacious (14). Amoxicillin with B-lactamase inhibitor, cefaclor, and the newer macrolides, azithromycin and clarithromycin are effective but expensive.

1. Mupirocin (Bactroban, Centany) is a safe and effective treatment for impetigo. Unlike other topical antibiotics, it has a very low rate of contact sensitization. Streptococci have not shown resistance, and the rates of resistance of *S. aureus* are very low.

   Mupirocin applied t.i.d. for 7 to 10 days may be superior to oral erythromycin in the eradication of *S. aureus*, including antibiotic-resistant *S. aureus*. Extensive impetigo should be treated with oral antibiotics.

   a. Topical antibiotics may be useful in preventing streptococcal pyoderma when applied t.i.d. for minor skin trauma, especially in children at increased risk for such infection.

   b. Recurrent disease is often secondary to colonization of the *S. aureus* in the nares or groin. Mupirocin applied t.i.d. to the nares has been shown to eliminate the carrier state for 90% of patients for greater than 6 months. In one long-term study, monthly 5-day applications of mupirocin reduced the nasal colonization in *S. aureus* carriers; an associated decrease in skin infections was noted (15).

2. Widespread or recalcitrant impetigo should be treated with oral antibiotics. Bullous staphylococcal impetigo should be treated with a semisynthetic penicillin (dicloxacillin, 250 mg q.i.d.), cephalosporin, or erythromycin if organisms are sensitive.

3. The lesions should be soaked three to four times a day in warm tap water or saline solution to remove the crusts. In addition, it might be useful to have both patient and family bathe at least once daily with a bactericidal iodine (e.g., Betadine skin cleanser) or bacteriostatic soap or solution containing hexachlorophene or chlorhexidine (Hibiclens) (see also Chap. 40, Antiinfective Agents).

4. Use of topical 0.3% triclosan (Bacti-Stat) eradicated an outbreak of methicillin-resistant *S. aureus* in a neonatal nursery (16). This soap was used for both hand washing for staff and visitors and bathing of the infants.

B. Superficial folliculitis may respond to aggressive topical hygiene and local antibiotics. Folliculitis on the male beard area is unusually recalcitrant and recurrent and should be treated with systemic antibiotics. Simple furunculosis needs to be treated with only moist heat. Local ophthalmic antibiotics should be instilled into the eye for sties (tobramycin, ciprofloxacin, erythromycin). Larger abscesses should be carefully and conservatively incised and drained. Afterwards, only topical antibiotics are needed. Furuncles or abscesses associated with a surrounding cellulitis or those associated with fever or located on the face should be treated with a semisynthetic penicillin, erythromycin, or clindamycin, and closely monitored. Because of the recent emergence of CA-MRSA, cultures should be obtained when possible and antimicrobial therapy tailored to the result. CA-MRSA is generally susceptible to clindamycin, trimethoprim-sulfamethoxazole, and rifampin (6).

Chronic folliculitis of certain areas, particularly the buttocks, may respond to the application of 6.25% aluminum chloride hexahydrate in absolute ethyl alcohol (Xerac A-C) once daily at bedtime (see also Chap. 40, Antiinfective Agents). This compound probably acts through a combination of direct antibacterial and antiperspirant effects. Antibacterial soaps such as chlorhexidine (Hibiclens), Dial, or Lever 2000 are helpful.

C. Recurrent furunculosis represents a difficult therapeutic problem, which should be approached as follows:

  1. Assess the organism's antibiotic sensitivity, and start on the appropriate drug (most often a semisynthetic penicillin). Continue treatment for 1 to 3 months and then later as necessary. Long-term systemic therapy will keep new lesions from erupting and sometimes causes the problem to disappear completely.

  a. Rifampin (600 mg PO daily for 7 to 10 days) is an alternative, albeit an expensive one, in especially stubborn cases. Addition of a semisynthetic penicillin, cephalosporin, minocycline, or ciprofloxacin help prevent rifampin resistance.

  2. Methods for maintaining rigorous topical hygiene are noted below. However, the use of such programs alone may not inhibit recurrent furunculosis, and it is not clear whether topical treatment is of substantial benefit.

  a. Patient and family should bathe and shampoo one to two times daily. Nails should be clipped short and scrubbed as in a surgical prep. Avoid occlusion or maceration (oils, impermeable clothing).

  b. Apply mupirocin (Bactroban, Centany) cream or ointment to the anterior nares twice daily.

  c. Precautions before and during shaving must be maintained whenever there are facial lesions. The beard should be soaked with hot water for 5 minutes before shaving. Brush-less shaving cream or soap alone should be used, and blades discarded daily. Electric razor heads should be soaked in alcohol for 1 to 2 hours between shaves. Seventy percent isopropyl alcohol may be used as an aftershave.

  d. Separate towels, washcloths, sheets, and clothing should be used; they should be laundered in hot water and changed daily.

  e. Dressings must be changed frequently and disposed of immediately. Paper tissues should be used instead of handkerchiefs.

D. Gram-negative folliculitis is best treated with isotretinoin (see Chap. 40, Acne Preparations, sec. II.A) (17). A dose of 0.5 to 1.0 mg/kg/day for 5 months resulted in clinical and bacteriologic cure in all of 21 patients, with only one recurrence observed during a 12-month follow-up (18). Alternatively, antibiotics targeted at the organism cultured from lesions may be used, although recurrences off therapy are common.

E. *Pseudomonas* folliculitis is self-limited and typically lasts 7 to 10 days. Although it may recur, ultimately, spontaneous resolution is the rule. For immunocompetent patients, no therapy has proved effective, and only symptomatic treatment is indicated.

F. Erythrasma responds best to oral erythromycin or tetracycline (250 mg q.i.d. for 0 to 21 days). Topical therapy with miconazole or clotrimazole creams or keratolytic compounds (e.g., Keralyt Gel, Whitfield's Ointment) can be effective, although the recurrence rate is higher. Clarithromycin in a one-time dose of 1 gm cleared three patients with erythrasma and the cost was equal to or less than alternative therapies (19).

References

1. Adachi J, Endo K, Fukuzumi T, et al. Increasing incidence of streptococcal impetigo in atopic dermatitis. *J Dermatol Sci* 1998;17:45–53.
2. Brook I, Frazier EH, Yeager JK. Microbiology of nonbullous impetigo. *Pediatr Dermatol* 1997;14:192–195.
3. Bloch AB, Smith JD, Facklam RR, et al. Poststreptococcal acute glomerulonephritis in Early County, 1982. *J Med Assoc Ga* 1987;76(12):839–844.
4. Crutchfield CE III. The causes and treatment of pseudofolliculitis barbae. *Cutis* 1998;61:351–356.
5. Frazee BW, Lynn J, Charlebois ED, et al. High prevalence of methicillin-resistant Staphylococcus aureus in emergency department skin and soft tissue infections. *Ann Emerg Med* 2005;45(3):311–320.
6. Kazakova SV, Hageman JC, Matava M, et al. A clone of methicillin-resistant Staphylococcus aureus among professional football players. *N Engl J Med* 2005;352(5):468–475.
7. Neubert U, Jansen T, Plewig G. Bacteriologic and immunologic aspects of gram-negative folliculitis: a study of 46 patients. *Int J Dermatol* 1999;38:270–274.
8. Hogan P. Pseudomonas folliculitis. *Australas J Dermatol* 1997;38:93–94.
9. Saltzer KR, Schutzer PJ, Weinberg JM, et al. Diving suit dermatitis: a manifestation of Pseudomonas folliculitis. *Cutis* 1997;59:245–246.
10. Maniatis AN, Karkavitsas C, Maniatis NA, et al. Pseudomonas aeruginosa folliculitis due to non-0:11 serogroups: acquisition through use of contaminated synthetic sponges. *Clin Infect Dis* 1995;21:437–439.
11. Weinberg JM, Mysliwiec A, Turiansky GW, et al. Viral folliculitis. Atypical presentation of herpes simplex, herpes zoster, and molluscum contagiosum. *Arch Dermatol* 1997;133:983–986.
12. Weimer MC, Neering H, Welten C. Preliminary report: furunculosis and hypoferremia. *Lancet* 1990;336:464–466.
13. Hedrick J. Acute bacterial skin infections in pediatric medicine: current issues in presentation and treatment. *Paediatr Drugs* 2003;5S1:35–46.
14. Feder HM, Pond KE Jr. Addition of rifampin to cephalexin therapy for recalcitrant staphylococcal skin infections—an observation. *Clin Pediatr (Phila)* 1996;35(4):205–208.
15. Raz R, Miron D, Colodner R, et al. A 1 year trial of nasal mupirocin in the prevention of recurrent staphylococcal nasal colonization and skin infection. *Arch Intern Med* 1996;156:1109–1112.
16. Zafar AB, Butler RC, Reese DJ, et al. Use of 0.3% triclosan (Bacti-Stat) to eradicate an outbreak of methicillin-resistant Staphylococcus aureus in a neonatal nursery. *Am J Infect Control* 1995;23:200–208.
17. James WD. Acne. *N Engl J Med* 2005;352:1463–1472.
18. James WD, Leyden JJ. Treatment of gram-negative folliculitis with isotretinoin: positive clinical and microbiologic response. *J Am Acad Dermatol* 1985;12:319–324.
19. Wharton JR, Wilson PL, Kincannon JM. Erythrasma treated with single-dose clarithromycin. *Arch Dermatol* 1998;134:671.

BITES AND STINGS
Melissa A. Bogle

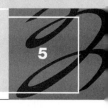

5

I. **DEFINITION AND PATHOPHYSIOLOGY.** Reaction to bites and stings is initiated by either a toxin or an allergen injected by the offending creature. Direct toxic mechanisms include contact with venoms, irritating hairs, salivary secretions, or vesicant fluids; indirect contact may result from inhalation or ingestion of debris, particles, body parts, or excretions. At least 30 to 50 people in the United States die each year from systemic reactions to stings. Approximately 50% of deaths attributed to venomous animals result from Hymenoptera (bee or wasp) stings, 20% from rattlesnake bites, and 14% from poisonous spiders. Spiders and snakes inject venoms that may be hemolytic, may disturb the clotting system, or act as neurotoxins. The black widow spider injects a neurotoxin called α-latrotoxin in its venom, which causes the release of acetylcholine and catecholamines at the neuromuscular junction. The brown recluse spider injects a phospholipase called *sphingomyelinase D* in its venom causing platelet aggregation, thrombosis, and severe intravascular hemolysis. The most serious reactions to biting insects, including bees, hornets, wasps, fleas, mosquitoes, fire ants, and bedbugs, are caused by an acquired hypersensitivity. Over 80% of deaths result from anaphylactic reactions and occur within an hour of the sting. Approximately 1% to 3% of adults in the United States have had a systemic allergic reaction to an insect sting. Many patients who develop generalized reactions to insect stings have no history of previous systemic or local reaction to a sting.

II. **SUBJECTIVE DATA**

    A. Spiders. The spiders that cause serious reactions in humans in the United States most commonly are the black widow (*Latrodectus mactans*) and the brown recluse spider (*Loxosceles reclusa*). The black widow spider is found throughout the United States. Systemic symptoms resulting from its bite include chills, nausea, tremors, muscle spasms, pain in the abdomen and legs, sweating, and cramps. Symptoms typically begin in 15 to 60 minutes and subside within hours. The brown recluse spider inhabits dark warm areas such as attics, closets, and woodsheds. This spider is endemic to the Midwest but can be found in eastern United States. Reactions to its bite are trivial approximately 90% of the time. Severe local pain and swelling may occur between 4 and 8 hours after a bite. Severe systemic symptoms include respiratory failure with pulmonary edema, anemia, renal failure, neurotoxicity, and rhabdomyolysis. In contrast to the bite of the black widow, there are no neurologic symptoms. Viscerocutaneous loxoscelism, with severe chills, vomiting, arthralgias, and severe intravascular hemolysis, is rare.

    B. Snakes. Of approximately 45,000 snakebites in the United States each year, only approximately 20% are by poisonous snakes. The Viperidae and Elapidae families of snakes are poisonous snakes of medical importance in the United States. The Viperidae family or pit viper snakes include the rattlesnake, cottonmouth, and copperhead varieties. The Elapidae family includes the coral snake. Increased interest in snakes as pets has brought the problem of snakebites to urban areas, and injuries are often associated with alcohol consumption. Bites from the diamondback rattlesnake account for 95% of fatalities. Local reactions to venomous snake bites include pain, swelling, ecchymosis, and lymphadenopathy, which may be accompanied by a tingling sensation around the lips, vertigo, muscular twitching, or bleeding (hematuria, hematemesis).

    C. Insects. By far the most important venomous insects are those belonging to the Hymenoptera family including bees, wasps, and ants. Venom from Hymenoptera contains serotonin, kinins, acetylcholine, lecithinase, hyaluronidase, phospholipase, and melittin; exposure to this venom has been shown to release histamine from leukocytes of patients allergic to Hymenoptera. Most stings result in instantaneous pain followed by a localized wheal and flare reaction with pruritus and variable edema. The harvester ant and fire ant cause most ant-sting reactions in humans. Both are associated with "fire" because of the intense burning and pain associated with their stings. Some patients may develop immediate systemic allergic reactions.

The immediate allergic reaction to the injected salivary fluids of mosquitoes is pruritus; the delayed reaction, occurring several hours later, is a more severe, intense, burning itch. Flies do not actually bite but pierce through the skin, thereby allowing salivary gland fluids to enter and cause toxic and allergic reactions. The black fly is renowned for inducing an extremely painful and long-lasting reaction. Fleabites manifest as scattered pruritic papules.

D. **Caterpillars.** Injury following contact from caterpillars usually involves contact with urticating hairs or venomous spines. The largest outbreaks have been associated with spines detached from live or dead caterpillars or cocoons. Direct contact with caterpillars with hollow spines containing venom glands can cause instantaneous pain, erythema, and swelling. Although nausea, vomiting, and fever may occur, systemic symptoms are rare. Caterpillar hairs may cause an erythematous, papular, or urticarial rash persisting for several days to 1 week. Conjunctivitis, upper respiratory tract irritation, and asthma-like symptoms may also occur.

E. **Animal bites.** Approximately 2 million animal bites occur yearly (mostly to children), with 300,000 emergency room visits, 10,000 hospitalizations, and 20 deaths per year. Dogs are responsible for 80% of the bites, although cat bites are more infectious. Dog and cat bites can become infected with a complex group of pathogens usually including the *Pasteurella* species (50% of dog bites and 75% of cat bites). *Pasteurella canis* is the most common dog isolate and *Pasteurella multocida* and *septica* in cat bites. Other aerobic isolates include streptococci, staphylococci, moraxellae, and neisseriae. Common anaerobes include fusobacteria, *Bacteroides*, *Porphyromonas*, and *Prevotella*. Human bites are usually deep puncture wounds and often result in a polymicrobial infection. The usual case scenario is a high force hand injury that is a result of a fistfight with a punch to the mouth. A clenched fist injury can lead to soft tissue infection and tendon or bone injury.

III. **OBJECTIVE DATA**

A. **Spiders.** The black widow spider can be identified by a distinct red to orange hourglass marking on its abdomen. Its bite leaves an urticarial papule with a white halo surrounding. In patients who develop systemic symptoms, neuromuscular symptoms can become quite severe with involuntary spasm and rigidity affecting large muscles predominantly in the abdomen and also in the extremities and lower back. Patient presentation may mimic that of an acute abdomen. Severely ill patients may also develop diaphoresis, ptosis, vomiting, pulmonary edema, rhabdomyolysis, hypertension, and a characteristic pattern of facial swelling known as *Lactrodectus* facies.

The brown recluse spider has a characteristic violin-like marking on its dorsal thorax. Local reactions to its bite range from mild skin irritation to severe local necrosis. Severe reactions generally begin as localized edema with an erythematous halo surrounding an irregularly shaped center of necrosis. If the edema is severe, serous or hemorrhagic bullae may arise over the underlying eschar. Multiple toxins released, including sphingomyelinase D, result in progressive necrosis resembling necrotizing fasciitis or pyoderma gangrenosum. Healing can take 3 weeks or more. Severe systemic symptoms include hemoglobinuria, anemia, fever, chills, a morbilliform rash, arthralgias, nausea, and vomiting. Death may result from renal failure or intravascular hemolysis.

B. **Snakes.** The pit viper family of snakes can be recognized by a triangular head, elliptical "cat's eye" pupils, and a single row of ventral scales. All have a depression, or heat-sensing facial pit, in the maxillary bone near the nostril on both sides of the head. The venom is anticoagulative and bites typically result in local pain immediately after the bite with fang puncta, weakness, swelling, paresthesias, nausea, and vomiting. Ecchymoses, hypotension, and damage to the vascular endothelium may ensue. The most dreaded complications are respiratory arrest, disseminated intravascular coagulation (DIC), acute renal failure, neurotoxicity, and/or rhabdomyolysis. Studies are in progress to develop a rapid enzyme-linked immunosorbent assay (ELISA) to determine the snake species to provide specific antivenom.

The Elapidae family of coral snakes can be identified by round eyes with red and yellow or white bands. Nonvenomous mimics tend to have red and black bands in the United States; however, this rule does not hold true south of Mexico City and in other foreign countries. Bites usually have little or no pain, local edema, or necrosis. The venom is primarily neurotoxic, causing a weak or numb feeling in the bitten extremity. Systemic symptoms may appear within hours including tremors, marked salivation, muscle fasciculations, bulbar paralysis manifested as dysphagia and dyspnea, and total flaccid paralysis. Paralysis of the diaphragm leads to respiratory paralysis and death.

C. Insects

1. **Hymenoptera.** The Hymenoptera family includes bees, wasps, and ants. Most localized stings result in mild wheal and flare reactions with variable edema persisting <24 hours. Multiple bee, wasp, yellow jacket, or hornet stings can result in systemic reactions including vomiting, diarrhea, generalized edema, dyspnea, hypotension, and collapse. Life-threatening allergic sting reactions may occur, characterized by the usual manifestations of anaphylaxis: urticaria, laryngeal edema, bronchospasm, abdominal cramps, and shock. Most fatalities occur within 1 hour of being stung. Delayed allergic reactions occur within hours to 2 weeks following the sting and have symptoms similar to those of serum sickness with urticaria accompanied by lymphadenopathy and polyarthritis.

    Solenopsis or fire ant stings develop as a wheal and evolve into small pustules. The venom contains phospholipase and hyaluronidase. Anaphylaxis and death have been reported.

2. **Mosquitoes.** The immediate reaction is production of a wheal; a swollen papular lesion may appear as a delayed reaction several hours later. The culex mosquito is medically important and can spread filariasis (elephantiasis) and dirofilariasis (dog heart worm). Mosquitoes can also harbor many viruses such as Eastern Equine Encephalitis (EEE), malaria, or yellow fever.

3. **Diptera (flies).** The bites of most two-winged flies cause immediate pruritic wheals followed by itchy, red papules. The botfly (*Dermatobia hominis*) can cause myiasis with painful furuncles that occur when a fly deposits parasitic larvae on human skin. The Simulium black fly is endogenous to parts of Mexico and South America causing onchocerciasis with facial edema, subcutaneous nodules, and iritis. The sand fly carries Leishmaniasis, which may cause mucocutaneous lesions or visceral disease.

4. **Siphonaptera (fleas).** These bites are typically grouped urticaria papules, some with a central punctum. Fleas medically important to the United States include the human flea (*Pulex irritans*) found in farms and urban area, the chigoe flea (*Tunga penetrans*) which is found in tropical areas of North and South America and causes intense itching and local inflammation as it burrows into the skin between the toes and under the toenails, and the oriental rat flea (*Xenopsylla cheopis*) which carries *Yersinia pestis* (plague) and *Rickettsia typhi* (endemic typhus).

5. **Hemiptera (true bugs).** The Hemiptera family includes the bed bug (*Cimex lenticularis*) and the Reduviid bug. The bed bug leaves linear pruritic papules in groups of two to three on the face and extremities. They are found most commonly in poor living conditions and unkempt hotels, living in mattresses and upholstery and coming out at night to feed. The Reduviid bug found in South America is the vector for Trypanosoma cruzi, causing American trypanosomiasis or Chagas' disease. The bug spreads disease-depositing stool on the skin as it bites. Local reactions include a chagoma or unilateral periorbital conjunctivitis and edema. Systemic reactions include myocardial damage, megacolon, or megaesophagus.

6. **Mites.** Cheyletiella mites, often called "walking dandruff," subsist by eating keratin off small mammals such as dogs and cats. They cause a pruritic dermatitis in humans who handle pets. The house mouse mite (*Liponyssoides sanguineus*) carries Rickettsial pox. The scabies mite (*Sarcoptes scabei*) can cause a pruritic eruption in humans as it burrows under the epidermis, leaving eggs and feces. The most commonly involved areas are the interdigital spaces, palms, flexor surfaces of the wrists, and genitalia. The red mite (Chigger or Trombiculidae) can cause extremely pruritic papular bites. The most common variety in the United States is *Eutrombicula alfreddugesi*. Chiggers can transmit scrub typhus (*Rickettsia tsutsugamushi*), leaving a black eschar at the bite site, pneumonitis, and constitutional symptoms. Demodex folliculorum mites are generally asymptomatic and can be found in the hair follicles and sebaceous glands of virtually all adult humans. They have been associated with rosacea and may cause folliculitis.

D. **Caterpillars.** Pain, erythema, and urtication are the most common reactions to bites of the caterpillar species. Atypical reactions include muscle spasms, paresthesias, and radiating pain. The most important urticating caterpillars in the United States are the *Automeris io* characterized by red and white lateral stripes, the *Megalopyge opercularis* or puss caterpillar resembling a tuft of cotton, and the *Sibine stimulea* or saddleback caterpillar resembling a brown or purple saddle on a green blanket.

E. **Animal bites.** Animal bites range from small scratches to severe bites which may involve muscle, tendons, or fractured bone. Cat bites have a high likelihood of infection due to puncture inoculation from their longer, pointed teeth.

IV. **ASSESSMENT.** Patients with severe systemic reactions should be cared for in facilities prepared to handle acute respiratory and cardiovascular emergencies.

V. **THERAPY**

A. **Spiders.** Mild local reactions to black widow spider bites should be treated by application of a cold pack and/or a topical corticosteroid. When there is a severe reaction, immediate treatment should include application of a proximal band to occlude venous return, administration of opiates for pain, muscle relaxants, calcium gluconate, and antivenom effective against bites of all spiders of the genus *Latrodectus* (Lyovac). Mild local reactions to brown recluse spider bites heal well with no specific therapy. Brown recluse bites have a more favorable prognosis if (i) the bites are treated with ice bags and elevation, (ii) strenuous exercise is avoided, (iii) localized heat, surgery, and intralesional steroids are avoided, and (iv) antibiotics (erythromycin or cephalosporins) and aspirin are given. Test for anemia and thrombocytopenia. Administer dapsone if the patient is not glucose 6-phosphate dehydrogenase deficient and the lesions are progressive. High-dose systemic corticosteroids are indicated in the treatment of severe bites and when hemolysis occurs. Dialysis may be required in patients with acute renal failure, anuria, and azotemia. Tetanus prophylaxis must be considered. Brown recluse spider antivenom is being developed, and there is early evidence that hyperbaric oxygen might help speed healing of the skin.

Dr Michael L. Smith, an entomologist and pediatric dermatologist, has a spider bite hot line for physicians that can be reached at 615-322-BITE.

B. **Snakes.** The best firstaid measures for snakebites are as follows: (i) Immobilize the injured part by splinting as if for a fracture. A constricting band may be applied proximal to the bite tightly enough to occlude veins and lymphatics but loosely enough to preserve a distal pulse. (ii) Incision and suction with a negative pressure device can remove a significant amount of venom; however, it must be applied within 3 to 5 minutes of the bite and left in place for 30 minutes. Ice is generally not recommended as vasoconstriction of already compromised tissue may contribute to necrosis. (iii) Get the victim to a physician or hospital as soon as possible. At that time, start an IV in the contralateral arm; type and cross match blood early, before venom action makes this impossible; and check for the presence of coagulopathy. (iv) In severely envenomized patients, administer horse-based antiserum. Two types of antivenom are commercially available, one for bites by rattlesnakes and other pit vipers and the other for coral snake bites. Antivenom reactions are common. Pit viper envenomation causes local platelet consumption, which can be ameliorated somewhat by antivenom but is worsened by steroids. Platelet and clotting factors should be restored by blood component therapy as indicated. Tissue necrosis and injury should be limited by debridement and mechanical removal of venom and local necrotic tissue. Locations of antivenom for rare species of poisonous snakes and the names and phone numbers of experts on venomous bites can be obtained 24 hours a day from the Arizona Poison Control Center (602-626-6016).

C. **Insects.** Insects should be flicked or brushed (not squeezed) off the skin. This action should also remove the venom sac. Forceps are not recommended to remove the stinger as it may squeeze the attached venom sac and worsen envenomation. Cold packs, systemic antihistamines, and a topical steroid may be useful for the pruritus and inflammation of local reactions.

The treatment of systemic allergic reactions and anaphylaxis to insect bites should follow conventional guidelines: (i) Inject 0.3 to 0.5 mg epinephrine HCl (0.3 to 0.5 mL of a 1:1,000 dilution) IM and repeat q15 to 30 min as needed. Lower doses should be used in the elderly and in patients with cardiovascular problems. Only in profound anaphylaxis with hypotension and poor peripheral circulation should intravenous administration be necessary. In such cases, use epinephrine in a 1:10,000 dilution (1 mg = 10 mL) and give 0.1-mg boluses until symptoms improve. (ii) Begin an intravenous line as soon as possible with a saline drip. If patients are not responsive to initial measures, critical care with fluids, oxygen, and pressors may become necessary. Cases of severe laryngeal edema may require intubation or tracheostomy. (iii) Persistent bronchospasm should be treated with intravenous aminophylline and inhaled bronchodilators such as albuterol, isoetharine, or isoproterenol. The recommended dose of aminophylline is a loading dose of 3 to 5 mg/kg followed by a drip of 0.5 to 0.9 mg/kg/hr. The dose should be lowered in elderly patients and in those with congestive heart failure or liver disease. Smokers may require higher doses. (iv) Antihistamines should be administered as an adjunct to epinephrine because their effect is not immediate. Use diphenhydramine 50 mg PO or IM, depending on the severity of the reaction. Treatment should continue as long as symptoms persist. (v) Steroids have a delayed onset of action and are not first-line drugs for treating a severe systemic reaction. However, unless medically contraindicated, they should be used to prevent continued reaction in all but the mildest allergic reactions. Begin with hydrocortisone 100 mg IV q6h and discharge on prednisone 30 mg/day, tapering over 3 to 7 days as symptoms dictate.

Sensitive patients should carry medications such as an epinephrine inhalation spray, ephedrine, and antihistamine tablets with them at all times. Commercial kits containing a syringe loaded with epinephrine (EpiPen) and antihistamine tablets (Ana-Kit) are available. Patients should also always carry an aerosol insecticide spray and avoid walking without shoes. They should dress in protective clothing and avoid wearing items that attract flying insects such as perfumes and other scented preparations; brightly colored clothing or jewelry; and wool, suede, or leather apparel. Insect venom immunotherapy is effective and should be considered mandatory for patients who have had an immediate systemic reaction to an insect sting. Commercial venoms and fire ant extract can be used for diagnosis (skin testing) and desensitization. Adults with a previous systemic reaction to a sting and a positive venom test will have a similar reaction in approximately 50% of instances if stung again. After immunotherapy, a resting will elicit a systemic reaction in <5% of patients.

Insect repellents containing diethyltoluamide (DEET) are the agents of choice for protection against mosquitoes, flies, fleas, mites, and ticks. These include Mosquitone lotion, OFF products, and Cutter insect repellent. Ethyl hexanediol, dimethyl phthalate, and dimethyl carbate butopyronoxyl are also effective but do not cover the wide spectrum that DEET does. A combination of two or more of these repellents is more effective than one alone. No product will protect against spiders, wasps, or bees. Factors that attract mosquitoes to skin include warmth, sweat, moisture, carbon dioxide, and other body emanations found in the convective air currents above or downwind of humans. Repellents do not mask these attractive stimuli but form a barrier against penetration that extends to <4 cm away from the skin. DEET blocks the ability of the mosquito to track the human's carbon dioxide vapor trail. At room temperature, protection time may last 10 to 12 hours. Approximately 10% of applied DEET evaporates from the skin in the first hour after application. There are many factors that will decrease the protection time, including heat, wind, friction against clothing, water, or sweat. Repellent-treated nets and clothing not only prevent mosquitoes from biting through clothes but also from biting adjacent areas. Repellents may remain effective for several days on fabric.

D. Caterpillars. Any spines or hairs from the caterpillar should be removed from the skin with adhesive tape, a commercial face peel, or a thin layer of rubber cement. Oral antihistamines and topical steroids should be administered to decrease urticaria and localized reactions. Severe dermatitis may benefit from oral prednisone 30 to 60 mg for adults and 1 mg/kg for children, tapered over 10 days.

E. Dog and Cat Bites. Wounds should be washed immediately with a non-tissue toxic soap. Pulsatile forced irrigation can be administered if available. Infected or necrotic tissue should be manually debrided. Primary closure of the wound should be avoided in high-risk wounds (the hand, deep penetrating wounds, immunocompromised patients, any wound showing signs of infection or devitalized tissue, and ferret and cat wounds). A delayed primary closure can be undertaken at 4 to 5 days if there is uncertainty about infection. Prophylactic antibiotics have not been shown to prevent infection although they are frequently used in dog and cat bites. Tetanus status should be updated and postexposure rabies prophylaxis should be considered. Human bites should be treated in a manner similar to dog and cat bites. They should never be sutured closed because of the high risk of soft tissue infection, especially on the hand.

Suggested Readings

Atlas E, Yee A. Bites of the brown recluse spider. *N Engl J Med* 2005;352:2029–2030.

Barth FG. Spider mechanoreceptors. *Curr Opin Neurobiol* 2004;14:415–422.

Brown M, Hebert AA. Insect repellents: an overview. *J Am Acad Dermatol* 1997;36:243–249.

Correira K. Managing dog, cat, and human bite wounds. *JAAPA* 2003;16:28–37.

Diaz JH. The epidemiology, syndromic diagnosis, management, and prevention of spider bites in the South. *J La State Med Soc* 2005;157:32–38.

Elston DM. Systemic manifestations and treatment of brown recluse spider bites. *Cutis* 2004;74:336–340.

Gold BS, Barish RA, Dart RC. North American snake envenomation: diagnosis, treatment, and management. *Emerg Med Clin North Am* 2004;22:423–443, ix.

Hogan CJ, Barbaro KC, Winkel K. Loxoscelism: old obstacles, new directions. *Ann Emerg Med* 2004;44:608–624.

Lalloo DG, Theakston RD. Snake antivenoms. *J Toxicol Clin Toxicol* 2003;41:277–290, 317–327.

Saucier JR. Arachnid envenomation. *Emerg Med Clin North Am* 2004;22:405–422, ix.

Steen CJ, Carbonaro PA, Schwartz RA. Arthropods in dermatology. *J Am Acad Dermatol* 2004;50:819–842.

Swanson DL, Vetter RS. Bites of brown recluse spiders and suspected necrotic arachnidism. *N Engl J Med* 2005;352:700–707.

Taplitz RA. Managing bite wounds. Currently recommended antibiotics for treatment and prophylaxis. *Postgrad Med* 2004;116:49–59.

Thorson A, Lavonas EJ, Rouse AM, et al. Copperhead envenomations in the carolinas. *J Toxicol Clin Toxicol* 2003;41:29–35.

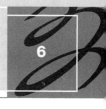

BURNS
John G. Hancox and Joseph L. Jorizzo

6

I. **DEFINITION AND PATHOPHYSIOLOGY.** Approximately 1.2 million individuals in the United States suffer burns each year, of whom 60,000 require hospitalization and 6,000 die. Thirty percent to 40% of those hospitalized are under the age of 15 (1), and burns are the second leading cause of death in children between the ages of 1 and 4 years. Scald burns (from spilled liquids or hot bath water) are the most common childhood burns (2). In addition, 10% to 15% of burns in children can be attributed to child abuse. Men suffer burns twice as often as women. The incidence of burns is high among the very young and very old, among nonwhites and members of lower socioeconomic groups, and in rural areas where space heaters or fireplaces are used for heat. Children's skin is thinner; therefore, severe burns will occur in less time and at a lower temperature than in adults. Electrical burns occur from toddlers putting metal objects into outlets or biting an electrical cord. These injuries are usually not life threatening, but a burn around the mouth could erode the labial artery and cause significant bleeding.

Thermal burns occur when infrared radiation (800 to 170,000 nm) exceeds 44°C (3). The degree of cutaneous damage caused by thermal injury to the skin is related directly to the duration and intensity of exposure to heat, the type of heat source, and the thickness of the exposed cutaneous surface. As the temperature increases, significantly less time is required to induce thermal damage. Necrosis of the epidermis occurs in approximately 45 minutes at 47°C, but in 1 second at 70°C (3). During burns, denaturation of cellular proteins and coagulation occur. Altered osmotic pressure and capillary permeability lead to edema. Chemical mediators, including prostaglandins, bradykinin, serotonin, oxygen radicals, and histamine are released, perpetuating tissue injury. In extensive burns, patients may enter a hypermetabolic state and catabolic hormones may be released, destroying fat and muscle.

Burn categories are based on depth, and are traditionally categorized as first, second or third degree (see sec. III for details). The depth of the burn is often related to its cause. Scalds from hot liquids are usually partial thickness, whereas injuries from contact with flames, hot metal, or electric current are usually full thickness in depth. The degree of chemical burn damage depends on the agent, and injury may progress for several days if untreated. Typically, alkaline substances produce more serious injury than acidic compounds. It is often difficult to determine the depth of injury during the first 2 weeks of healing.

II. **SUBJECTIVE DATA.** First- and second-degree burns are generally painful, whereas deeper damage destroys nerves and may render the tissue insensitive to pain.

III. **OBJECTIVE DATA**
   A. First-degree burn (epidermal involvement)
   1. **Clinical.** First-degree burns appear erythematous and edematous. Patients with such burns present with erythema, pain, tenderness, and edema. Desquamation may occur after a few days.
   2. **Histopathology**
      a. Epidermis. Loss of intercellular cohesiveness with cleft formation.
      b. Dermis. Vasodilatation and edema.
   3. **Course.** The lesions normally heal within several days with postinflammatory pigmentary alteration, but without scarring unless secondarily infected.
   B. Second-degree burn (partial-thickness burn)
   1. **Clinical.** Superficial second-degree burns display nonblanchable erythema, edema, serous or hemorrhagic bullae, erosion, and exudation. Patients with such deeper burns may present with red to pale skin with serosanguineous bullae

43

and erosions. Deeper second-degree burns may be difficult to differentiate from third-degree lesions.

  2. Histopathology
   a. Epidermis. Coagulative necrosis with bulla formation at dermoepidermal junction.
   b. Dermis. Marked vasodilatation and edema; destruction of adnexae may occur; evidence of continued capillary circulation may be observed.

  3. Course. For superficial second-degree burns, reepithelialization takes place from adnexal structures (hair follicles) and, if left undisturbed, lesions will heal within 2 to 3 weeks without scarring. For deeper burns, adnexal structures are often damaged or destroyed, and, therefore, healing is delayed and scarring will result.

 C. Third-degree burn (full-thickness burn)
  1. Clinical. The cutaneous surface assumes a dry, firm, nonblanching, translucent appearance, often resembling parchment paper. A charred or ulcerated wound surface with extensive tissue necrosis may also be present.

  2. Histopathology
   a. Epidermis. Full-thickness necrosis of epidermis.
   b. Dermis. Variable dermal and subcutaneous necrosis with destruction of adnexae.

  3. Course. Such burns heal slowly, often over months, with significant scarring.

IV. ASSESSMENT. For adults, the rule of nines is a useful technique to assess the percentage of body surface area (BSA) involved: the head, neck, and each upper extremity represent 9% of the BSA; the anterior trunk, posterior trunk, and each lower extremity comprise 18% of the BSA. The palm of the hand is approximately 1% of the total BSA and may be used as a guide to measure by surface area, especially in pediatric patients. Evaluators often overestimate the size of a burn by >50%.

Partial-thickness burns that involve <15% of BSA and spare the face, hands, feet, and perineum or full-thickness burns of <2% of the body surface are classified as minor burns. Such burns can often be managed in an ambulatory setting. Second-degree burns involving <5% of the total BSA and third-degree burns affecting <1% of BSA in children may also be managed as an outpatient. Burns in the elderly may be more serious and require individualized evaluation. Any burn can become secondarily infected, leading to cellulitis and/or sepsis.

V. THERAPY. The pathophysiology and therapy of moderate and severe burns will not be discussed. Such burns require intensive specialized care in hospitals. Expert management of the wound and of the severe cardiopulmonary disturbances caused by fluid and electrolyte changes associated with extensive cutaneous damage is always necessary. Survival rates of burn patients have doubled over the last 20 years, owing to improved resuscitation methods and the use of artificial skin and skin-equivalent allografts or homografts.

 A. Immediate therapy. Treatment of less severe burns should be started as soon as possible (within the first hour of injury). The affected area should be gently cleansed with soap and water to remove foreign material. Cool compresses should be applied to the site or the burned area should be immersed in static cool tap water (72 to 77°F). Ice should not be directly applied, as it can convert a superficial partial-thickness burn into a deeper burn. Cooling is an effective therapy because burnt skin still retains enough heat to extend coagulation to surrounding tissues. Cool compresses also relieve pain and reduce edema and reactive hyperemia. Warm blankets may be used to cover uninvolved areas to prevent systemic hypothermia.

 B. Continued therapy
  1. First-degree burns. The most superficial burns may require no dressing or medications, although the application of an emollient such as petrolatum may be soothing. Patients should consider tetanus prophylaxis as indicated and be given analgesics as required (see Table 6-1 for recommendations on tetanus prophylaxis). Although they lessen pain, topical anesthetics such as benzocaine add the risk of allergic contact dermatitis and are normally not indicated. Topical antibiotics, such as silver sulfadiazine (Silvadene), are effective in preventing

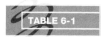

TABLE 6-1   Tetanus Prophylaxis

History of tetanus toxoid doses	Clean, minor wounds		All other wounds[a]	
	Td[b]	TIG[c]	Td	TIG
Unknown or <3	Yes	No	Yes	Yes
Three or more	No[d]	No	No[e]	No

[a]Such as, but not limited to, wounds contaminated with dirt, feces, soil, saliva and so on, puncture wounds, avulsions, and wounds resulting from crushing, burns, and frostbite.
[b]Tetanus toxoid, diphtheria toxoid (active immunization).
[c]Tetanus immune globulin (passive immunization).
[d]Yes, if >10 years since last dose.
[e]Yes, if >5 years since last dose. (More frequent boosters are not needed and can accentuate side effects.)

infection and creating a proper healing milieu. Leukopenia has been reported when silver sulfadiazine is extensively used.

2. **Second-degree burns.** Careful examination is necessary. Deeper burns require debridement of necrotic tissue. However, caution must be exercised, as it may be difficult to delineate the extent of the damage for several days. Debridement performed too early may remove living tissue. Comfortable, occlusive dressings are important for such burns. If oozing or weeping is present, application of an ointment or petrolatum-impregnated (Xeroform) gauze next to the wound will prevent adherence of the bandage to the wound. Absorptive material such as fluffed gauze pads should be placed over the initial gauze layer, and a final layer of elastic bandage should be applied with even compression. Dressings should remain in place for several days unless there is copious exudate, in which case they need to be changed more often. Adherent dressings should be moistened, or the affected cutaneous surface should be bathed in warm water before the dressings are removed to ease removal and limit trauma. Newer skin substitutes, such as acellular dermal matrix (AlloDerm), glycosaminoglycan-modified bovine collagen matrix covered with silicon (Integra), and synthetic bilaminate biocomposite of nylon mesh bonded to silicon film membrane (Biobrane) are gaining popularity. Topical antibiotic agents such as silver sulfadiazine are important adjuncts in the treatment of second-degree burns.

3. **Chemical burns.** Such injuries require immediate and prolonged irrigation with water. The depth of the injury may be reduced by 2 to 4 hours or more of washing. Do not rinse acid burns with alkali, and vice versa; doing this causes an exothermic reaction, which leads to further tissue damage. Industrial toxicity texts should be consulted regarding specific therapy for offending chemicals.

4. **Rehabilitation.** Rehabilitation of burn patients may require years of therapy. Reepithelialized or grafted skin is prone to blister formation, dryness, pruritus, contact dermatitis, photosensitivity, and hypertrophic scar formation. Burn scars, like chronic wounds, are prone to the development of skin cancer, particularly squamous cell carcinoma. Such malignancies are more aggressive than those occurring in actinically damaged skin.

References
1. Ramzy PI, Barret JP, Herndon DN. Thermal injury. *Crit Care Clin* 1999;15:333–352.
2. Morrow SE, Smith DL, Cairns BA, et al. Etiology and outcome of pediatric burns. *J Pediatr Surg* 1996;31(3):329–333.
3. Page EH, Shear NH. Temperature dependent skin disorders. *J Am Acad Dermatol* 1988;18:1003–1019.

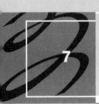

CORNS AND CALLUSES
Adrienne M. Feasel

7

I. **DEFINITION AND PATHOPHYSIOLOGY.** Corns (clavi) and calluses are acquired areas of thickened skin that appear over sites of repeated or prolonged trauma to the epithelium. Neither soft corns nor hard corns occur in normal feet. These lesions arise because of pressure, friction, and shearing forces of bone (through the overlying skin) against adjacent digits, metatarsal heads, or footwear. They are associated with poorly fitting footwear, underlying anatomic deformities, and high levels of activity. The severity and type of growth are related to the degree and chronicity of the local irritation. The formation of the center (nucleus, radix) of a corn is secondary to vascular changes and fibrosis underlying the point of maximum stress. In both conditions, there is marked hyperkeratosis of the stratum corneum overlying an epidermis that has otherwise the same thickness as the adjacent skin.

Some studies show that the structure of keratin in callus differs from that of the normal stratum corneum. The individual cells are thicker and much more highly interdigitated, and a dense cement material occupies the intercellular spaces. All signs of desquamation are absent. The keratin appears to be similar in structure to that of finger pad and nail. Differences in plantar callosities may be explained by altered epidermal differentiation due to an increased rate of epidermal cell production.

Corns are more symptomatic and better demarcated than calluses. Hard corns (heloma durum) are located most frequently over the dorsolateral aspect of the fifth toes but may be seen commonly at any point under the metatarsal ends. Small "seed corns" may be found anywhere on the plantar surface. Poorly fitting shoes are the most frequent cause of corns. Soft corns (heloma mole) that result from pressure of the head of the proximal phalanx of the fifth toe on the base of the proximal phalanx of the fourth toe or those that result from interdigital maceration are most often located in the fourth interdigital web; 65% of a series of more than a thousand patients occurred in the fourth interspace. Congenital factors including a short first metatarsal, a short fifth metatarsal, or third and fourth metatarsals of equal length predispose the foot to corn formation; other factors include hallux valgus, hammer toe deformities, and curling of the smaller toes.

Calluses are more diffuse hyperkeratotic areas present most commonly under the first and/or fifth metatarsal heads. They are also seen as occupational marks, for example, the callused palms of a laborer or the callused fingers of a violinist.

Callosities on the dorsum of the hand overlying the metacarpophalangeal and interphalangeal joints can be seen in individuals with bulimia. Repeated contact of the incisors with the skin during induced vomiting produces this finding, which is called *Russell's sign.*

II. **SUBJECTIVE DATA.** Corns may cause a constant dull discomfort or a severe knife-like pain on downward pressure. Calluses are either asymptomatic or painful on pressure, causing a feeling somewhat akin to walking with a pebble in one's shoe. Lateral pressure elicits pain in a wart; direct pressure produces pain in a corn.

III. **OBJECTIVE DATA**

   A. Corns are sharply delineated, hyperkeratotic, small (several millimeters in diameter or smaller) areas with a central translucent pit. They are conical in shape, with the apex pointing into the tissue. Soft corns are less discrete, whitish thickenings found in the interdigital webs. If one palpates these lesions, an underlying bone prominence will always be found.

B. Calluses are large (millimeters to centimeters in diameter), diffuse areas of thickened skin with indefinite borders.

IV. ASSESSMENT. If a suspect lesion is pared down (debrided), a number of differential features become apparent.

A. Corns. A central nucleus becomes evident; with continued debridement, this clear area becomes smaller and eventually disappears, at which point the normal skin markings can again be followed through the lesion.

B. Soft corns. These are often confused with simple maceration or an interdigital fungal infection. Paring the lesion will reveal a central nucleus and at times a small sinus tract at the base of the interdigital web. This sinus may close intermittently and result in recurrent bouts of bacterial infection.

C. Calluses. The normal skin markings remain evident, and no nucleus is found.

D. Plantar warts. A central area composed of red and black dots, punctate bleeding, and obliteration of skin markings will be revealed on debridement. The dots represent thrombosed capillaries in the highly vascularized wart. A callus will commonly overlie a wart and be responsible for the associated discomfort.

V. THERAPY

A. Therapy to allay symptoms

1. With both corns and calluses, the cause of pain is thickened hyperkeratotic areas of skin. The pain caused by such a mass may be completely eradicated simply by reducing the lesion by debridement with a curette, a No. 15 blade, a No. 86 Beaver, or No. 313 Gillette chisel blade. To ensure satisfactory results with a corn, it is often advisable to anesthetize the area (to remove the entire central nucleus). The patient may then carry out intermittent debridement as follows:

   a. Cut out a piece of 40% salicylic acid plaster slightly larger than the lesion and apply it to the skin, sticky side down.

   b. Apply a felt pad fashioned to fit around the lesion to relieve the pressure.

   c. Leave overnight or for as long as 5 to 7 days for very thick lesions.

   d. Remove the dressing and soak the foot in water.

   e. Remove whitened, soft, and macerated skin with a rough towel, pumice stone, or callus file.

   f. Reapply plaster as often as necessary to keep the lesion flat.

   g. As a corn thins, protective felt padding is all that is necessary.

2. At times, injection of a small amount of corticosteroid (Aristocort, Kenalog) beneath a painful corn will result in dramatic relief of symptoms.

3. Topical urea or salicylic acid preparations may soften the hyperkeratosis.

4. Caution should be exercised in the treatment of corns and calluses in the foot of a patient with diabetes because of the increased risk of infection, ulceration, and sepsis. Removal of calluses in a patient with diabetes will reduce plantar pressures and reduce the chance of developing neuropathic foot ulceration.

B. Definitive therapy

1. Removal of the lesion treats only the result and not the cause of the difficulty. Poorly fitting footwear, anatomic malformations, faulty weight distribution, or similar factors must be corrected; otherwise, the hyperkeratoses will rapidly recur. Both corns and calluses will disappear after the causative factors have been removed. Corrective shoe supports, orthotics, x-ray studies for anatomic defects, and referral to a podiatrist or orthopedic surgeon are warranted in difficult cases.

2. Corrective surgery is associated with resolution of the hyperkeratosis and decreased pain in many patients, but lesions may recur.

Suggested Readings

Cambiaghi S, Morel P. Hereditary painful callosities with associated features. *Dermatology* 1996;193:47–49.

Coughlin MJ, Kennedy MP. Operative repair of fourth and fifth toe corns. *Foot Ankle Int* 2003;24(2):147–157.

Day RD, Reyzelman AM, Harkless LB. Evaluation and management of the interdigital corn: a literature review. *Clin Podiatr Med Surg* 1996;13:201–206.

Freeman DB. Corns and calluses resulting from mechanical hyperkeratosis. *Am Fam Physician* 2002;65(11):2277–2280.

Murray HJ, Young MJ, Hollis S, et al. The association between callus formation, high pressures and neuropathy in diabetic foot ulceration. *Diabet Med* 1996;13:979–982.

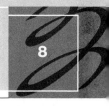

DERMATITIS/ECZEMA

Peter C. Schalock

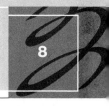

8

I. DEFINITION AND PATHOPHYSIOLOGY. The word eczema is derived from Greek, "ek" meaning out and "zein" meaning to boil. The Greek word therefore defines the superficial inflammatory diseases of the skin which represent the most common reaction pattern seen by the dermatologist. The morphologic and histopathologic changes in all forms of dermatitis and eczema are similar. The earliest and mildest changes are erythema and edema. These early changes may progress to vesiculation and oozing and then to crusting and scaling. Finally, if the process becomes chronic, the skin will become lichenified (thickened, with prominent skin markings), excoriated, and either hypo- or hyperpigmented.

The microscopic changes in this process show (i) initially, inter- and intracellular fluid accumulation, with resultant vesicle formation and associated dermal vasodilatation and infiltration with chronic inflammatory cells and (ii) later, thickening of the epidermis and altered keratinization patterns, with retention of nuclei in the stratum corneum. The factors that may initiate dermatitis are numerous, and the patterns of the dermatitis will dictate both the clinical classification and therapy.

The following categories of dermatitis will be discussed separately:
1. Atopic dermatitis
2. Circumscribed chronic dermatitis
3. Contact dermatitis
4. Hand dermatitis
5. Nummular dermatitis

 ATOPIC DERMATITIS

I. DEFINITION AND PATHOPHYSIOLOGY. Atopic dermatitis (AD) is an intensely pruritic, chronic skin disease that can affect all age-groups. It is the most common type of infantile eczema; approximately 3% of infants have some evidence of AD during the first few months of life. Increased risk of AD has been linked to a parental history of atopy and duration of breast-feeding. Maternal smoking during pregnancy and maternal body mass index and the gender, socioeconomic status, immunizations, and antibiotic usage of the infant during the first year of life were not associated with an increased risk of an infant having AD. Approximately 90% of affected children manifest their disease by 5 years of age, and 10% to 15% of children are affected. Approximately 70% of patients with AD have a family history of atopy (polygenic inheritance with an environmental influence appears most likely), and approximately 50% of children with AD develop either rhinitis or asthma. If one parent has AD, the prevalence of AD among their children is 56% to 60%; it is 81% if both parents have AD. There is a higher correlation between siblings for atopic disease than between parent and child.

Although AD may disappear with time, it is estimated that 30% to 80% of atopic patients will continue to have intermittent exacerbations throughout life, often when under physical or emotional stress. Eyelid dermatitis, retroauricular dermatitis, and hand eczema are the most common adult residuals of childhood atopic disease.

Severe, easily triggered itching is the outstanding feature of this disease. Many of the clinical signs are secondary to scratching and rubbing of the skin. AD may be particularly devastating in its effects on the patient's mental well-being and emotional development, because it is frequently present during the most critical periods of life.

In infancy, it interferes with a healthy mother–child relationship; in adolescence and early adulthood, it plagues and disfigures patients during a crucial formative period. Emotional stress and altered family interactions play an important role in its course.

Patients with AD have immunologic abnormalities, including elevated serum immunoglobulin E (IgE) levels, reduced cell-mediated immune responses, and slowed chemotaxis of neutrophils and monocytes. There is usually a correlation between IgE serum level and the severity, duration, and amount of body surface affected by dermatitis. There are, however, many facts that argue against IgE playing an important role in the causation of this entity. Approximately 20% of adults with AD have normal or low IgE levels; others have no IgE at all, whereas there are some patients with enormous elevations of IgE but no dermatitis. Further, in infantile eczema, IgE levels are consistently low or normal. IgE has been suggested to play a role in causing AD reactions caused by cross-reaction between a fungal and human manganese superoxide dismutase (MnSOD).

Skin testing, hyposensitization, and special diets are usually unrewarding. In one study, despite limiting exposure to common allergens before 2 years of age, by age 7 there was no difference among all measured factors including AD and asthma. (i) House dust mites are felt to be an etiologic role in patients with AD, and measures to reduce dust mites in the environment can improve symptoms of AD. (ii) *Pityrosporum ovale*, a lipophilic yeast, may play a role in AD of the face, scalp, and neck; patients have a high frequency of positive skin prick tests and two thirds of patients may have IgE antibodies against *P. ovale*.

There are multiple theories regarding the mechanism of inflammation in AD:

A. AD is secondary to excessive T-cell stimulation. Supporting evidence includes high levels of activated T cells in lesional skin and increased interleukin-4 (IL-4) production by T cells.

B. AD is secondary to hyperstimulated antigen presenting cells (APCs). Langerhans cells (LCs) of patients with AD, stimulated by IL-4, have an increased capacity to stimulate T cells. Macrophages in AD secrete IL-10, which stimulates a Th2 cytokine response.

C. Macrophages in AD have an increase in phosphodiesterase activity that degrades cyclic adenosine monophosphate (cAMP). Decreased cAMP levels result in impaired cell function and hyperactivity of immune competent cells. Experimental phosphodiesterase isoenzyme type 4 (PDE4) inhibitors clinically improve patients with AD.

D. A recent study examined specific IgE activity against human and fungal MnSOD. Twenty-nine out of 67 patients were reactive with serum IgE that reacted with both fungal and human MnSOD. The human protein was able to induce *in vitro* T-cell reactivity and eczematous reactions in sensitized patients. These reactions may support MnSOD as a human autoallergen in a subset of patients sensitized, potentially, to fungal MnSOD. In these patients, IgE could play an important role in AD pathogenesis.

Although certainly not an infectious disease *per se*, both the uninvolved and dermatitic skin of atopic individuals often harbor large numbers of *Staphylococcus aureus*, which may secondarily exacerbate the condition. Sensitization to *S. aureus* superantigens may be involved in disease exacerbation. Thirty percent of relapses are due to a secondary bacterial infection. Topical steroids alone can be effective in the eradication of *S. aureus* because inflammation plays a key role in colonization by the bacteria. Atopic patients react in an aberrant fashion to many environmental and physiologic factors; they demonstrate heightened and prolonged pruritus in response to normally subthreshold stimuli and an altered vascular response to pressure and injections of histamine, serotonin, and cholinergic and sympathomimetic agents, as well as abnormal reactions to heat and cold. Fifty percent of children with human immunodeficiency virus infection have evidence of AD and adults can commonly have an "AD-like" syndrome.

II. SUBJECTIVE DATA. The primary and predominant symptom of AD is itching. This often sets up a vicious cycle: itching leads to scratching, scratching causes lichenification and other changes, and lichenification lowers the threshold for renewed itching. Children with AD often have disrupted sleep and daytime irritability related to lack of sleep (1). Thirty percent of women report a premenstrual flare of their AD; 50% of pregnant women note worsening of their symptoms (2).

III. OBJECTIVE DATA

A. In the infantile phase of AD (age 2 months to 2 years), there is involvement primarily of the chest, face, scalp, neck, and extensor extremities with erythematous papulovesicles and oozing. At age 2 months, purposeful scratching begins and by 18 months, flexural lichenification can be observed. Some infants also have very dry skin that predisposes them to itching and recurrent inflammation.

B. In the childhood phase (between the ages of 4 and 10 years), the lesions are less acute and exudative, more scattered, and often localized in the flexor folds of the neck, elbows, wrists, and knees. Dry papules, excoriations, lichenification, and periorbital erythema and edema are common.

C. In the adolescent and adult phase (from the early teens to the early twenties), the lesions are primarily dry, lichenified, hyperpigmented plaques in flexor areas and around the eyes. Persistent hand dermatitis may be the only remnant of an atopic diathesis.

D. These three phases may imperceptibly blend together, or any of the changes may be seen at any time.

E. Essential features for the diagnosis of AD include pruritus and eczematous changes in a typical and age-specific pattern (as previously described) and a chronic or relapsing course. The presence of these features is enough for diagnosis. Other important and frequently seen features include early age of onset, IgE reactivity (atopy), and xerosis. Other associated features include ichthyosis vulgaris, hyperlinear palms, white dermographism, nipple eczema, Dennie-Morgan lines (extra infraorbital skin folds), and keratosis pilaris (this finding improves in one third of patients by adulthood).

F. A Swedish study of 105 patients with AD found the following criteria to be of diagnostic value: cheilitis, pityriasis alba, white dermatographism, wool intolerance, nipple eczema, and fissures under the ear (3).

G. In one study, 90% of atopic children had evidence of cervical lymphadenopathy (4).

IV. ASSESSMENT

A. A detailed personal, family, environmental, and psychological history is mandatory for delivering proper care.

B. Factors that often trigger pruritus include the following: extreme heat or cold, rapid changes in temperature, sweating, irritating or occlusive medications or clothing (especially wool and synthetic fibers), fragrances, greases, oils, soaps, and detergents, and at times, inhalants or other environmental allergens. Patch testing is helpful in the assessment of individuals with worsening AD.

C. Concomitants of AD include pathologic changes in the eye (posterior cataract, keratoconus, and retinal detachment) and lowered resistance to viral infections—especially infections with herpes simplex (eczema herpeticum) and vaccinia viruses—resulting in the dissemination of usually localized infections. Eczema herpeticum (Kaposi's varicelliform eruption) is often clinically confused with bacterial superinfection.

Patients with AD should not be vaccinated or be close to family or friends who have had recent vaccinations for vaccinia (smallpox) or have active herpes simplex infections. One third of patients with eczema herpeticum had a history of herpes labialis present in one parent the previous week. If vaccination for vaccinia is mandatory, it should take place immediately after administering vaccinia immune globulin (0.3 mL/kg IM) or should utilize newer strains of vaccinia virus that reduce the risk of eczema vaccinatum. Routine vaccinations should not be avoided, and these have actually been suggested to be protective against the development of AD (Gruber, 2004). Other retrospective studies have suggested higher rates of AD in children following routine vaccinations.

D. Fungal infections occur three times more often in atopic than in nonatopic patients. Molluscum contagiosum and verruca vulgaris may spread more extensively in atopic patients.

V. THERAPY. The aims of therapy are to decrease trigger factors and pruritus, suppress inflammation, lubricate the skin, and alleviate anxiety.

A. **Preventive measures**
   1. The environment should be kept at a constant temperature, and excess humidity or extreme dryness should be avoided. Clothing worn next to the skin should be absorbent and nonirritating (cotton), laundered with bland, fragrance-free soaps, and rinsed thoroughly. High levels of stress have been linked to a decrease in barrier permeability recovery kinetics after barrier disruption by cellophane tape stripping. There was recovery of barrier function during periods of lower stress. Adequate rest and relaxation are important and a vacation in a warm, dry climate is often beneficial.
   2. Eliminate excessive bathing and other factors that promote xerosis. Keep the skin moist and supple. Use a bland, nonirritating soap or just a nonfragranced bath oil. The ideal time to apply a topical steroid is on a b.i.d. basis after bathing or application of wet compresses or a spray mist of water.
   3. Emollients or medications should be applied immediately after bathing, within 3 minutes, to "trap" water in the skin. Frequent application of bland lubricants both soothes and physically protects the skin and is the most important single measure in the therapy of AD. Ointments are preferable to creams.
   4. Scratch and intradermal allergy tests are not useful. Patch tests for contact allergies may be productive. A decrease in environmental allergens and trial elimination diets might be considered if the more usual therapeutic measures fail.
   5. The patient's emotional stability is essential. Continued contact with an optimistic and reassuring physician will allay much anxiety. Occasionally, formal psychological consultation or therapy will be beneficial.
   6. Short-term hospitalization is often efficacious, and improvement in the skin may appear before medications are applied. This complete but temporary environmental and emotional rearrangement will often suffice to break the itch-scratch cycle.

B. **Treatment for active dermatitis**
   1. Exudative areas should be compressed with aluminum acetate (Burow's) for 20 minutes four to six times a day, or the patient should be placed in a tub with antipruritic and/or emollient additives such as oatmeal (Aveeno or Oilated Aveeno) or lubricating bath additives.
   2. The primary and most important therapeutic tool in eczema is the frequent use of topical corticosteroids. They should be applied in small amounts two to three times a day. If the skin remains dry, use emollients between steroid applications. This therapy will suppress inflammation and stop pruritus, thereby interrupting the inflammation-itch-scratch-inflammation cycle. High-potency topical steroids help decrease colonization of the skin with *S. aureus*, by eliminating the organism after 2 weeks of treatment. Treatment should be initiated with a high-potency steroid to quickly quell inflammation and pruritus. Once the acute eruption subsides, the goal should be to use topical steroids only a few days per week.
      If maintenance therapy is needed, 1% hydrocortisone or a low-potency steroid is more appropriate. Ointments are superior for all but the most acute, exudative lesions. Alternating the application of corticosteroids with lubricants will lessen the risks of prolonged steroid use and tachyphylaxis. The ultimate height of the patient may not be affected by topical steroids, but impaired growth and delayed puberty are well described in atopic patients. Growth should be closely monitored in children receiving topical steroids (5). Parents are often reluctant to use topical steroids on their children, and they often need significant counseling and reassurance.
   3. Calcineurin inhibitors are a relatively new class of topical therapy for AD. This is a class of immunomodulatory drugs that are used in an oral form in the transplant population and are now widely used for the treatment of AD. These agents compete for calcineurin binding sites with calmodulin. Binding of the calcineurin inhibitor decreases calcium-dependent signaling, which

subsequently regulates cell division, triggers early steps of T-cell activation, and decreases gene transcription of IL-2 and its receptor.

There are two forms currently approved for cutaneous usage, tacrolimus ointment (Protopic) and pimecrolimus cream (Elidel). Tacrolimus is derived from the fungus *Streptomyces tsukubaensis* and pimecrolimus is derived from macrolactam ascomycin. Studies have shown a dramatic decrease in the severity of AD, in children and adults, with the ability to tolerate this therapy even on facial skin. Protopic and Elidel are both significantly more effective than vehicle control in all cases. Protopic 0.1% is as effective as potent corticosteroids and 0.03% of it is more effective than hydrocortisone acetate but less effective than hydrocortisone butyrate. Elidel is far less effective than betamethasone valerate. Reported side effects occurring at >5% that occurred significantly more often than vehicle control include significant skin burning or tingling on application compared with corticosteroid application, flu-like symptoms, headache, tingling, acne, flushing with EtOH consumption, hyperesthesia, folliculitis, and rash. There were no reports of skin thinning or adrenal suppression with Protopic or Elidel.

The U.S. Food and Drug Administration (FDA) has recently reviewed the safety profile of calcineurin inhibitors. Owing to the mechanism of their action and the concerns for local impairment of immunosuppression, an advisory and a "Black Box" warning were issued in March 2005. Their concern was due to 19 postmarket cases of cancer of any type in patients treated with calcineurin inhibitors. Nine of these cases were lymphoma and 10 cutaneous tumors (7 at the site of application). There is evidence in animals of a dose-dependent increase in lymphoma with the use of calcineurin inhibitors. The data in humans are currently unclear and an estimated 10 years will be needed before the risks will be defined with more certainty. The FDA has issued the following guidelines for the use of calcineurin inhibitors:

- Use Elidel/Protopic only as second-line agent for short-term and intermittent treatment of AD.
- Avoid use of Elidel/Protopic in children younger than 2 years of age. The effect of Elidel on the developing immune system in infants and children is not known. In clinical studies, infants and children younger than 2 years old treated with Elidel had a higher rate of upper respiratory infections than those treated with placebo cream.
- Use Elidel/Protopic only for short periods of time, not continuously. The long-term safety of Elidel is unknown.
- Children and adults with a weakened or compromised immune system should not use Elidel/Protopic.
- Use the minimum amount of Elidel/Protopic needed to control the patient's symptoms. In animals, increasing the dose resulted in higher rates of cancer.

4. Tar compounds T-gel, liquor carbonis detergens 5% to 10% in hydrophilic ointment, or others are useful as adjunctive therapy in patients with chronic dermatitis. Their use may be alternated with the corticosteroids (i.e., tars overnight, corticosteroids during the day), or they may be applied at the same time to affected skin or used in the bath.

5. Other topical agents: Polidocanol in a concentration of 3% to 12% has been shown to have an antipruritic effect in AD. The only side effect noted was allergic contact dermatitis (ACD) to the agent in some patients. Topical capsaicin has been used with some success in AD. It inhibits substance P in the C-nerve fibers, thereby inhibiting itch and pain after 6 weeks of continuous usage. A starting concentration of 0.025% is suggested. Side effects of stinging and burning can be problematic.

6. The efficacy of antihistamines in AD is controversial. Antihistamines taken by mouth will often suppress pruritus, allay anxiety, and allow sleep. First-generation antihistamines cross the blood-brain barrier, whereas the subsequent generations do not. The effect in AD is believed to be mainly due to the sedative effect of first-generation antihistamines. The dose administered

should be increased gradually to an effective level. In acute cases, these drugs should be given on a continuous basis. Hydroxyzine is often the drug of choice to promote sleep. Multiple other classic and nonsedating antihistamines are available, but no controlled studies have shown their efficacy against the itch of AD. Nonsedating second- or third-generation antihistamines are useful for treating infants and children with coexistent allergies, urticaria, or allergic rhinoconjunctivitis but are usually not helpful for diminution of pruritus.

7. Long-term administration of systemic corticosteroids plays no part in the therapy of AD. Acute flare-ups may be suppressed by a short-term course of prednisone (40 to 60 mg PO everyday, tapering to 0 in 10 to 14 days) or one injection of 6 mg betamethasone sodium phosphate and betamethasone acetate suspension (Celestone), 40 to 80 mg methylprednisolone (Depo-Medrol), or 40 mg triamcinolone acetonide (Kenalog) or triamcinolone diacetate (Aristocort). Occasionally, the dermatitis will flare up after cessation of steroids, but usually the eczematous disease will not reappear for months after one such course.

8. Phototherapy can induce remission in select patients with recalcitrant chronic AD. Light therapy should be instituted when the skin disease has stabilized or the patient is being tapered off a systemic medication. Ultraviolet B (UVB) phototherapy used along with emollients or tars is also very effective. A combination of Ultraviolet A (UVA) and UVB phototherapy has been shown to be more effective than UVB alone (6). Narrowband UVB (311 nm) is a useful and effective treatment for AD. Psoralen plus UVA (PUVA) can control severe AD but because of its slow onset of action, aging, and carcinogenic effects, it is usually not the first choice, especially for children.

9. Secondary *S. aureus* infection should be treated with appropriate oral antibiotics, which may often be helpful even without clinical evidence of infection.

10. Recombinant γ-interferon (which inhibits IgE synthesis by promoting proliferation of the Th1 cells) administered by weekly subcutaneous injections may have a role in patients with severe AD and elevated IgE levels, although some patients experience flu-like side effects (7). Owing to the high cost, a 20% nonresponse rate, and adverse events, γ-interferon is not recommended for the first-line treatment of AD. It may be a reasonable treatment option for patients with otherwise recalcitrant moderate-to-severe AD.

11. Thymopentin, whose mechanism of action is likely the decreased production of histamine-releasing factor, has shown promise in severe AD with minimal adverse reactions (8).

12. Mast cell stabilizers such as topical sodium cromoglycate were found to be very effective in the relief of pruritus, with decrease in AD when studied in children (9). Neocromil sodium has also been used for the treatment of AD, showing no benefit in several clinical trials (Roos, 2004).

13. Acyclovir (IV) or other antiviral treatments can lead to rapid improvement of eczema herpeticum, although untreated cases may improve without antiviral therapy.

14. Cyclosporin A (5 mg/kg/day) significantly improved the extent and severity of disease in adults with severe AD. Patients are usually started at 2.5 to 5 mg/kg/day to obtain clearance and then tapered; low-dose therapy is often required to maintain clinical remission. Ultraviolet light can be introduced once stabilized and dose reduction begins. Patients should not be treated with a course longer than 12 months. The risks versus benefits of this drug must be taken into consideration; hypertension and decreased renal function are the two most common adverse reactions. Frequent laboratory monitoring is recommended. There are multiple drug interactions relating to the cytochrome P-450 3A microsomal enzymes that need to be taken into consideration.

15. Azathioprine (Imuran) at doses of 0.7 to 2.5 mg/kg/day is an effective treatment for adult patients with AD; one of its major drawbacks is the slow onset of action (6 to 8 weeks). Nausea and vomiting are the most frequent side effects. The risk of myelosuppression can be minimized by screening patients

for thiopurine methyltransferase (TPMT) activity. One in 300 individuals have TPMT deficiency as an autosomal recessive trait. The long-term toxicity of this drug is unclear, with possible increased risk of hematologic malignancies.

16. Evening primrose oil, a plant oil rich in γ-linolenic acid, modulates prostaglandin levels and has been advocated as a treatment for AD. Fifteen studies of evening primrose oil or borage oil (another plant oil rich in γ-linolenic acid) were recently analyzed. There was no clinical benefit in any of the studies, even with high doses compared with control. This agent is not recommended for use in AD.

17. Zonalon cream, topical doxepin (an antihistamine), was released in 1994 and may be helpful with the symptoms of pruritus associated with AD and localized eczematous dermatitis. Side effects such as sedation and dry mouth have been reported, usually when the application exceeds >10% of the total body surface area. Zonalon is indicated for short-term (up to 8 days) management of moderate, localized pruritus. Cases of ACD to this drug have been well documented, and systemic doxepin should be avoided if cutaneous hypersensitivity exists.

18. Traditional Chinese herbal therapy has been found to be helpful in several studies, with long-term use being associated with a sustained remission. Standardization of the herbs is problematic in addition to the palatability and a risk of hepatotoxicity and cardiomyopathy.

19. Hypnotherapy and massage therapy have been found to be helpful in children with AD.

 CIRCUMSCRIBED CHRONIC DERMATITIS

(Lichen Simplex Chronicus)

I. DEFINITION AND PATHOPHYSIOLOGY. Circumscribed chronic dermatitis (lichen simplex chronicus) is a localized, chronic pruritic disorder resulting from repeated scratching and rubbing. Patients with this disease often have other atopic manifestations (asthma, allergic rhinitis) and frequently have a positive personal and family history of atopic disorders. The original pruritogenic stimulus usually remains undefined; it could have been an insect bite, constricting clothing, contact or seborrheic dermatitis, or psoriasis. Once the itch-scratch-lichenification cycle is established, it makes little difference what initially incited the problem. In these patients, scratching seems to be a conditioned response; one that becomes a fixed pattern and has a relative specificity for certain areas of skin, all in areas easily accessible to the patient. Lichenified skin tends to be itchier than normal skin following minor stimuli, thereby leading to further scratching. It must be emphasized that the scratching of these lichenified areas is not always unpleasant—it is sometimes very pleasurable—and this secondary gain may interfere with conscientious application of therapy by the patient. Scratching is often vigorously accomplished with the heels, nails, combs, or other implements. Repeated trauma to the skin results in an increased number of cells undergoing mitosis, an increased transepidermal transit time, and hyperplasia involving all components of the epidermis. Within nodular lesions, there may also be thickened nerve fibers, axon and Schwann cell proliferation, neuroma-schwannoma formation, and axon swelling. The extreme pruritus in chronic lesions may be related to the increased number of dermal nerves.

II. SUBJECTIVE DATA. Continuous, spasmodic, or paroxysmal pruritus is the only symptom.

III. OBJECTIVE DATA. These well-circumscribed, lichenified plaques, at times with psoriasiform scaling, are located most frequently on the ankles and anterior tibial and nuchal areas. The inner thighs, sides of the neck, extensor surfaces of the forearms, and anogenital areas may also be affected. Dry keratotic papules and giant "scratch papules" or prurigo nodules are also a response to repeated scratching. Patients will usually have only one area of involvement.

IV. ASSESSMENT. Detailed questioning regarding the itch stimulus is worthwhile but often fruitless. Psychogenic factors are important. Secondary infection or sensitization to topical therapeutic agents is not uncommon. One study found a significant number of positive patch tests in a group of patients with prurigo nodularis.

V. THERAPY. Despite the chronicity of these lesions, effective therapy will usually induce remission of the pruritus and the lichenification within 1 to 2 weeks.

- **A.** High-potency topical corticosteroids, usually applied under plastic, biosynthetic, or hydrocolloid dressings (DuoDerm Extra Thin, Actiderm) overnight or for continuous 3- to 7-day periods, are extremely effective (10). Cordran tape, which is impregnated with a mid-potency steroid, can be applied daily; it helps moisturize the area, decrease inflammation, and prevent the patient's hands from being in contact with the area.
- **B.** Intralesional injection of corticosteroids will induce involution most rapidly and is often the therapy of choice. Steroids such as triamcinolone acetonide (Kenalog) in concentration of 3.3 to 10 mg/mL are injected in 0.1 mL amounts in a checkerboard pattern throughout the lesion.
- **C.** Topical photochemotherapy with psoralens and UVA may induce remission in those responding poorly to other forms of treatment.
- **D.** Antihistamines or ataractic agents are occasionally of value, especially Atarax 25 to 50 mg before bed. Topical doxepin (Zonalon), an H1 and H2 antihistamine, can be helpful for localized areas and as an adjunct to topical steroids, but should only be used for a maximum of 8 days of therapy owing to the risk of sensitization and ACD. Oral doxepin should be avoided if cutaneous allergy occurs.
- **E.** Emollients containing antipruritic agents (menthol, phenol), such as Sarna lotion, PrameGel, or tar, can also be useful. Agents with phenol should not be given to pregnant women.
- **F.** Liquid nitrogen cryotherapy provided dramatic relief of prurigo nodularis in a single uncontrolled case report.
- **G.** Pulsed dye laser has also been reported to be useful for prurigo nodules.

 CONTACT DERMATITIS

I. DEFINITION AND PATHOPHYSIOLOGY. Contact dermatitis may be produced by primary irritants or allergic sensitizers. Irritant contact dermatitis is a nonallergic reaction of the skin caused by exposure to irritating substances. Any person would react to an irritant if the concentration and duration of contact were sufficient. Most primary irritants are chemical substances, although physical and biologic (infectious) agents may produce the same picture. Irritants account for 80% of occupational contact dermatitis and also cause the most frequent type of nonindustrial contact reaction. The two types of irritants are (i) mild, relative, or marginal irritants, which require repeated and/or prolonged contact to produce inflammation, and include soaps, detergents, and most solvents and (ii) strong or absolute irritants, which are such damaging substances that they will injure skin immediately on contact (strong acids and alkalis). If daily exposure to mild irritants is continued, normal skin may become "hardened" or tolerant to this trauma, and contact may be continued without further evidence of irritation. Water and soap from frequent hand washing can be sufficient to produce irritant dermatitis, especially in patients with an atopic background.

ACD is a manifestation of delayed hypersensitivity (type IV) and results from the exposure of sensitized individuals to contact allergens. The sequence leading to inflammation is initiated by the binding of relatively simple chemical group(s) to an epidermal protein on or in the vicinity of LCs to form a complete antigen (the afferent limb or sensitization phase). The ensuring events include the following:

1. Exposure of the antigen (Ag) to an antigen presenting cell (APC), usually an LC.
2. The LC internalizes the antigen and processes in the lysosomes.
3. The Ag binds noncovalently to an MHC II (HLA-DR) molecule intracellularly.
4. The Ag/MHC complex is transported to and expressed on the LC cell membrane.

5. The LC migrates the lymph nodes and presents this complex to MHC-restricted CD4 T cells with specific Ag recognition sites.

The second response is the efferent limb or response phase and consists of the following:

1. Ag-specific T cells are activated.

2. IL-1 from LC and keratinocytes also activate T cells.

3. Stimulated T cells secrete IL-2 and interferon-γ (IFN-γ).

4. IL-2 nonspecifically stimulates other T cells to proliferate.

5. IFN-γ induces intercellular adhesion molecule -1 (ICAM-1) and HLA-DR expression, promotes tumor necrosis factor (TNF) and transforming growth factor (TGF) α production, increases IL-1 production, activates cytotoxic T cells, and recruits memory effector T cells.

6. ICAM-1 is an adhesion molecule that is seen on APC, keratinocytes, and endothelial cells within 24 to 96 hours after Ag exposure. Some allergens such as poison ivy can directly induce ICAM-1.

7. The released mediators attract an inflammatory infiltrate including macrophages, neutrophils, basophils, and eosinophils that are involved in the eczematous response.

The last phase is the resolution phase and includes the following:

1. CD4 cells decline and CD8 suppressor cells predominate.

2. Basophils and macrophages increase.

3. Macrophages produce prostaglandins that inhibit IL-2 and therefore downregulate inflammation.

Most contact allergens produce sensitization in only a small percentage of those exposed. Poison oak and poison ivy, which induce sensitization in >70% of the population, are notable exceptions to this rule. The incubation period after initial sensitization to an antigen is 5 to 21 days, whereas the reaction time after subsequent reexposure is 12 to 48 hours. Mild exposure of a sensitized person to poison oak or poison ivy, for example, will result in appearance of the rash in 2 to 3 days and clearing within the following 1 to 2 weeks; with massive exposure, lesions will appear more quickly (6 to 12 hours) and heal more slowly (2 to 3 weeks). Autoeczematization can occur in sites remote from the allergen exposure.

Factors that contribute to the development of contact dermatitis include genetic predisposition, local concentration of antigen, duration of exposure, site variation in cutaneous permeability, and the development of immune tolerance. Other contributing factors may be friction, pressure, occlusion, maceration, heat and cold, and the presence of other skin diseases.

Several specific types of contact dermatitis deserve mention.

A. Latex and rubber hypersensitivity is a growing medical problem, with 6% to 10% of hospital physicians and nurses affected. Patients requiring frequent bladder catheterization, such as patients with spina bifida and quadriplegia, are also at high risk for latex allergy. Allergic reactions to the additives in latex rubber may be delayed. Rubber accelerators are the most frequent cause of ACD in glove dermatitis. Chemicals such as carbamates, thiurams, and mercaptobenzothiazole are added to speed the processing of latex and other nonlatex gloves. Immediate hypersensitivity, with symptoms of tachycardia, flushing, burning, or erythema of the exposed skin, and urticaria can also occur owing to a reaction to the natural rubber latex protein. A radioallergosorbent test (RAST) to latex allergens can be done to determine whether a person is latex allergic; prick testing should only be done in a doctor's office that is equipped for a possible anaphylactic reaction. Extensive cross-reactions can occur between latex and foods including bananas, avocados, potatoes, tomatoes, chestnuts, and kiwis. Most skin reactions to gloves are a primary irritant reaction rather than contact dermatitis/urticaria.

B. Topical corticosteroid contact dermatitis should be suspected if dermatitis worsens with steroid applications. The allergy may be to the steroid itself or the vehicle; cross-reactivity may occur between corticosteroids. Tixocortol pivalate, budesonide, and hydrocortisone-17-butyrate are good screening agents for the subgroups of topical steroids. Clobetasol propionate and betamethasone valerate have the lowest frequency of positive reactions (11). Mometasone furoate (Elocon) also has a low rate of contact allergy.

C. Sunscreens may cause an irritant, allergic contact, or photoallergic contact dermatitis. Para-aminobenzoic acid (PABA), PABA derivatives, benzophenones, and cinnamates may be implicated in the reaction.

D. Eyelid dermatitis, significantly more common in women, is caused by ACD in 46% of individuals, 15% have an irritant reaction, and 23% have AD. Epoxies and tosylamide formaldehyde resins are common allergens, often found in fingernail care products.

E. Preservatives are found in almost all cosmetic and topical products with which our skin comes in contact. The role of the preservatives is to prevent overgrowth of bacteria in water-based products. In Britain, a recent study found that 23% of women and 14% of men had an adverse reaction to personal care products over the course of 1 year. Ten percent of these cases were ACD. Often, the culprit allergens in these products are preservatives. Increased rates of contact allergy have been reported to the following substances:

1. Formaldehyde
2. Formaldehyde releasers
   a. Quaternium 15 (no. 1 sensitizer)
   b. Imidazolidinyl urea (no. 2 sensitizer)
   c. Methylchloroisothiazolinone/methylisothiazolinone (Kathon CG)
   d. 2-Bromo-2-nitropropane-1,3-diol (Bronopol)
3. Nonformaldehyde releasers
   a. Parabens
   b. Thimerosal (found in vaccines)
   c. Methyldibromoglutaronitrile (MDGN)/Phenoxyethanol (PE)

F. Occupationally acquired skin disease is caused most commonly by irritant contact dermatitis; the prognosis of the dermatitis is often poor, even if a job change is undertaken. Physicians are often called on to make a determination regarding reasonable probability for worker's compensation settlement.

1. Hairdressers are at high risk for hand dermatitis from exposure to paraphenylenediamine (PPD) used in hair dyes and glycerol monothioglycolate (GMTG) used in perms. Many of these individuals also become sensitized to nickel. Twenty percent of those tested will have an irritant dermatitis with negative patch tests (12).
2. Dentists are at risk for contact dermatitis to natural rubber latex, rubber accelerators, acrylates (dental cement), ester anesthetics, epoxies/epoxy acrylates, and glutaraldehyde (a cold sterilant). Acrylates, epoxies, and glutaraldehyde are able to rapidly pass through natural rubber latex gloves and do not provide protection from exposure, sensitization, and chronic dermatitis.
3. Florists develop reactions to sesquiterpene lactone–containing plants, with the chrysanthemum being the most common flower in the compositae family. Other compositae flowers include marigolds, daisies, and sunflowers as well as many common weeds and wildflowers. Tulips and Peruvian lilies contain tuliposid-A, which can cause a characteristic dermatitis often on the medial thumb and lateral index finger. Irritant dermatitis occurs with exposure to Narcissus, Hyacinth, and Dieffenbachia.
4. Nail technicians and customers who use applied artificial nails can develop allergic reactions. Contact with glues such as epoxy and acrylates as well as tosylamide formaldehyde resin in nail polishes can cause dermatitis, especially of the eyelids.

G. Phototoxic and photoallergic contact dermatitis requires ultraviolet light to induce a reaction. Phototoxic reactions can be caused by psoralens in various plants, perfumes, and in tar-related products. Common plants with the potential to cause phototoxic dermatitis include carrots and celery, parsley, wild parsnip, lemons and limes, and figs. Photoallergic reactions require prior systemic sensitization to an allergen (e.g., PABA in sunscreens). The cutaneous manifestations of phototoxic contact dermatitis are generally erythematous and bullous, sometimes with hyperpigmentation. It will appear in minutes to days. Photoallergic contact dermatitis tends to appear eczematous in nature and will develop usually with 24 to 72 hours of exposure. Patch testing is necessary for the accurate diagnosis of a photoallergic eruption, but not with phototoxic agents.

H. Systemic contact dermatitis may be caused by food or drugs; a high index of suspicion is required to make this difficult diagnosis in a patient with an eczematous skin eruption. The skin lesions are usually symmetrical, often affecting the face and anogenital region. The most common allergens are metal salts such as nickel, drugs, phytoallergens, and Balsam of Peru. A review of edible causes of systemic dermatitis reported myriad potential allergens.

I. Pediatric patients were previously thought to have a low level of contact sensitization. Twenty percent to 37% of patients have been found to have significant contact allergens in individual studies. The actual prevalence is not known. Patch testing can be undertaken in children younger than 2 years of age using the standard adult allergens. Nickel is the most common sensitizer, followed by thimerosal, rubber compounds, fragrance, and preservatives. Facial and hand dermatitis may be a clue to the diagnosis of contact dermatitis in this age-group.

J. Airborne Contact Dermatitis (ABCD) is caused when an allergen that is aerosolized comes into contact with sensitized individuals. Frequently, involvement will be in a characteristic distribution on the face, 'V' of neck, hands and forearms, and hand dermatitis. In the United States, compositae plant pollen is a frequent cause of ABCD. In India, *Parthenium hysterophorus* is the most common cause of ABCD. Skin manifestations of ABCD include pruritic, erythematous, papular, papulovesicular, or confluent lesions on exposed areas of the body. Infrequently, parthenium dermatitis may present as actinic reticuloid or photocontact dermatitis.

II. SUBJECTIVE DATA. Irritants will cause an inelastic and stiff-feeling skin; discomfort related to dryness; pruritus secondary to inflammation; and pain related to fissures, blisters, and ulcers. As with other forms of acute and chronic dermatitis, the primary symptom of ACD is pruritus.

III. OBJECTIVE DATA (SEE COLOR INSERT.)

A. Mild irritants produce erythema, microvesiculation, and oozing that may be indistinguishable from ACD. Chronic exposure to mild irritants or allergens results in dry, thickened, and fissured skin.

B. Strong irritants cause blistering, erosion, and ulcers.

C. ACD, in its mild form, is similar in appearance to the irritant eruption. A more typical allergic contact reaction will consist of grouped or linear tense vesicles and blisters. If involvement is severe, there may be marked edema, particularly on the face and in the periorbital and genital areas. The allergen is frequently transferred from the hands to other areas of the body, where the rash then appears. Palms, soles, and scalp, however, are relatively resistant to contact reactions because of thicker stratum corneum and greater barrier function. The gradual appearance of the allergic contact eruption over a period of several days reflects the amount of antigen deposited on the skin and the reactivity of the individual site. Vesicle fluid, as in poison ivy, is a transudate and will not spread the eruption elsewhere on the body or to other people.

It is not the specific morphology of lesions that clinically distinguishes contact dermatitis from other types of eczema, but their distribution and configuration. The eruption is in exposed or contact areas and typically has a bizarre or artificial pattern, with sharp, straight margins, acute angles, and straight lines. Any eruption with such an unusual appearance should suggest contact dermatitis. Subacute contact dermatitis may evidence only crusting; chronic contact dermatitis resembles a chronic eczematous reaction with lichenification.

IV. ASSESSMENT. Exact diagnosis is very important, because successful therapy depends on avoidance of contact with irritants and elimination of contact with allergens. The patient must be questioned about his or her total environment: home, work, hobbies, medications, clothing, cosmetics, and any other contactants. Inquiry must be detailed, imaginative, and frequently repetitive if the necessary details are to be elicited. Sensitization to components of topical medications is not uncommon and must be considered when an eruption is slow to disappear while being treated with what would seem to be appropriate therapy. Having the patient bring with them EVERY personal care item that touches their skin or the material safety data sheet (MSDS) sheet for potential work-related cases can be helpful.

Patch testing for contact allergens is essential for specific identification of causative agents. This test, in effect, attempts to reproduce the disease in diminutive form. There are no clinically useful methods available to evaluate patients thought to have an irritant dermatitis, although application of a suspected substance to the antecubital fossa twice a day for 10 days is helpful if irritation develops.

V. THERAPY

A. Preventive measures—for primary irritant or hand dermatitis

    1. Decrease exposure to household and work irritants such as frequent water contact, soaps, detergents, solvents, bleaches, ammonia, and moist vegetables such as onions or garlic.

    2. Avoid abrasive soaps. Remove all rings that occlude the underlying skin before doing any work. Waterless hand cleansers will remove stubborn soils and greases without significant damage to the skin. (Use of solvents to cleanse the skin is one of the most frequent predisposing factors.)

    3. Lubricate the skin frequently. An ointment such as Vaseline is preferable, but when this is not practical, a cream/lotion such as Aveeno Daily Moisturizer or Curel Fragrance Free cream should be used. Fragrance-free products are preferable.

    4. If possible, wear heavy-duty vinyl gloves or plastic gloves while working. Allerderm Protective Glove System provides vinyl, cotton, and disposable vinyl gloves that are very helpful for patients with hand dermatitis (www.allerderm.com). Spontex Bluettes cotton knit-lined gloves also contain no rubber and are suitable for "heavy-duty" use. Lined rubber gloves (Playtex) are acceptable, but occasionally patients become allergic to the rubber. Gloves provide excellent protection against mild irritants, but some antigens such as nickel may penetrate rubber-based gloves. High concentrations of irritants such as 10% potassium hydroxide will also penetrate. Gloves should be chosen carefully and changed frequently. Tru-Touch plastic gloves are very helpful, for they permit freer use of the hands while working. Thin white cotton liners should be worn next to the skin to absorb sweat and prevent maceration.

    5. Barrier protective creams designed to be used against aqueous compounds (Kerodex No. 71, SBS-44), solvents (Kerodex No. 51, SBS-46), or dusts, dirt, and grime (West No. 211) will be moderately useful. They should be applied in the morning and then reapplied at lunchtime and at work breaks. Barrier creams are manufactured for industrial use and are available through industrial supply sources. They are not stocked in community pharmacies.

B. Preventive measures—for ACD

    1. Avoidance of the allergen is of paramount importance. Being aware of which products contain the allergen and using appropriate barrier protection can help prevent dermatitis. Gloves do not protect the user from all allergens; barrier creams must be applied frequently. Wash thoroughly as soon as possible after exposure to antigens.

    2. If exposure to poison oak/ivy is possible, prior application of Ivy Block (www.ivyblock.com) has been very successful in preventing allergic dermatitis.

    3. The results of hyposensitization to allergic contact antigens such as poison oak and poison ivy are usually of negligible, if any, benefit. Unpleasant and dangerous adverse effects can occur with currently available preparations.

C. Treatment for active dermatitis

    1. Acute, mild to moderate, exudative, and vesicular

        a. Aluminum acetate (Burow's solution) (diluted 1:20) cold compresses for 20 to 30 minutes four to six times a day.

        b. Soothing shake lotions, e.g. calamine.

        c. After vesiculation subsides, a topical corticosteroid aerosol, cream, or lotion will help.

        d. Antihistamines PO. Avoid topical antihistamines such as Benadryl spray or Zonalon cream.

2. Acute, absolute irritant
   a. Forceful and prolonged irrigation with water.
   b. Then treat as for a burn.
3. Acute, severe, marked edema, and bullae
   a. Topical therapy as in sec. C.1.a.
   b. Tepid tub baths with Aveeno, 1 cup to 1/2 tub, b.i.d.–t.i.d., or cornstarch.
   c. Early and aggressive treatment with systemic corticosteroids. Initial pred-
      nisone dosage should be at least 60 mg everyday; the course should be no
      shorter than 2 to 3 weeks. Alternatives to oral prednisone include 6 mg
      betamethasone sodium phosphate and betamethasone acetate suspension
      (Celestone), 40 to 80 mg methylprednisolone (Depo-Medrol), 40 mg triam-
      cinolone acetonide (Kenalog), or 40 mg triamcinolone diacetate (Aristocort),
      all of which are equally effective. Treatment with inadequate amounts of
      steroid for inadequate periods of time is unfortunately too common. Sys-
      temic corticosteroids should be withdrawn gradually to prevent a flare-up
      or rebound reaction. If the process is suppressed for too short a time, a
      generalized exacerbation of rash and symptoms may result when steroids are
      stopped. Inhibition of the rash and symptoms will be seen within 48 hours of
      therapy is initiated. It is essential that secondary infection such as impetigo,
      cellulitis, or erysipelas be diagnosed and treated before corticosteroid therapy
      being initiated. The clinical picture of erysipelas can at times be quite similar
      to that of an ACD.
4. Chronic contact or hand dermatitis
   a. Soak the hands or other affected areas for 5 to 20 minutes in water and then
      immediately apply a hydrophobic emollient (e.g., petrolatum) and/or topical
      corticosteroid ointment with or without occlusion. Cotton or plastic gloves
      work well for occlusion.
   b. High-potency corticosteroids are needed in the treatment of chronic hand
      dermatitis. In lesions recalcitrant to the usual therapies, intralesional corti-
      costeroid injections may induce limited remissions.
   c. Tar and/or iodochlorhydroxyquin preparations are useful adjuncts in chronic
      cases.
   d. UVB phototherapy or topical photochemotherapy can be extremely useful in
      cases of chronic hand dermatitis.
   e. If available, superficial Grenz ray therapy can be used in cases of recalcitrant,
      chronic dermatitis that does not respond to other therapy.
5. Bacterial superinfection is not uncommon and should be treated with topical
   and systemic antibiotics.

HAND DERMATITIS

I. DEFINITION AND PATHOPHYSIOLOGY. Hand dermatitis is a common, chronic
pruritic disorder that is perplexing and frustrating to patients and physicians alike.
The clinical changes are not specific and may be a manifestation of one or several
precipitating or predisposing factors. It is most commonly a reaction to repeated events.
The eruption itself is common in those exposed to wet work, especially new mothers,
food handlers, bartenders, nurses, dentists, and surgeons. Those with an atopic history
are especially prone to hand dermatitis when exposed to frequent wetting and drying of
the hands. It is the most frequent dermatitis seen in industry. Hairdressers are especially
prone to hand dermatitis, often requiring a job change.

   Chronic hand dermatitis is often a remnant or part of atopic or nummular
dermatitis. Hand dermatitis is four to ten times more common in patients with a history
of AD, especially childhood eczema, than among controls with no personal or family
history of atopy.

   ACD will tend to involve the sides of the fingers and the dorsa of the hands more
than the palms and show a more bizarre configuration.

1. In individuals with chronic refractory hand eczema, patch testing should be routine. Many of these patients will have a positive reaction to nickel. Allergy to the accelerator chemicals used in the manufacture of natural rubber latex is another common reactant owing to the sensitization from the regular use of rubber gloves to protect the hands.
2. Patients with refractory foot eczema should be tested for shoe allergies through patch testing. The most common allergens are rubber, chromate, butyl phenol formaldehyde resins, and colophony.

   Primary fungal infection or dermatophytid (id) reactions to tinea pedis must always be considered in the differential diagnosis and fungal scrapings and cultures obtained. The "two-foot one-hand syndrome" consists of bilateral tinea pedis with dermatitis of only one hand. The etiology is unknown and not related to hand dominance. The eruption on the hand clears with treatment of the tinea pedis.

   Dyshidrotic eczema preferentially involves the sides of the fingers and palms and may affect the soles of the feet as well. Hyperhidrosis, when present, is only coincidental but is an aggravating factor. Fifty percent of patients may have an atopic history; 20% may have a positive patch test to nickel.

   Pustular psoriasis and hand involvement with other cutaneous eruptions, such as drug reactions, may also appear as hand dermatitis. The appearance of palmoplantar pustulosis is that of sterile pustules admixed with yellow to brown macules.

   It is often impossible to find a specific etiology for chronic hand dermatitis.
II. **SUBJECTIVE DATA.** Pruritus is the primary symptom, but dryness, fissuring, inelasticity, and superinfection often lead to inability to use the hands at all. Hand dermatitis is a predictor of a poor skin-related quality of life and is the cause of much social, personal, and financial grief.
III. **OBJECTIVE DATA**
   A. Erythema, dryness, and chapping are the mildest changes.
   B. The most characteristic lesions are myriads of small "bubbles"—intraepidermal spongiotic vesicles—scattered on the sides of the fingers and, less often, throughout the palms.
   C. More severe changes include bulla formation and extreme hardening and inelasticity of the skin, with deep fissures.
   D. Hyperhidrosis and secondary bacterial infections are common.
IV. **ASSESSMENT.** A detailed history and physical examination must include inquiry about a personal or family history of atopy or psoriasis or other cutaneous diseases, factors that precipitate and alleviate the dermatitis, and occupational, household, and hobby contactants. Patch testing, using a screening tray as well as properly diluted occupational or other agents that the patient has supplied, may identify a causative agent.
V. **THERAPY.** See Contact Dermatitis
   A. Nickel-sensitive patients with vesicular hand eczema may benefit from a nickel-elimination diet (13).
   B. Topical psoralen photochemotherapy (PUVA) and superficial radiotherapy (Grenz rays) are beneficial in chronic unresponsive hand eczema.

 NUMMULAR DERMATITIS

I. **DEFINITION AND PATHOPHYSIOLOGY.** Nummular dermatitis, characterized by coin-shaped eczematous plaques, is a chronic, often very pruritic, but nonspecific reaction pattern found most commonly in older patients. It may also be a manifestation of AD in children, a reaction to topical irritants, or a manifestation of xerosis, particularly in wintertime. IgE levels are usually not elevated. Emotional stress has been emphasized as a contributing factor. The course tends to be chronic, with remission occurring frequently during the summer.
II. **SUBJECTIVE DATA.** Pruritus is the primary symptom, although patients may complain of a burning sensation.

III. OBJECTIVE DATA. Dry to inflammatory papular, vesicular, exudative, and/or crusted, round plaques 1 to 5 cm in diameter are located most commonly on the dorsa of the hands and forearms, lower legs, and buttocks. Over time, the plaques may demonstrate central clearing.

IV. ASSESSMENT. Questioning should be directed toward eliciting a history of predisposing environmental factors (i.e., dryness), occupational or household work habits, other cutaneous diseases, and any recent or chronic emotionally stressful situation.

V. THERAPY

A. Decrease exposure to irritants. If dryness is a factor, see the items outlined under Dry Skin in Chap. 11. Decrease the amount of bathing, and add bath oils and emollients.

B. For acute dermatitis, use Burow's solution compresses for 20 minutes t.i.d.

C. Use topical corticosteroids one to three times a day. Ointments are often preferable. Overnight application under occlusion, coupled with the use of emollients during the day, is often effective.

D. Intralesional corticosteroid injection will rapidly eliminate lesions.

E. Tar compounds (10% liquor carbonis detergens in hydrophilic ointment, tar ointments) and iodochlorhydroxyquin are occasionally useful. Daily application of topical corticosteroids and nightly use of the tar compounds and/or iodochlorhydroxyquin may work when either medication used alone is not wholly effective.

F. Phototherapy may be effective in nummular dermatitis, as it is in other chronic inflammatory dermatoses.

G. Antihistamines, particularly hydroxyzine (Atarax, Vistaril), will diminish itch and anxiety. Topical antihistamines (doxepin; Zonalon) can also be useful.

References

1. Dahl RE, Bernhisel-Broadbent J, Scanlon-Holdford S, et al. Sleep disturbances in children with atopic dermatitis. *Arch Pediatr Adolesc Med* 1995;149:856–860.
2. Kemmett D, Tidman MJ. The influence of the menstrual cycle and pregnancy on atopic dermatitis. *Br J Dermatol* 1991;125:59–61.
3. Mevorah B, Frenk E, Wietlisbach V, et al. Minor clinical features of atopic dermatitis. Evaluation of their diagnostic significance. *Dermatologica* 1988;177:360–364.
4. Ballin A, Kenet G, Senetzky J, et al. Cervical lymphadenopathy as a sign of atopy in children. *J Allergy Clin Immunol* 1996;96:264–265.
5. Patel L, Clayton PE, Jenney ME, et al. Adult height in patients with childhood onset atopic dermatitis. *Arch Dis Child* 1997;76:505–508.
6. Jekler J, Larko O. Combined UVA-UVB versus UVB phototherapy for atopic dermatis: a paired-comparison study. *J Am Acad Dermatol* 1990;22:49–53.
7. Stevens SR, Hanifin JM, Hamilton T, et al. Long-term effectiveness and safety of recombinant human interferon gamma therapy for atopic dermatitis despite unchanged serum IgE levels. *Arch Dermatol* 1998;134:799–804.
8. Stiller MG, Shupack JL, Kenny C, et al. A double-blind, placebo-controlled clinical trial to evaluate the safety and efficacy of thymopentin as an adjunctive treatment in atopic dermatitis. *J Am Acad Dermatol* 1994;30:597–602.
9. Moore C, Ehlayel MS, Junprasert J, et al. Topical sodium cromoglycate in the treatment of moderate to severe atopic dermatitis. *Ann Allergy Asthma Immunol* 1999;81:452–458.
10. Kragballe K, Larsen FG. A hydrocolloid occlusive dressing plus triamcinolone acetonide is superior to clobetasol cream in palmo-plantar pustulosis. *Acta Derm Venerol (Stockh)* 1991;71:40–42.
11. Dooms-Goossens A, Andersen KE, Brandao FM, et al. Corticosteroid contact allergy: an EECDRG multicentre study. *Contact Dermatitis* 1996;35:40–44.
12. Conde-Salazar L, et al. Contact dermatitis in hairdressers: patch test results in 379 hairdressers (1980–1993). *Contact Dermatitis* 1995;33:226–230.
13. Nielsen GD, Jepsen LV, Jorgensen PJ, et al. Nickel-sensitive patients with vesicular hand eczema: oral challenge with a diet naturally high in nickel. *Br J Dermatol* 1990;122:299–308.

Suggested Readings

Ashcroft DM, Dimmock P, Garside R, et al. Efficacy and tolerability of topical pimecrolimus and tacrolimus in the treatment of atopic dermatitis: meta-analysis of randomised controlled trials. *BMJ* 2005;330:516.

Brancaccio RR, Alvarez MS. Contact allergy to food. *Dermatol Ther* 2004;17(4):302–313.

FDA Alert for Healthcare Providers. http://www.fda.gov/cder/drug/InfoSheets/HCP/ProtopicHCP.htm. Accessed on May 9, 2005.

Garg A, Chren MM, Sands LP, et al. Psychological stress perturbs epidermal permeability barrier homeostasis: implications for the pathogenesis of stress-associated skin disorders. *Arch Dermatol* 2001;137:53–59.

Gruber C, Illi S, Lau S, et al. MAS-90 Study Group. Transient suppression of atopy in early childhood is associated with high vaccination coverage. *Pediatrics* 2003;111(3): e282–288.

Hanifin JM. Defining AD and assessing its impact: seeking simplified, inclusive and internationally applicable criteria. *Paper presented at the International symposium on Atopic Dermatitis*. Portland, OR: National Eczema Association for Science and Education, September 6–9, 2001.

Orton DI, Wilkinson JD. Cosmetic allergy: incidence, diagnosis, and management. *Am J Clin Dermatol* 2004;5(5):327–337.

Purvis DJ, Thompson JM, Clark PM, et al. Risk factors for atopic dermatitis in New Zealand children at 3.5 years of age. *Br J Dermatol* 2005;152(4):742–749.

Roos TC, Geuer S, Roos S, et al. Recent advances in treatment strategies for atopic dermatitis. *Drugs* 2004;64(23):2639–2666.

Schmid-Grendelmeier P, Fluckiger S, Disch R, et al. IgE-mediated and T cell-mediated autoimmunity against manganese superoxide dismutase in atopic dermatitis. *J Allergy Clin Immunol* 2005;115(5):1068–1075.

Simpson D, Noble S. Tacrolimus ointment: a review of its use in atopic dermatitis and its clinical potential in other inflammatory skin conditions. *Drugs* 2005;65(6):827–858.

Williams HC. Evening primrose oil for atopic dermatitis. *BMJ* 2003;327(7428):1358–1359.

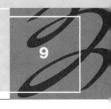

DIAPER DERMATITIS
Ethel Ying
9

I. DEFINITION AND PATHOPHYSIOLOGY. Diaper dermatitis refers to any eruption that occurs in areas covered by diapers caused by either direct effect of wearing diapers or indirectly as an exacerbation of a rare underlying condition. Irritant diaper dermatitis is the end result of constant exposure to an adverse local environment, particularly an exposure to moisture. Other irritants include feces and fecal enzymes. Elevated pH may also cause damage to the epidermis, further subjecting it to irritation with the loss of its barrier function. Risk factors for diaper dermatitis include diarrhea as well as the use of antibiotics. Once established, diaper dermatitis may be colonized by organisms (*Staphylococcus aureus, Candida albicans*) that may induce secondary changes and potentially result in superinfections.

Diaper dermatitis is unusual during the first month of life as fecal enzymes are present in low levels during this period. It peaks between 6 and 12 months of age, but may continue until diapers are no longer needed. Underlying atopic, seborrheic, or psoriatic diatheses may predispose the infant to this eruption.

II. SUBJECTIVE DATA. The baby is uncomfortable and irritable.

III. OBJECTIVE DATA

    A. Irritant diaper dermatitis. Mild cases present with erythema over convex surfaces in contact with the diaper including the buttocks, genitalia, lower abdomen, and upper thighs. Creases are generally spared. With prolonged irritation, it can progress to a shiny deep erythema followed by the development of erythematous papules, erosions, and ulcers. Jacquet's erosive diaper dermatitis is a specific eruption that consists of punched-out ulcers and erosions primarily involving the labia.

    B. Candida diaper dermatitis. The classical presentation of this eruption is a "beefy-red" rash with satellite pustules. However, a more common presentation is a diffuse erythematous patch with peripheral scale and satellite lesions, which consist of small erythematous papules. Creases are also involved. Oral thrush may also be present. There may be a history of recent antibiotic use.

    C. Seborrheic dermatitis. This appears as well-circumscribed erythematous plaques with varying degrees of scale. Greasy yellow scale is more commonly seen with involvement of scalp and face. It can be difficult to distinguish from the infantile presentation of psoriasis.

    D. Staphylococcal pustulosis. This presents within the first few weeks of life, earlier than other common causes of diaper rash. Multiple thin-walled pustules are present primarily over the lower abdomen and diaper region. They are easily ruptured, leaving a collarette of scale with a shallow erythematous base.

IV. ASSESSMENT

    A. A detailed history concerning skin and diaper care is necessary to discover any immediate predisposing factors.

    B. A complete skin examination should be performed to evaluate for any underlying conditions (e.g., atopic dermatitis, zinc deficiency).

    C. Further consideration must be given to intractable cases of diaper dermatitis including various infectious (scabies, congenital syphilis, human immunodeficiency virus), metabolic, or nutritional deficiencies as well as immunologic etiologies.

    D. The diagnosis is made primarily by clinical findings. Swabs of pustule contents can be examined by Gram's stain/KOH prep and cultured for confirmation of infection and for assistance in selecting therapeutic agents, particularly in resistant cases.

V. THERAPY

A. **Preventive.** Skin in the diaper area should be kept as dry and as free from irritants as possible. Frequent diaper changes and the use of diapers with absorbent gel material are useful means to prevent diaper dermatitis. An emollient or paste (e.g., petrolatum, zinc oxide) may be applied as a barrier from irritants with diaper changes.

B. **Treatment**

1. **Irritant diaper dermatitis.** An emollient or paste with every diaper change may be sufficient in the treatment of mild cases of diaper dermatitis. It protects the skin from direct contact with irritants. In moderate to severe cases, a mild, non-fluorinated corticosteroid (1% hydrocortisone) can be applied three times a day, followed by an emollient. An emollient should also be used with the rest of the diaper changes throughout the day. The corticosteroid should be discontinued once the inflammation has resolved. Moderate-strong potency corticosteroids should not be used in this region.

2. **Candida diaper dermatitis.** Candida infections are treated with topical anti-fungals such as nystatin, clotrimazole, and ketoconazole three times a day. This can be used in conjunction with a mild corticosteroid (1% hydrocortisone) as an antiinflammatory to decrease symptoms and to promote healing. An emollient should be used following the application and with all other diaper changes as a barrier to further irritation.

3. **Seborrheic dermatitis.** In this region, seborrheic dermatitis can be treated with a mild corticosteroid such as 1% hydrocortisone three times a day along with preventative skin care measures.

4. **Staphylococcal pustulosis.** In an otherwise well neonate (afebrile, no evidence of cellulitis), an oral β-lactamase–resistant antibiotic such as cephalexin, cloxacillin, or dicloxacillin can be administered for 10 days. In more complicated staphylococcal infections, the patient requires admission to hospital for a complete sepsis work-up and intravenous antibiotics. Cultures should be used to select therapeutic agents particularly in suspected cases of methicillin-resistant *S. aureus*.

Suggested Readings

Atherton DJ. The aetiology and management of irritant diaper dermatitis. *J Eur Acad Dermatol Venereol* 2001;15(Suppl 1):1–4.

Atherton DJ. A review of the pathophysiology, prevention and treatment of irritant diaper dermatitis. *Curr Med Res Opin* 2004;20(5):645–649.

Baldwin S, Odio MR, Hains SL, et al. Skin benefits from continuous typical administration of a zinc oxide/petrolatum formulation by a novel disposable diaper. *J Eur Acad Dermatol Venereol* 2001;15(Suppl 1):5–11.

Boiko S. Treatment of diaper dermatitis. *Dermatol Clin* 1999;17:235–240.

Eichenfield L, Frieden U, Esterly NB, eds. *Textbook of neonatal dermatology*, 1st ed. Philadelphia, PA: WB Saunders, 2001.

Gupta A, Skinner AR. Management of diaper dermatitis. *Int J Dermatol* 2004;43(11): 830–835.

Hoppe JE. Treatment of oropharyngeal candidiasis and candidal diaper dermatitis in neonates and infants: review and reappraisal. *Pediatr Infect Dis J* 1997;16:885–894.

Odio MR, O'Connor RJ, Sarbough F, et al. Continuous topical administration of a petro-latum formulation by a novel disposable diaper? Effect on skin condition. *Dermatology* 2000;200:238–243.

Rodriguez-Poblador J, Gonzalez-Castro U, Herranz-Martinez S, et al. Jacquet erosive diaper dermatitis after surgery for Hirschsprung disease. *Pediatr Dermatol* 1998;15:46–47.

Singalavanija S, Frieden I. Diaper dermatitis. *J Pediatr Rev* 1995;16:142–147.

Sires UI, Mallory SB. Diaper dermatitis. How to treat and prevent. *Postgrad Med* 1995;98:79–86.

Zimmerer RE, Lawson KD, Calvert CJ, et al. The effect of wearing diapers on skin. *Pediatr Dermatol* 1986;3:95–101.

DRUG ERUPTIONS, ALLERGIC
Karen Chen

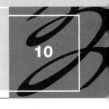

10

I. **DEFINITION AND PATHOPHYSIOLOGY.** Cutaneous drug reactions may occur on an immunologic or a nonimmunologic basis. It is usually the former when one is confronted by a "drug rash," though nonimmunologic drug reactions are, in fact, more common. Pseudoallergic reactions occur by causing direct mast cell release, complement activation, or alteration of arachidonic acid metabolism, inducing a reaction that clinically mimics a true allergy. Examples of drugs and agents that may cause pseudoallergic reactions include opiates, aspirin, vancomycin, and radiocontrast media.

The most common cutaneous drug eruptions are hypersensitivity reactions with an underlying immunologic basis. Hypersensitivity drug reactions may be grouped according to the Gell-Coombs classification:

A. Type I, immunoglobulin E (IgE)-dependent reactions (urticaria, angioedema, anaphylaxis). Type I reactions may be immediate or may take >72 hours to occur.

B. Type II, cytotoxic reactions (drug-induced pemphigus, petechiae secondary to drug-induced thrombocytopenia).

C. Type III, immune-complex formation (vasculitis, serum sickness-like reaction).

D. Type IV, delayed type hypersensitivity, cell-mediated mechanism (exanthems, fixed drug eruption, lichenoid eruption, acute generalized exanthematous pustulosis (AGEP), erythema multiforme, Stevens-Johnson syndrome (SJS), toxic epidermal necrolysis (TEN), drug-induced hypersensitivity syndrome (DHS), and pseudolymphoma).

Adverse drug reactions occur in 6.7% of all hospitalized patients, with cutaneous drug reactions occurring in >2% of hospitalized patients (1). The incidence of skin reactions to antibiotics in outpatients is approximately 1%, with trimethoprim-sulfamethoxazole (Bactrim) being the highest, followed by the penicillins, and then the fluoroquinolones. Penicillins cause most drug reactions among hospitalized patients. Drug reactions can occur in complex medical situations where multiple drugs are involved and a detailed review of all medications must be undertaken with the most likely culprits being discontinued.

II. **CLINICAL PRESENTATION.** In addition to skin findings, drug reactions may be manifested as fever or as abnormal reactions of one or many organ systems (e.g., hemolysis, thrombocytopenia, and renal damage).

A. **Urticaria** is the second most common type of cutaneous drug eruption. A few to multiple pruritic wheals are widely scattered on the body. Individual lesions last <24 hours. Angioedema may result in eyelid, lip, and mucous membrane swelling. Urticarial eruptions may be due to pseudoallergic, type I-, or type III-mediated reactions. Angiotensin-converting enzyme (ACE) inhibitors are frequent causes of angioedema, often without urticaria, with the reaction occurring with an hour or within several months of its administration.

B. Serum sickness-like reaction (SSLR). Serum sickness-like eruptions consist of fever, a rash with usually urticarial features, and arthralgias occurring within 1 to 3 weeks of initiation of the drug. Lymphadenopathy and eosinophilia may also be found. Two of the most common drugs to induce this reaction are cefaclor and minocycline. A short course of oral corticosteroids may be necessary if symptoms are severe.

C. Exanthematous eruptions, the most common type of reaction, usually appear within 1 week of the causative drug being started; sensitization may occur after the first exposure or may develop to an antigen that the patient has been intermittently exposed to for years. Other adjectives used to describe this eruption include morbilliform and maculopapular. A rash may also start within 4 to 7 days of the offending drug being stopped (some antibiotics, particularly semisynthetic penicillins and allopurinol, may produce a rash 2 or more weeks after initiation). Lesions most often start first and clear first from the head and upper extremities. Lesions of the trunk and lower legs often follow in succession. Whenever the eruption starts, whether it is while the patient is taking the drug or after its discontinuation, the cutaneous lesions will become more severe and widespread over the following several days to a week and will then clear over the next 7 to 14 days. This slow and constant evolution of the eruption makes it difficult to single out the offending agent from among numerous drugs, and to judge whether the correct one has been stopped; the rash will go through its 2- to 3-week course.

Multiple drugs are associated with an exanthematous eruption including the penicillins, sulfonamides, barbiturates, and seizure medications. Amoxicillin-induced morbilliform eruptions are mediated by a T-cell–immune reaction, which may explain the increased incidence of this eruption when a patient is infected with the Epstein-Barr virus (acute mononucleosis) (2).

D. DHS consists of an exanthem, hepatitis, and fever. Eighty percent of patients have an exanthem-type eruption, where others will develop a more serious SJS. DHS may be life threatening and requires prompt discontinuation of the drug and systemic corticosteroids. DHS usually occurs within the first 1 to 6 weeks of the initial exposure to the drug, with a reaction rate of 1:3,000. A metabolite that is unable to be detoxified by the epoxide hydroxylases is thought to be the offending agent. A familial occurrence of this reaction has been reported. Cross-reaction occurs between the three aromatic anticonvulsants (phenytoin, carbamazepine, and phenobarbital) in 75% of patients. Lamotrigine (Lamictal) does not cross-react with this group of drugs, but is also associated with cases of DHS. Minocycline, allopurinol, sulfonamides, and dapsone have been associated with a similar syndrome. Erythromycin can cause elevated liver function tests, eosinophilia, and fever.

If a DHS is suspected, the clinician should obtain liver function tests, urinalysis, serum creatinine, and complete blood count (CBC). Hypothyroidism may develop in a subset of these patients, usually within 2 months of the incident. A baseline thyroid-stimulating hormone (TSH) should be measured at the time of diagnosis and rechecked in 2 to 3 months.

E. AGEP is characterized by the sudden onset of fever, leukocytosis, and a generalized eruption of monomorphous sterile pustules on a background of edema and erythema. The most common offending drugs are the β-lactam and macrolide antibiotics. Discontinuation of the drug is usually all that is necessary, and 2 weeks later, a generalized desquamation occurs.

F. Drug-induced lupus is associated with arthralgias, arthritis, fever, weight loss, pleuritis, and pericarditis. Skin findings are rare. A positive antinuclear antibody (ANA) is usually found in a subset of patients having antihistone antibodies but not anti-deoxyribonucleic acid (DNA) antibodies. The drugs involved in this reaction include procainamide, hydralazine, isoniazid, penicillamine, methyldopa, and minocycline.

Drug-induced cutaneous lupus is distinct and presents with photodistributed diffuse erythema, subacute cutaneous lupus erythematosus–type lesions without systemic complaints. ANA, anti-Ro/SSA, and anti-La/SSB antibodies may be present. Hydrochlorothiazide, calcium channel blockers, ACE inhibitors, statins and terbinafine have been associated with drug-induced cutaneous lupus.

G. Erythema multiforme, SJS/TEN. Erythema multiforme major and SJS/TEN are most frequently caused by drugs and are discussed in Chap. 12. Less common forms of drug reactions, which will not be discussed in detail, include fixed drug eruptions, erythema nodosum (see Chap. 13), leukocytoclastic vasculitis, bullous and pustular drug eruptions, lichen planus–like eruptions, abnormal pigmentary reactions, neutrophilic eccrine hidradenitis secondary to chemotherapeutic agents, pseudolymphoma, and exfoliative dermatitis. Drugs may exacerbate underlying dermatoses (e.g., β-blockers can worsen psoriasis and lithium can exacerbate acne).

TEN, with extensive sheet-like shearing of epidermis, may be life threatening, as may drug-induced vasculitis.

III. EVALUATION

A. Clinical presentation. Mild to severe pruritus is the predominant symptom of urticarial and exanthematous drug eruptions. Enquire about symptoms of fevers, chills, malaise, arthralgias, myalgias, and dyspnea. Evaluate for extracutaneous signs such as fever, tachycardia, hypotension, lymphadenopathy, synovitis, and tachypnea. A complete skin examination should be performed. Is the primary lesion exanthematous, urticarial, blistering, or pustular? Are palms, soles, and mucous membranes involved? Mild petechiae or frank nonpalpable purpura on the lower extremities is commonly associated with a vigorous eruption, but this does not imply that vasculitis or thrombocytopenia is present. More serious and violent reactions may include bullae, erosions, extensive purpura, or exfoliation. Palpable purpuric lesions that do not blanch on pressure (diascopy) suggest vasculitis. Many types of drugs can produce identical eruptions; the morphology of the rash usually gives little clue as to the causative agent

B. Other differential diagnoses. Consider differential diagnoses such as infections, collagen-vascular disease, primary skin conditions and neoplasia.

C. Detailed drug history. Questions about offending drugs must be detailed and direct. In general, any new drug started within the past 8 weeks should be considered. Drug-induced lupus (e.g., minocycline) may not manifest until after a year of therapy. Any substance that enters any body orifice, with the exception of most foods and water, is suspect. Specific questioning concerning eye or ear drops, nasal sprays, suppositories, injections, immunizations, nerve pills, vitamins, laxatives, sedatives, and analgesics, including even aspirin, must be pursued. Nonmedical items such as preservatives, tonics, toothpaste, and topical lotions must also be considered. Penicillin is present in small amounts in some biologic products (such as poliomyelitis vaccine) and in dairy products from cows treated for mastitis. The possibility of illicit drugs must be considered. A review of medical literature may provide information about the frequency of specific types of drug eruptions associated with a given drug. However, all drugs need to be considered a possible cause of any reaction. Patients given ampicillin during the course of infectious mononucleosis will quite frequently experience an exanthematous type of reaction, although they might be given ampicillin again without ill effects once the viral illness has resolved. In a similar vein, sulfamethoxazole-trimethoprim reactions are exceptionally common in patients with acquired immunodeficiency syndrome (AIDS).

Penicillin drugs, sulfonamides, and blood products are the most common causes of cutaneous reactions to drugs (Table 10-1). Amoxicillin, for instance, can be expected to incite an eruption in approximately 5% of courses of drug therapy. Drug-specific quantitative data are available to help evaluate which agents are most likely causes of drug-induced rash, itching, or hives. This information gives reaction rates for all commonly used drugs and allows one to calculate which drug might have caused an adverse reaction (3).

D. Diagnostic Workup. Skin biopsies may help distinguish between a drug-induced condition and another skin disease, e.g. differentiating between TEN and staphylococcal scalded skin syndrome. Blood workup may also aid in the clinical diagnosis. In a patient with systemic symptoms or signs, blood workup may be needed to determine extent of internal organ involvement. A CBC with differential may show atypical lymphocytosis, leukopenia, leukocytosis, eosinophilia, and so on. Liver function tests, serum creatinine, urinalysis, and TSH may be indicated in patients with suspected drug-induced hypersensitivity syndrome. Abnormal blood tests should be repeated during the convalescent period and TSH rechecked in 3 months. Cultures of skin/blood/tissue, erythrocyte sedimentation rate (ESR), ANA, and other tests may be ordered to help confirm or rule out other conditions. If palpable purpuric lesions are present, a complete physical and laboratory examination is required with an eye toward ruling out vasculitic involvement of other organ systems and other causes of vasculitis such as infection or collagen-vascular disease. A skin biopsy should be considered to confirm the diagnosis.

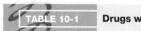

Drug	Reaction rate (reactions/ 1,000 recipients)
Amoxicillin	51
Trimethoprim-sulfamethoxazole	34
Ampicillin	33
Blood	22
Cephalosporins	21
Semisynthetic penicillin	21
Erythromycin	20
Penicillin G	19
Cyanocobalamin	18
Quinidine	13
Cimetidine	13
Phenylbutazone	12

TABLE 10-1   Drugs with Reaction Rates <1%

Source: Bigby M, Jick S, Jick H, et al. Drug-induced cutaneous reactions: a report from the Boston Collaborative Surveillance Program on 15,438 consecutive inpatients, 1975 to 1982. *JAMA* 1986;256:3358–3363. Copyright 1986, American Medical Association. Reproduced with permission.

E. Apart from clinical challenge, there is no consistently reliable test to confirm that a drug is the cause of an adverse reaction. Oral provocation tests under closely monitored conditions can be undertaken if the prior reaction consisted of urticaria or an exanthematous eruption (4), but are not recommended for patients who have had severe reactions. Given the laboriousness and the medical (and legal) risks, oral provocation tests are rarely performed. A topical rechallenge with the suspected drug may be helpful in patients with fixed drug eruptions. Skin testing with penicilloyl-polylysine (PPL, Pre-Pen) and a "minor determinant mixture" (usually diluted aqueous penicillin G) can accurately predict reactions to all penicillins. Skin prick testing with major and minor determinants is useful for confirmation of an IgE-mediated allergic reaction to penicillin (5). Of note, only one third of patients who report a penicillin allergy will have a positive intradermal or patch test reaction (6). Radioallergosorbent test (RAST) tests on serum for penicillin allergy will give similar data without the danger of injecting an allergenic drug.

The use of patch testing for cutaneous drug eruptions is not standardized, and its diagnostic value in this situation is unproven. Patch testing may be particularly helpful in patients with a systemic contact-type drug eruption, originally sensitized by topical application, and in AGEP, where the offending agent may illicit an isomorphic pustular reaction. Patch testing may occasionally be helpful in fixed drug eruptions. The frequency of positive patch test reactions in patients with a history of a drug exanthema to any medication is approximately 10% to 11%. In patients with a history of an exanthematous drug eruption to antibiotics, 31% to 83% may have positive patch test reactions (7).

IV. THERAPY

A. Discontinue the offending drug.

B. Use antihistamines PO.

C. Soothing tepid water baths with Aveeno or cornstarch and/or cool compresses may be useful.

D. A drying antipruritic lotion (calamine with or without 0.25% menthol and/or 1% phenol) or lubricating antipruritic emollients (Eucerin, Keri Lotion with 0.25%

menthol and 1% phenol, Sarna Lotion, Prax Lotion, Neutrogena Soothing Relief Moisturizer) applied p.r.n. will help relieve the pruritus. Lotions with phenol should not be given to pregnant women.

E. Topical steroids may provide some relief.

F. If signs and symptoms are severe, a 2-week course of systemic corticosteroids (prednisone, starting at 60 mg) or injection of a repository corticosteroid preparation (see Chap. 8, Contact Dermatitis) will usually stop the symptoms and prevent further progression of the eruption within 48 hours of the onset of therapy.

G. Sulfamethoxazole-trimethoprim desensitization with a strict protocol and close observation can be undertaken in patients with human immunodeficiency virus (HIV) who have a high cutaneous reaction rate to this drug.

H. Cephalosporins rarely cross-react in a penicillin-allergic patient. The overall incidence of allergic reactions to cephalosporins is low and usually mild (rash, urticaria). The incidence of drug reactions in penicillin-allergic patients was 0.04% (8).

I. Review warnings about cross-reacting drugs and risk of family members for patients who have had severe reactions such as DHS and SJS/TEN.

References

1. Lazarou J, Pomeranz BH, Carey PN. Incidence of adverse drug reactions in hospitalized patients. A Meta-analysis of prospective studies. *JAMA* 1998;279:1200–1205.
2. Barboud AM, Bene MC, Schmutz JL, et al. Role of delayed cellular hypersensitivity and adhesion molecules in amoxicillin-induced morbilliform rashes. *Arch Dermatol* 1997;133:481–486.
3. Bigby M, Jick S, Jick H, et al. Drug-induced cutaneous reactions: a report from the Boston Collaborative Surveillance Program on 15,438 consecutive inpatients, 1975 to 1982. *JAMA* 1986;256:3358–3363.
4. Stubbs S, Heikkila H, Kauppinen K. Cutaneous reactions to drugs: a series of in-patients during a five-year period. *Acta Derm Venereol (Stockh)* 1994;74:289–291.
5. Sogn D, Evans R III, Shephard GM, et al. Results of the National Institute of Allergy and Infectious Diseases Collaborative Clinical Trial to test the predictive value of skin testing with major and minor penicillin derivatives in hospitalized adults. *Arch Intern Med* 1992;152:1025.
6. Romano A, Difonso M, Papa G, et al. Evaluation of adverse cutaneous reactions to aminopenicillins with emphasis on those manifested by maculopapular rashes. *Allergy* 1995;50:113–118.
7. Cham P, Warshaw EM. A review of patch testing for the evaluation of drug exanthems due to systemic antibiotics. *Dermatitis* Accepted for publication.
8. Ann S, Reisman RE. Risk of administering cephalosporin antibiotics to patients with histories of penicillin allergy. *Ann Allergy Asthma Immunol* 1995;74:167–170.

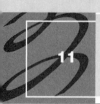

DRY SKIN (CHAPPING, XEROSIS) AND ICHTHYOSIS VULGARIS

11

Jennifer Hunter-Yates

I. **DEFINITION AND PATHOPHYSIOLOGY.** Dry skin and ichthyosis vulgaris are often indistinguishable, and because the clinical findings blend together, it is useful to discuss the two entities together. Dry skin, a dehydration of the stratum corneum, is a very common condition and is especially prevalent among the elderly and in arid climates. Xerosis is more commonly found on the lower legs but may affect any area of skin. When xerosis is severe enough to be associated with inflammation and pruritus, it has been termed *asteatotic eczema* or *winter itch*. The sequence leading to dry skin varies considerably from person to person, and in many cases, remains obscure. Some individuals will note a familial tendency to excessive dryness and chapping. Others will state that xerosis appeared only with increasing age or illness. Environmental factors are extremely important. Repeated exposure to solvents, soaps, and disinfectants will remove lipids from the skin and decrease the natural moisturizing factor (NMF), thereby damaging the cutaneous barrier and increasing the water loss up to 75 times normal. Decreasing relative humidity and exposure to dry air or seasonal cold can lead to water loss from the stratum corneum and will literally "pull" water from the skin. Factors that act to decrease relative humidity include increasing room heat and ventilating with cold, dry, winter air, which holds little moisture when cool and becomes drier when warmed and expanded inside the house.

The typical patient with xerosis is an elderly person who comes in with localized or generalized pruritus. Dryness and itching of the lower extremities may be particularly notable. Symptoms frequently start in early winter soon after the heat goes on, the relative humidity indoors decreases, and exposure to cold, dry wind increases. Rubbing and scratching cause increased irritation, thereby leading to more pruritus and inflammation. If untreated, the symptoms often subside spontaneously the following spring.

Ichthyosis vulgaris is a dominantly inherited disorder of keratinization that is estimated to occur in 1 in 300 individuals. Skin changes are usually not present at birth, are typically noted by 5 years of age, and often improve during adulthood. Clinical findings include dry skin with small white to brown scales, hyperlinear palms, and prominent keratotic follicles. Those with ichthyosis vulgaris also have a high incidence of atopic diseases (atopic dermatitis, rhinitis, asthma) and keratosis pilaris. The primary abnormality in dry skin and in ichthyosis vulgaris is greater-than-normal corneocyte cohesion resulting in a thicker stratum corneum and a decrease in the normal rate of desquamation. In ichthyosis vulgaris, decreased or absent expression of profilaggrin with a resultant reduction in keratohyaline granules has been found.

II. **SUBJECTIVE DATA.** Lesions are usually asymptomatic. If symptoms are present, the chief complaint is most often pruritus, at times severe.

III. **OBJECTIVE DATA**

A. In xerosis, dry skin covered with a fine scale is seen most often on the anterior tibial areas, the dorsal hands, and the forearms. The distribution may be generalized or in round patches. With more severe involvement, the skin loses its suppleness, cracks, and becomes fissured. The superficial reticulated cracking takes on an uneven diamond pattern similar to that of cracked porcelain, and erythema appears in and around the involved areas (eczema or erythema craquele). Nummular plaques of eczema may also be present.

B. In ichthyosis vulgaris, scaling is most prominent over the extensor aspects of the extremities. Flexural areas are typically spared. Milder forms appear as dryness present only during the winter months or in dry climates. Follicular accentuation and keratinization (keratosis pilaris) may be prominent over arms, thighs, and buttocks. The palms and soles may have accentuation of the dermatoglyphic lines and a wrinkled appearance.

IV. ASSESSMENT. A detailed family history and history of the home and work environment are needed both to help make an educated etiologic diagnosis and to outline a therapeutic program that will eliminate or counteract any causative factors. Many diseases have been associated with xerosis, including hypothyroidism, human immunodeficiency virus (HIV) infection, Sjögren syndrome, and various eating disorders, and the possibility of an associated disorder may need to be investigated. Acquired ichthyosis can be secondary to drugs (cholesterol-lowering agents, cimetidine, hydrochlorothiazide, etc.), malignancy (most commonly, Hodgkin's lymphoma), HIV infection, sarcoidosis, autoimmune disease, chronic renal failure, thyroid disease, hyperparathyroidism, or metabolic/nutritional disorders.

V. THERAPY. Skin is dry not because it lacks grease or skin oils but because it lacks water. All therapeutic efforts are aimed at replacing water in the skin and in the immediate environment.

A. Preventive

1. Room temperatures should be kept as low as is consistent with comfort.

2. The use of humidifiers is encouraged. These may be either portable or installed in the ducts of forced-air heating systems. However, unless the house is relatively airtight with proper insulation, the moisture will either disperse rapidly to the outside or be caught within the walls and cause eventual damage to the house or paint.

3. Although bathing frequently without moisturization may contribute to xerosis, it is now recognized that bathing once or twice daily with postbath application of emollients to damp skin can improve the water content of the skin and aid in the prevention and treatment of this condition. Bath water should be warm but not hot. Bath oils may be added (Alpha Keri, Aveeno, or others). However, these may make the bathtub slippery and difficult to clean. An alternative instruction to the patient is to add one teaspoon of bath oil to one quarter cup of warm water and to use the mixture as a rubdown either after the bath or as a substitute for a bath.

4. Excessive exposure to soap and water, solvents, or other drying compounds should be eliminated. Use of a mild soap such as Dove or a nonsoap skin cleanser (Cetaphil, Purpose, or others) is recommended. Patients should be counseled that it is the very mild irritants, often used casually and without thinking, that are often causative. Mechanical trauma from rough (often wool) or constricting clothing must also be avoided.

5. Frequent use of emollients should be encouraged. The lubricating agents may range from lotions (Keri, Lubriderm, Moisturel) and creams (Cetaphil, Eucerin, Keri, Neutrogena) to thicker preparations (Aquaphor, hydrated petrolatum, petrolatum). They are best applied when the skin is moist. Many elderly patients seem to tolerate petrolatum better than some of the more elegant preparations.

6. Change of venue to a subtropical environment, especially for the winter, although helpful, is not without its cost.

B. Treatment of preexisting dryness

1. The primary means of correcting dryness is to first add water to the skin and then apply a hydrophobic substance to keep it there. *In vitro*, the stratum corneum can absorb as much as five to six times its own weight and increase its volume threefold when soaked in water. *In vivo*, this hydration is accomplished by either soaking the affected area or bathing for 5 to 10 minutes and then immediately applying water-in-oil or fatty hydrophobic medications (Aquaphor, Eucerin, lanolin, petrolatum). Use of the latter ointments alone is only moderately effective; they hydrate the skin simply by preventing the normal transepidermal water loss rather than replenishing the water deficit.

2. Topical corticosteroid ointments are the most effective and rapid therapy for symptomatic xerosis with associated eczematous changes.

3. If emollient products have been used without success, it is necessary to use "high-potency" agents. These formulations include chemicals that have the ability to hold water in the skin (humectants) or that affect desquamation of the stratum corneum. The α-hydroxyacids glycolic and lactic acid (Lac-Hydrin or Am-Lactin [12% lactic acid]) are humectants that decrease corneocyte cohesion, increase water content of the stratum corneum, and increase dermal glycosaminoglycans. They are effective therapy for dry skin, ichthyosis, and callosities. Urea creams or lotions (Carmol [20% to 40% urea], Ultra Mide [25% urea]) may increase desquamation as well as promote hydration. Urea provides a sustained decrease in transepidermal water loss and tendency toward irritation, even after three applications.

4. Maximum hydration can be accomplished by the use of 40% to 60% propylene glycol in water applied under plastic occlusion overnight. If 6% salicylic acid is added to this formula, an extremely effective keratolytic and hydrating gel is obtained. Used overnight once or twice weekly initially and then only as often as needed thereafter, this product is the therapy of choice for removing the dark scales from the dry, scaly skin of ichthyosis vulgaris.

Suggested Readings

Berardesca E, Distante F, Vignoli GP, et al. Alpha hydroxyacids modulate stratum corneum barrier function. *Br J Dermatol* 1997;137:934–938.

DiGiovanna J, Robinson-Bostom L. Ichthyosis: etiology, diagnosis, and management. *Am J Clin Dermatol* 2003;4(2):81–95.

Glorio R, Allevato M, De Pablo A, et al. Prevalence of cutaneous manifestations in 200 patients with eating disorders. *Int J Dermatol* 2000;39(5):348–353.

Harding CR. The stratum corneum: structure and function in health and disease. *Dermatol Ther* 2004;17:6–15.

Heymann WR, Gans EH, Manders SM, et al. Xerosis in hypothyroidism: a potential role for the use of topical thyroid hormone in euthyroid patients. *Med Hypotheses* 2001;57(6):736–739.

Lodén M. Urea-containing moisturizers influence barrier properties of normal skin. *Arch Dermatol Res* 1996;288:103–107.

Okulicz JF, Schwartz RA. Hereditary and acquired ichthyosis vulgaris. *Int J Dermatol* 2003;42:95–98.

Strumia R. Dermatologic signs in patients with eating disorders. *Am J Clin Dermatol* 2005;6(3):165–173.

Utter W, Gefeller O, Schwanitz HJ. An epidemiological study of the influence of season (cold and dry air) on the occurrence of irritant skin changes of the hands. *Br J Dermatol* 1998;138:266–272.

ERYTHEMA MULTIFORME

Peter C. Schalock

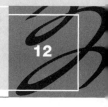

12

I. DEFINITION AND PATHOPHYSIOLOGY. Erythema multiforme (EM) is a reaction pattern with diverse clinical manifestations that usually affects children and young adults. Most cases run a relatively short, benign course (bullous EM), but a more severe form with extensive blistering and widespread mucosal involvement (Stevens-Johnson syndrome [SJS]) may be associated with significant morbidity and mortality. Toxic epidermal necrolysis (TEN) is regarded by some as the most extreme form of EM and by others, as a totally separate entity.

The nomenclature regarding the naming within the EM spectrum is unclear at best, with EM being a term used to refer to an entire spectrum of diseases. To help clarify expected clinical course and outcomes, precision in terminology is desirable. After review of the relevant literature regarding classification of EM, the newest classification system by Bastuji-Garin et al. is used. EM minor is classified as bullous EM and EM major, as SJS. TEN is also considered in this system and was broken down into three subcategories. For the sake of clarity, only the term TEN will be used. Skin involvement is required for all these diagnoses and the number of mucosal surfaces involved does not play a diagnostic role in this system.

Lesional morphology is highly variable: true iris or target lesions with three rings of color are very characteristic and most commonly found in an acral location in bullous EM. Atypical target lesions with two zones and often with a purpuric quality usually predominantly on the trunk characterize SJS. Recurrent episodes of varying severity occur in 22% to 37% of patients, especially in those with mucous membrane involvement. The mild form of EM heals spontaneously in 2 to 3 weeks; the severe forms, SJS and TEN, may last 6 to 8 weeks and are life-threatening diseases. Full thickness epidermal necrosis occurs rapidly; most cases do not evidence typical target lesions. All mucosal surfaces may be involved and the nails shed. Ocular involvement can occur with TEN, SJS, and EM (1). Pulmonary involvement can occur in the presence of a negative chest x-ray with involvement of the bronchial epithelium causing dyspnea, bronchial hypersecretion, and hypoxemia (2).

Drugs are implicated as the cause in 75% of the cases of TEN. The relative risk for short-term drugs in decreasing order of risk are sulfonamides, chlormezanone, aminopenicillins, quinolones, cephalosporins, and acetaminophen. For drugs that had been used for months to years, the relative frequency in decreasing order are carbamazepine, phenobarbital, phenytoin, valproic acid, oxicam nonsteroidal antiin- flammatory drugs (NSAIDs), allopurinol, and corticosteroids (3). Though drugs are the most common cause of TEN, other causative agents include recent infections, ulcerative colitis, and lymphoma.

The earliest histologic findings of EM are endothelial cell swelling, dermal papil- lary edema, and a perivascular lymphohistiocytic infiltrate. Later, epidermal necrosis, dermal–epidermal interface alteration, subepidermal or, less frequently, intraepidermal separation, and bulla formation occur. Necrotic keratinocytes concentrated within the eccrine ducts have been observed, implicating direct toxic effects of higher concentra- tions of drugs in the acrosyringeal unit (4).

TEN is remarkable for its lack of inflammatory reaction, apoptotic cell death, and separation of the dermoepidermal junction. Elevated levels of Fas, a cell surface death receptor, and its ligand have been documented in TEN. Patients with SJS and TEN have been shown to have increased levels of soluble Fas ligand (sFasL), produced by peripheral blood monocytes. sFasL binds to Fas receptors on keratinocytes, inducing caspases and, subsequently, apoptosis of the cell. This elevation of sFasL was not found in patients with bullous EM or normal controls (5).

The pathophysiology of the EM spectrum remains unclear. Several reports have documented the presence of complement and immunoglobulin in the superficial cutaneous microvasculature in early lesions, as well as circulating immune complexes in serum. These studies suggest that deposition of immune complexes in vessel walls plays a primary role. Other researchers have found evidence favoring a cell-mediated immune response. Though an association with HLA-B62, HLA-B35, HLA-DQ3, HLA-DQB1, and HLA-DR53 antigen has been reported, the importance of this finding is uncertain, and human leukocyte antigen (HLA) typing is not diagnostically useful.

At least for herpes-associated EM, it is possible that herpes antigen, present within the epidermis, activate the alternative complement pathway. Herpes simplex deoxyribonucleic acid (DNA) is found primarily in the skin lesions of recurrent EM, with the viral antigens being present for as long as 3 months with no evidence of clinical disease. The herpes simplex DNA is found in peripheral white blood cells only during an acute episode of EM (6).

Multiple precipitating factors have been associated with EM, including infections, drugs, endocrine changes, contact dermatitis, radiation therapy, and underlying malignancy. Herpes simplex infections are the most frequent cause (implicated in 15% to 79% of cases) of bullous EM, especially the recurrent type. Direct links with *Mycoplasma pneumoniae* and both bullous EM and SJS have been documented. A large study of 70 patients demonstrated that *M. pneumoniae* is involved in the pathogenesis of SJS (7). All patients had oral lesions, three fourths had genital lesions, and two thirds had ocular lesions. Bullous EM is a rare complication of *M. pneumoniae* infection and has been reported in 31 patients. It is of note that *M. pneumoniae* infection can cause an SJS-like syndrome with disease confined to the mucous membranes. This has been defined as *M. pneumoniae*–related mucositis. Diagnosis of SJS requires skin involvement. Antibiotics and/or steroids had little effect on the clinical course with symptoms lasting usually for 2 weeks (7).

Many other viral, bacterial, and fungal agents may elicit EM. Penicillin, barbiturates, sulfonamides, and many other drugs may initiate the same picture. In approximately 50% of cases, no etiologic factor can be identified. Recurrent EM in both children and adults is highly associated with herpes simplex; the antigen has been detected by polymerase chain reaction in biopsy specimens of active lesions and inactive sites. Bullous EM is most often infection related, especially herpes simplex, and not related to drug exposure. SJS is almost always related to drugs and not to the herpesvirus (8), but can be caused by *M. pneumoniae* infections.

II. SUBJECTIVE DATA. Mild prodromal symptoms of malaise and sore throat often precede the eruption, and drugs given for these symptoms are often inadvertently blamed for the EM. Individual lesions may sting or burn and large bullae may be painful. In severely ill patients, there is high fever, cough, sore throat, myalgias, malaise, and severe pain in mucosal areas with secondary photophobia and inability to ingest food or fluids.

III. OBJECTIVE DATA (See color insert.)

    A. In the mild and typical case, the patient will usually have lesions distributed symmetrically on extensor surfaces, distal limbs, palms and soles, and face. Bright red-purple annular, macular, and papular areas and some urticaria-like lesions may be seen. The iris or target lesion is seen most often on the hands and consists of a central vesicle or livid erythema surrounded by a concentric pale and then red ring. The eruption usually occurs in crops; therefore, lesions are seen in different stages of evolution. Mucosal lesions are present in 25% to 90% of cases and usually start at the same time as the skin lesions, though only mucous membrane lesions may be seen. The number of mucous membrane areas involved is not useful for diagnosis or prognosis. Suprainfection with *Candida* should be considered and treated.

    B. With SJS, there are usually generalized lesions (with and without bullae or hemorrhage) with severe involvement of ocular, oral, and other mucous membranes. A copious and often purulent discharge from the eyes and mouth may be present with red painful conjunctiva and photophobia. A characteristic hemorrhagic crust occurs on the lips, resulting in difficulty in eating and possible dehydration. Balanitis and vulvovaginitis may cause difficulty with urination and possible scarring and stenosis. Associated symptoms may include malaise, pruritus, fever, myalgias, and prostration. Widespread vesicles occur that arise on an erythematous or purpuric base and atypical targets are seen predominantly on the trunk.

C. Most cases of recurrent EM are associated with herpes simplex virus (HSV) infection, either type 1 or 2, and the skin lesions occur 7 to 10 days after the oral, genital, or other site outbreak of HSV.

D. Complications are usually confined to the more severe forms such as SJS and TEN. These include dehydration, esophagitis, pneumonia, sepsis, and death. Ocular injury is particularly frequent and may result in permanent visual impairment. Conjunctival scarring occurs in 10% of patients with severe disease. Respiratory tract involvement is also common.

IV. ASSESSMENT

A. Workup. Antecedent infection, drug administration, or illness for up to 3 weeks before the rash should be detailed. Every attempt should be made to identify and eliminate any precipitating factors. For a complete workup, the following should be considered:

1. Cultures for streptococci, HSV, and deep fungi (e.g., histoplasmosis, coccidioidomycosis). *M. pneumoniae* cultures are not useful because of specialized media and long duration (approximately 3 weeks) necessary for growth.

2. Serologic studies for hepatitis-associated antigens, histoplasmosis, mononucleosis, and *M. pneumoniae* infection.

3. Chest x-ray (to rule out *M. pneumoniae*, deep fungal infection, or tuberculosis).

4. Skin biopsy will demonstrate a characteristic histopathologic picture. This test is worthwhile, particularly when the clinical presentation is not typical. Direct immunofluorescence studies are helpful primarily to rule out other diseases such as bullous pemphigoid, linear immunoglobulin A (IgA) disease, or dermatitis herpetiformis.

5. Has the patient been vaccinated recently, had a "cold sore," or had x-ray therapy for a tumor? Is she pregnant, or has she been taking birth control pills? The causes of EM are so numerous that they cannot all be listed here, and the direct cause may escape detection.

B. Differential diagnosis includes (i) other vascular reaction pattern diseases (urticaria, erythema nodosum, vasculitis), (ii) blistering eruptions (pemphigus, bullous pemphigoid), (iii) TEN, (iv) mucocutaneous syndromes (Behçet's syndrome, hand-foot-and-mouth disease, aphthous stomatitis, acute herpetic gingivostomatitis), (v) drug reactions or serum sickness, (vi) Kawasaki's disease, (vii) Sweet's syndrome, and (viii) graft versus host disease.

V. THERAPY

A. Mild involvement (bullous EM)

1. Antihistamines PO.

2. Antibiotics (azithromycin) if there is suspected mycoplasma infection.

3. The use of prophylactic oral antiviral antibiotics in frequently recurrent herpes-associated EM will decrease recurrent attacks.

4. Open wet compresses, Burow's solution (Domeboro compresses, one packet in 1 pt of water), followed by silver sulfadiazine cream (Silvadene) b.i.d. for bullous or erosive lesions.

5. Mouth care
   a. Half-strength aqueous hydrogen peroxide (1.5%) mouthwash for cleanliness two to five times a day.
   b. Dyclone solution, viscous lidocaine, or a mixture of Kaopectate in elixir of diphenhydramine applied directly to the lesions for pain p.r.n.
   c. Chloraseptic mouthwash may be used for both purposes as needed t.i.d.
   d. Peridex mouth rinse q.i.d. has antibacterial properties.

6. Bland foods are preferable.

7. Analgesics (aspirin, 600 mg q4h).

B. Severe involvement (SJS and TEN)

1. Immediate hospitalization and institution of intravenous fluid administration. Extensive involvement is best treated in burn units, and delay can be associated with increased risk of sepsis and death (9).

2. The usefulness of systemic corticosteroids is quite controversial. Their effectiveness in affecting the course and outcome of SJS has been prospectively examined. Treatment of ten patients with methylprednisolone (4 mg/kg/day) was successful in decreasing periods of fever and shortened the course of disease by 2.8 days when compared with six patients not being treated (Kakorou, 1997). Patients receiving steroids subjectively reported feeling better and did not have complications from steroid use. Steroids were not useful in TEN. Another study prospectively treated 67 patients with methylprednisolone, finding that treatment decreased symptoms and mortality in SJS (Tripathi, 2000). No control group was examined as the investigators felt that not treating would be unethical. A "Special Symposium" of 17 pediatric dermatologists were split in their recommendations. Nine would not use corticosteroids and eight would consider their use in SJS. In a series of patients with TEN, 7.6% were on long-term corticosteroids for other reasons. The steroids appeared to delay the onset of the TEN but did not affect the final course of the disease (10). Prospective studies of TEN have demonstrated decreased survival in the group treated with systemic corticosteroids. Retrospective studies also suggest that steroids may be associated with a worse prognosis, and their use is contraindicated. Many clinicians avoid using corticosteroids in the treatment of EM altogether.

    For those who still believe this therapy may be of benefit, prednisone 80 to 120 mg PO or methylprednisolone 4 mg/kg bolus infusion everyday is given until the disease responds and is then tapered over 2 to 3 weeks.

3. Human intravenous immunoglobulin (IVIg) administration for SJS and TEN is controversial. There are multiple studies stating that IVIg is useful for shortening the course, morbidity, and mortality for both these conditions. Other studies have failed to show significant efficacy with use of IVIg. Doses ranging from 0.2 to 0.75 g/kg of body weight per day for 4 days (5) to a single infusion at 1.5 to 2 g/kg have been suggested. Use early in the course of disease is necessary. While further prospective studies are needed to clarify the efficacy of this expensive therapy, its use may be justified by a mortality rate as high as 10% for SJS and 30% to 40% in some series for TEN patients.

4. Plasmapheresis has been shown in small case series to be effective with fairly rapid cessation of necrolysis. The same group subsequently reported on 13 more cases of TEN treated with plasmapheresis. Seventy-seven percent of patients had full recovery and 23% died. This is an expensive therapy, and a large-scale controlled study is needed to show the advantages of this therapy (11).

5. Local care as previously described for mild involvement; bullae may be drained, but the blister roof should be left intact.

6. An ophthalmologist should be consulted if there is any evidence of eye involvement.

C. Recurrent bullous EM

1. Acyclovir (400 mg PO b.i.d. or 200 mg PO five times a day) or other antiviral antibiotics can suppress herpes-associated EM. It is of no value once the EM has started. Not all episodes of a herpes simplex recurrence are associated with EM, but in recurrent cases, a 6-month trial of suppressive therapy can be helpful.

2. Cyclosporine 4 mg/kg PO q.d. for 1 to 2 weeks has been reported to be effective in aborting severe recurrent bullous EM episodes, when started on day 1 or 2 of the episode. Screening laboratory tests including urinalysis, creatinine, and blood pressure should be evaluated every 14 days.

3. Fixed drug eruption should be considered in the differential diagnosis of recurrent EM-like lesions, because the clinical and histologic pictures may be similar.

4. One study has documented positive patch tests to benzoic acid, and a benzoate-free diet eliminated the recurrences in all positive patients (12).

References

1. Power WJ, Ghoraishi M, Merayo-Lloves J, et al. Analysis of the acute ophthalmic manifestations of the erythema multiforme/Stevens-Johnson syndrome/toxic epidermal necrolysis disease spectrum. *Ophthalmology* 1995;102:1669–1676.
2. Lebargy F, Wolkenstein P, Gisselbrecht M, et al. Pulmonary complications in toxic epidermal necrolysis: a prospective clinical study. *Intensive Care Med* 1997;23:1237–1244.
3. Roujeau J-C, Kelly JP, Naldi L, et al. Medication use and the risk of Stevens-Johnson Syndrome or toxic epidermal necrolysis. *N Engl J Med* 1995;333:1600–1607.
4. Zohdi-Mofid M, Horn TD. Acrosyringeal concentration of necrotic keratinocytes in erythema multiforme: a clue to drug etiology. Clinicopathologic review of 29 cases. *J Cutan Pathol* 1997;24:235–240.
5. Abe R, Shimizu T, Shibaki A, et al. Toxic epidermal necrolysis and Stevens-Johnson syndrome are induced by soluble Fas ligand. *Am J Pathol* 2003;162(5):1515–1520.
6. Brice SL, Leahy MA, Ong L, et al. Examination of non-involved skin, previously involved skin, and peripheral blood for herpes simplex virus DNA in patients with recurrent herpes-associated erythema multiforme. *J Cutan Pathol* 1994;21:408–412.
7. Tay YK, Huff JC, Weston WL. Mycoplasma pneumoniae infection is associated with Stevens-Johnson Syndrome, not erythema multiforme (Hebra). *J Am Acad Dermatol* 1996;35:757–760.
8. Assier H, Bastuji-Garin S, Revuz J, et al. Erythema multiforme with mucous membrane involvement and Stevens-Johnson Syndrome are clinically different disorders with distinct causes. *Arch Dermatol* 1995;131:539–543.
9. McGee T, Munster A. Toxic epidermal necrolysis syndrome: mortality rate reduced with early referral to regional burn center. *Plast Reconstr Surg* 1998;102:1018–1022.
10. Guibal F, Bastuji-Garin S, Chosidow O, et al. Characteristics of toxic epidermal necrolysis in patients undergoing long-term glucocorticoid therapy. *Arch Dermatol* 1995;131:669–672.
11. Chaidemenos GC, Chrysomallis F, Sombolos K, et al. Plasmapheresis in toxic epidermal necrolysis. *Int J Dermatol* 1997;36:218–221.
12. Lewis MA, Lamey PJ, Forsyth A, et al. Recurrent erythema multiforme: a possible role of foodstuffs. *Br Dent J* 1989;166:371–373.

Suggested Readings

Bakis S, Zagarella S. Intermittent oral cyclosporin for recurrent herpes simplex-associated erythema multiforme. *Australas J Dermatol* 2005;46(1):18–20.

Bamichas G, Natse T, Christidou F, et al. Plasma exchange in patients with toxic epidermal necrolysis. *Ther Apher* 2002;6(3):225–228.

Bastuji-Garin S, Rzany B, Stern RS, et al. Clinical classification of cases of toxic epidermal necrolysis, Stevens-Johnson syndrome, and erythema multiforme. *Arch Dermatol* 1993;129(1):92–96.

Kakourou T, Klontza D, Soteropoulou F, et al. Corticosteroid treatment of erythema multiforme major (Stevens-Johnson syndrome) in children, *Eur J Pediatr* 1997;156(2):90–93.

Lam N, Yang YH, Wang LC, et al. Clinical characteristics of childhood erythema multiforme, Stevens-Johnson syndrome and toxic epidermal necrolysis in Taiwanese children. *J Microbiol Immunol Infect* 2004;37:366–370.

Morici MV, Galen WK, Shetty AK, et al. Intravenous immunoglobulin therapy for children with Stevens-Johnson syndrome. *J Rheumatol* 2000;27(10):2494–2497.

Schalock PC, Brennick JB, Dinulos JG. Mycoplasma pneumoniae infection associated with bullous erythema multiforme. *J Am Acad Dermatol* 2005;52(4):705–706.

Schalock PC, Dinulos JG. Mycoplasma pneumoniae-induced Stevens-Johnson syndrome without skin lesions: fact or fiction? *J Am Acad Dermatol* 2005;52(2):312–315.

Tripathi A, Ditto AM, Grammer LC, et al. Corticosteroid therapy in an additional 13 cases of Stevens-Johnson syndrome: a total series of 67 cases. *Allergy Asthma Proc* 2000;21(2):101–105.

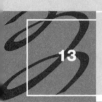

13 ERYTHEMA NODOSUM
Peter C. Schalock

I. **DEFINITION AND PATHOPHYSIOLOGY.** Erythema nodosum (EN), a cutaneous reaction pattern, consists of tender red nodules on the legs and occasionally elsewhere. The most common form is acute and self-limited. It is a reactive process generally associated with a variety of underlying diseases. It will generally resolve, with the acute course running 3 to 6 weeks. Chronic EN has a chronic course and should be distinguished from acute EN.

EN is the most common form of panniculitis (inflammation of the fat). It represents a hypersensitivity response, perhaps involving immune complex formation, to any of numerous factors. Activated polymorphonuclear neutrophils produce reactive oxygen intermediates and these exert their effects by oxidative tissue damage and by promoting tissue inflammation. A polarized Th1 immune response occurs in the skin lesions of EN with production of interleukin (IL)-2 and interferon-γ (IFN-γ) (1).

A family has been described with four sisters who had acute or recurrent EN; human leukocyte antigen (HLA) typing demonstrated a common haplotype. EN appears most commonly in young women but may be seen in patients of any age. It indicates a need for an investigation of underlying precipitating disorders and should not be viewed as a disease in itself.

In adults, women are three to six times more commonly affected than men; the peak incidence is between 20 and 30 years of age. The most common cause of EN in the United States is a preceding streptococcal infection, especially in children. Reactions to medications, particularly sulfonamides and birth control pills, are also frequent causes. Iodides and bromides have been implicated. In Spain, the most common etiologies of EN in children were tuberculosis followed by *Salmonella enteritidis* and Group A β-hemolytic *Streptococcus*. Similar results were seen in adults in Turkey, with the most common causes being primary tuberculosis (18%) followed by a poststreptococcal phyrngitis (16%), sarcoidosis (12%), inflammatory bowel diseases (IBDs) (4%), Behçet's disease (2%), and pregnancy (2%).

Acne fulminans and EN developed in a man after 3 weeks of isotretinoin therapy and responded to Dapsone without oral steroids (2). EN and bilateral hilar adenopathy (Lofgren's syndrome) may be the presenting sign of sarcoidosis, although hilar adenopathy may be associated with EN without evidence of sarcoidosis. Other etiologic considerations should include tuberculosis, secondary syphilis, hepatitis, viral, and deep fungal infections (coccidioidomycosis, blastomycosis, histoplasmosis). *Mycoplasma pneumoniae, Salmonella, Campylobacter, Chlamydia,* and *Yersinia* infections, leukemia, and lymphoma should also be considered. EN was present in 3% of patients with Crohn's disease and can be seen in other IBDs (ulcerative colitis or regional enteritis). EN has developed in patients with septicemia due to *Neisseria meningitides* and *Pseudomonas aeruginosa*. EN-like lesions can occur in Behçet's syndrome and Sweet's syndrome. In as many as 55% of cases, the etiology remains unknown (3).

EN will usually subside spontaneously in 3 to 6 weeks, temporarily leaving an area resembling a deep bruise "erythema contusiformis." Chronic EN or EN migrans refers to a syndrome differing from acute EN because of a persistent course, peripherally expanding lesions, tendency for unilateral distribution, and a painless or of a mild degree of tenderness; 50% of patients will have arthralgias. It is not associated with any underlying diseases.

Other diseases can mimic chronic EN. Syphilitic gummas and sporotrichosis are unilateral in nature. Erythema induratum is commonly seen on the posterior calves and not the shins, but will have a chronic course and can ulcerate. Other forms of panniculitis such as subcutaneous fat necrosis associated with pancreatitis or nodular vasculitis can occur on the shins. A skin biopsy can be helpful in sorting out these diagnostic possibilities.

II. SUBJECTIVE DATA. A 1- to 2-week period of malaise and arthralgias with or without fever may precede the outbreak of lesions. The overriding characteristic of these lesions is their exquisite sensitivity, which is so severe that even contact with bed clothing or sheets may be intolerable.

III. OBJECTIVE DATA (See color insert). Single to numerous, bright red, hot, oval or round, slightly raised nodules, several centimeters in diameter, with diffuse borders and surrounding edema, are seen distributed unilaterally or bilaterally, although not necessarily symmetrically, on the pretibial surfaces. Other sites may include the thighs, arms, face, and neck. The extent of the lesions is easier to determine by palpation than by inspection. After 1 to 2 weeks, the redness will become blue and then yellow green as the nodules subside. Mild scaling will be seen as the lesions heal. Ulceration or scarring is never a part of the syndrome. A fever of 38 to 39°C and conjunctivitis may appear with the skin lesions.

IV. ASSESSMENT

A. Workup

  1. A detailed history concerning travel, present illness, and drug administration.

  2. A thorough physical examination.

  3. Laboratory studies should include complete blood count (CBC), erythrocyte sedimentation rate (ESR), urinalysis, chest x-ray, throat culture, and antistreptolysin-O (ASO) titer.

B. Differential diagnosis. Other entities that may resemble the lesions of EN include erythema induratum, nodular vasculitis, cutaneous polyarteritis nodosa, superficial thrombophlebitis, Weber-Christian disease, Churg-Strauss syndrome, giant cell arteritis, fungal granuloma, bite reactions, or fat necrosis produced by lipolytic enzymes liberated in acute or chronic pancreatic disease.

C. Histopathology. Biopsy of EN will reveal a septal panniculitis. Although a specific histologic diagnosis may not be possible in all instances, many of the foregoing conditions have distinctive clinicopathologic patterns. An adequate deep incisional biopsy should be considered part of a thorough investigation. Punch biopsies frequently provide insufficient information to make a diagnosis and should be avoided.

V. THERAPY

A. Treat the underlying disease as indicated.

B. Bed rest with elevation of the patient's legs will gradually reduce pain and edema. A bed cradle will keep sheets and blankets from direct skin contact.

C. Analgesics (aspirin, 600 mg q4h).

D. Nonsteroidal antiinflammatory drugs may be useful.

E. Very symptomatic patients may be treated with potassium iodide 360 to 900 mg [or saturated solution of potassium iodide, 0.36 to 0.90 mL (6 to15 drops) in fruit juice] daily for 3 or 4 weeks. Decrease in pain and swelling should occur within 24 to 48 hours and complete resolution within 2 weeks. Early cessation of therapy may result in relapse. The mechanism of action of potassium iodide is unknown, but heparin release from mast cells can suppress a delayed hypersensitivity reaction and this drug inhibits neutrophil chemotaxis. Long-term therapy can produce a hypothyroid state in the patient. Potassium iodide is contraindicated in pregnancy, as it can produce a goiter in the fetus.

F. Some patients may respond to a course of colchicine, 0.6 to 1.2 mg twice a day.

G. In chronic or recurrent cases unresponsive to these treatments, there is often a therapeutic dilemma. The most detailed investigation may not uncover the cause in most cases, yet some patients may be disabled, in pain, and unable to work. In such instances, the injection of small amounts of a corticosteroid suspension into the middle of each nodule will cause involution of the lesion within 48 to 72 hours. A 1- to 2-week course of oral corticosteroids is also effective (40 mg/day); the possibility of an underlying primary tuberculous infection must never be overlooked. Other infectious etiologies must also be ruled out.

References
1. Llorente L, Richaud-Patin Y, Alverado C, et al. Elevated Th1 cytokine mRNA in skin biopsies and peripheral circulation in patients with erythema nodosum. *Eur Cytokine Netw* 1997;8:67–71.
2. Tan BB, Lear JT, Smith AG. Acne fulminans and erythema nodosum during isotretinoin therapy responding to dapsone. *Clin Exp Dermatol* 1997;22:26–27.
3. Cribier B, Caille A, Heid E, et al. Erythema nodosum and associated diseases. A study of 129 cases. *Int J Dermatol* 1998;37:667–672.

Suggested Readings
Arndt KA, Harrist T. Fever and subcutaneous masses in an elderly man (Case Records of the Massachusetts General Hospital). *N Engl J Med* 1982;306:1035–1043.
Mert A, Ozaras R, Tabak F, et al. Erythema nodosum: an experience of 10 years. *Scand J Infect Dis* 2004;36(6–7):424–427.
Ozdil S, Demir K, Boztas G, et al. Crohn's disease; analysis of 105 patients. *Hepatogastroenterology* 2003;50(Suppl 2):cclxxxvii–cclxccxci.
Sota Busselo I, Onate Vergara E, Perez-Yarza EG, et al. Erythema nodosum: etiological changes in the last two decades. *An Pediatr (Barc)* 2004;61(5):403–407.

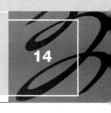
 CANDIDIASIS

I. DEFINITION AND PATHOPHYSIOLOGY. *Candida albicans* is a normal inhabitant of mucous membranes, skin, and the gastrointestinal tract, which can evolve from a commensal organism to a pathogen to cause mucocutaneous infection. Factors that predispose to infection include (i) a local environment of moisture, warmth, and occlusion, (ii) systemic antibiotics, corticosteroids and other immunosuppressive agents, or birth control pills, (iii) pregnancy, (iv) diabetes, (v) Cushing's disease, and (vi) debilitated states. Immune reactivity to Candida is reduced in infants up to 6 months of age and in patients with lymphoproliferative diseases or acquired immunodeficiency syndrome (AIDS). However, most women with recurrent vulvovaginal candidiasis have normal cellular immunity. Recently, nonalbicans Candida strains have been recognized as an important pathogen, particularly in recurrent infections (1).

   The resident bacteria on skin inhibit the proliferation of *C. albicans*. Cell-mediated immunity plays a major role in the defense against infection. In addition, *C. albicans* can activate complement through the alternative pathway. The innate immune system appears to respond to mannan, a *C. albicans* cell wall polysaccharide, through toll-like receptors 2 and 4 (2).

II. SUBJECTIVE DATA. In chronic paronychia, the area surrounding the nail is tender, and there is often a history of frequent wetting of the hands. Candida intertrigo, perlèche, and vulvovaginitis are often accompanied by pruritus and burning. The discomfort of oropharyngeal candidiasis may interfere with eating.

III. OBJECTIVE DATA

   A. Paronychia is associated with rounding and lifting of the proximal nail fold, disruption of the cuticle, and erythema and swelling of the fingertip. The nail plate may display transverse ridging or greenish-brown discoloration.

   B. Intertriginous lesions (inframammary, axillary, groin, perianal, interdigital) are red, macerated, and sometimes fissured. The lesions are well demarcated, with peeling borders, and often surrounded by satellite erythematous papules or pustules.

   C. The white plaques of thrush can be scraped from mucous membranes with a tongue blade, in contrast to the fixed lesions of oral hairy leukoplakia. The underlying mucosa is bright red. Lesions may extend into the esophagus.

   D. Perlèche presents with fissured erythematous moist patches at the angles of the mouth. Poorly fitting dentures or mouth breathing may be associated.

   E. Candida vulvovaginitis is frequently associated with a vaginal discharge. There may be severe vulvar erythema and edema.

IV. ASSESSMENT

   A. Direct examination of scrapings from lesions with potassium hydroxide (KOH) will reveal budding yeasts with or without hyphae or pseudohyphae. Hyphae are almost always seen in mucous membrane infection, but may be absent in skin infection. A rapid latex agglutination test is also available for diagnosis but offers little advantage over KOH in terms of sensitivity and specificity (3).

   B. *C. albicans* grows readily within 48 to 72 hours on fungal or bacterial media. Specific identification is based on the presence of chlamydospores when the organism is subcultured on cornmeal agar.

   C. Gram-negative rods may play a synergistic role in infection of intertriginous areas; Gram's stain and culture of these areas can be helpful.

D. It is important to address predisposing medical conditions and physical factors. For example, spermicide use increases susceptibility to recurrent vulvovaginal candidiasis.

V. THERAPY. The imidazoles and broader-spectrum triazoles are used most often in the treatment of candidal infections. The pyridone derivative ciclopirox (Loprox) and the polyene antibiotic nystatin are also effective. The allylamines naftifine (Naftin) and terbinafine (Lamisil) and the benzylamine butenafine (Mentax) are fungistatic against Candida. Tolnaftate (Tinactin; see Chap. 40, Antiinfective Agents, sec. II.C.6) and undecylenic acid (Cruex; Desenex) are not effective against Candida.

Systemic treatment of vaginal infections has become widespread. Oral imidazoles and triazoles are also useful in chronic mucocutaneous candidiasis and recalcitrant candidal onychomycosis. Ketoconazole and, to a lesser degree, itraconazole have many drug–drug interactions owing to the inhibition of cytochrome P-450 3A4. Their use is contraindicated with simvastatin, lovastatin, cisapride, triazolam, midazolam, quinidine, dofetilide, and pimozide (4).

A. Paronychia

1. Successful treatment of a chronic paronychia often requires weeks to months, and nails will grow out normally within 3 to 6 months of the paronychia healing.

2. An imidazole such as ketoconazole (Nizoral), sertaconazole (Ertaczo), clotrimazole (Lotrimin, Mycelex), ciclopirox olamine (Loprox), or miconazole should be applied several times a day. Other effective agents include naftifine (Naftin), haloprogin (Halotex), or nystatin. If there is associated pain or edema, use a combined steroid-nystatin ointment (e.g., Mycolog II) or a topical corticosteroid cream along with the antifungal agent for the first several days. Overnight application under occlusion may increase effectiveness. Oral therapy may be helpful as well. In addition, the area should be protected during wet work by wearing waterproof gloves and cotton liners.

3. Two percent to 4% thymol in chloroform or absolute alcohol is a simple and effective alternative that is applied b.i.d. to t.i.d.

4. Amphotericin B (Fungizone) lotion or cream or 1% alcoholic solution of gentian violet may also be used. Because Amphotericin B and imidazole agents counteract one another, they should not be used simultaneously.

B. Intertriginous lesions

1. Education about the role of moisture and maceration is important. The following techniques may be recommended: (i) drying affected areas after bathing using a handheld hair dryer on low heat, at least once a day; (ii) supportive clothing and weight reduction; (iii) air conditioning in warm environments; and (iv) regular application of a plain or medicated powder (nystatin or miconazole) to the areas.

2. For very inflammatory lesions, open compresses three to four times a day with water or Burow's solution (Domeboro) will expedite relief of symptoms.

3. A topical antifungal cream or nystatin or miconazole powder should be applied to the dried skin.

4. Gentian violet 0.25% to 2.0% and Castellani's paint (fuchsin, phenol, and resorcinol) are older remedies which are effective but may sting and will stain clothing, bed linen, and skin.

C. Thrush

1. Clotrimazole buccal troches (10 mg) five times a day for 2 weeks are usually effective for oropharyngeal candidiasis in adults and older children. The dose for infants has not been well established.

2. Alternatively, nystatin oral suspension (400,000 to 600,000 units) q.i.d. is held in the mouth for several minutes before swallowing. The dosage for infants is 2 mL (200,000 units) q.i.d.

3. Oral fluconazole (50 mg daily) has been the mainstay of systemic therapy in the past (5). However, with frequent use in immunocompromised hosts, fluconazole-resistant candidiasis has been reported. In this situation, itraconazole 200 mg PO q.d. for 2 to 4 weeks may prove effective (4). Voriconazole (Vfend), a second-generation triazole antifungal, may also be useful (6). Anidulafungin, a member of the novel class of antifungals, echinocandins, is equal in efficacy to fluconazole in the treatment of esophageal candidiasis, has few significant drug–drug interactions, and is well tolerated (7).

4. Amphotericin B (80 mg/mL) may be used as a rinse.

5. Gentian violet solution 1% to 2% may be tried in difficult or recurrent cases.

D. Vulvovaginitis

1. Imidazoles or triazoles are the first-line drugs. Fluconazole has the least potential for drug interactions and is considered the least toxic. Monthly treatment in women with chronic vulvovaginal candidiasis increases the time to recurrence, but long-term remission remains elusive (8).

2. Resistance to therapy may be due to infection with nonalbicans strains such as *Candida glabrata* and *Candida tropicalis*.

3. Topical therapies

a. Imidazole compounds are effective and are available in a wide array of formulations: 500-mg clotrimazole vaginal tablet as a single dose (Gyne-Lotrimin), 200-mg miconazole tablet at bedtime for 3 days (Monistat-3), 100-mg vaginal tablet or suppository at bedtime for 7 days (Gyne-Lotrimin, Mycelex, Monistat-7), 2% butoconazole (Gynazole, Femstat) or miconazole (Monistat-7) cream daily at bedtime for 3 to 7 days, or 1% miconazole cream for 7 to 14 days (Gyne-Lotrimin, Mycelex). Prophylactic treatment may be helpful in chronic infection (see sec. 5c). Miconazole is pregnancy category C and clotrimazole, category B.

b. Terconazole (Terazol) is a fungicidal triazole topical preparation effective against many Candida strains. It is used as either a 3-day or a 7-day course (Terazol 7—0.4% cream for 7 days or Terazol 3—0.8% cream for 3 days). Terconazole is pregnancy category C and is not recommended for use during the first trimester.

c. Nystatin vaginal suppositories (100,000 units) may be slightly less effective. They are dosed twice daily for 7 to 14 days and then nightly for an additional 2 to 3 weeks. Topical nystatin is pregnancy category A.

d. Boric acid, 600 mg in a gelatin capsule, used intravaginally daily for 14 days, has been reported effective even in resistant Candida infections. It may cause local irritation or toxicity from systemic absorption.

e. In severe or very symptomatic Candida vulvitis, a topical corticosteroid for the first 3 to 4 days may be used.

4. Systemic therapies

a. A single oral dose of 150 mg of fluconazole has been U.S. Food and Drug Administration (FDA)-approved for the treatment of vaginal candidiasis. Its efficacy is equivalent to topical therapy and to oral itraconazole 200 mg at two doses 12 hours apart (9). Slightly greater efficacy may be achieved with fluconazole 100 mg/day for 5 to 7 days or itraconazole 200 mg/day for 3 to 5 days (10).

b. In a randomized controlled trial, neither oral nor intravaginal use of yogurt-containing *Lactobacillus acidophilus* was shown to decrease candidal infection (11).

c. Recurrent infection is defined as greater than three episodes/year in the absence of antibiotic use. Prophylactic regimens include clotrimazole (Gyne-Lotrimin) two 100-mg tablets intravaginally BIW, terconazole (Terazol) 0.8% cream one applicator/week, and fluconazole (Diflucan) 150 mg PO each month (12).

 DERMATOPHYTE INFECTIONS

I. DEFINITION AND PATHOPHYSIOLOGY. The dermatophyte fungi are unique; having evolved to live on humans, they cannot survive elsewhere. However, what clinically resembles a dermatophyte infection can occasionally be caused by saprophytic or zoophilic fungi. In addition, although some dermatophyte species may tend to produce a specific clinical picture, reliable identification based on clinical characteristics alone is usually not possible.

Dermatophytes live in the superficial layers of the epidermis, nails, and hair. The presence of serum fungal inhibitory factor prevents them from invading living tissue. Poor nutrition and hygiene, a tropical climate, debilitating disease, atopy, and contact with infected animals, people, or fomites all predispose to fungal infection. Although pathogenic fungi are common in our environment, the overall incidence of infection is low, implying that host resistance is key. Acute infection tends to be associated with the rapid development of a delayed hypersensitivity to intradermal Trichophyton antigen. Protective cell-mediated immunity is acquired by 80% of patients after primary infection. Those who develop chronic infection tend to have poor cell-mediated immunity *in vitro* and immediate, as opposed to delayed, hypersensitivity to Trichophyton antigen.

II. CLINICAL TYPES OF INFECTION

A. Tinea capitis may be transmitted by contact from child to child in an epidemic setting. Children between the ages of 3 and 7 are primarily affected. Pediatric infection has no gender predilection, but in the unusual case of adult infection, women outnumber men (13,14). Organisms have been cultured from such objects as barbers' instruments, hairbrushes, theater seats, and hats. Crowded living conditions and low socioeconomic status may contribute to a high incidence in some urban areas. *Trichophyton tonsurans* has surpassed *Microsporum audouinii* as the primary causative organism in the United States.

   1. Subjective data. Tinea capitis may be asymptomatic. Kerion, which is a deep, boggy swelling caused by an exaggerated host response to infection, is often painful.

   2. Objective data. Patchy hair loss and broken hairs, inflammation, and scaling are characteristic. In kerion, a pustular folliculitis within an area of purulence and swelling is present which may heal with scarring.

B. Tinea barbae, infection of the beard area, is seen in adult men, much less commonly now than in decades past. It is typically acquired from animals.

   1. Subjective data. Pruritus or pain may occur.

   2. Objective data

      a. Superficial infection is scaly, slightly to moderately erythematous, and may have an annular border (see sec. C.2).

      b. Deeper infection is associated with kerion formation. Loss of facial hair is common, and commonly involves the angle of the jaw.

C. Tinea corporis, or infection of glabrous skin, affects all ages, but children are most susceptible. It is more prevalent in hot, humid climates and in rural areas.

   1. Subjective data. Tinea corporis may be either asymptomatic or mildly pruritic.

   2. Objective data. The typical lesions start as erythematous macules or papules that spread outward and develop into annular and arciform lesions with well-defined scaling or vesicular borders and central clearing. Tinea corporis is most common on the face, arms, and shoulders.

D. Tinea cruris, or "jock itch," is often accompanied by tinea pedis. Friction and maceration predispose to infection, which is most common in warm climates.

   1. Subjective data. Symptoms may be absent or may include pruritus and irritation from rubbing.

   2. Objective data (see color insert). The eruption affects both the groin and upper inner thigh symmetrically with clearly defined borders. Lesions often extend into the gluteal fold and onto the buttocks.

E. Tinea of the hands (tinea manuum) and feet (tinea pedis). Tinea pedis is the most common of all fungal diseases, with 30% to 70% of the population having been infected at some time. Unlike other tinea infections, tinea pedis is generally a disease of adults. Like the others, it is seen more often in warm climates or seasons. The causative fungi may be found in shoes, flooring, and socks. Occlusive footwear is a predisposing factor. Simple contact is not sufficient for infection; concomitant disruption of the skin barrier is necessary. Various bacteria and yeasts can also produce symptomatic intertriginous scaling and maceration. For example, *Scytalidium dimidiatum* and *Scytalidium hyalinum* produce an infection that is clinically indistinguishable from the moccasin or interdigital types of tinea pedis (14).

1. **Subjective data.** Pruritus is the most common symptom. Fissures may be painful and also predisposed to secondary bacterial infection. This is of particular importance in patients with diabetes, chronic lymphedema, and venous stasis.

2. **Objective data**

   a. Tinea pedis may take several forms.

      i. Interdigital scaling and maceration with fissures is most common.

      ii. Widespread fine scaling in a "moccasin" distribution is also frequent. The scaling usually extends up onto the sides of the feet and lower heel, where it exhibits a characteristic, well-defined, polycyclic scaling border.

      iii. A highly inflammatory, vesicular, or bullous eruption is uncommon and caused by a small subset of often zoophilic dermatophytes.

   b. Tinea manuum is most often a mild erythema with hyperkeratosis and scaling over the palmar surfaces. Hand infection almost always accompanies foot involvement. Inflammatory lesions on the feet may cause a sterile vesicular "id" reaction on the hands, which may be confused with a primary fungal infection. Unilateral involvement of one hand and both feet is so characteristic that it immediately suggests this diagnosis.

F. Onychomycosis, or fungal infection of the nails, is seen in approximately 40% of patients with fungal infections in other locations. Clinical subtypes of infection include distal subungual, proximal subungual, white superficial, and candidal onychomycosis. The most common subtype, distal subungual, fungi spread from the distal lateral nail fold through the hyponychium to the nail. Fingernails are less commonly involved than toenails. Nondermatophyte molds such as *Scopulariopsis brevicaulis, Fusarium* sp., *Acremonium*, and *Aspergillus* sp. can account for up to 17% of cases (15).

1. **Subjective data.** The nails become brittle, friable, and thickened. Patients may be disturbed by the appearance, experience tenderness, or report that the nails catch on clothing.

2. **Objective data.** In distal subungual infection, changes are first seen at the free margin or distal lateral border of the nail as a white or yellow discoloration and progresses proximally. The nail may become thickened, crumbly, and lifted by accumulated debris. In some cases, the nail plate becomes entirely replaced by this keratinaceous debris.

III. ASSESSMENT

A. Definitive diagnosis is made by the microscopic identification of hyphae in scales or hair. In nails, the presence of hyphae usually indicates dermatophyte infection; however, secondarily invading saprophytic fungi may also be present. The sensitivity of the KOH can be enhanced with the addition of dyes or a fluorescent brightener (e.g., calcofluor white).

B. Histologic evaluation of nails using a periodic acid-Schiff (PAS) stain and fungal culture of nail clippings may be even more useful than KOH, depending on the clinical situation. Of the three methods, PAS is the most sensitive, and fungal culture, the most specific (16).

C. In the past, examination with a Wood's lamp was routine in the assessment of tinea capitis, because fluorescing *Microsporum* species were the most common causative agents in the United States. Nonfluorescent *T. tonsurans* is now most common. Wood's lamp examination is still helpful in certain circumstances.

IV. THERAPY

A. Prophylactic measures

1. Intertriginous or interdigital areas should be dried thoroughly after bathing and a talc or antifungal powder should then be applied.

2. Footwear should fit well and be nonocclusive (avoid sneakers and plastic or rubber footwear).

3. Patients with hyperhidrosis should wear absorbent cotton socks and avoid wool and nonwicking synthetic fibers. Control of the hyperhidrosis is vital to the therapy of concomitant fungal infection.

4. Clothing and towels should be changed frequently and laundered in hot water.

B. Local therapy. Limited infections can be usually treated with topical therapy alone.

  1. Acute, inflammatory lesions with blistering and oozing should be treated with open wet compresses at least three times a day.

  2. Many effective topical antifungals are available. The most effective classes include the imidazoles sertaconazole (Ertaczo), econazole (Spectazole), ketoconazole (Nizoral), clotrimazole (Lotrimin, Mycelex), miconazole (Micatin), oxiconazole (Oxistat), and sulconazole (Exelderm); the allylamines naftifine (Naftin) and terbinafine (Lamisil); the benzylamine butenafine (Mentax); and the pyridone derivative ciclopirox olamine (Loprox). Other useful topicals include haloprogin (Halotex) and tolnaftate (Tinactin). All but tolnaftate are also active against *C. albicans* infections.

    a. Apply one of the medications mentioned in the preceding text b.i.d. Most lesions will respond in 1 to 3 weeks, but treatment should continue for at least 4 weeks to prevent relapse. Most topical antifungal agents have a high initial cure rate (80% to 90%), but relapse or reinfection is very common.

  3. Undecylenic acid and its salts (Desenex and others) are modestly effective.

  4. In thick, hyperkeratotic infection, such as on acral skin, concomitant therapy with keratolytic agents such as salicylic acid is helpful. This allows for more effective penetration of the antifungal agent as well as decreasing the burden of organisms through exfoliation. One regimen is to apply salicylic acid or lactic acid under occlusion overnight and to use an antifungal agent at another time of the day.

  5. Severe interdigital tinea pedis is often associated with bacterial overgrowth. Aluminum chloride hexahydrate 20% applied b.i.d. for 7 to 10 days will decrease odor, itching, and maceration in most cases, because it is both drying and bactericidal.

  6. Topical treatment of the nails is significantly less effective than oral therapy for onychomycosis from dermatophytes. It may be helpful in decreasing the chance of relapse after a course of systemic therapy. One small study showed relapse in 22% of patients at 36 months of follow-up after systemic treatment (17). More long-term studies need to be performed to properly evaluate relapse rates with various antifungal regimens.

    a. Ciclopirox solution, 8%, in a nail lacquer formulation (Penlac) is applied daily to the entire nail surface and surrounding skin. The accumulated lacquer is removed weekly, and unattached nail and debris are trimmed regularly. The clinical cure rate is 5.5% after a 48-week course of therapy.

    b. Naftifine (Naftin), terbinafine (Lamisil), and ciclopirox (Loprox) creams have some efficacy in onychomycosis. One study demonstrated clinical improvement in 8 of 10 patients after 6 months of therapy with 1% naftifine gel (18).

    c. Urea ointment may be a useful adjunct to topical antifungal therapy. In one placebo-controlled study of 60 patients, 20% urea and 2% butenafine hydrochloride were used twice daily under occlusion to chemically avulse the nail. Clinical and mycologic cure by culture were achieved in 73%, with no relapses in 36 weeks of follow-up (19).

    d. Reduction of a thickened, crumbling nail with an emery board or electric rotary sandpaper drill may reduce cosmetic and mechanical problems.

C. Systemic therapy

  1. Allylamines

    a. Terbinafine (Lamisil), a second-generation allylamine, is FDA approved for the treatment of onychomycosis and is considered the treatment of choice for this indication. Efficacy has also been demonstrated in tinea capitis and in certain deep fungal infections. It is well absorbed and rapidly delivered to the stratum corneum and nails where therapeutic levels are achieved within hours and days, respectively. Levels remain therapeutic in the nails for up to 36 weeks after drug discontinuation. It is metabolized by the liver, necessitating dose adjustment in liver failure. The dose should be halved in patients with a creatinine clearance <50 mL/min. The recommended dose for the treatment of onychomycosis is 250 mg q.d. for 6 weeks for fingernails and for 12 weeks for toenails. Studies comparing pulse therapy of 250 mg b.i.d. 1 week of each month to continuous therapy over 3 months showed no difference in efficacy. For the treatment of tinea capitis, recommended doses are 250 mg q.d. for weight >40 kg, 125 mg q.d. for weight 20 kg to 40 kg, and 62.5 mg q.d. for weight <20 kg. Adverse effects include gastrointestinal disturbance (4.9%), taste disturbance, cutaneous eruptions including (rarely) Stevens–Johnson syndrome/toxic epidermal necrolysis, hepatobiliary dysfunction, visual disturbance, and rare hematologic disturbance including neutropenia. Liver enzyme abnormalities are typically asymptomatic and reversible. Symptomatic liver injury may occur in approximately 1 in 50,000 exposures, and fulminant liver failure has been reported (25). As with itraconazole, liver function testing is recommended in patients treated for longer than 6 weeks. Drug interactions through cytochrome P-450 enzymes include rifampin, cimetidine, terfenadine, caffeine, and cyclosporine. Terbinafine may be more efficacious than either pulse-dose or continuous-dose itraconazole (26).

2. Triazoles

   a. Fluconazole (Diflucan) is FDA approved for the treatment of vaginal, oropharyngeal, and systemic candidiasis and cryptococcosis. It has also been effective in dermatophyte infections and onychomycosis. It has good oral absorption, is well tolerated, and is preferentially taken up in keratinized tissues, reaching concentrations up to 50 times that in plasma. This allows for once-weekly dosing in most cases. Drug interactions are less likely to be significant than with itraconazole (20). Doses for treating tinea corporis, cruris, and pedis are 150 mg/week for up to 4 weeks. For onychomycosis, recommended doses are 200 to 400 mg qwk for 3 months for fingernails and for 6 months for toenails. For kerion, the dose is 50 mg/day for 20 days. It is FDA approved for use in children and infants as young as 6 months, albeit for invasive infection, and is available as a liquid that may be given as 6 mg/kg day for 20 days or 8 mg/kg each week for 4 to 6 weeks in the treatment of tinea capitis.

   b. Itraconazole (Sporanox) is effective in the treatment of histoplasmosis, blastomycosis, candidiasis, and dermatophyte infection. Its efficacy in the treatment of tinea capitis in children is equal to griseofulvin, and it is usually better tolerated (21). It is metabolized by the cytochrome P-450 system and may increase the levels of warfarin, cyclosporine, and digoxin among others. Its use is contraindicated with certain medications. Adverse effects include nausea, vomiting, and elevated aminotransferase levels in 5% to 10% of patients, and monitoring of liver function tests is recommended if therapy exceeds 6 weeks. The suggested daily dose is 200 mg q.d. for 7 days for tinea corporis/cruris and 200 mg b.i.d. for 7 days for tinea pedis/manus (22). For onychomycosis, pulse therapy with 200 mg b.i.d. for 1 week out of each month may be used instead of continuous therapy with 200 mg daily for 3 months (4). Two monthly pulses are recommended for fingernails, and three for toenails. Despite the lower overall dose drug during pulse therapy, there has been a case report of fulminant hepatic failure requiring transplantation associated with this dosing method (23). Levels of drug are higher in the epidermis than in the plasma, although not as high as with fluconazole. Therapeutic concentrations of itraconazole remain present in the nails up to 11 months following a three-pulse course. Itraconazole is also effective in onychomycosis due to nondermatophyte molds (24).

3. Imidazoles

   a. Ketoconazole (Nizoral) is a broad-spectrum imidazole antifungal which is excreted in eccrine sweat. Therefore, methods to promote delivery of the drug to the skin, such as exercise 1 hour after dosing, are helpful. Although usually well tolerated, there is a definite risk of hepatic injury (incidence between 1 in 10,000 and 1 in 15,000), including fatal hepatic necrosis. Other adverse side effects include anaphylaxis, interference with anabolic steroid synthesis, interaction with oral anticoagulants, and inhibition of hepatic metabolism of cyclosporine.

    i. Therapy for dermatophyte infections is 200 mg (occasionally up to 400 mg) daily for the same period of time noted earlier for griseofulvin.

    ii. Use of ketoconazole in the treatment of dermatophyte infections has been largely replaced by the triazoles and allylamines because of their better safety profile.

4. Griseofulvin, a fungistatic antibiotic derived from *Penicillium* species, is effective against all dermatophyte fungi but not against bacteria, *Malassezia*, or *Candida*. The oral triazoles and allylamines are broader spectrum, better tolerated, and usually more cost effective and, therefore, have become the treatments of choice for most fungal infections requiring oral therapy (27). Griseofulvin is still useful in treating tinea capitis in children, particularly as it is the only systemic therapy currently FDA approved for this indication in this age-group. However, ongoing trials and accumulated data may soon make the use of griseofulvin even for this indication obsolete (28).

    a. Tinea capitis requires griseofulvin administration for 6 weeks or longer. The recommended daily dose is 10 to 11 mg/kg for children. In general, children weighing 14 to 23 kg may take 125 to 250 mg/day of the oral suspension, and children weighing over 23 kg, 250 to 500 mg/day. Alternatively, a single dose of 1.5 to 2.0 g (which may be repeated in 3 to 4 weeks) will be effective in most children. In general, infections with *Microsporum* species require longer courses of treatment than those due to *Trichophyton*. Therapy should be continued for at least 2 weeks after clinical and mycologic cure. Shampooing with ciclopirox (Loprox), ketoconazole, or 2% selenium sulfide shampoo is recommended as adjuvant therapy.

 TINEA VERSICOLOR

I. DEFINITION AND PATHOPHYSIOLOGY. Tinea versicolor is a chronic superficial fungal infection caused by members of the fungal genus *Malassezia* (*Pityrosporum*). These organisms are a part of normal skin flora and only produce color changes when they flourish beyond normal levels. Although historically *Malassezia furfur* has been implicated as the cause, recent evidence suggest that *Malassezia globosa* may be the predominate species in most cases. The eruption is found worldwide, is seen most commonly in young adults in temperate zones, and accounts for approximately 5% of all fungal infections. Factors predisposing to clinical infection include (i) pregnancy, (ii) serious underlying diseases, (iii) a genetic predisposition, (iv) high plasma cortisol, as in patients taking corticosteroids, and (v) a warm and humid climate. Tinea versicolor often persists for years because of inadequate treatment, reinfection, or an inherent predisposition to infection.

Tinea versicolor has a unique propensity to present either hyper- or hypopigmented lesions, hence its name. Hypopigmentation has been attributed to the causative organism's production of azelaic acid, a dicarboxylic acid that interferes with melanin synthesis and may also be directly cytotoxic to melanocytes (29). The cause of hyperpigmented lesions remains obscure, although these lesions have a thicker keratin layer, and more organisms are present.

II. SUBJECTIVE DATA. The eruption is usually asymptomatic, and most patients object to its appearance.

III. OBJECTIVE DATA. Lesions vary in color from white and pink to brown but usually consist of round, coalescing macules and patches with fine scale found primarily on the trunk and neck. Facial lesions are more common in children than in adults and in women than in men, and these usually involve the forehead. Hypopigmented lesions are often noted by patients during summer months when they are accentuated by tanning of surrounding normal skin.

IV. ASSESSMENT

A. Examination of a KOH preparation will reveal numerous short, straight, and angular hyphae and clusters of thick-walled, round, and budding yeasts (see Chap. 38, Cytologic Smears, sec. II.G). In contrast to dermatophyte infections, a negative microscopic examination virtually excludes the diagnosis.

B. The causative organism can only be cultured on media enriched in C12- to C14-sized fatty acids.

C. Wood's light examination will intensify the pigmentary changes and allow the extent and margins of involvement to be seen more readily. Affected areas may show a gold-to-orange fluorescence.

V. THERAPY

A. There is an abundance of treatment options. Topical treatments should be applied to the entire torso from the neck to the waist, because lesions may be widespread as well as clinically unapparent. The appearance of the rash will improve within days, but to achieve a durable response, therapy should be continued for several weeks. The pigmentary changes resolve much more slowly, over months. Despite seemingly adequate therapy, relapse or reinfection is common, but typically responds to retreatment. The frequency of relapse has led some to recommend that therapy be continued for two consecutive nights each month for 1 year.

B. Useful agents

1. Topical

a. Ketoconazole (Nizoral) 2% shampoo applied to the skin, allowed to dry, and left on overnight either as a single dose or daily for 3 consecutive days (30).

b. Ciclopirox (Loprox) shampoo is effective when left on for several minutes before rinsing for 2 weeks.

c. Antifungal creams or solutions, including all imidazoles, allylamines, haloprogin, and tolnaftate, should be applied b.i.d. for 2 weeks.

d. Zinc pyrithione is found in many shampoos (DHS-Zinc, Head and Shoulders) and should be applied for 5 minutes daily for 2 weeks.

e. Selenium sulfide suspension (Selsun) applied and left in place for 5 to 10 minutes before rinsing is used for 7 to 14 consecutive days.

f. Keratolytic creams, ointments, or lotions containing 3% to 6% salicylic acid (Sebulex shampoo, 3% to 6% sulfur and salicylic acid ointment, 6% salicylic acid cream, 3% salicylic acid in 70% alcohol) applied overnight for 1 to 2 weeks in addition to a salicylic acid–containing soap may be helpful.

g. Sodium hyposulfite 25% should be applied to lesions b.i.d. for several weeks.

h. Retinoic acid cream (Retin-A cream) applied b.i.d. for 2 weeks will treat the tinea versicolor and may lighten pigmentation where it is applied. It is therefore useful in those particularly distressed by hyperpigmentation.

2. Systemic

a. Fluconazole given as a single oral dose of 400 mg cleared 65% of 20 patients treated at 8 weeks (31). A higher cure rate may be achieved by giving a second dose of 200 to 400 mg 1 week after the first dose.

b. Itraconazole 200 mg daily for 5 to 7 days is also effective (32).

c. Ketoconazole given as a 400-mg dose repeated in a week is equivalent in efficacy to 300 mg of fluconazole dosed in the same manner (33).

References

1. Richter SS, Galask RP, Messer SA, et al. Antifungal susceptibilities of Candida species causing vulvovaginitis and epidemiology of recurrent cases. *J Clin Microbiol* 2005;43(5):2155–2162.
2. Roeder A, Kirschning CJ, Rupec RA, et al. Toll-like receptors and innate antifungal responses. *Trends Microbiol* 2004;12(1):44–49.
3. Reed BD, Pierson CL. Evaluation of a latex agglutination test for the identification of Candida species in vaginal discharge. *J Am Board Fam Pract* 1992;5(4):375–380.

4. Huang DB, Ostrosky-Zeichner LO, Wu JJ, et al. Therapy of common superficial fungal infections. *Dermatol Ther* 2004;17:517–522.
5. Hay RJ. The management of superficial candidiasis. *J Am Acad Dermatol* 1999;40: S35–S42.
6. Kofla G, Ruhnke M. Voriconazole: review of a broad spectrum triazole antifungal agent. *Expert Opin Pharmacother* 2005;6(7):1215–1229.
7. Vasquez JA. Anidulafungin: a new echinocandin with a novel profile. *Clin Ther* 2005;27(6):657–673.
8. Sobel JD, Wiesenfeld HC, Martens M, et al. Maintenance fluconazole therapy for recurrent vulvovaginal candidiasis. *N Engl J Med* 2004;351(9):876–883.
9. Edelman DA, Grant S. One-day therapy for vaginal candidiasis. *J Reprod Med* 1999;44:543–547.
10. Mikamo H, Kawazoe K, Sato Y, et al. Comparative study on the effectiveness of antifungal agents in regimens against vaginal candidiasis. *Chemotherapy* 1998;44:364–368.
11. Pirotta M, Gunn J, Chondros P, et al. Effect of lactobacillus in preventing post-antibiotic vulvovaginal candidiasis: a randomised controlled trial. *BMJ* 2004;329(7465):548.
12. Ringdahl EN. Treatment of recurrent vulvovaginal candidiasis. *Am Fam Physician* 2000;61:3306–3312.
13. Elewski BE. Tinea capitis: a current perspective. *J Am Acad Dermatol* 2000;42:1–20.
14. Ungpakorn R, Lohaprathan S, Reangchainam S. Prevalence of foot diseases in outpatients attending the Institute of Dermatology, Bangkok, Thailand. *Clin Exp Dermatol* 2004;29(1):87–90.
15. Tosti A, Piraccini BM, Lorenzi S. Onychomycosis caused by nondermatophytic molds: clinical features and response to treatment of 59 cases. *J Am Acad Dermatol* 2000;42(2 Pt 1):217–224.
16. Weinberg JM, Koestenblatt EK, Tutrone WD, et al. Comparison of diagnostic methods in the evaluation of onychomycosis. *J Am Acad Dermatol* 2003;49(2):183–187.
17. Tosti A, Piraccini BM, Lorenzi S. Relapses of onychomycosis after successful treatment with systemic antifungals: a three-year follow-up. *Dermatology* 1998;197:162–166.
18. Meyerson MS, Scher RK, Hochman LG, et al. Open-label study of the safety and efficacy of naftifine hydrochloride 1 percent gel in patients with distal subungual onychomycosis of the fingers. *Cutis* 1993;51:205–207.
19. Syed TA, Ahmadpour OA, Ahmad SA, et al. Management of toenail onychomycosis with 2% butenafine and 20% urea cream: a placebo-controlled, double-blind study. *J Dermatol* 1998;25(10):648–652.
20. Elewski BE. Once-weekly fluconazole in the treatment of onychomycosis: introduction. *J Am Acad Dermatol* 1998;38:S73–S76.
21. Lopez-Gomez S, Del Palacio A, Van Cutsem J, et al. Itraconazole versus griseofulvin in the treatment of tinea capitis: a double-blind randomized study in children. *Int J Dermatol* 1994;33:743–747.
22. Lesher JL. Oral therapy of common superficial fungal infections of the skin. *J Am Acad Dermatol* 1999;40:S31–S34.
23. Srebrnik A, Levtov S, Ben-Ami R, et al. Liver failure and transplantation after itraconazole treatment for toenail onychomycosis. *J Eur Acad Dermatol Venereol* 2005;19(2):205–207.
24. De Doncker PR, Scher RK, Baran RL, et al. Itraconazole therapy is effective for pedal onychomycosis caused by some nondermatophyte molds and in mixed infection with dermatophytes and molds: a multicenter study with 36 patients. *J Am Acad Dermatol* 1997;36:173–177.
25. Gupta AK, Shear NH. Terbinafine: an update. *J Am Acad Dermatol* 1997;37:979–988.
26. Sigurgeirsson B, Billstein S, Rantanen T, et al. L.I.ON. Study: efficacy and tolerability of continuous terbinafine (Lamisil) compared to intermittent itraconazole in the treatment of toenail onychomycosis. Lamisil vs. itraconazole in onychomycosis. *Br J Dermatol* 1999;141:S5–14.
27. Gupta AK, Shear NH. A risk-benefit assessment of the newer oral antifungal agents used to treat onychomycosis. *Drug Saf* 2000;22:33–52.
28. Roberts BJ, Friedlander SF. Tinea capitis: a treatment update. *Pediatr Ann* 2005;34(3): 191–200.

29. Galadari I, el Komy M, Mousa A, et al. Tinea versicolor: histologic and ultrastructural investigation of pigmentary changes. *Int J Dermatol* 1992;31:253–256.
30. Lange DS, Richards HM, Guarnieri J, et al. Ketoconazole 2% shampoo in the treatment of tinea versicolor: a multicenter, randomized, double-blind, placebo-controlled trial. *J Am Acad Dermatol* 1998;39:944–950.
31. Partap R, Kaur I, Chakrabarti A, et al. Single-dose fluconazole versus itraconazole in pityriasis versicolor. *Dermatology* 2004;208(1):55–59.
32. Delescluse J. Itraconazole in tinea versicolor: a review. *J Am Acad Dermatol* 1990;23: 551–554.
33. Farschian M, Yaghoobi R, Samadi K. Fluconazole versus ketoconazole in the treatment of tinea versicolor. *J Dermatolog Treat* 2002;13(2):73–76.

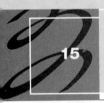

HERPES SIMPLEX
Danielle M. DeHoratius

15

I. DEFINITION AND PATHOPHYSIOLOGY. Cutaneous herpes simplex infections take two distinct forms: (i) the painful and disabling primary infection of previously uninfected individuals and (ii) the common, bothersome recurrent form colloquially known as cold sores or fever blisters. These infections are asymptomatic in up to 80% of patients. The mode of transmission is by close personal contact. The virus is inoculated either through mucous membranes or through small cracks in the skin. By 4 years of age, approximately 50% of the population has antibodies to herpes simplex virus (HSV) indicative of prior exposure. This percentage increases to 60% to 70% by age 14. Following primary infection, effective immunity develops in some individuals, but 20% to 45% will have recurrent disease. Seven percent of the general population has at least two episodes of recurrent facial herpes per year.

Herpes simplex is a deoxyribonucleic acid (DNA) virus, infects humans alone, and has an almost universal distribution. There are two types of HSV: type 1, which is usually responsible for nongenital herpetic infections, and type 2, which is usually the agent involved in genital infections in both men and women. It is important to recognize that the herpesvirus has three unique properties. It has the capacity to invade and replicate within the nervous tissue. The virus then remains latent within the neural tissue, most commonly the trigeminal ganglia for HSV-1 and the sacral nerve root ganglia for HSV-2. Lastly, the latent virus has the capacity to reactivate and replicate, causing cutaneous disease. There are certain biologic differences between the two types. For example, HSV-2 genital infections recur more frequently than genital herpes due to HSV-1, whereas nongenital HSV-1 infections recur more frequently than nongenital herpes due to HSV-2. Genital HSV infections recur sixfold more frequently than oral-labial HSV infections. Previous infection with one type of HSV does not appear to provide effective immunity to subsequent infection with the other.

True primary infection occurs in a person with no previous exposure to HSV and is usually quite severe. First-episode genital infections can occur in persons who either had previous nongenital HSV infection or have serologic evidence of prior subclinical exposure to the virus. Although not sufficient to prevent reinfection, this degree of immunity at least confers partial protection such that first-episode genital infection is less severe than a true primary one. The primary infection, which has an incubation period of 3 to 12 days following exposure, runs a clinical course of 1 to 3 weeks; recurrent lesions heal more quickly (7 to 10 days). Viral excretion persists for 15 to 42 days after the primary infection. Viral titer in recurrent orofacial disease decreases dramatically by 2 days, and most lesions are negative by 5 days. In women with recurrent genital herpes, virus is present for a mean of 4.8 days, while 16% may continue to shed virus from lesions after 6 days. Asymptomatic shedding of HSV has also been demonstrated from both oropharyngeal and genital sites at low rates without evident lesions. The most recent studies suggest that most transmission of genital herpes occurs from persons who asymptomatically shed virus. The annual risk of transmission from a sexual partner with genital herpes in a heterosexual relationship is approximately 10%.

Genital herpes simplex is one of the most common sexually transmitted diseases (STDs). The prevalence of HSV-2 infection in the United States ranges from 20% to 60%. The average man in the United States has a 40% to 60% chance of having been infected with this virus. Even without considering its sometimes-significant psychosocial impact, genital herpes simplex infection may pose other health problems for female patients. Pregnant women with a history of genital herpes must be carefully monitored.

The risk of HSV infections in neonates exposed to the virus at the time of vaginal delivery to mothers with a history of recurrent genital HSV infections is very low ($\leq 8\%$). The presence and titer of neutralizing antibody to HSV contribute to this low rate. Infants born to women who have primary HSV infection are at more than 50% risk of developing a clinical infection, and a C-section is indicated in this situation. Neonatal herpes is a serious disease with up to a 50% mortality rate and a significant chance of permanent sequelae among its survivors. Perinatal HSV infection is part of the TORCH (toxoplasmosis, other agents, rubella, cytomegalovirus, herpes simplex) syndrome. Up to 60% to 80% of babies infected with HSV are delivered by women with no evidence of clinical HSV on examination. Disease during early pregnancy may produce malformations that are clinically indistinguishable from those produced by cytomegalovirus. In addition to the potential threat to the fetus when HSV infects the reproductive tract during pregnancy, an etiologic role in cervical dysplasia and carcinoma has been proposed, although not proved. Women with genital herpes simplex infections appear to have a five to ten times greater likelihood of developing cervical carcinoma than uninfected women, and HSV-2 antigens have also been found in a high percentage of atypical epithelial lesions of the vulva. These findings may reflect infection by a ubiquitous agent. Alternatively, an HSV infection may be a covariable. Anorectal herpes is being recognized with increased frequency. When caused by HSV-2, it is usually transmitted by anal intercourse. HSV-1 causes perianal infections in immunosuppressed patients, presumably by autoinoculation from orofacial lesions.

After primary infection, the virus appears to remain latent in sensory ganglia. In patients with recurrent herpes, the virus is periodically reactivated and conducted to the epidermis through peripheral nerve fibers. It then replicates in the skin, producing the recurrent herpetic lesion. Trigger factors include emotional stress, physical trauma (including genital trauma), sunburn, menses, fever, and systemic infections. The long-term natural history of recurrent nongenital herpes infection is not well characterized. The virus type influences the recurrence rate of genital herpes, as does gender, with men being at greater risk for recurrent disease. There is a great deal of variation in recurrence rates among individuals. Over time, most patients experience clinically significant reductions in disease severity. Rates of recurrence begin to decline by the second year after initial outbreaks (1).

Patients with atopic dermatitis risk the development of generalized lesions (eczema herpeticum), regardless of whether their eczema is active. Diseases or drugs that interfere with host response, particularly with cell-mediated immunity, also predispose to widespread, slowly healing, and more destructive infections. Those with lymphoreticular malignancies or thymic defects and immunosuppressed transplant or acquired immunodeficiency syndrome (AIDS) are most prone to severe HSV infections.

II. SUBJECTIVE DATA

A. Primary symptomatic oral or genital infections

1. Infections on mucosal surfaces are preceded by a day or two of local tenderness.
2. The lesions are accompanied by severe and disabling pain and tender lymphadenopathy, often making it impossible for those with gingivostomatitis to eat or drink or patients with extensive genital involvement to walk or urinate.
3. High fever and purulent malodorous secretions accompany oral and vaginal infections.
4. Primary infection in men usually results in painful penile lesions. It may also cause urethritis with dysuria and discharge.
5. Anorectal infection may be complicated by tenesmus, constipation, and urinary retention.

B. Recurrent lesions are preceded by several hours of a burning or tingling sensation in 80% of patients. They are uncomfortable, but much less than the lesions of the primary infection. Virus is present in the lesion at the time of prodromal symptoms.

III. OBJECTIVE DATA (See color insert.)

A. Primary infection

1. Acute herpetic gingivostomatitis is the most frequent manifestation of primary infection, usually seen in young children. It is usually abrupt at onset and is

associated with a high fever, anorexia, and listlessness. This acute episode lasts from 5 days to 1 week.

   a. Vesicles, erosions, and maceration are seen over the entire buccal mucosa; this can involve the perioral skin because of contamination.

   b. Marked erythema and edema of the gingiva are typical.

   c. Submandibular adenopathy is usually present and is tender.

  2. Acute herpetic pharyngotonsillitis is usually seen in adults and is an oropharyngeal infection of HSV-1. Symptoms are usually a sore throat, fever, malaise, and headache. HSV-2 can be an etiologic agent; however, this usually involves an orogenital contact.

  3. Vulvovaginitis is seen most frequently in girls and young women.

   a. It consists of widespread vesicles, erosions, and edema in the vulva, labia, and surrounding skin.

   b. These areas become very edematous, erythematous, and extremely tender.

   c. A profuse vaginal discharge is present, and some women develop urinary retention.

   d. Bilateral, tender, inguinal adenopathy is usually present.

  4. Urethritis in men is accompanied by a watery discharge and the occasional presence of vesicles around the urethral meatus.

  5. Inoculation herpes is commonly found on the paronychial area (herpetic whitlow) of nurses and physicians, particularly those involved with mouth care, and may also be found on previously traumatized or burned skin. The lesions are characterized by the sudden appearance of vesicles and are accompanied by extreme local pain, sometimes a sterile lymphangitis, and rarely a systemic reaction. The first episode may last up to 28 days. Recurrent infections most often occur in adults with HSV-2 infection. Herpetic whitlow is often misdiagnosed as a bacterial paronychia and mistreated with incision and drainage of lesions, with subsequent implantation of the virus into the incised tissue.

  6. Cervicitis is often asymptomatic but nevertheless important to recognize in pregnant women because of the associated risk of fetal infection and spontaneous abortion. Pregnant women who acquire genital herpes during the first 20 weeks of pregnancy have an increased risk of abortions, whereas the infants of those who acquire an infection after 20 weeks have an increased incidence of prematurity and birth defects.

  7. Anorectal herpes is characterized by the typical cutaneous lesions as well as rectal ulcerations. Extensive indolent lesions are not uncommon in patients with AIDS.

  8. In the United States, genital ulcers are most commonly caused by HSV-2. These ulcers may contain multiple pathogens, and the patient should be evaluated for coexisting STDs. Most of the episodes of primary genital herpes are asymptomatic and up to 80% have no history of symptomatic genital herpes.

  9. Herpes gladiatorum occurs among wrestlers, secondary to contact with opponents with active herpesvirus infection.

B. Recurrent infection is termed **herpes labialis** or **recurrent genital herpes**. Most individuals have two recurrences each year.

  1. Multiple small vesicles, clustered together, appear at the site of premonitory symptoms.

   a. The vesicles may arise from normal skin or from an area that has a slight erythematous blush.

   b. Vesicles are initially clear, then become cloudy and purulent, dry, and crusty, and heal within 7 to 10 days.

   c. The mature lesion consists of grouped vesicles and/or pustules on an erythematous, edematous base.

  2. The presence of a yellow or golden crust on older lesions indicates bacterial superinfection.

  3. Regional, often tender, adenopathy is almost always present. Lymphangitis and lymphadenitis may be seen, particularly with recurrent lesions of the hands.

4. The most common sites for lesions are on the face (lips, perioral area, cheeks, and nose) and neck. The next common site is the anogenital area and then the sacrum and buttocks. However, recurrent herpes can be seen anywhere on the skin. It is uncommon for recurrent lesions to be located inside the oral cavity except in the immunocompromised host.

5. Recurrent erythema multiforme is often associated with HSV infection and responds to antiviral prophylaxis.

IV. ASSESSMENT. Any doubt concerning the presence of a herpes simplex infection may be clarified by any of the several diagnostic procedures that follow:

A. Skin biopsy of a typical viral vesicle will reveal a characteristic picture: (i) intraepidermal lesion located in the mid-to-upper epidermis, (ii) ballooning degeneration of cells, (iii) acantholytic cells floating free, and (iv) large, multinucleated viral giant cells. Intranuclear inclusions may be seen in the giant cells as well as in other infected epidermal cells.

B. A cytologic smear of the vesicle, to look for giant cells and inclusion bodies, is easily and quickly done. The smears are positive in approximately 75% of virus culture-positive recurrent facial herpes but in only approximately 40% of ulcerative genital lesions. It is important that the earliest vesicle be chosen for biopsy or cytologic smears. Cells from the base of the vesicle will afford the best opportunity to detect the virus. Lesions of herpes simplex, herpes zoster, and varicella will have an identical appearance on biopsy and tissue smear. Exfoliative cytology may be used to detect asymptomatic cervical or vaginal infection, but in pregnant women, it is no substitute for actual viral culture.

C. The virus may be easily and rapidly grown in culture from the vesicle fluid (24 to 48 hours).

D. Specific neutralizing antibody titers will rise after the first week of primary infection and peak at 2 to 3 weeks. Change in antibody titer cannot be used to diagnose recurrent disease.

E. If the appropriate facilities and reagents are available, the following procedures may be carried out if indicated:

1. The virus may be easily identified under the electron microscope.

2. The virus can be demonstrated in tissue specimens using immunofluorescent or immunoperoxidase techniques; both techniques can differentiate herpes type 1, herpes type 2, and varicella-zoster virus.

3. The virus may be typed by appropriate serologic tests.

4. The polymerase chain reaction (PCR) is a very rapid and sensitive technique that is also available for use in certain clinical situations.

5. A new, rapid HSV-2 POCkit is commercially available and is quoted to have high sensitivity.

6. Western Blot assays are also very sensitive and specific; however, they are only available for research purposes.

V. THERAPY

A. Specific measures

1. Valacyclovir (Valtrex), a valine ester prodrug of acyclovir (see following text), has a bioavailability three to five times that of acyclovir. This is due to its improved gastrointestinal absorption compared to acyclovir. Valacyclovir is rapidly and almost completely converted to acyclovir after oral administration, with levels comparable to those of intravenous acyclovir. This allows for twice-daily dosing, which may improve compliance and ultimate clinical efficacy. It is more costly than acyclovir. Valacyclovir is the only antiviral agent approved for herpes labialis, for a 3-day course in the episodic treatment of recurrent genital herpes (2). Valacyclovir is indicated for recurrent genital herpes and is administered at 500 mg twice daily for 3 days at the onset of prodromal symptoms or at the first sign of infection. This dosage regimen is as effective as five-times-daily acyclovir in the treatment of recurrent genital herpes in immunocompetent patients (3). Valacyclovir use is contraindicated in immunocompromised patients. Thrombotic thrombocytopenic purpura and hemolytic uremic syndrome have occurred in patients with advanced human immunodeficiency virus (HIV) disease, renal

transplant, and bone marrow transplant. The most commonly reported adverse events are headache and nausea.

2. Famciclovir (Famvir) undergoes extensive first-pass metabolism to penciclovir after oral administration. Penciclovir is another nucleoside analog that has a mechanism of action similar to that of acyclovir. Compared with oral acyclovir, famciclovir has improved bioavailability as well as a significantly prolonged intracellular half-life, allowing for less frequent dosing. Valacyclovir and famciclovir are similar in their high absorption, bioavailability, renal elimination, minimal drug interaction profiles, safety profiles, and efficacy. Famciclovir is indicated for recurrent genital herpes infections and is administered at 125 mg twice daily for 5 days beginning at the onset of prodromal symptoms or at the first sign of infection. At recommended doses, treatment efficacy is similar to that with acyclovir (4,5). Recent research has shown that oral famciclovir of 250 mg twice daily is effective for the suppression of genital HSV infection (6).

3. Acyclovir, a purine nucleoside analog, revolutionized the treatment of herpes simplex infections. Its safety and specificity are dependent on two factors: (i) a viral enzyme, thymidine kinase, is necessary for the conversion of the drug to its active form and (ii) once activated, acyclovir inhibits a virus-specific DNA polymerase required for viral replication (mammalian DNA polymerase is more substrate specific and therefore unaffected).

   a. Intravenous acyclovir (500 mg/m^2 IV q8h) is indicated mainly for the treatment of potentially catastrophic herpes infections in the normal (e.g., herpes encephalitis) or immunocompromised host. Treatment promptly aborts new lesion formation, reduces viral titers, promotes healing, and ameliorates pain. Intravenous acyclovir also effectively prevents reactivation of HSV in seropositive immunocompromised patients undergoing chemotherapy or transplantation. Eczema herpeticum and initial herpes infections in immunocompetent patients respond favorably as well.

   b. Oral acyclovir (200 mg PO five times daily or 400 mg t.i.d. for 10 days) promotes resolution of primary and first-episode genital herpes infections if begun within 3 days of onset. Acyclovir treatment of the initial attack does not reduce recurrence rates. Patient-initiated early treatment of recurrent genital herpes (<48-hour duration) with acyclovir 800 mg t.i.d. or 200 mg five times a day for 5 days may shorten healing times and reduce the duration and formation of new lesions. If administered as a continuous dosage (400 mg b.i.d.) in patients who have frequent recurrences, acyclovir has been clearly shown to reduce or even prevent outbreaks. Because viral latency is unaffected by therapy, on discontinuation of such "prophylaxis," recurrent attacks can be expected to resume as before treatment.

      i. Prophylactic oral acyclovir of 400 mg b.i.d. started 7 days before or 5 minutes after ultraviolet light exposure in patients with a history of sun-induced herpes labialis has been shown to prevent the development of delayed-onset (2 to 7 days) herpes simplex. If oral acyclovir is started 48 hours after ultraviolet exposure, delayed lesions develop but are less severe. Application of topical acyclovir 5 minutes after light exposure does not reduce the lesion frequency or severity. Recurrent labial herpes in the 26% of individuals who develop immediate (within 48 hours) lesions was unaffected by oral acyclovir therapy. Famciclovir is effective as well (7).

         (1) Topical acyclovir applied q3h while awake shows a modest effect on primary and first-episode genital herpes infection if begun within 72 hours of onset. It does not abort recurrent episodes even if applied at the first sign of prodromal symptoms. In multiple clinical trials, topical acyclovir was found ineffective.

         (2) Except for transient renal dysfunction if the intravenous form is administered too rapidly, acyclovir is remarkably free of side effects. The greatest concern is that with widespread use resistant viral strains will render this drug ineffective, especially in the treatment of the more serious infections. Resistance may occur through three mechanisms:

(i) mutant viruses deficient in thymidine kinase, (ii) mutants with altered substrate specificity of thymidine kinase, or (iii) mutants with altered viral DNA polymerase enzymes. Thymidine kinase–deficient mutants have been isolated, primarily from immunocompromised hosts. Indiscriminate or inappropriate dispensing of acyclovir should be discouraged.

4. Vidarabine, another nucleoside analog, is effective in the treatment of serious herpes infections. However, it has no apparent superiority over acyclovir, may be less effective in some circumstances (e.g., herpes encephalitis), and has more potential side effects, including anemia and neurotoxicity.

5. Therapy with interferon reduces the virus yield but is ineffective against the latent stage in ganglia.

6. Foscarnet is the only antiviral approved by the FDA for the treatment of acyclovir-resistant HSV infections, a growing problem in the AIDS population. Foscarnet does not require HSV-encoded thymidine kinase. Foscarnet therapy reduces the healing time, pain, and viral shedding. It is administered intravenously, 40 mg/kg every 8 to 12 hours within 7 to 10 days in patients suspected of having acyclovir-resistant herpes simplex infection. Foscarnet is administered for 10 days. Associated side effects include azotemia secondary to nephrotoxicity, hyperphosphatemia, hypocalcemia, anemia, nausea, vomiting, and genital ulceration. Patients may eventually develop resistant strains. Preliminary trials indicate that topical 1% foscarnet cream may have some benefit for the treatment of acyclovir-resistant mucocutaneous HSV infection in patients with AIDS (8).

7. Cidofovir, a monophosphorylated nucleotide analog, does not require viral thymidine kinase phosphorylation to act and therefore has activity against herpes simplex infections with deficient or altered thymidine kinase activity. It is ineffective against rare strains with mutations in DNA polymerase. It is administered intravenously, 5 mg/kg/week for acyclovir-resistant infections in immunocompromised hosts. Associated side effects include nephrotoxicity and neutropenia. Concomitant administration of cidofovir with probenecid and saline hydration decreases the nephrotoxicity. Cidofovir resistance has not been documented.

8. Topical 1% penciclovir cream (Denavir) can reduce the time for healing of recurrent sunlight-induced herpes labialis by 2 days. Pain and discomfort are also diminished (9).

9. Topical 1.8% tetracaine cream can reduce the time for healing of recurrent herpes labialis by 2 days. Significant relief from itching is obtained (10).

10. Docosanol 10% cream (Abreva) was approved by the U.S. Food and Drug Administration (FDA) for over-the-counter topical use for recurrent herpes labialis. In clinical trials, use of docosanol decreased the healing time by 0.7 days, which is similar to the modest benefit obtained with the use of topical penciclovir cream (Denavir) in clinical trials. Docosanol is commonly used as a filler in lipsticks and other cosmetics. Docosanol acts by inhibiting fusion between the human cell membrane and the HSV envelope, thereby preventing viral entry into cells and viral replication.

B. General measures

1. The primary infection is extremely painful, and adequate analgesia is important. If salicylates or nonsteroidal anti-inflammatory drugs (NSAIDs) are inadequate, opiates may be needed for the first 7 to 10 days.

2. When lesions are vesicular, apply cool compresses with tap water or Burow's solution for 10 minutes t.i.d. to q.i.d.

3. Cleansing mouthwashes [with benzalkonium chloride (Zephiran) 1:1,000 or tetracycline suspension 250 mg/60 mL H_2O] both clean and soothe the involved mucous membranes and decrease secondary bacterial superinfections.

4. Vulvovaginitis and genital lesions may be aided by sitz baths in tepid water with or without Aveeno colloidal oatmeal. Women unable to void may sometimes be able to do so while in a bath. If not, intermittent catheterization or a temporary indwelling Foley catheter is necessary.

5. Apply topical antibacterials such as mupirocin (Bactroban), povidone-iodine ointment, or bacitracin ointment to prevent bacterial superinfection.
6. Early and repeated application of a potent corticosteroid to recurrent lesions will often decrease its severity by inhibiting the inflammatory response. If this modality is used, the periorbital area must be avoided.
7. If a consistent trigger factor for recurrent episodes can be identified, specific measures may be taken to counteract the stimulus (e.g., use of sunscreens). Treatment of primary infections is one of the few instances in which topical anesthetics are justified. Dyclonine hydrochloride (Dyclone), Benadryl elixir, or viscous Xylocaine may be used for oral lesions and benzocaine aerosol (Americaine) or Tronothane ointment may be beneficial symptomatically for the vulvar area. Application should be as frequent as necessary to keep the patient comfortable. The benzocaine preparations may sensitize the skin and should not be used routinely.
8. Prophylactic systemic antivirals should be given before facial surgical procedures (chemical peels, laser surgery, dermabrasion, etc.) if the anatomic area involves the site of a previous HSV infection.
9. Agents that have been shown to be ineffective or that have not been clearly shown to be useful include ethyl ether, chloroform, alcohol, idoxuridine (IDUR), adenine arabinoside (Vira-A), vitamins C, E, and B_{12}, lactobacillus, 2-deoxy-d-glucose, zinc, lysine, povidone-iodine, dye-light (photodynamic inactivation), silver sulfadiazine (Silvadene), nonoxynol-9 cream, and dimethyl sulfoxide (DMSO).
10. Many HSV vaccines have been under investigation; however, most have not shown effectiveness in either the treatment or the prevention of herpes genitalis.
C. **Ocular infection.** Patients with symptoms of corneal involvement (photophobia, pain) should be examined with a slit lamp. Herpes simplex keratitis is treated with trifluridine (Viroptic), idoxuridine (Herplex, Stoxil), or adenine arabinoside monophosphate (Vira-A); however, herpetic lesions of the lids and the immediate periorbital area, in the absence of ocular involvement, need not be treated with intraocular medication.

Disease/etiologic agent	Initial disease	Recurrent disease
Herpes simplex labialis	Valacyclovir 1 g b.i.d. × 10 d	Valacyclovir 2 g b.i.d. × 1 d
	Acyclovir 400 mg t.i.d. × 10 d	Famciclovir 500 mg t.i.d. × 5 d
		Acyclovir 800 mg t.i.d. × 5 d
		Topical 1% penciclovir q2h × 4 d
Herpes simplex genitalis	Valacyclovir 1 g b.i.d. × 10 d	Episodic therapy: famciclovir 125 mg b.i.d. × 5 d
	Famciclovir 250 mg t.i.d. × 10 d	Valacyclovir 500 mg b.i.d. × 3 d
	Acyclovir 400 mg t.i.d. × 10 d	Suppressive therapy: famciclovir 250 mg b.i.d.
		Valacyclovir 500 mg q.d. (if <10 episodes/year)
		Valacyclovir 500 mg b.i.d. (if 10 or more episodes/year)
		Acyclovir 800 mg t.i.d. × 5 d
		For immunosuppressed: famciclovir 500 mg b.i.d.

Adapted from Lin P, Torres G, Tyring SK. Changing paradigms in dermatology: antivirals in dermatology. *Clin Dermatol* 2003;21:426–446; Lin et al. (11).

References

1. Benedetti JK, Zeh J, Corey L. Clinical reactivation of genital herpes simplex virus infection decreases in frequency over time. *Ann Intern Med* 1999;131:14–20.
2. Wu JJ, Brentjens MH, Torre G, et al. Valcyclovir in the treatment of herpes simplex, herpes zoster, and other viral infections. *J Cutan Med Surg* 2003;7:372–381.
3. Tyring SK, Douglas JM Jr, Corey L, et al. A randomized, placebo-controlled comparison of oral valacyclovir and acyclovir in immunocompetent patients with recurrent genital herpes infections. The Valaciclovir International Study Group. *Arch Dermatol* 1998;134:185–191.
4. Wald A, Corey L. Antiviral therapies for long-term suppression of genital herpes. *JAMA* 1999;281:1169–1170.
5. Diaz-Mitoma F, Sibbald RG, Shafran SD, et al. Oral famciclovir for the suppression of recurrent genital herpes: a randomized controlled trial. Collaborative Famciclovir Genital Herpes Research Group. *JAMA* 1998;280:887–892.
6. Tyring SK, Diaz-Mitoma F, Shafran AD, et al. Oral famciclovir for the suppression of recurrent genital herpes: the combined data from two randomized controlled trials. *J Cutan Med Surg* 2003;7:449–454.
7. Spruance SL, Rowe NH, Raborn GW, et al. Perioral famciclovir in the treatment of experimental ultraviolet radiation-induced herpes simplex labialis: a double-blind, dose-ranging, placebo-controlled, multicenter trial. *J Infect Dis* 1999;179:303–310.
8. Javaly K, Wohlfeiler M, Kalayjian R, et al. Treatment of mucocutaneous herpes simplex virus infections unresponsive to acyclovir with topical foscarnet cream in AIDS patients: a phase I/II study. *J Acquir Immune Defic Syndr* 1999;21:301–306.
9. Boon R, Goodman JJ, Martinez J, et al. Penciclovir cream for the treatment of sunlight-induced herpes simplex labialis: a randomized, double-blind, placebo-controlled trial. Penciclovir Cream Herpes Labialis Study Group. *Clin Ther* 2000;22:76–90.
10. Kaminester LH, Pariser RJ, Pariser DM, et al. A double-blind, placebo-controlled study of topical tetracaine in the treatment of herpes labialis. *J Am Acad Dermatol* 1999;41:996–1001.
11. Lin P, Torres G, Tyring SK. Changing paradigms in dermatology: antivirals in dermatology. *Clin Dermatol* 2003;21:426–446.

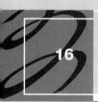

16

HERPES ZOSTER AND VARICELLA

Danielle M. DeHoratius

I. DEFINITION AND PATHOPHYSIOLOGY. Infection with the varicella-zoster virus (VZV), a double-stranded deoxyribonucleic acid (DNA) virus, will produce one of two clinical entities. Generalized, highly contagious, and usually benign chickenpox represents primary infection in a nonimmune host, whereas localized and painful zoster (shingles) is recurrence of a latent infection in the partially immune host. Clinical manifestations reflect the interaction between this virus and the host immune mechanisms.

Chickenpox, usually acquired through respiratory droplets, is seen primarily in the winter and spring, has an incubation period of 10 to 23 days, begins abruptly, and the lesions heal or even disappear within 7 to 10 days. Ninety percent of reported cases occur in children <10 years of age. Four percent of infections are subclinical. Almost every individual would have been infected by young adulthood. The disease is communicable 1 day before the appearance of the exanthem to 6 days after; crusts are noninfectious. Signs, symptoms, and complications often become more severe with age; adolescents and adults may become severely ill, particularly with pulmonary involvement. VZV infections during pregnancy can cause a distinct clinical syndrome. There is a 5% risk of fetal damage if intrauterine infection occurs during the first semester or early second trimester, producing the congenital varicella syndrome characterized by limb hypoplasia, muscular atrophy, skin scarring, cortical atrophy, microcephaly, cataract formation, and rudimentary digits. HIV-infected patients may experience atypical varicella, with a small number of disseminated pox-like lesions (1). Viral transmission may also occur through direct contact with the vesicles because of the high viral titers found within.

Zoster results from the reactivation of latent virus in dorsal root or cranial nerve ganglion cells. It is suspected that the virus is transported from the dorsal root or trigeminal ganglia through the myelinated nerves to the skin. As these nerves may terminate at the isthmus of hair follicles, primary infection first occurs in the follicular and sebaceous epithelium and then spreads to the rest of the epidermis. Histologic evidence reveals that herpes infection may occur exclusively in the folliculosebaceous units before the clinical appearance of vesicles (2).

The incidence of zoster shows no seasonal variation. Two thirds of patients are older than 40 years. Lesions erupt for several days and are usually gone within 2 to 3 weeks in children and 2 to 4 weeks in adults. Zoster is a self-limited, localized disease that causes discomfort for several days but usually heals without complications. Postherpetic neuralgia (PHN) is seen with increasing frequency in those older than 60 years of age and can be extremely painful, chronic, and, at times, unremitting.

In patients with serious underlying conditions that alter immunologic competence, more severe disease develops. Lesions may be greater in number and persist for up to 7 months in the immunosuppressed; visceral dissemination can occur in 8% of untreated immunocompromised patients. For children with lymphoma or leukemia, varicella is a life-threatening infection; adults with such diseases often develop zoster, which may then disseminate. Dissemination occurs in only 2% to 4% of zoster cases in normal hosts. However, of all cases of disseminated zoster, approximately two thirds of the patients have malignant disease, including approximately 40% with lymphoproliferative disorders. In Hodgkin's disease, dissemination occurs in approximately 25% of cases, with a mortality approaching 25%. In patients with any type of malignant disease and in particular Hodgkin's disease, localized dermatomal zoster also develops more frequently than in age-matched controls. The location of the affected dermatome is often related to a site of prior radiation therapy or to the presence of neoplastic lesions either centrally (lesions in or around the spinal column), causing neural irritation, or peripherally, as metastatic deposits. Immunosuppressive therapy for lymphoproliferative diseases or that used in transplantation programs predisposes to recurrence of varicella-zoster infection but not necessarily to dissemination. In patients known to be at risk for AIDS, the occurrence of zoster may be one sign that heralds depression of cellular immunity and may be the first sign of human immunodeficiency virus (HIV) infection.

II. SUBJECTIVE DATA

A. Varicella

1. Varicella in children is preceded by little or no prodrome; there may be only 24 hours of malaise and fever. In adolescents and adults, fever and constitutional symptoms almost always precede the exanthem by 24 to 48 hours. Patients are usually infectious for 1 to 2 days before the development of the rash and for 4 to 5 days following the beginning of the eruption, which is usually when the last vesicular crop has crusted over. Oftentimes, patients experience intense pruritus with the vesicular stage.

2. The appearance of cough, dyspnea, and chest pain within 2 to 5 days after the onset of the rash is indicative of severe pulmonary involvement.

3. Pruritus is the primary and most troublesome feature of chickenpox. Excoriation contributes to secondary bacterial infection and scarring.

B. Zoster.
The appearance of zoster lesions is frequently preceded by a mild to severe pre-eruptive pruritus, tenderness, or pain; the last may be generalized over the entire nerve segment, localized to part of it, or referred. Depending on the location, this pain may be confused with that of pleural or cardiac disease, cholecystitis or other abdominal catastrophe, renal or ureteral colic, sciatica, or other ailments. Neurologic changes within the affected dermatome include hyperesthesia, dysesthesia, or hypoesthesia. The interval between pain and eruption may be as long as 10 days but averages 3 to 5 days. In some patients, particularly children, there are no sensory changes. The pain will usually subside within several weeks, but 73% of patients older than 60 years of age have discomfort that persists beyond 8 weeks.

III. OBJECTIVE DATA (See color insert.)

A.
Chickenpox begins abruptly with the appearance of discrete, erythematous macules and papules located primarily over the thorax, scalp, and mucous membranes; the face and distal extremities remain less involved. Lesions progress rapidly from erythematous macules to 2- to 3-mm clear, tense, fragile vesicles surrounded by an erythematous areola. This appearance is often descriptively coined as "dew drops on a rose petal." As the lesions progress, they first become umbilicated and then within hours become cloudy and purulent, with crusts forming in 2 to 4 days. Varicella lesions appear in 3 to 5 distinct crops for up to a 5-day period, and lesions in all stages of development may be seen within one area. This is an important difference from smallpox. Crusts fall off in 1 to 3 weeks. Lesions usually heal without scarring. The most common complications are secondary bacterial infection of the skin lesions, usually staphylococci and streptococci. Adults often have a more complicated course with a more widespread rash, a prolonged fever, and an increased chance of complications, most commonly varicella pneumonia.

B.
Zoster lesions first appear posteriorly and progress to the anterior and peripheral distribution of the nerve involved (see dermatome charts on the inside covers). Only rarely will the eruption be bilateral. Erythematous macules, papules, and plaques are seen first, and in most instances grouped vesicles appear within 24 hours, although occasionally blisters never develop. Plaques may be scattered irregularly along a dermatomal segment or may become confluent. Mucous membranes within the dermatomes are also affected. The vesicles become purulent, crust, and fall off within 1 to 2 weeks. The presence of a few vesicles (10 to 25) outside the affected dermatome can occur and does not imply dissemination.

In >50% of individuals, zoster will involve the thoracic nerves; cervical or lumbar nerve involvement occurs in 15% to 20% of cases. Lesions on the tip of the nose herald involvement of the nasociliary branch of the ophthalmic division of the trigeminal nerve, implying a strong possibility of concomitant keratoconjunctivitis. Paresis and permanent motor damage are more common than previously thought and are found mostly with involvement of the trigeminal and upper cervical and thoracic nerves. Shingles may appear in multiple dermatomes both contiguous and noncontiguous and this is termed **zoster multiplex** (3), which is more common in immunocompromised individuals. VZV may reactivate without causing cutaneous vesicles but instead present with other symptoms and is termed **zoster sine herpete**. Overall incidence is 10% to 20%, with >66% of individuals affected with zoster being older than 50 years of age. Twenty-five percent of patients with HIV and 7% to 9% of patients with renal and cardiac transplant experience at least one episode of zoster. Ninety-five percent to 100% of individuals are seropositive for VZV antibodies. The disseminated form of zoster occurs in 2% to 20% of patients with herpes zoster; in contrast, up to 35% of patients with herpes zoster will have a few scattered vesicles in remote sites.

C. Those patients predisposed to more severe disease may show hemorrhagic, bullous, and infarctive-gangrenous lesions, which will heal slowly with scarring.

D. Persistent varicella zoster in an immunocompromised host may present with atypical hyperkeratotic papules.

IV. ASSESSMENT

A. Infection may be confirmed by cytologic smear of the vesicle, viral culture, direct immunofluorescence with a monoclonal antibody, biopsy, or serologic methods (see Chap. 15, sec. IV.B). Of 56 patients with typical clinical herpes zoster, 64% had positive Tzanck smears, 55% had positive immunofluorescence assays, and 26% had positive cultures (4).

B. Patients who are more at risk for severe varicella or those with disseminated zoster should be hospitalized and kept under strict precautions—in private rooms and away from seriously ill patients and those with lymphoproliferative disease or on immunosuppressive therapy. All patients with disseminated zoster or those severely ill with varicella should be investigated for underlying neoplastic or immunologic disease.

C. Approximately 50% of adults with varicella show nodular pulmonary infiltrates, but not all will manifest clinical respiratory disease. A chest x-ray is indicated for evaluation.

D. Nonimmune hospital employees who have been exposed to varicella should avoid patient contact for 8 to 21 days following exposure.

V. THERAPY

A. Varicella. Most patients with varicella require only symptomatic therapy.

   1. Localized itching may be alleviated by application of a drying antipruritic lotion (calamine alone or with 0.25% menthol and/or 1.0% phenol). Lotions with phenol should not be given to pregnant women. Powdered oatmeal baths are also helpful for the itching.

   2. Antihistamines may help pruritus. Salicylates should not be used for fever control to avoid Reye's syndrome.

   3. The patient should cut nails short and keep hands clean, and children should wear gloves, if necessary, to prevent excoriation.

   4. Mouth and perineal lesions may be treated by rinses or compresses with 1.5% hydrogen peroxide, saline, or other agents (see Chap. 15, sec. V.B).

   5. Apply topical antibiotic ointments to locally infected lesions. If infection is widespread, it is most often due to group A β-hemolytic *Streptococcus* or *Staphylococcus*, and systemic antibiotics should be used.

   6. The American Academy of Pediatrics does not recommend oral acyclovir routinely for the treatment of uncomplicated varicella in otherwise healthy children. This is due to the marginal therapeutic effect, the cost of the drug, and the feasibility of drug administration in the first 24 hours. Acyclovir [20 mg/kg (not to exceed 800 mg) PO q.i.d. for 5 days] is indicated for children over 24 months with chronic cutaneous or pulmonary disorders, as well as adolescents, who are found to have more severe diseases than young children. If the child is over 40 kg, the adult dose is appropriate. Administration of oral acyclovir within 24 hours of onset for 5 to 7 days has been demonstrated to reduce the maximum number of lesions, shorten the time to healing, decrease the number of patients with fever by the second day, and decrease severe itching.

7. Severe varicella, especially in the immunocompromised patient, should be treated with acyclovir as done for disseminated zoster.

8. Antiviral treatment of varicella (800 mg PO q.i.d. for 5 days) in healthy adults, initiated the first day of illness, decreases the time of illness, decreases the time to healing, and lessens symptoms. Valacyclovir and famciclovir have not been extensively studied for use in primary varicella infection.

9. In the immunocompromised or immunosuppressed population, intravenous acyclovir therapy is recommended. This is generally done to decrease the likelihood of life-threatening complications associated with severe disseminated disease such as pneumonia, encephalitis, thrombocytopenia, and purpura. This population may also be complicated by acyclovir-resistant strains of VZV; foscarnet is a potential alternative therapy. The varicella-zoster immune globulin (VZIG) may be indicated in highly susceptible individuals. If given within 96 hours of exposure, the disease is not prevented but the course may be modified. VZIG is indicated for infants born to mothers who experience the onset of chickenpox 5 days before delivery or within 2 days after delivery.

10. In March 1995, the U.S. Food and Drug Administration (FDA) approved the use of the live attenuated varicella vaccine for use in susceptible healthy children and adults. Recommendations include one-dose vaccination for healthy children 12 to 18 months of age and two-dose vaccination, in a 4- to 8-week interval, in adolescents aged 13 years or older who are at high risk for varicella exposure. Prophylactic immunization for all children and adolescents susceptible to varicella is recommended. Long-term immunity of children having received the varicella Oka vaccine strain has been observed to persist 10 years after administration. Nonetheless, the duration of immunity to varicella after childhood vaccination is not yet determined. Similarly, the risk of herpes zoster after vaccination needs to be established. The possibility of vaccine-induced primary varicella or herpes zoster infection is low. Vaccination of susceptible adults, particularly health care workers, international travelers, day care workers, family contacts of immunocompromised patients, and nonpregnant women of childbearing age, should be performed. Adverse reactions to the vaccine include fever, infection-site reactions, and rash. Although rare, the occurrence of vaccine-induced zoster infection in both immunocompetent and immunocompromised individuals has been reported. Two studies found that there is an increased risk of breakthrough varicella if the person has been vaccinated 5 or more years previously (5,6). An ongoing case–control study in Connecticut reported that vaccine effectiveness was 97% within the first 12 months but decreased to 84% thereafter (7). Concerns remain whether varicella vaccine in young children will create a cohort of adults at risk for potentially life-threatening varicella. At present, fewer than 2% of adults older than 30 years in the United States are susceptible to varicella. Mathematic models indicate that if varicella vaccine coverage in children exceeds 90%, a greater proportion of cases will occur at older ages, but the varicella disease burden will decrease for children and adults. The American Academy of Pediatrics strongly encourages physicians to support varicella immunization requirements for childcare and school entry. The effectiveness of a single dose of the vaccine in children under 13 is approximately 80%. A second booster dose may be considered for increased effectiveness, as is done with the measles-mumps-rubella vaccine. Certainly, a combination vaccination of varicella, measles, mumps, and rubella would increase the chances of this booster; however, the immunogenic formulation has been difficult up until this point (8). Kuter et al. showed that over 10 years of follow-up, children who received two doses of vaccine were three times less likely to develop breakthrough varicella as compared with the patients who received a single dose (9). Interestingly, even though there has been a decrease in vaccination-associated varicella, this has not resulted in increased incidence of herpes zoster (10).

B. Zoster

1. Acyclovir, a purine nucleoside analog, has been proved effective in both localized and disseminated zoster.

   a. Administered intravenously for acute zoster, it decreases the duration of pain and the healing time. In the immunocompromised patient, it can also prevent or abort dissemination. Side effects are rare but include a transient recurrence of pain on discontinuing therapy and impaired renal function following rapid infusion.

   b. Topical acyclovir (5% in polyethylene glycol applied q4h for 10 days) promotes healing of localized zoster in immunocompromised patients. However, it is ineffective in reducing pain and preventing postherpetic neuralgia.

   c. Oral acyclovir (800 mg q4h, five times daily for 7 to 10 days), if started within the first 24 to 48 hours, is capable of shortening the time to lesion crusting, healing, and cessation of pain, and reducing new lesion formation. Treatment within 72 hours at onset may halve the incidence of residual neuropathic pain at 6 months in immunocompetent patients (11). Acyclovir-resistant VZV infection has been reported in patients with AIDS; clinically, they have persistent, generalized hyperkeratotic papules. Two of the drugs listed below (Valtrex and Famvir) are more bioavailable prodrugs of Acyclovir and are therefore more effective. A comparison study between Valtrex and Famvir showed no difference in effectiveness (12).

2. Valacyclovir (Valtrex) is the L-valyl ester and prodrug of acyclovir. It displays improved bioavailability and prolonged half-life compared with acyclovir (see Chap. 15, sec. V.A.1). The current recommended dose of valacyclovir is 1,000 mg by mouth three times a day for 7 days. Valacyclovir is superior in decreasing the duration or PHN and zoster-associated pain compared with acyclovir. Valacyclovir is as effective as famciclovir. The use of valacyclovir is contraindicated in immunocompromised patients. Thrombotic thrombocytopenic purpura and hemolytic uremic syndrome have occurred in patients with advanced HIV disease, renal transplant, or bone marrow transplant.

3. Famciclovir (Famvir), another purine nucleoside analogue, was approved for use in herpes zoster in 1994. It displays improved availability compared with acyclovir and valacyclovir (see Chap 15, sec. V.A.2.). The dose is 500 mg three times a day for 7 days; the cost is similar to that of acyclovir. Famciclovir was effective in reducing PHN in individuals older than 50 years old when compared with placebo. Valacyclovir and famciclovir appear to be equally efficacious for the treatment of herpes zoster and both may be superior to acyclovir in decreasing the duration of acute pain as well as PHN. This suggests that both cost and prescription plan availability should be taken into consideration when selecting between the two newer antiviral agents.

4. Foscarnet is a pyrophosphate antagonist that inhibits DNA polymerase. It is approved for use in the treatment of acyclovir-resistant herpes zoster infections. It is administered intravenously, 40 mg/kg every 8 to 12 hours within 7 to 10 days in patients suspected of having acyclovir-resistant herpes zoster infection. Foscarnet is administered for 10 days. The associated side effects include azotemia secondary to nephrotoxicity, hyperphosphatemia, hypocalcemia, anemia, nausea, vomiting, and genital ulceration.

5. Analgesics should be given as necessary. Opiates may be needed.

6. For the vesicular stages, one of the following may be effective:

   a. Application of cool compresses with 1:20 Burow's solution.

   b. Painting of lesions with equal parts of tincture of benzoin and flexible collodion or with flexible collodion q12h.

   c. Application of a drying lotion containing alcohol, menthol, and/or phenol.

   d. Splinting the area with an occlusive dressing is often very useful in relieving pain. Lesions should be covered with cotton and then wrapped with an elastic bandage as for a fractured rib.

7. When lesions are crusted and/or secondarily infected, Burow's solution compresses should be applied (see Chap. 40, Wet Dressings, Baths, Astringents, sec. I.B.1) and systemic antibiotics used if appropriate.

8. Ocular involvement should be evaluated by an ophthalmologist. Herpes zoster keratoconjunctivitis is treated with topical ophthalmic corticosteroids. The distinction from herpes simplex keratitis is crucial, because the treatment is quite different (see Chap. 15, sec. V.C).

9. When herpes zoster occurs along the facial nerve and involves the geniculate ganglion—it may be accompanied by symptoms such as hearing loss and a rapid onset of facial pain—one must consider the diagnosis of herpes zoster oticus, also called **Ramsay Hunt Syndrome**. On physical examination, there may be a unilateral herpetic rash of the pinna and peripheral facial paralysis. Patients may also experience a loss of taste and vertigo.

10. Systemic corticosteroids are thought to decrease the incidence of PHN presumably by inhibiting perineural inflammation and fibrosis in patients older than 50 years of age. The effectiveness of this treatment remains unclear. Several regimens have been proposed, all advocating that treatment is started early (within 5 to 7 days of the eruption), adequate doses are used (40- to 60-mg prednisone PO daily or its equivalent), and treatment be continued for 3 to 4 weeks in a tapering fashion. Acyclovir with prednisone has been shown to be at least as effective as acyclovir alone in reducing the time to healing of the acute eruption (13). While the additional benefit of adding systemic corticosteroids is not significant, the doses used do not increase the risk of dissemination. Corticosteroids decrease the severity of edema and pain and are very useful in patients with severe facial swelling either with or without ocular involvement. The risk–benefit ratio must be determined for each patient. Two larger studies reported that the addition of oral steroids to an antiviral course showed no protective effect against PHN (13,14).

11. Intralesional injections of corticosteroids and/or anesthetics into the affected dermatome may be useful in decreasing the pain of acute zoster. Intralesional corticosteroids also might reduce the incidence of PHN in a fashion similar to their systemic usage. Use of the treatment techniques for injecting the involved skin is an innovative and useful approach (15).

12. Therapy with levodopa and benserazide (a peripheral decarboxylase inhibitor) has been reported to ameliorate the pain of acute zoster and, in elderly patients or those with ophthalmic zoster, to promote healing. Its effect on PHN is unclear.

13. Emetine or its derivative, dehydroemetine, with or without systemic corticosteroids, has also been reported to decrease the pain of acute zoster. Given their cardiotoxic side effects, these agents should be used with caution.

14. The use of a live attenuated vaccine (Oka/Merck) in older adults to prevent herpes zoster and PHN was recently reported in the New England Journal of Medicine. Previous studies show that VZV vaccines can significantly increase a person's cell-mediated immunity to VZV in immunocompetent older adults (16). In the subpopulation of hematopoietic-cell transplant recipients, the VZV vaccine reduced the incidence and severity of herpes zoster (17). Oxman et al. showed that the burden of illness, defined as the incidence, severity, and duration of the associated pain and discomfort, was reduced by 61.1% (p <0.001) and the incidence of PHN was decreased by 66.5% (p <0.001). The incidence of herpes zoster was reduced by 51.3% (p <0.001). In conclusion, the zoster vaccine markedly reduced morbidity from herpes zoster and PHN among older adults (18).

C. PHN is defined as pain persisting longer than 1 month up to at least 120 days following resolution of the vesicles. When the pain starts within 120 days of the rash, it is defined as subacute herpetic neuralgia. With acute infection there is direct viral damage and inflammatory neuritis of the peripheral nerve fibers, dorsal route ganglia, and the spinal cord. When the inflammatory phase decreases, fibrosis and destruction on nerve tissue begins and affects all levels of the pain pathway (19).

PHN occurs in 9% to 14% of patients. Its incidence and severity are directly related to age. The incidence in patients between ages 30 and 50 is 4%, in contrast to 50% in patients over the age of 80. The pain improves from severe to mild in two thirds of cases. Preexisting postherpetic pain is extremely difficult to alleviate, in testimony to which multiple approaches have been suggested. The most important strategy is prevention. Evidence supports the use of low doses of tricyclic antidepressants and phenothiazines. Local physical modalities can be helpful, and neurosurgical procedures remain an option in failed medical cases. Pain clinics can be very helpful in the long-term management of these patients. Researchers in the United Kingdom reported that after 3 months, 15% of patients still had pain and at 1 year roughly 5% to 10% still reported pain. Spontaneous resolution after 1 year is limited (20).

1. Application of capsaicin cream 0.025% or 0.075% (Zostrix) t.i.d. to q.i.d. may cause complete pain relief in 25% and reduction of pain in as many as 80% of patients with PHN. Capsaicin is a derivative of hot chilli peppers and depletes and prevents reaccumulation of the chemomediator substance P in peripheral sensory resources.

2. The use of a combination of a tricyclic antidepressant and a substituted phenothiazine medication may lead to relief of pain within 1 to 2 weeks after institution of therapy. Amitriptyline (Elavil) 75 to 100 mg daily should be used in combination with either perphenazine (Trilafon) 4-mg t.i.d. to q.i.d., fluphenazine hydrochloride (Permitil) 1 mg t.i.d. to q.i.d., or thioridazine (Mellaril) 25 mg q.i.d. Nortriptyline (Aventyl, Pamelor) may be substituted for amitriptyline, with the former being as effective but associated with fewer unpleasant side effects (21). It may be necessary to continue medication for months.

3. Chlorprothixene (Taractan) has been reported twice to be effective in the treatment of PHN. For severe pain, an initial 50 to 100 mg IM injection has been advocated. Otherwise, the dosage is 25 to 50 mg PO q6h. The recommended duration of therapy is 4 to 10 days. Higher doses are unwarranted and frequently result in side effects.

4. Gabapentin (Neurontin) significantly decreases pain scores and sleep interference associated with PHN. An initial dose of 300 mg/day is increased over 4 weeks (900, 1,800, 2,400, 3,600 mg/day divided t.i.d.) until efficacy is obtained or side effects become intolerable. Dose-limiting adverse effects include somnolence, dizziness, ataxia, peripheral edema, and infection (22).

5. Beneficial results have been reported with the combined use of either carbamazepine (Tegretol) 600 to 800 mg/day or phenytoin sodium (Dilantin) 300 to 400 mg/day with 50 to 100-mg nortriptyline (Aventyl, Pamelor) and with the combined use of carbamazepine (Tegretol) up to 1,000 mg/day and clomipramine up to 75 mg/day.

6. Opioids are effective in controlling neuropathic pain; therefore, oxycodone may provide some relief from PHN. In one study, patients treated with oxycodone experienced greater pain relief ($p <0.0001$) and reduced allodynia ($p <0.0004$) as compared with the placebo group. The initial dose was oxycodone 10 mg every 12 hours and was increased over 4 weeks to a maximum of 30 mg every 12 hours. Across the oxycodone group, the average dose was 45 mg/day (23).

7. Daily intralesional or subcutaneous injection of triamcinolone 0.2 mg/mL into the affected dermatome achieves pain relief in some patients with acute herpes zoster and in many patients with postzoster neuralgia. Up to 30 mL of the drug diluted in saline can be administered at each session. Injection by tumescent technique may be particularly helpful. Some authors report that when combined with local anesthetic and given over days or weeks the duration of pain is reduced (24).

8. Topical EMLA cream applied for a 24-hour period of time significantly decreased pain scores in PHN.

9. Lidocaine (5%) adhesive patch (Lidoderm) significantly reduces pain intensity. Several of the 10 × 14 cm patches can be used simultaneously to cover the affected area. Minimal systemic absorption of lidocaine occurs (25).

10. Repeated cryosurgery to limited areas affected by PHN has been reported to reduce the sensitivity of trigger areas and produce long-term relief from pain.
11. Transcutaneous electrical stimulation has brought pain relief to a high percentage of patients.
12. Neurosurgical intervention is occasionally necessary in patients with intractable pain.
13. Pain clinics at major medical centers can be helpful in evaluating and treating these patients. They often employ the use of nerve blocks (26).
14. Intrathecal methylprednisolone has been reported to relieve pain and allodynia. Potential toxicities include arachnoiditis or other neurotoxic event. This treatment may be most appropriately administered by a pain clinic or neurologist (27).

References

1. Perronne C, Lazanas M, Leport C, et al. Varicella in patients infected with the human immunodeficiency virus. *Arch Dermatol* 1990;126:1033–1036.
2. Walsh N, Boutilier R, Glasgow D, et al. Exclusive involvement of folliculosebaceous units by herpes. *Am J Dermatopathol* 2005;27:189–194.
3. Vu AQ, Radonich MA, Heald PW. et al. Herpes zoster in seven disparate dermatomes (zoster multiplex): report of a case and review of the literature. *J Am Acad Dermatol* 1999;40:868–869.
4. Sadick NS, Swenson PD, Kaufman RL, et al. Comparison of detection of varicella-zoster virus by the Tzanck smear, direct immunofluorescence with a monoclonal antibody, and virus isolation. *J Am Acad Dermatol* 1987;17:64–69.
5. Lee BR, Feaver SL, Miller CA, et al. An elementary school outbreak of varicella attributed to vaccine failure:policy implications. *J Infect Dis* 2004;190:477–483.
6. Tugwell BD, Lee LE, Gillette H, et al. Chickenpox outbreak in a highly vaccinated school population. *Pediatrics* 2004;113:455–459.
7. Vazquez M, LaRussa PS, Gershon AA, et al. Effectiveness over time of varicella vaccine. *JAMA* 2004;291:851–855.
8. Watson B. expert review of antinfective therapy—varicella-zoster vaccine in the USA: success for control of disease severity, but what next? *Future Drugs* 2005;3:105–115.
9. Kuter BH, Matthews H, Shinefield H, et al. Ten year follow-up of healthy children who received one or two injections of varicella vaccine. *Pediatr Infect Dis J* 2004;23:132–137.
10. Jumaan AO, Yu O, Jackson LA, et al. Incidence of herpes zoster, before and after varicella-vaccination-associated decreases in the incidence of varicella, 1992–2002. *J Infect Dis* 2005;191:2002–2007.
11. Jackson JL, Gibbons R, Meyer G, et al. The effect of treating herpes zoster with oral acyclovir in preventing postherpetic neuralgia. A meta-analysis. *Arch Intern Med* 1997;157:909–912.
12. Tyring SK, Beutner KR, Tucker BA, et al. Antiviral therapy for herpes zoster. Randomized, controlled trial of valacyclovir and famciclovir therapy in immunocompetent patients 50 years and older. *Arch Fam Med* 2000;9:863–869.
13. Whitley RJ, Weiss H, Gnann JW Jr, et al. Acyclovir with and without prednisone for the treatment of herpes zoster. A randomized, placebo-controlled trial. The National Institute of Allergy and Infectious Diseases Collaborative Antiviral Study Group. *Ann Intern Med* 1996;125:376–383.
14. Wood MJ, Johnson RW, McKendrick MW, et al. A randomized trial of acyclovir doe 7 days of 21 days with and without prednisolone for treatment of acute herpes zoster. *N Engl J Med* 1994;330:896–900.
15. Chiarello SE. Tumescent infiltration of corticosteroids, lidocaine, and epinephrine into dermatomes of acute herpetic pain or postherpetic neuralgia. *Arch Dermatol* 1998;134:279–281.
16. Levin MJ, Smith JG, Kaufhold RM, et al. Decline in varicella-zoster virus (VZV)-specific cell-mediated immunity with increasing age and boosting with high-dose VZV vaccine. *J Infect Dis* 2003;188:1336–1344.

17. Hata A, Asanuma H, Rinki M, et al. Use of an inactivated varicella vaccine in recipients of hematopoietic-cell transplants. *N Engl J Med* 2002;347:26–34.
18. Oxman MN. A vaccine to prevent herpes zoster and postherpetic neuralgia in older adults. *N Engl J Med* 2005;352:2271–2284.
19. Johnson RW. Herpes zoster in the immunocompetent patient: management of postherpetic neuralgia. *Herpes* 2003;10:38–45.
20. Bowsher D. The lifetime occurrence of herpes zoster and prevalence of postherpetic neuralgia: a retrospective survey in an elderly population. *Eur J Pain* 1999;3:335–342.
21. Watson CP. A new treatment for postherpetic neuralgia. *N Engl J Med* 2000;343:1563–1565.
22. Rowbotham M, Harden N, Stacey B, et al. Gabapentin for the treatment of postherpetic neuralgia: a randomized controlled trial. *JAMA* 1998;280:1837–1842.
23. Watson CP, Babul N. Efficacy of oxycodone in neuropathic pain: a randomized trial in postherpetic neuralgia. *Neurology* 1998;50:1837–1841.
24. Pasqualucci A, Pasqualucci V, Galla F, et al. Prevention of post-herpetic neuralgia: acyclovir and prednisolone versus epidural local anaesthetic and methylprednisolone. *Acta Anaesthesiol Scand* 2000;44:910–918.
25. Rowbotham MC, Davies PS, Verkempinck C, et al. Lidocaine patch: double-blind controlled study of a new treatment method for post-herpetic neuralgia. *Pain* 1996;65:39–44.
26. Wu CL, Marsh A, Dworkin RH. The role of sympathetic nerve blocks in herpes zoster and postherpetic neuralgia. *Pain* 2000;87:121–129.
27. Kotani N, Kushikata T, Hashimoto H, et al. Intrathecal methylprednisolone for intractable postherpetic neuralgia. *N Engl J Med* 2000;343:1514–1519.

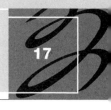

I. DEFINITION AND PATHOPHYSIOLOGY. Patients with pigmentary changes on their skin seek advice primarily for cosmetic reasons; they complain of having either too much or too little pigmentation, or they are unhappy with its distribution. Pigment changes are usually asymptomatic and of no medical consequence. However, they may signify underlying systemic disease. Treatment of diffuse and circumscribed hyper- and hypomelanotic disorders are the focus of this section.

A. Hyperpigmentation

1. Melasma (chloasma) is an acquired reticulated hyperpigmentation found most often on sun-exposed skin of women and men. Historically known as the "mask of pregnancy," its pathogenesis is now thought to be multifactorial. These factors include genetic predisposition, ultraviolet (UV) light exposure, oral contraceptive use, and pregnancy. Melasma may be found in men or women with no apparent endocrine abnormalities. It is present more frequently in darkly pigmented races.

2. Freckles (ephelides), like melasma, are present only on light-exposed skin; neither is found on mucous membranes. Freckling is genetically determined; usually appears by age 5 to 7 years; and is seen most commonly in redheads, blondes, and other fair-skinned individuals. Paradoxically, there are fewer melanocytes in a freckle than in normal surrounding skin, but those that are present are large and are able to form more melanin than usual. Freckles, like melasma, darken considerably during summertime and may fade almost completely in winter.

3. A lentigo (pl. lentigines) is most often confused with a freckle. These hyperpigmented spots, which may appear at any age, are usually darker than freckles and neither increase in darkness in the summer nor fade in the winter. Histologically, an increased number of melanocytes are present in the basal layer, and the epidermal rete ridges are elongated and clubbed.

   a. Solar lentigines (informally and inaccurately known as **liver or age spots**) appear on sun-exposed surfaces of fair-skinned people, usually in association with other changes from sun damage, including wrinkling, dryness, and actinic keratoses.

   b. Lentiginous pigmentation has been observed following prolonged psoralen plus ultraviolet A (PUVA) therapy, although these lesions, as opposed to solar lentigines, display melanocytic cytologic atypia.

   c. Lentigines associated with systemic disorders: multiple lentigines, especially if present on the palms, soles, mucous membranes, or non–sun-exposed skin, are often indicative of syndromes with significant internal abnormalities. Examples of such associations are the Peutz-Jeghers syndrome (lentigines, intestinal polyposis, ovarian tumors), the LEOPARD syndrome (lentigines, EKG changes, ocular hypertelorism, pulmonic stenosis, abnormal genitalia, retardation, and deafness), and the LAMB syndrome (lentigines, atrial myxoma, mucocutaneous myxomas, and blue nevi).

   d. Mucosal lentigines may occur on the lips, vulva, and penis. Labial melanotic macules occur most commonly on the lower lip of young women.

   e. Longitudinal pigmented streaks of the nails are common in darker-skinned individuals. However, they should be examined carefully for the possibility of an acral melanoma. Single pigmented bands, increasing in size with or without pigmentation of the nail fold, should be biopsied.

4. Postinflammatory hyperpigmentation is common in more darkly pigmented persons and is more related to the nature of the insult than to the degree of

111

previous inflammation; it is severe following some conditions, such as thermal burns, and mild after others. There is an increase in epidermal melanin, but melanin granules may also be present in dermal macrophages. Postinflammatory hyperpigmentation may persist for months to years.

B. Hypopigmentation

1. Vitiligo is a common, acquired disease affecting 1% to 2% of the population with women being more affected than men. Fifty percent develop their lesions before the age of 20 and 25%, before the age of 10. Localized or generalized areas of the skin completely lack melanin pigmentation. Melanocytes cannot be detected in depigmented areas, even on inspection by electron microscopy. This finding is in contrast to albinism, in which melanocytes are present but there is little or no pigmentation because of faulty or absent melanin synthesis. The cause of vitiligo is unknown; an abnormal neurogenic stimulus, intrinsic genetic defect of melanocytes, aberrant catecholamine response, an enzymatic self-destruction mechanism involving a deficiency of a melanocytic growth factor, a breakdown in epidermal free radical defense, and an autoimmune mechanism have been postulated as pathogenetic factors. Because of the association with other autoimmune diseases, an autoimmune etiology is favored. Serum of patients with active vitiligo has been found to be cytotoxic to normal melanocytes.

   Vitiligo appears to have a familial incidence of 20% to 30% and is found with increased frequency in patients with endocrinopathies. These include thyroid disease, Addison's disease, gonadal atresia, and pernicious anemia. In patients with vitiligo, there is also an increased incidence of halo nevi, diabetes mellitus, alopecia areata, and ocular abnormalities. Complete spontaneous repigmentation is rare.

2. Postinflammatory or posttraumatic hypopigmentation may be profound enough to mimic vitiligo but frequently appears as slightly scaly, slightly lighter areas of skin. It is often seen following cutaneous diseases such as psoriasis and atopic dermatitis and in those instances may be related to the inability of altered epidermal cells to accept melanin granules rather than to the decreased production of pigment in melanocytes. Pityriasis alba is found most frequently on exposed areas (e.g., face) in children with atopic backgrounds. Postinflammatory hypopigmentation repigments slowly but may be permanent in rare instances, especially if scarring has occurred.

II. SUBJECTIVE DATA. There are no symptoms associated with melasma, freckles, lentigines, or postinflammatory changes. The depigmented areas of vitiligo sunburn easily.

III. OBJECTIVE DATA

A. Melasma appears on sun-exposed skin as brown, gray, or even blue macules with irregular outlines or in a reticulated pattern on the cheeks, upper lip, and forehead.

B. Freckles (ephelides) are small (usually 2 to 5 mm), pale to dark macules scattered irregularly on the face, shoulders, back, and other sun-exposed areas. There is usually a sharp line of demarcation between freckled and unexposed skin.

C. Lentigines may be the same size as freckles or larger; they may be found anywhere on the cutaneous surface. Solar ("senile") lentigines are pale to dark-brown macules found on the dorsum of the hand and on the face. They vary in color and size (from millimeters to centimeters in diameter).

D. Vitiligo—There are three subtypes of vitiligo: localized (<20% of the body surface area, either focal or unilateral/segmental); generalized, also known as *vitiligo vulgaris*; and universal (complete or near complete depigmentation). Segmental vitiligo is much more common in children than adults and tends to spread rapidly within the segment of skin.

   The lesions of vitiligo are completely depigmented except in the rare case of trichrome vitiligo, which has both depigmented and hypopigmented areas. They usually have sharp borders and are found symmetrically over bone prominence such as the wrists and around body orifices (lips, eyes, and anogenital areas). Injury to the skin of these patients may cause a temporary or permanent loss of pigment in that area. Scars, scratch marks, and bruises may therefore heal with no pigment present. Hair growing from vitiliginous skin may or may not be depigmented.

E. Postinflammatory pigment changes vary in size and are present only at the site of previous inflammation and trauma. The degree of hyper- or hypopigmentation may be mild or marked.

IV. ASSESSMENT. It is useful to examine pigmentary lesions under Wood's light (see also Chap. 38, Wood's Light Examination). When pigment is present in the epidermis, the contrast between normal and hyperpigmented skin is enhanced. When pigment is present in the dermis, the contrast is not enhanced compared with ambient visible light. Thirty percent of patients with melasma will have pigment in the dermis, which makes treatment more difficult.

Patients with generalized lentigines and those with vitiligo deserve a thorough history and physical examination to search for related systemic findings. Patients with vitiligo, especially those in older age-groups, need to be checked periodically for incipient or clinically apparent thyroid disease, particularly hypothyroidism. T_4 and thyroid-stimulating hormone (TSH) determinations provide adequate screening. Phenolic germicidal agents present in household and industrial products may cause a chemical depigmentation indistinguishable from that of vitiligo.

V. THERAPY

A. Treatment of hyperpigmentation

1. Cryosurgery. Hyperpigmented macules and patches may be removed or their intensity of pigmentation diminished by light cryosurgical freezing (5 to 7 seconds of intermittent freeze) with liquid nitrogen. Melanocytes are more sensitive to cold injury than keratinocytes and may be selectively damaged by this technique.

2. Laser/light therapy. Treatment with the Q-switched ruby, Q-switched alexandrite, and Q-switched Nd:YAG are very effective. Latest studies show that laser with longer pulse width, such as long-pulse Nd:YAG or pulsed dye laser (PDL) may also be helpful. These lasers all target melanocytes and decrease hyperpigmentation, theoretically leaving the skin intact without scarring. However, they also carry a risk of postinflammatory hypo- or hyperpigmentation, scarring, and even keloid formation. Intense pulsed light (IPL) is a noncoherent, filtered, broad-spectrum light (500 to 1,200 nm) emitted from a pulsed flashlamp. IPL and PDL handpieces usually offer larger spot sizes, making them useful for treating large areas.

3. Topical bleaching agents

a. Hydroquinone (HQ) alone. The intensity of pigmentation in melasma, ephelides, lentigines, and the epidermal component of postinflammatory hyperpigmentation may be decreased by the regular application of 2% to 5% HQ cream or lotion b.i.d. for weeks to months. HQ over the counter is usually 2%; 4% is the typical concentration prescribed by dermatologists although pharmacists can mix concentrations up to 10%. HQ is thought to act by (i) competing with tyrosine oxidation by acting as an alternate substrate for tyrosinase, the enzyme that converts tyrosine to melanin and (ii) selective damage to melanosomes and melanocytes. Four to 6 weeks of monotherapy are required before depigmenting effects are seen. The hyperpigmented areas fade more rapidly and completely than the surrounding normal skin. The most common side effects are skin irritation and contact dermatitis which can be treated with topical steroids. A rare side effect is the development of exogenous ochronosis which can be extremely difficult to reverse. It is thought to result from the extended use of HQ, with the greatest risk in dark-complected individuals living in sunny climates. Alternating HQ in 4-month cycles with other depigmenting agents can prevent or reduce side effects.

b. Monobenzyl ether of hydroquinone (MBEH/Benoquin) is melanocidal. It is selectively taken up by melanocytes and metabolized into free radicals that can destroy melanocytes permanently, leading to irreversible depigmentation. As a result, MBEH is usually reserved for generalized depigmentation in patients with extensive vitiligo and should not be used under any other circumstances. This process requires 9 to 12 months of continuous daily application to achieve complete depigmentation.

c. **Kligman's formula.** Kligman and Willis in 1975 observed an enhanced efficacy of 5% HQ, 0.1% tretinoin and 0.1% dexamethasone in hydrophilic ointment in the treatment of melasma, ephelides, and postinflammatory hyperpigmentation. In contrast, they noted poor results using each of the aforementioned agents as monotherapies. A similar formulation is available as TRI-LUMA cream (fluocinolone acetonide 0.01%, HQ 4%, tretinoin 0.05%). The medications should be applied once at night and an SPF 30 sunscreen and protective clothing should be worn during the day.

d. Azelaic acid is a naturally occurring dicarboxylic acid derived from *Pityrosporum ovale*. It is available in strengths of 15% to 20% in the United States by prescription. It is applied b.i.d. for 3 to 12 months and is generally well tolerated.

e. Mequinol (4-hydroxyanisole) is a substrate of the enzyme tyrosinase and acts as a competitive inhibitor of melanogenesis. The combination of mequinol 2% and tretinoin 0.01% is available as Solagé and is indicated for twice-daily dosing.

f. Other treatments that are advocated for the treatment of hyperpigmentation include topical kojic acid, glycolic acid (either in topical preparations or peels in concentrations of 30% to 70%), topical Jessner's solution, and microdermabrasion. Multiple naturally occurring or alternative agents with potential therapeutic effects include aloesin (derivative of aloe vera), arbutin (found in bearberry fruits), licorice extract (Glabridin), soy, and vitamin C. These treatments have not been supported by rigorous clinical studies and represent a more theoretical and anecdotal experience.

g. **Combination therapy.** Numerous formulations are available on the market combining HQ together with sunscreens, vitamins, and α-hydroxy acids. Some of these products include Lustra, Lustra-AF, Lustra-Ultra, Glyquin, Eldoquin, Eldoquin Forte, Epiquin, and Soloquin Forte.

4. **Sun protection.** Because the ability of the sun to darken lesions is much greater than that of HQ to "bleach" the pigment, strict avoidance of sunlight is imperative. Although sunscreens help, even visible light will cause some pigment darkening, and to be totally adequate, sun protection must be opaque (e.g., Clinique Continuous Coverage). Some HQ products are available in an opaque base (Eldopaque, Eldopaque Forte) or with nonopaque sunscreens (Solaquin). Alternatively, a broad-spectrum sunscreen with sun protection factor (SPF) 15 or greater may be applied followed by makeup of the patient's choice.

B. **Treatment of vitiligo.** There are multiple methods that may be useful, including repigmentation methods, in addition to depigmentation in patients with widespread disease. All patients with vitiligo should practice aggressive sun protection measures. Avoidance of the sun during peak hours and/or conscientious use of broad-spectrum sunscreens should be stressed in all patients. Sun avoidance helps fade normal pigmentation in the fair-skinned individual, thereby making the vitiligo less noticeable. Patients with vitiligo should routinely use sunscreens with SPF 15 or greater that are effective against UVB when outside to prevent sunburn in nonpigmented areas.

1. **Psoralen plus ultraviolet A (PUVA)**

a. Systemic psoralen plus phototherapy attempts to repigment skin with the topical or systemic use of psoralen compounds. As a general guide, if the vitiliginous skin is <6 cm² (the size of a quarter or half-dollar), topical psoralens may be used; if a large portion of the body surface is involved, systemic psoralens and sunlight are indicated; if the area involved is extremely widespread (>50% of the body surface area), depigmentation with MBEH may be considered (see preceding text).

Psoralen compounds are tricyclic furocoumarin–like molecules found naturally in a variety of plants throughout the world and are also produced synthetically. They radically increase the erythema response of skin to long-wave ultraviolet light (UVA) after either topical application or systemic administration. Seventy-five percent of patients will have partial repigmentation when treated twice a week for more than a year. For this reason, therapy must be initiated gradually and monitored carefully.

The most commonly used oral psoralen is 8-methoxypsoralen (8-MOP). 8-MOP (Oxsoralen-Ultra) at a dose of 0.4 to 0.6 mg/kg, taken at least 1 hour before carefully monitored indoor UVA light source achieves some repigmentation in 70% of patients. Pigment reappears first as dots around hair follicles and then spreads slowly, becoming confluent. Dots of pigment should be seen within 25 exposures with facial lesions and 50 exposures with involvement elsewhere; if not, treatment should be discontinued. Treatments should be given one to two times weekly and never for 2 days in a row. Patients should be instructed to wear plastic-lens sunglasses known to block UVA before and after exposure on treatment days (UVA passes through glass). On nontreatment days, sun exposure should be restricted for patients on 8-MOP. Following treatment, a sunscreen effective against UVA should be applied to all exposed skin; this will provide partial protection. Those who sunburn easily may benefit from using a UVB sunscreen all day, even during treatment. Prolonged exposure to sunlight beyond the treatment period should be avoided for 8 hours after the medication has been ingested. Nontender, minimal pink coloration of the patches of vitiligo is acceptable, but if increasing redness develops, discontinue treatment until only faint pinkness remains.

To be successful, therapy must continue for 9 to 18 months. The age of the patient and duration of vitiligo do not affect the response rate. Lesions on the face and neck repigment more easily than those over an osseous prominence such as the dorsa of the hands, the elbows, and the knees. If treatment is discontinued before an area has completely filled in, the lesion is likely to gradually become white again. Psoralen therapy also increases the tolerance of vitiligo skin to sunlight, perhaps through thickening of the stratum corneum.

Psoralens may produce pruritus, nausea, corneal burns, and an acute and painful erythema. Long-term therapy with PUVA may produce premature aging, cataracts, photoallergic dermatitis, freckling of the skin, and an increased risk of skin cancer, including melanoma.

b. Bath PUVA. Dilute 1 mL of 8-MOP solution (1 mg/mL standard solution) in 2 L of warm water in a basin or dilute 10 mL of 0.1 mg/mL trioxsalen (trimethylpsoralen in 95% ethyl alcohol) in 2 L of warm water which must be agitated during soaking. The patient soaks the affected area of the body to be treated for 15 minutes, pats the skin dry, and then protects the nonaffected skin from the UV light. The initial dose for bath PUVA for all skin types is 0.5 J/cm^2 of UVA. The frequency is one to two times a week.

c. Paint PUVA. The patient should receive a compounded lotion containing 0.01% of 8-MOP or if prepared using an ointment base, the concentration should be 0.1% of 8-MOP. The compound is applied to the affected skin for 30 minutes. The initial dose of UVA for paint PUVA is 0.5 J/cm^2. After treatment, the area should be washed and protected from ambient UV exposure. The frequency is one to two times a week.

2. Narrowband UVB (NB-UVB) has demonstrated effectiveness as monotherapy (1). The initial starting dose is approximately 300 mJ/cm^2 with increments of 10% to 20% at each subsequent exposure. Treatment is administered 2 days a week. The advantages of NB-UVB over PUVA include shorter treatment times; no drug costs; reduced phototoxic reactions; and use in children, pregnant women, and patients with hepatic and kidney dysfunction.

a. The excimer laser (intense NB-UVB light at a wavelength of 308 nm) appears to be effective in repigmentation after at least six sessions. However, the results are temporary and must be maintained with retreatment.

3. Other phototherapies. Khellin and phenylalanine plus UVA have also been proposed for the treatment of vitiligo. There have been conflicting reports regarding these treatment strategies, including concern of hepatic toxicity with khellin, and, therefore, these are not considered first-line therapies for vitiligo (2). In addition, a combination of topical pseudocatalase and UVB has demonstrated conflicting results (3,4). Further studies are necessary.

4. Depigmenting the surrounding skin to blur the margins of the lesion or removing all remaining pigmentation in extensive cases may lead to cosmetic improvement. Blurring of the margins of the lesion may be attempted with HQ compounds. Permanent removal of pigment requires the use of MBEH (Benoquin) cream.

5. Camouflage the lesions using Covermark or Dermablend; Dy-O-Derm, a stain that contains aniline dyes and dihydroxyacetone; Vitadye, a cosmetic cover containing FD and C dyes and dihydroxyacetone; or quick-tan preparations containing dihydroxyacetone. These latter agents do not provide protection against sunburn, and psoralen phototherapy can take place through such stains.

   An aloe-based synthetic melanin product (Melasyn) is helpful in covering depigmented areas of vitiligo. This product offers protection against UV light and can be made waterproof by applying a spray-on sealant. (Vitiligo Solution Inc www.vitiligosolution.com.)

6. Topical immunomodulators may induce some repigmentation in up to 90% of patients. Application of 0.1% tacrolimus ointment twice daily for 2 months has been shown to be nearly as effective as superpotent topical corticosteroids and does not carry with it the risk of adverse effects (5,6).

7. Topical and intralesional corticosteroids have yielded very mixed results in the treatment of vitiligo, although for localized lesions, a trial of a potent topical steroid administered on a b.i.d. basis is worthwhile. The potential adverse reactions—particularly atrophy, glaucoma (if used near the eyes), and, for intralesional therapy, treatment-related depigmentation—must be kept in mind. Treatment is continued for 3 to 4 months. When topical corticosteroid treatment is contraindicated, calcipotriol and tacrolimus therapy can be considered.

   Low-dose oral corticosteroids (0.3 mg/kg/day) over a 4-month course were found to be helpful in patients with actively spreading vitiligo (7).

8. Permanent dermal micropigmentation using a nonallergenic iron oxide pigment can permanently tattoo recalcitrant areas of vitiligo (i.e., hands, perioral region, and the hairline).

9. Surgical techniques to transplant autologous melanocytes or cultured epidermal autografts to nonpigmenting areas have been found promising (8,9). Epithelial sheet grafting (after dermabrasion or suction blister formation), minigrafting, and "flip-top" procedure have been successful in stable vitiligo patients (10).

C. **Postinflammatory hypopigmentation.** Treatment is usually neither necessary nor rewarding. If any inflammation persists, antiinflammatory therapy is obviously advisable. Otherwise, the best approach is education, reassurance, and, if appropriate, concealing cosmetics.

References

1. Westerhof W, Nieuweboer-Krobotova L. Treatment of vitiligo with UV-B radiation vs topical psoralen plus UV-A. *Arch Dermatol* 1997;133:1525–1528.
2. Siddiqui AH, Stolk LM, Bhaggoe R, et al. L-Phenylalanine and UVA irradiation in the treatment of vitiligo. *Dermatology* 1994;188:215–218.
3. Patel DC, Evans AV, Hawk JL. Topical pseudocatalase mousse and narrowband UVB phototherapy is not effective for vitiligo: an open, single-centre study. *Clin Exp Dermatol* 2002;27:641–644.
4. Schallrueter KU, Wood JM, Lemke KR, et al. Treatment of vitiligo with a topical application of pseudocatalase and calcium in combination with short-term UVB exposure: a case study on 33 patients. *Dermatology* 1995;190:223–229.
5. Silverberg NB, Lin P, Travis L, et al. Tacrolimus ointment promotes repigmentation of vitiligo in children: a review of 57 cases. *J Am Acad Dermatol* 2004;51(5):760–766.
6. Lepe V, Moncada B, Castanedo-Cazares JP, et al. A double-blind randomized trial of 0.1% tacrolimus vs 0.05% clobetasol for the treatment of childhood vitiligo. *Arch Dermatol* 2003;139(5):581–585.

7. Kim SM, Lee H-S, Hann S-K. The efficacy of low-dose oral corticosteroids in the treatment of vitiligo patients. *Int J Dermatol* 1999;38:546–550.

8. Falabella R, Arrunategui A, Barona MI, et al. The minigrafting test for vitiligo: detection of stable lesions for melanocyte transplantation. *J Am Acad Dermatol* 1995;32:228–232.

9. Kim HU, Yun SK. Suction device for epidermal grafting in vitiligo: employing a syringe and a manometer to provide adequate negative pressure. *Dermatol Surg* 2000;26:702–704.

10. McGovern TW, Bolognia J, Leffell DJ. Flip-top pigment transplantation: a novel transplantation procedure for the treatment of depigmentation. *Arch Dermatol* 1999;135(11):1305–1307.

Suggested Readings

Guerra L, Capurro S, Melchi F, et al. Treatment of "stable" vitiligo by timed surgery and transplantation of cultured epidermal autografts. *Arch Dermatol* 2000;136:1380–1389.

Halder RM, Young CM. New and emerging therapies for vitiligo. *Dermatol Clin* 2000;18:79–89.

Nijoo MD, Westerhof W, Bos JD, et al. The development of guidelines for the treatment of vitiligo. *Arch Dermatol* 1999;135:1514–1521.

Nijoo MD, Bos JD, Westerhof W. Treatment of generalized vitiligo in children with narrow-band (TL-01) UVB radiation therapy. *J Am Acad Dermatol* 2000;42:245–253.

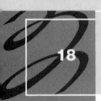

IMMUNOCOMPROMISED PATIENTS: HUMAN IMMUNODEFICIENCY VIRUS- AND NON-HUMAN IMMUNODEFICIENCY VIRUS POSITIVE

18

Elaine S. Gilmore and Wanla Kulwichit

 HUMAN IMMUNODEFICIENCY VIRUS

The human immunodeficiency virus (HIV) is an enveloped ribonucleic acid retrovirus that infects CD4$^+$ T lymphocytes as well as both macrophages and monocytes. The multiple dermatologic manifestations of HIV disease are secondary to these immunologic changes. Up to 92% of HIV-positive patients display skin signs at some point during their illness. As the number of CD4$^+$ cells decreases and acquired immunodeficiency develops, skin diseases become more common and often more difficult to treat. These patients may have common skin diseases with both typical and atypical presentations and uncommon skin diseases that may be the initial presentation of a serious systemic infection. Preexisting diseases such as psoriasis may worsen in HIV-infected individuals. The sudden onset of previously inactive acne in an adult may indicate immunosuppression from HIV.

Triple antiretroviral therapy, a combination of a nonnucleoside reverse transcriptase inhibitor (NNRTI) or a protease inhibitor (PI) plus two nucleoside reverse transcriptase inhibitors (NRTIs), has had a large impact on the natural history of HIV disease. This regimen is also referred to as highly active antiretroviral therapy (HAART). Many patients have partial restoration of immune function and very low viral loads on this therapy with fewer cutaneous diseases reported. However, owing to the immune reconstitution syndrome, patients starting HAART are at a fivefold increased risk of developing herpes zoster. While molluscum contagiosum and Kaposi's sarcoma (KS) regress, eosinophilic folliculitis (EF) can appear and worsen particularly within the first 3 to 6 months of treatment. Human papillomavirus (HPV) infections do not respond favorably to HAART, with some evidence that prevalence or severity may worsen. Itraconazole and isotretinoin can interact with HAART.

The main treatment for HIV-related skin disease is maximal suppression of the virus. Emergence of any new HIV-related skin disease while on antiretroviral therapy may be a clue that the current regimen is inadequate.

The following is a compilation of HIV-related skin diseases and is designed as a general overview. Refer to related chapters in this text and others that are referenced for in-depth discussion of these disorders and for specific treatment protocols.

I. OVERVIEW: HIV-RELATED SKIN DISEASES

A. Acute exanthem. An acute retroviral syndrome occurs in most individuals 3 to 6 weeks after successful infection by the HIV virus (1). The symptoms are similar to a mononucleosis-like syndrome with fever, headache, sore throat, malaise, and lymphadenopathy. Leukopenia, thrombocytopenia, and a decrease in CD4$^+$ cells can occur. This syndrome is secondary to viral antigenemia with seroconversion from 1 to 12 weeks after the onset of symptoms. The exanthem consists of a morbilliform eruption present predominantly on the trunk, face, and neck and usually resolves spontaneously. The individual lesions may resemble pityriasis rosea lacking peripheral scale but with focal hemorrhage. A Gianotti-Crosti–like syndrome with monomorphous papules over joints may occur. These rashes are usually asymptomatic, although pruritus may occur. Urticaria, vesicles, and desquamation have been described. Associated findings in the oral mucosa consist of erythema, petechiae, stomatitis, and erosions that may resemble aphthae in the mouth, esophagus, and anus. Dysphagia may be a prominent symptom. The greater the number of signs and symptoms at the time of acute seroconversion, the more rapid the disease progression, especially if oral candidiasis is present (2). HIV testing should be performed on febrile patients with poorly defined cutaneous and mucosal signs and symptoms.

B. Allergic reactions. Patients with HIV have a high incidence of drug eruptions; 50% to 80% of patients with HIV have allergic reactions to trimethoprim-sulfamethoxazole, usually with a macular and papular eruption; 50% of these patients will also develop a rash with dapsone and/or pentamidine. Erythroderma, Stevens-Johnson syndrome, and toxic epidermal necrolysis have also occurred with this drug. This high incidence of drug eruptions may be analogous to the rash that occurs with ampicillin and mononucleosis; either cytomegalovirus (CMV) or Epstein-Barr virus (EBV) may be interacting with the drug.

C. Viral infections: herpesviruses

1. CMV. CMV is the most common postmortem infection found in patients with HIV infection. Although cutaneous findings are rare and there are no characteristic mucocutaneous lesions, the presence of this pathogen should be considered in patients with persistent anogenital and oral ulcerations. Clinical presentations can vary from ulcers, vesicles, and verrucous lesions to digital infarcts. Because of the ubiquitous nature of this virus, it may be only an associated finding when detected in a culture or biopsy. CMV is often cocultured with herpes simplex virus (HSV) or varicella-zoster virus. Systemic CMV infection may cause a severe retinitis with blindness.

2. EBV. In HIV-infected individuals, EBV is associated with the development of classic Burkitt's lymphoma, large cell lymphoma, and Hodgkin's disease. EBV has selectivity for mucosal epithelial cells, making the oropharynx the usual route of primary infection. It acts as a cofactor and has been shown to enhance the growth of the HIV virus.

3. Oral hairy leukoplakia (OHL) is caused by EBV as a form of lytic replication of the virus. OHL is essentially specific for HIV disease, and its presence correlates with a moderate-to-severe degree of immunodeficiency. It rarely occurs in other immunosuppressed populations and children with HIV disease. This asymptomatic plaque is found most commonly on the lateral border of the tongue but has also been observed on the buccal mucosa. The surface is verrucous with white to gray parallel, vertical rows that have a corrugated appearance. OHL is not a premalignant condition and therefore often left untreated. However, topical podophyllin, topical retinoids, or oral acyclovir (200 mg five times a day or 400 mg b.i.d.) may improve the clinical appearance or dysphagia, if present (3).

4. HSV. Classically, HSV-1 is the agent responsible for herpes labialis and HSV-2, for herpes genitalis. However, there is increasing evidence of crossover infection, with HSV-1 implicated in 5% to 30% of primary genital herpes. Genital herpes infection is likely to enhance the sexual transmission of HIV owing to the break in the normal skin barrier function. HSV infection is common in patients with acquired immunodeficiency syndrome (AIDS), with a prevalence of 18% to 27%. The severity of symptoms parallels a decrease in the number of CD4$^+$ cells. Hematogenous dissemination of the virus is rare, although the virus may disseminate widely, especially if there is an extensive cutaneous disease present such as atopic dermatitis (Kaposi's varicelliform eruption). Additionally, HSV can manifest as herpes keratoconjunctivitis, herpetic whitlow, and herpes keratitis. HSV lesions can be zosteriform in arrangement. An unusual clinical variant with chronic deep ulcerations in periorificial areas (most commonly perianal) has been described. These ulcers may become impetiginized and require long-term oral acyclovir administration to prevent relapse. Failure of routine antiviral therapy may be indicative of an acyclovir-resistant virus requiring foscarnet or other antiviral therapy.

5. Herpes zoster. Herpes zoster occurs with 7 to 15 times the expected incidence in HIV-positive patients (25% of adults). Consequently, HIV risk factors should be addressed in patients developing herpes zoster. The eruption occurs as the CD4$^+$

cell count decreases and may be dermatomal, multidermatomal, recurrent, or disseminated; all forms may be associated with severe pain and a high incidence of postherpetic neuralgia. Herpes zoster ophthalmicus can be associated with acute retinal necrosis in HIV-positive patients. A chronic verrucous cutaneous herpes zoster with necrotic lesions resembling ecthyma has been described. Acyclovir-resistant herpes zoster is well described and can be treated with intravenous foscarnet until clearance of lesions. The risk of herpes zoster increases with the immune reconstitution syndrome after the initiation of triple antiretroviral therapy (4).

Primary varicella in patients with AIDS may be severe; prolonged; and complicated by pneumonia, hepatitis, encephalitis, and death. HIV-positive patients with exposure to varicella may require prophylactic treatment with varicella immune globulin or acyclovir. Children with AIDS can develop herpes zoster soon after a primary varicella infection. The incidence of unusual clinical features and severe, persistent varicella infections is greater in HIV-infected children than in the normal population.

D. Other viral infections
   1. Molluscum contagiosum. Molluscum contagiosum is caused by a deoxyribonucleic acid pox virus and occurs in 18% of patients with AIDS. The lesions may be quite extensive, especially in the beard area. Giant lesions occur as grape-like clusters of multiple small lesions. The morphology is not as distinctive as in immunocompetent patients. If a central umbilication is noted after lightly touching a lesion with liquid nitrogen, the diagnosis is clear. Disseminated infections by *Penicillium marneffei, Mycobacterium spp., Pneumocystis jiroveci, Histoplasma, Cryptococcus,* and rarely *Toxoplasma* in immunocompromised patients may mimic molluscum contagiosum. It is best to avoid shaving affected areas to prevent spread. Treatment options include liquid nitrogen, curettage, and imiquimod 5% cream.
   2. HPV. Anogenital warts are present in as many as 40% of HIV-infected homosexual men. Large, difficult-to-treat lesions may develop, and squamous cell carcinoma (SCC) *in situ* has been well described secondary to HPV subtypes 6, 11, 16, 18, 31, and 33. Multiple common warts on the face and hands are more common and difficult to treat. Facial lesions may have a hemorrhagic morphology, and plantar warts may be quite large and recalcitrant to therapy.
E. Yeast infections
   1. Candida albicans. Almost 100% of patients with AIDS have candidiasis at some point in their disease. The most common form is oral mucosal involvement, and this may be the presenting complaint before the diagnosis of HIV infection. Oral candidiasis may be asymptomatic or have symptoms of burning. The common subtypes of oral candidiasis include white exudative, erythematous, hyperplastic (commonly on the tongue), and angular cheilitis. As the number of CD4 cells decreases, more erosive changes can occur with a subsequent loss of taste. *Candida esophagitis,* a sign of AIDS, will present with dysphagia. Disseminated candidiasis is very uncommon. Vaginal candidiasis is a common initial presentation of HIV disease in women (more common than oral involvement). Children with AIDS may have extensive diaper dermatitis secondary to *Candida.* Young children may also develop a *Candida* onychodystrophy. Oral candidiasis in children is an indication of disease progression and poor prognosis. Patients with HIV have an increased incidence of achlorhydria, and therefore, ketoconazole and itraconazole are less well absorbed.
   2. Malassezia furfur complex. *M. furfur* complex, a group of superficial yeasts, can cause a folliculitis on the trunk and upper arms in patients with HIV. This is also the organism related to the pathogenesis of seborrheic dermatitis. Intravenous catheter sepsis from this ubiquitous organism has also been reported. A special olive oil media is required for culture of *Malassezia.* Tinea versicolor, also caused by this organism, is common, more extensive, and difficult to treat in patients with AIDS. Oral antifungal therapy is often required. A KOH preparation is diagnostic, with both yeast and spore forms identified.

3. **Superficial mycoses.** The prevalence of tinea pedis in patients with HIV is 29% to 37%, only slightly higher than controls. However, the severity and type of infection vary. Infection of the nails may present as proximal subungual onychomycosis or superficial white onychomycosis. *Trichophyton rubrum*, rather than *Trichophyton mentagrophytes*, is the most common pathogen. Tinea faciale should be included in the differential diagnosis of patients with difficult-to-treat "seborrheic dermatitis."

F. **Deep mycoses**

1. **Cryptococcus.** The most common deep fungal infection in patients with AIDS is cryptococcosis; cutaneous lesions may be found in 2% to 9% of patients. Disseminated disease may present with 1- to 4-mm molluscum contagiosum–like papules; necrotic ulcerating centers may occur. The infection may be polymorphic with nodules, pustules, abscesses, ulcers, vegetating lesions, and herpetiform patterns described. The hard palate may also be involved and ulcerated. A skin biopsy with special stains is diagnostic. Once systemic involvement has been determined, antifungal agents (intravenous amphotericin B, flucytosine, and fluconazole) can be lifesaving. Maintenance therapy until improved immune status is achieved is recommended especially in patients with AIDS.

2. **Histoplasmosis.** Eleven percent of patients with pulmonary or disseminated histoplasmosis will have cutaneous involvement. As with *Cryptococcus*, the skin lesions may resemble molluscum contagiosum. Other manifestations include ulcers, plaques, cellulitis, a diffuse dermatitis, and perianal ulceration. The oral mucosa is commonly involved. Biopsy, culture, and special stains will help in the diagnosis.

G. **Sporotrichosis.** Systemic sporotrichosis has been described in patients with HIV who have no history of exposure to soil or plants; the presumed portal of entry is the lung, with subsequent hematogenous dissemination. Skin lesions, although uncommon, may present as enlarging, crusted, violaceous nodules. Erosive arthritis and osteomyelitis are seen in 80% of these patients. Pulmonary disease may be difficult to treat, requiring amphotericin B for an effective response. Itraconazole can be used for cutaneous lesions or prophylaxis after amphotericin B treatment in patients with AIDS and with disseminated disease.

H. **P. marneffei.** Endemic to Southeast Asia and China, this is a fairly new opportunistic infection in HIV disease. Papular skin lesions with central necrotic umbilication on the face and extremities can be seen in two thirds of patients. Other symptoms of generalized dissemination include generalized lymphadenopathy, hepatomegaly, splenomegaly, anemia, and thrombocytopenia (5). Treatment involves itraconazole in mild cases and amphotericin B in severe infection, followed by maintenance azole therapy (6).

I. **Bacterial infections.** With advancing immunosuppression in HIV disease, B cell function is also affected with loss of specific antibody function including the eradication of encapsulated organisms such as *Streptococcus pneumoniae* and *Haemophilus influenzae*. Patients often have a functional neutropenia making them more susceptible to infection.

Pyodermas are very common in patients with AIDS, especially children, including folliculitis, cellulitis, hidradenitis, and abscesses. *Staphylococcus aureus* is the most common pathogen. Impetigo, bullous impetigo, ecthyma, staphylococcal scalded skin syndrome (SSSS), and toxic shock syndrome have all been reported in patients with AIDS. A toxic streptococcal syndrome caused by group A β-hemolytic *Streptococcus* includes symptoms of lymphadenitis, fever, diarrhea, hypotension, and a scarlatiniform rash. Nasal carriage of *S. aureus* is increased in HIV-positive patients, and nasal septal abscesses can occur. Chlorhexidine gluconate washes and topical antibiotic treatment of the nares can help reduce colonization.

J. **Nonbacterial folliculitis.** EF is a pruritic follicular eruption that resembles Ofuji's disease (a condition seen primarily in Japanese patients). The skin findings include urticarial and/or follicular papules on the head, trunk, and proximal extremities. Most of the lesions are above the anterior nipple line, extending down the midline of the back toward the lumbar spine. Pustules are rarely found, but are usually on the forehead and trunk. An associated eosinophilia and elevated serum immunoglobulin E level are frequently seen. The CD4$^+$ cell count is usually <200/mL. Therapy with systemic antibiotics, itraconazole, ultraviolet B phototherapy, and isotretinoin (Accutane) has been reported to be effective in this disorder. However, cases can be resistant to treatment.

K. Mycobacterial infections

1. *Mycobacterium avium* complex is present in 50% of autopsies of patients with AIDS; skin involvement is very rare but has been described as follicular, crusted papules, as well as ulcers and verrucous plaques. Lymph nodes may be infiltrated, with the organism causing matting and erythema of the overlying skin.

2. **Tuberculosis.** Active tuberculosis is present in 10% of patients with AIDS, and with 50% having at least one extrapulmonary site involved. Cutaneous forms of the disease are rare, but can present with nodules, erythematous papules, and vesiculopustules. The use of HAART has decreased the incidence of this form of the disease.

L. Spirochete infections. Seventy percent of homosexual patients with HIV have a history of syphilis, caused by *Treponema pallidum*. Syphilitic chancres and other genital ulcers alter the cutaneous barrier and predispose individuals to being coinfected with HIV. Progression from primary to tertiary syphilis or rapid progression to central nervous system (CNS) syphilis in patients with AIDS can occur in several months. Characteristic lesions of the papulosquamous variety are observed, in addition to noduloulcers. Lues maligna, a papulopustular eruption associated with fever, headache, and myalgias, is seen more often in patients with HIV. Standard penicillin regimens have failed to cure syphilis in some patients with AIDS, thereby requiring a longer duration of therapy. The spirochetal reservoirs include the CNS, lymph nodes, spinal cord, and liver. Recurrent secondary syphilis has been described in addition to one case of biopsy-proven secondary syphilis with negative serologies.

M. Infestations. Scabies, resulting from infestation with *Sarcoptes scabiei*, may be more severe and extensive in patients with AIDS, with involvement of the face and scalp described in adults. The distribution may also be atypical without classic intertriginous involvement, sometimes resembling pityriasis rosea. Burrows are less commonly observed in patients with HIV than in those with intact immune systems. With advanced immunosuppression, crusted (Norwegian) scabies is more common, with thick, crusted plaques often on the hands and feet containing a large number of mites. Patients with AIDS have an increased incidence of postscabietic dermatitis and pruritus. Scabies should be considered in all immunocompromised patients with unexplained pruritus. Treatment includes both topical agents (Permethrin cream 5% overnight on days 1 and 8; Lindane lotion 1% overnight) and oral antiparasitic agents (Ivermectin 250 to 400 μg/kg) (3).

N. Bacillary angiomatosis is a potentially fatal disease that is presumed to be caused by a gram-negative organism, *Bartonella quintana*, the causative agent of trench fever. The clinical manifestations include the presence of rubbery, red, firm, papules and nodules, often on the upper trunk and face. Infection usually involves the liver and spleen. They clinically resemble pyogenic granulomas, with red-purple papules, nodules, and ulcers that bleed easily. Biopsy of a skin lesion with a Warthin-Starry stain performed can identify the organism. Treatment is with oral erythromycin 2 g/day or doxycycline 200 mg/day for 3 months (7). Without effective treatment, pulmonary and hepatic failures can develop.

O. Neoplasias. As many as 40% of patients with AIDS will develop one or more malignancies in their lifetime.

1. **KS.** KS occurs in 11% to 15% of patients with AIDS; 95% of KS has occurred in homosexual men, although the incidence has decreased possibly due to safe sex practices. The causative agent of KS and primary effusion (body cavity) B cell lymphoma is the human herpesvirus 8. This virus infects the general population, with the highest seroprevalence in the young adult years presumably secondary to sexual transmission. Children rarely have KS, although when present it has an aggressive course.

The skin is the most common site of involvement, although 5% of patients have no cutaneous lesions. In its early stages, the morphology is variable but marked by unusual symmetry of lesions. Early lesions can present as violaceous papules and plaques to ulcerated nodules. The differential diagnosis includes purpura, a hematoma, a melanocytic lesion, or a fixed drug eruption. Variations in arrangement include linear, perifollicular, and dermatomal. Mucosal lesions are common especially on the palate; examination of the oral mucosa often helps support the diagnosis if both cutaneous and mucosal lesions are present. KS may rapidly progress to tumors and ulcerations, but it also may regress spontaneously.

Treatment is recommended if functional or cosmetic improvements are of concern (8). Radiation therapy causes remission of lesions in 93% of patients, but should be avoided for oral mucosal lesions because of side effects of severe radiation-induced stomatitis. Local destruction can be effective with liquid nitrogen; surgical excision, oral thalidomide, and intralesional injection of vinblastine or bleomycin are all treatment options. Systemic chemotherapy does not alter survival, may compromise an already impaired immune system, and should be considered only in selected cases. Use of systemic interferon-α may bring about tumor shrinkage. AIDS-related KS can respond well to triple antiretroviral therapy.

2. **Lymphoma.** The presence of HIV infection increases the risk of development of lymphoma. Non-Hodgkin's B cell type lymphomas are the second most frequent neoplasm in patients with AIDS. The skin is involved in 15% of patients. The disease is usually diagnosed at an advanced stage, after other opportunistic infections have occurred. The median survival is only 5 months. Other B cell processes seen in patients with AIDS include primary B cell lymphoma of the brain, Burkitt's lymphoma, chronic lymphocytic leukemia, and multiple myeloma.

Hodgkin's disease in this setting has an aggressive course with a median survival of 14 months. Cutaneous involvement, both contiguous and noncontiguous spread, is more common in HIV-infected patients than in noninfected patients. Cutaneous T-cell lymphoma has also been reported in patients with AIDS with both indolent disease resembling mycosis fungoides and Sézary syndrome. Large cell lymphomas have a poor prognosis; these cells are usually CD30 positive and harbor the EBV. Adult T-cell leukemia and lymphoma are observed in this population and testing for human T lymphotrophic virus type 1 (HTLV-1) infection should be pursued.

3. **SCC.** The rate of SCC is increased in HIV-positive patients, as in other immunocompromised patients. The number of lesions does not appear to correlate with the degree of immunosuppression. HIV-positive patients develop SCC at an earlier age than the general population and often involve unexposed sites. Periungual SCC has been seen in patients with HIV and is associated with high-risk HPV subtypes.

Women with HIV disease have a significantly higher incidence of cervical SCC with higher degrees of dysplasia than controls. The incidence of cervical carcinoma parallels the decrease in CD4 cell number. More widespread involvement is common with extension to the vagina and vulva; the recurrence rate is 36% versus 8% of non–HIV-infected patients.

Anogenital SCC is seven times more common in homosexual men with HIV disease than in those without. Approximately 64% of specimens have been found to contain HPV, most commonly subtypes 16, 18, and 33. Replication of more oncogenic HPV subtypes is associated with increased immunosuppression. The HIV tat protein has been shown to increase expression of HPV. Velvet-like plaques that may be white or hyperpigmented with erosions can involve the entire perianal area including the anal canal. Cloacogenic carcinoma, arising in the transitional mucosa of the anal canal, occurs in individuals who practice receptive anal intercourse. These patients experience rectal bleeding, constipation, and occasionally perirectal erythema and induration. There is also an increased incidence of condyloma acuminatum in this population.

4. **Basal cell carcinoma (BCC).** BCC has been seen with increased frequency in HIV-infected patients. The most common presentation is a multifocal BCC on the trunk in fair-skinned men between the ages of 20 to 60 years. There have been rare reports of metastases.

5. **Malignant melanoma (MM).** The incidence of MM in HIV-positive patients has not been established; however, melanomas, including multiple primary tumors, have been reported. At the time of diagnosis, the melanomas tend to be thicker (average Breslow measurement of 2.61 mm), and metastases are common. Seven patients have been described with multiple eruptive dysplastic nevi, and some had coexisting melanoma.

P. Side effects of HIV therapy

1. PI therapy has been associated with the induction of cervical fat pad development resembling Cushing's syndrome. Computed tomography scans demonstrated nonencapsulated adipose tissue. Submandibular fat accumulation and central obesity are also described (9). Patients with HIV not taking PI have also developed this "buffalo hump."

2. Lipodystrophy syndrome, with localized loss of adipose tissue in the cheeks, forehead, and extremities is also described in patients with HIV receiving long-term antiretrovirals (10).

3. Foscarnet can lead to painful oral and genital ulcers in 30% of patients who are on high-dose therapy.

4. Liposome-encapsulated doxorubicin used in the treatment of KS has been associated with a painful hand and foot syndrome. The initial swelling and painful extremities may ultimately develop erosions, fissures, and desquamation.

5. Azidothymidine (AZT) is associated with linear pigmented bands of the nails, a morbilliform eruption, and a rare dermatomyositis-polymyositis–like syndrome.

Q. Other cutaneous disorders associated with HIV infection (Table 18-1)

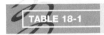

TABLE 18-1	**Cutaneous Disorders Associated with HIV Infection**

Vascular diseases	Aphthous ulcerations
Periarteritis nodosa	Acute necrotizing gingivitis
Granulomatous angiitis	Pigmentation secondary to AZT
Leukocytoclastic vasculitis	Hair diseases
Telangiectasias	Alopecia areata
Angiomas	Telogen effluvium
Papulosquamous diseases	Premature graying
Psoriasis	Elongated eyelashes
Palmoplantar keratoderma	Nail diseases
Reiter's syndrome	Linear hyperpigmentation: AZT
Dermatitis	Leukonychia
Xerotic eczema	Splinter hemorrhages
Ichthyosis	Yellow nail syndrome
Miscellaneous skin diseases	Loss of lunulae
Granuloma annulare	Ridging
Redistribution of fat	Nutritional deficiencies
Bullous diseases	Scurvy
Porphyria cutanea tarda	Pellagra
Oral mucosal diseases	Zinc deficiency

AZT, azidothymidine.

IMMUNOCOMPROMISED PATIENTS (NON-HUMAN IMMUNODEFICIENCY VIRUS INFECTED)

The number of immunocompromised individuals has increased significantly in the last decade owing to the increase in immunosuppressive therapies for organ transplantation and malignancies and for disease states such as autoimmune diseases. Each patient has specific immunodeficiencies based on his or her underlying disease and/or therapies. Skin lesions may be the first sign of systemic disease in such patients. Skin infections have been reported in 22% to 33% of severely immunocompromised patients. Because of the underlying immunodeficiency, dermatologic diseases may present in atypical forms or with difficulty in treatment. Unexplained skin eruptions should be biopsied for routine histology and culture in this population.

I. OVERVIEW
A. Bacterial infections
1. **Pseudomonas aeruginosa.** *P. aeruginosa* is part of the normal skin flora of the external ear canal, skin folds, and umbilicus. In neutropenic patients, this bacteria gains entry through adnexal structures such as hair follicles. Ecthyma gangrenosum is an enlarging necrotic plaque, anywhere on the cutaneous surface, secondary to a *Pseudomonas* septic vasculitis with an associated bacteremia. Diagnosis is made by direct culture of the wound or lesional biopsy which shows gram-negative rods within the medial and adventitial walls of deeper vessels. In immunocompromised patients, this infection is associated with a 10% to 20% mortality rate and should be treated with a combination of antipseudomonal antimicrobials.

B. Superficial fungal infections
1. **Tinea.** In immunocompromised patients, especially solid organ transplantation patients, extensive cutaneous areas may be involved. Tinea faciale is often misdiagnosed as seborrheic dermatitis, lupus erythematosus, or eczema. Topical antifungals are useful in treating localized infection; however, systemic agents, although associated with a higher incidence and severity of side effects, may be needed for extensive disease.
2. **Candida.** In recent years, there have been increasing reports of invasive candidiasis, usually secondary to *C. albicans* or *Candida tropicalis*. The risk of azole resistance may be as high as 20%. The yeast colonizes the gastrointestinal tract or intravenous sites and gains access to the systemic circulation. Approximately 10% to 15% of patients with systemic candidiasis will have cutaneous lesions (papules or nodules). The response rate to amphotericin B therapy is 50% to 75%.
3. **Trichosporonosis.** *Trichosporon beigelii*, in the normal host, causes a superficial infection of the hair shaft known as white piedra. Factors that predispose to systemic trichosporonosis include cytotoxic chemotherapy, systemic corticosteroids, prosthetic valve surgery, and HIV disease. Signs of systemic infection include purple papules or nodules with central ulceration, pulmonary and renal failure, and hypotension. Diagnosis is made by biopsy and culture of a skin lesion or blood cultures. Treatment can be difficult with breakthrough disease observed during the use of amphotericin B, itraconazole, fluconazole, and voriconazole.

C. Deep fungal infections
1. **Aspergillosis.** *Aspergillus fumigatus* and *Aspergillus flavus* are the two most common deep invasive mycoses in immunocompromised hosts. Solid organ transplantation patients and individuals on high-dose corticosteroids or with prolonged granulocytopenia are at the greatest risk. Primary cutaneous disease can result from inoculation at sites of burns, trauma, or intravenous catheters. More commonly, secondary cutaneous aspergillosis results from pulmonary infection that disseminates widely. The skin lesions consist of erythematous nodules that rapidly ulcerate, leaving a black eschar. Involvement of the CNS, heart, lungs, and kidneys can be seen with disseminated disease. A lesional skin biopsy with touch prep will demonstrate the septate hyphae with acute angle

branching. Surgical debridement and treatment with amphotericin B are the treatments of choice. Additionally, voriconazole and caspofungin can be used if side effects of amphotericin toxicity are of concern. A combination of antifungals may be of potential benefit.

2. **Mucormycosis.** Mucormycosis results from infection with fungi in the genera *Rhizopus, Mucor,* and *Absidia,* among others. Infection occurs most commonly in diabetic patients with ketoacidosis and in individuals on high-dose corticosteroids or those with prolonged neutropenia. Cutaneous mucormycosis may occur in burn sites or be acquired from contaminated dressings at surgical or minor trauma sites; the skin lesions extend rapidly with progressive necrosis. A rapidly spreading cellulitis may occur over the sinuses and orbits as a sign of rhinocerebral mucormycosis; these patients are usually quite ill and can subsequently develop coma, proptosis, and ophthalmoplegia. The diagnosis of mucormycosis is made by biopsy with a touch prep and culture to demonstrate the broad, nonseptate hyphae branching at right angles, resembling ribbons. The mortality rate is high despite amphotericin therapy. Oral therapy with posaconazole is a promising addition to the mucormycosis therapeutic armamentarium.

D. **Viral infections**
   1. **Herpesviruses**
      a. **HSV.** Immunocompromised patients are more likely to develop chronic herpetic ulcers and disseminated HSV infection. Reactivation of HSV occurs in 70% to 80% of HSV-seropositive bone marrow transplantation patients; these patients are often placed on prophylactic acyclovir. Rapid fluorescent antibody tests of lesional exudate can be performed at the bedside to diagnose HSV or herpes zoster. Treatment with oral or intravenous acyclovir or famciclovir is indicated until lesions have crusted. Emergence of acyclovir-resistant HSV is a concern in immunocompromised patients not responsive to typical therapies. Foscarnet is approved for treatment of acyclovir-resistant HSV.
      b. **Varicella zoster.** The incidence of herpes zoster in the immunocompromised adult is very high; the virus is shed for a longer time than in the healthy host, and the risk of dissemination is significantly higher (visceral dissemination occurs in 8% of patients). Approximately 25% of children with acute lymphocytic leukemia will develop herpes zoster. Intravenous acyclovir is indicated for treatment of immunocompromised individuals.
      c. **CMV.** CMV is the most common opportunistic pathogen in transplantation patients; one third of renal transplantation patients develop complications of CMV infection. Transplantation patients may have reactivation of a latent virus or transplantation of a new infection along with the organ. CMV most commonly causes interstitial pneumonia and affects the gastrointestinal tract; skin findings are rare but have a predisposition for the formation of perineal ulcerations. Prevention of development of infection is key; pre- and posttransplantation patients receive CMV prophylaxis with interferon, ganciclovir, or CMV immunoglobulin. Antiviral therapies for active infection, including ganciclovir, valganciclovir, foscarnet, and cidofovir, are variably effective.
   2. **HPV.** HPV infections can be more extensive and respond less readily to conventional therapies in immunocompromised patients. Twenty percent to 70% of renal transplantation patients will experience extensive warts after renal transplantation. A number of different HPV subtypes, including epidermodysplasia verruciformis and novel ones, can be detected in nonmelanoma skin cancers. Cutaneous and genital warts are often resistant to typical therapies in immunosuppressed patients. Topical treatment with imiquimod 5% cream has produced effective results in reducing the burden of genital warts in immunocompromised patients.

E. **Cutaneous neoplasms**
   1. **KS.** KS is associated with Hodgkin's disease, non-Hodgkin's lymphoma, leukemia, myeloma, hairy cell leukemia, and cutaneous T-cell lymphoma. The

incidence of KS in renal transplantation patients has increased two to four times since the introduction of cyclosporine. The risk of KS is 150 to 200 times higher in renal transplantation patients than the general population. On average, KS develops 2.5 years after transplantation and shows increased involvement of internal organs. KS related to iatrogenic immunosuppression should be treated by reduction of the immunosuppressant dose; 25% of the cases will resolve with drug dosage adjustment.

2. **Nonmelanoma skin cancer.** Thirty percent to 70% of organ transplantation patients will develop skin cancer within 20 years of their transplantation. The two major risk factors for the development of nonmelanoma skin cancer in immunocompromised patients are cumulative ultraviolet exposure and infection with HPV strains. p53 gene mutations are important in the biology of these tumors. The ratio of SCC to BCC (2.3:1) is reversed in immunocompromised patients as compared with the normal host. The overall incidence of SCC in transplantation patients can be as great as 40 to 250 times higher than in the general population (3). Heart transplantation patients have the highest incidence because of an average older age at the time of transplant and higher doses of immunosuppressive agents. SCCs in immunosuppressed patients behave more aggressively and are more likely to metastasize. The period of immunosuppression is directly related to the increased risk of cutaneous malignancies. This group of patients should be examined at least every 6 months for skin cancers and be instructed in the need for stringent photoprotection. Low-dose acitretin appears to be helpful in reducing the number of SCC in the high-risk transplantation population. Topical retinoids are impractical to apply to large body surface areas.

The risk of MM in this population is not as clear as the nonmelanoma skin cancers but one estimate is three times the normal population.

Posttransplantation lymphoproliferative disorders occur during marked immunosuppression and are B cell malignancies driven by the EBV. The gastrointestinal tract and CNS are most commonly involved. The skin lesions are ulcers, nodules, or plaques. Patients with the highest degree of immunosuppression are at the highest risk (i.e., heart transplantation patients) and the lymphoma usually occurs within 3 years of the transplant.

References

1. Kahn JO, Walker BD. Acute human immunodeficiency virus type 1 infection. *N Engl J Med* 1998;339:33–39.
2. Vanhems P, Lambert J, Cooper DA, et al. Severity and prognosis of acute human immunodeficiency virus type 1 illness: a dose-response relationship. *Clin Infect Dis* 1998;26:323–329.
3. Cocherell CJ, Chen TM. Cutaneous manifestations of HIV and HIV-related disorders. In: Bolognia J, Jorizzo J, Rapini R. *Dermatology*. Philadelphia, PA: Mosby, 2003.
4. Martinez E, Gatell J, Moran Y, et al. High incidence of herpes zoster in patients with AIDS soon after therapy with protease inhibitors. *Clin Infect Dis* 1998;27:1510–1513.
5. Sirisanthana V, Sirisanthana T. Disseminated Penicillium marneffei infection in human immunodeficiency virus-infected children. *Pediatr Infect Dis J* 1995;14:935–940.
6. Supparatpinyo K, Perriens J, Nelson KE, et al. A controlled trial of itraconazole to prevent relapse of Penicillium marneffei infection in patients infected with the human immunodeficiency virus. *N Engl J Med* 1998;339:1739–1743.
7. Foucault C, Brouqui P, Raoult D. Bartonella Quintana characteristics and clinical management. *Emerg Infect Dis* 2006;12:217–223.
8. Hengge UR, Ruzicka T, Tyring SK, et al. Update on Kaposi's sarcoma and other HHV8 associated diseases. Part 1: epidemiology, environmental predispositions, clinical manifestations, and therapy. *Lancet Infect Dis* 2002;2:281–292.
9. Miller KK, Daly PA, Sentochnik D, et al. Pseudo-Cushing's syndrome in human immunodeficiency virus-infected patients. *Clin Infect Dis* 1998;27:68–72.
10. Rodwell GE, Maurer TA, Berger TG. Fat redistribution in HIV disease. *J Am Acad Dermatol* 2000;42:727–730.

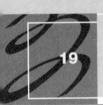

INFESTATIONS: PEDICULOSIS, SCABIES, AND TICKS

19

Melissa A. Bogle

I. DEFINITION AND PATHOPHYSIOLOGY

A. Pediculosis. There are two species of blood-sucking lice specific to the human host: *Phthirius pubis* and *Pediculus humanus*. These wingless, six-legged insects are obligate parasites and are host-specific for humans. The lice that inhabit the head or body are both types of *P. humanus* (*P. humanus humanus* and *P. humanus capitis*); only the body louse is capable of transmission of disease-endemic typhus (*Rickettsia prowazekii*), trench fever (*Bartonella quintana*), and relapsing fever (*Borrelia recurrentis, Borrelia duttoni*). *P. capitis* is not known to be a disease vector. Head and body lice look similar to one another and will interbreed; however, they do have different physiologic feeding habits and head lice prefer to confine themselves to the scalp. The head louse is transmitted through shared clothing and brushes; the body louse, by bedding or clothing; and the pubic louse, from person-to-person contact and not infrequently through clothing, bedding, or towels.

The adult body louse (*Pediculosis humanis*) is 2- to 4 mm-long, has three pairs of legs with delicate hooks at the tarsal extremities, and is gray-white in appearance. The adult female louse has a lifespan of approximately 25 days, lays up to 10 eggs each day, and will die after 10 days away from a host. Body lice prefer to live in clothing, particularly seams, and move to the body to feed. As the lice feed, they inject their digestive juices and fecal material into the skin; it is this, plus the puncture wound itself, that causes pruritus. Their saliva also contains a unique anticoagulant and vasodilator that produce some of the symptoms of irritation and pruritus. Heavy infestation is common in crowded, unhygienic surroundings such as military personnel and refugees during wartime, prisons, chronic health care institutions, and homelessness. Chronic infection may lead to lichenification and hyperpigmentation from repeated scratching.

Head lice (*P. capitis*) most commonly affect white children, between the ages of 3 and 11. Head lice prefer clean healthy heads and will leave a host if conditions are not optimal. Lice transmission usually begins at home in larger families and is then spread to the school environment. Straight hair is more vulnerable than curly hair and African American children are less commonly affected, presumably secondary to the oval-shaped hair shaft. However, new head lice variants have been found with a stronger cuticle and angular curved claws as an adaptation to the variety of hair structure. The incubation period from exposure to pruritus is approximately 30 days. The ova (nits), which are oval, 1-mm long and gray, and firmly attached to the hair, hatch in approximately 7 to 9 days and become mature in another week. Ova are laid very close to the scalp and hatch before the hair grows more than 1/4 in. If no nits are found within 1/2 in. of the scalp and no lice are seen, treatment is not necessary because nits more than 1/2 in. from the scalp are eggshells from a past infection. Head lice do not jump or fly from one person to another. They adapt to their surroundings; darker skin types and hair color have red/black lice whereas lighter skin or hair types have gray/white lice. Egg production occurs ideally at 84°F; in warmer climates, the viable eggs can be found further down the hair shaft.

The crab or pubic louse (*P. pubis*), which usually inhabits the genital region, is short (1 to 2 mm) and broad, and the first pair of legs is shorter than the claw-like second and third pairs. Infestation may occur in other areas including the moustache, beard, axillae, chest, and even scalp hair. Pediculosis palpebrarum or "phthiriasis palpebrarum" is the name given to infestation of the eyelashes. Pubic lice are found in most ethnic groups except Asians, perhaps because of sparser pubic hair. Homosexual men have a high rate of infestation. Crab lice usually lay only three eggs per day. Adult lice can live off the host for up to 36 hours and viable eggs, for 10 days. The chance of acquiring pediculosis pubis from one sexual exposure with an infected person is approximately 95%. Transmission of crab lice can occur without body contact, especially in warmer environments. Through the use of polymerase chain reaction (PCR), the previous host of a crab louse can be identified (a possible forensic tool). The human immunodeficiency virus (HIV) has also been detected by PCR in collected crab louse specimens, but it is unclear whether any of the louse subtypes can transmit the virus.

B. Scabies is caused by infestation with the mite *Sarcoptes scabiei* var *hominis*. *S. scabiei* has four pairs of legs and transverse corrugations and bristles on its dorsal aspect. The 1.3-mm by 0.4-mm female mite, just visible to the human eye, excavates a burrow in the stratum corneum and travels as much as 5 mm everyday for 1 to 2 months before dying. Each female lays a total of 10 to 38 eggs, which hatch in approximately 1 week, reach maturity in approximately 3 weeks, and start a new cycle. Mating occurs only once, after which the male dies. Fewer than 10% of deposited eggs produce adult mites. Most infected adults will harbor 10 to 12 mites. Live mites have been recovered from dust and fomites. Twenty-five percent of surveyed chronic-care facilities reported problems with scabies outbreaks over a 1-year period.

Crusted or Norwegian scabies occurs in debilitated or immunocompromised patients and patients with adult T-cell lymphoma associated with human T lymphotrophic virus type I (HTLV-1); the infestation often presents as a generalized dermatitis with crusted hyperkeratosis of the palms and soles. Deep fissures between the crusted plaques are a source for bacterial invasion of the blood and also allow for the penetration of antiscabetic treatments into the blood. This variant of scabies is highly contagious, because the skin is infested with thousands of mites. Patients with HIV disease may present with scabies as their first acquired immunodeficiency syndrome (AIDS) defining illness, especially as the CD4 count drops below 200.

Scabies is acquired principally through close personal contact but may be transmitted through clothing, linens, furniture, or towels. The female can survive away from humans for at least 96 hours. The incubation period is usually <1 month but can be as long as 2 months. The severe pruritus is probably caused by an acquired sensitivity to the organism and its saliva, eggs, and feces and is first noted 3 to 4 weeks after primary infestation but sooner (24 to 48 hours) in subsequent infections. *S. scabiei* has cross-antigenicity with the house dust mite; this may play a role in the susceptibility to scabies and its clinical manifestations. Immunofluorescent studies suggest a cutaneous vasculitis-like pattern in dermal vessels, with the presence of immunoglobulin M (IgM) and C3 conjugates; skin-biopsy specimens can demonstrate immunoreactants indistinguishable from bullous pemphigoid. The delayed host response and these findings suggest a humoral component to the disease. Canine scabies (sarcoptic mange) causes crusting and hair loss over the ear margins, legs, and abdomen of dogs. This is highly communicable and may result in small epidemics in humans, although the mite is unable to reproduce in the human host.

C. Ticks are large mites covered by a tough integument. These ectoparasites live by sucking blood from mammals, birds, and reptiles. They are found in trees, grass, bushes, or on animals (dogs, cattle). After attaching to the human skin, the female tick feeds, becomes engorged after 7 to 14 days, and then drops off. The three most medically important ticks in the United States are the Lone Star tick (*Amblyomma americanum*), Dermacentor, and Ixodes ticks. The Lone Star and Dermacentor ticks can transmit Rocky Mountain spotted fever (*Rickettsia rickettsii*), ehrlichiosis (*Ehrlichia chaffeensis*), and tularemia (*Francisella tularensis*). Ixodes ticks can transmit Lyme disease (*Borrelia burgdorferi*) and babesiosis.

Lyme disease is often overdiagnosed and overtreated because of its protean manifestations and unreliable serologic tests. The risk of Lyme disease is low from deer tick bites that are attached for <24 hours. Early Lyme disease can be divided into localized (Stage 1) and disseminated (Stage 2) types. The localized rash develops in 60% to 80% of patients, usually at the tick bite site within days to 1 month of the bite. The tick bite is often not recognized. Systemic symptoms are present in most patients with erythema migrans (EM) (fatigue, arthralgias, myalgia, headache, stiff neck, and anorexia). Forty-two percent of patients will have either lymphadenopathy or fever. Disseminated disease indicates spread of the disease to other organs, usually with central nervous system (CNS), cardiac, or rheumatologic symptoms. Late disease (Stage 3) occurs in untreated individuals with manifestations involving the CNS and/or the musculoskeletal system.

II. SUBJECTIVE DATA

A. Extreme pruritus is the primary characteristic of pediculosis. It takes 4 to 6 weeks for the pruritus to develop in a nonsensitized individual and only 24 to 48 hours with repeat exposures. In some sensitized patients, generalized pruritus, urticaria, and eczematous changes may develop. In some cases, children may be totally asymptomatic. Sleeplessness may be reported, because lice are more active during nocturnal hours.

B. Scabies is noted for severe itching, which becomes most marked shortly after the patient goes to bed or for children during naptime. Pruritus may be delayed or overlooked in the immunocompromised or elderly patient. Early in the course, only the sites of burrows are pruritic; later, the itching may become generalized.

C. Tick bites are painless; ticks are often discovered several days later when itching develops or the engorged tick is found. Occasionally, symptoms of fever, headache, and abdominal pain may occur while the feeding tick remains attached. Minor or major constitutional symptoms can be associated with early-stage Lyme disease. Multiple symptoms can accompany both the early-disseminated disease and late-stage disease, depending on which system is involved (CNS, cardiac, or musculoskeletal). Very rarely, children can develop a reversible flaccid paralysis that starts after the tick has been attached for several days.

III. OBJECTIVE DATA

A. Pediculosis

1. Scalp

a. Nits may be found most easily on the hairs on the occiput and above the ears. The nits are attached to the hair with protein-containing cement and need to be removed with nit combs or fingernails or trimmed. It is often difficult to differentiate a viable from a nonviable nit. Pseudonits are desquamated epithelium encircling the hair but are more readily removed than true nits. If uncertain, the patient can put the specimen in 70% rubbing alcohol for microscopic examination. Erythematous macules, papules, and urticaria may be present.

b. Adult lice are fast and avoid light and are often impossible to find as they blend in with the skin and hair. In the average case, there will be fewer than 10 mature insects present. Parents or school nurses can screen the posterior scalp with tongue blades or lice combs.

c. Secondary impetigo and furunculosis with associated cervical lymphadenopathy are frequent complications. In severe cases, fever and anemia may be found. Feeling "lousy" was a term developed to describe the symptoms of pediculosis.

2. Body

a. Scratch marks, eczematous changes, lichenification, urticaria, and persistent erythematous papules may be seen. Lesions are often most noticeable on the back.

b. The lice will be found in the seams of clothing and only rarely on the skin. They can move as much as 3.5 cm in 2 hours.

3. Pubic

a. Pubic, perianal, and thigh hair can be infested by only a few or by uncountable numbers of nits. The infection load may be particularly severe at the base of the eyelashes.

b. The yellow-gray adults may be difficult to find and are usually located at the base of the hairs, resembling small freckles, scabs, or moles.

c. Small blue-black dots (macula cerulea) present in infested areas represent either ingested blood in adult lice or their excreta.

d. Body and axillary hair as well as the eyelashes and beard should also be examined for nits; the scalp may rarely be involved. Pubic lice can move 10 cm a day and live <20 hours if away from the host. Eggs continue to hatch for 1 week after treatment.

e. Shaving of the pubic area should be discouraged because folliculitis and irritation may develop.

B. Scabies

1. Multiple straight or S-shaped ridges or dotted lines, 5 to 20 mm long, which frequently resemble a black thread and end in a vesicle, represent the characteristic burrow, although this need not be present. Mites are also in papules and vesicles, the most common lesions.

2. Sites of involvement are chiefly the interdigital webs of the hands, wrists, antecubital fossae, points of the elbows, nipples, umbilicus, lower abdomen, genitalia, and gluteal cleft. Lesions of the glans penis are characteristic in males. Infants and small children often have lesions on the palms, soles, head, and neck.

3. Generalized urticarial papules, excoriations, and eczematous changes are secondary lesions caused by sensitization to the mite.

4. Indurated erythematous nodules, most noticeable on the male genitalia, are more common than discrete burrows and are slow to resolve after treatment.

5. Secondary bacterial infection with impetiginization and furunculosis is common. Sepsis has been described in AIDS patients with Norwegian scabies. Nephritogenic strains of *Streptococcus*, mainly in topical areas, have colonized scabietic lesions.

6. Canine scabies lesions are papules or vesicles without burrows seen on the trunk, arms, or abdomen.

C. Ticks. The engorged tick, often the size of a large pea, may resemble a vascular tumor or wart.

1. Previously sensitized hosts may develop a localized urticarial response.

2. The usual bite reaction shows a small dermal nodule surmounted by a necrotic center.

3. The site of a tick bite may also be marked by an eschar (a round crusted ulcer).

4. The rash of localized Lyme disease, EM, starts as a localized erythematous macule/papule that gradually expands over days taking on an annular configuration up to many centimeters in diameter. The outer border is very red and flat; the center can be dusky, violaceous, and rarely vesicular or necrotic. Multiple secondary lesions can be observed in addition to a diffuse urticaria or erythema. Mucosal and palm and sole involvement do not occur. Regional lymphadenopathy and conjunctivitis have been described.

   Cardiac abnormalities occur in 6% to 10% of individuals within 1 month of the tick bite in disseminated disease. Self-limited atrioventricular block, pericarditis, and left ventricular dysfunction can occur.

5. Granulomatous response to tick bites causes lesions that resemble dermal fibromas (dermatofibroma, histiocytoma).

IV. ASSESSMENT

A. Unexplained pyoderma of the scalp, inflammatory cervical or occipital adenopathy, or itching with mild inflammation of the occipital scalp and nuchal area should be attributed to pediculosis until proved otherwise. It is necessary to be persistent in searching for nits. If suspicion is high, a therapeutic trial or reexamination in 2 to 3 days is indicated.

   Unexplained pubic pruritus is very often a manifestation of pediculosis. In fastidious individuals, few adult lice and nits will be found, and a careful search—ideally employing a hand lens—should be made, with special attention to the genital area. The possibility of other coexisting venereal diseases must be kept in mind.

B. The diagnosis of scabies is made by demonstrating the presence of the organisms, the eggs, or the oval, brown-black fecal concretions called **scybala** in a burrow or papule. A superficial epidermal shave biopsy is the best method. The best papules for examination are often small but very itchy. Raise the burrow or papule between the forefinger and thumb and use a No. 15 scalpel blade to "saw" off the top of the papule or entire burrow. This procedure is almost painless. Place the material on a glass slide, cover with immersion oil, and examine under scanning power. Burrows or papules are found most often between the fingers, on the flexor aspect of the wrists, or on the ulnar aspect of the hands. It may sometimes be difficult to find either the burrow or the mite, especially in elderly or infirm patients, and in such cases, the clinical picture of intense pruritus and papular and excoriated lesions will lead one to the correct diagnosis. The addition of potassium hydroxide (KOH) to the preparation can be helpful in removing the keratinous debris in crusted scabies; prompt microscopic examination is required as the KOH also dissolves the mites and eggs. The mite of canine scabies is easily demonstrated in scrapings from the dog but rarely seen in preparations taken from human lesions. Epiluminescence microscopy may help detect the mite *in vivo*.

C. Lyme disease is often diagnosed with the EM skin lesion. The presence of other acute symptoms (fever, myalgia, arthralgias, headache, and stiff neck) is helpful. A history of a tick bite is not required. Laboratory confirmation is established with isolation of the spirochete from serum or cerebrospinal fluid (CSF), or a change in antibody levels in acute and convalescent serum. Skin-biopsy culture or PCR can also be useful.

Serologic testing is not helpful in early disease because of the low sensitivity. Positive or equivocal results of an enzyme-linked immunosorbent assay (ELISA), immunofluorescent assay (IFA), or immunodot assay require supplemental testing with a Western blot assay.

V. THERAPY. There have been increasing reports of resistance of head lice to traditional pediculicides. Resistance can increase if the same formulation has been used for an extended period of time. Resistance has been found to permethrin, synthesized pyrethrins, and lindane. Most treatment failures can be attributed to poor technique, noncompliance, or reinfection. Insecticides work by damaging the nervous system of the louse; because the newly laid eggs have no nervous system, ovicidal properties are also ideal. There are no products that kill 100% of the eggs; therefore, all patients should be retreated in 1 week's time to eradicate the matured eggs. The eggs also have a thick lipid layer that is difficult to penetrate; a 10-minute application is likely not sufficient to penetrate this membrane. A lice comb with an intertooth space less than the width of the nit is necessary between and after the treatment. Many parents prefer shampoo preparations but, overall, they are less effective than the cream rinse and lotion preparations. A great deal of counseling is required with any infestation as many patients feel socially stigmatized, confused, and distressed with the diagnosis.

A. The treatment of choice for pediculosis capitis or pubis is pyrethrins with piperonyl butoxide (RID, A-200 Pyrinate), permethrin (Nix), or lindane (Kwell).

1. Pyrethrins, rapid-acting compounds, derived from chrysanthemum plants, are the leading over-the-counter louse remedy. These compounds interfere with neural transmission, leading to paralysis and death. Piperonyl butoxide (PBO) potentiates the pyrethrins by inhibiting the hydrolytic enzymes responsible for pyrethrin metabolism in arthropods. When the compounds are combined, the insecticidal activity of the pyrethrin is increased 2 to 12 times. Medication is applied for 10 minutes and then rinsed off. It should not be used more than twice within a 24-hour period. As tested against head lice, these agents are more effective than lindane in terms of the rapidity with which they kill lice (10 to 23 minutes vs. 3 hours). Their ovicidal effect is about equal to that of lindane. These agents should not be used near the eyes or on mucous membranes. They are also toxic to houseflies, fleas, chiggers, and mosquitoes. Rid and R&C are 0.33% pyrethrin shampoos; A-200 is a 0.33% Pyrinate shampoo and is less ovicidal than the pyrethrins. These products are unstable in heat and light and contraindicated in individuals with known allergy to ragweed, chrysanthemums, or other pyrethrin products, but these reactions are rare.

2. Permethrin is a synthetic pyrethroid active against lice, ticks, mites, and fleas. It acts on neural cell membranes, delaying repolarization and causing paralysis. The compound has no reported adverse properties, is heat and light stable, has 70% to 80% ovicidal activity, and leaves an active residue on the scalp. Permethrin is 26 times less toxic than lindane and 3 times less toxic than pyrethrins. A 1% permethrin cream rinse (Nix) preparation with a single application was determined to be more effective than treatment with RID. Permethrin-treated military uniforms are effective against human body lice. Apply the cream rinse for 10 minutes and rinse off with water. Localized pruritus may be reported with use of this product.

3. Gamma-benzene hexachloride (GBH) (Kwell), a pesticide also known as lindane, is an organochlorine with very slow onset of action and poor ovicidal activity; it takes over 3 hours to kill the lice during which increased lice crawling and twitching can cause increased pruritus for the patient. Lindane is available as a shampoo for the treatment of pediculosis capitis and/or pubis and in cream and lotion form for treating scabies and all forms of pediculosis. GBH also repels ticks and other arthropods and kills chiggers. Up to 10% of the topically applied drug may be absorbed percutaneously, and therefore it should be applied to the skin after it has completely dried; alternative treatments should be considered in infants, young children, pregnant women, and individuals with significant alteration in epidermal barrier function (i.e., erythroderma). However, good toxicologic data about other treatment methods are lacking. Most adverse reactions to lindane, including aplastic anemia, are secondary to improper usage, especially repeated (and unnecessary) applications.

   a. For pediculosis capitis or pubis, 1 oz of shampoo is worked into a lather and left on the scalp or genital area for 4 minutes. After thorough rinsing, the hair should be cleaned with a fine-toothed comb to remove nit shells. Retreatment is usually not necessary.

   b. Pediculosis pubis should be treated with an application of lindane cream or lotion to infested and adjacent areas for 8 to 12 hours. In hairy individuals, the thighs, trunk, and axillae should also be treated, because involvement of these sites is not infrequent. Alternatively, the shampoo can be used as described previously. Eyelash infestation with pediculosis pubis may be treated by applying a thick layer of petrolatum b.i.d. for 8 days with mechanical removal of nits or physostigmine 0.025% ophthalmic ointment with a cotton-tipped applicator.

4. Malathion lotion 0.5% is rapidly effective against lice (5 minutes) and ovicidal (95% killed). This organophosphate is one of the least toxic agents, as it is rapidly metabolized by mammalian carboxylesterase. This formulation is now being re-marketed in the United States under the name Ovide and is available by prescription; it was previously available as a 1% preparation. It binds slowly to hair but can maintain a residue for 2 to 6 weeks, which helps protect against reinfestation. This product is flammable until dry, and hair dryers and open flames should be avoided.

5. Trimethoprim-sulfamethoxazole (Bactrim, Septra) PO once daily for 3 days, repeated in 10 days, seems effective in the treatment of pediculosis capitis. This therapy is not useful for treating scabies.

6. Carbaryl (Sevin), a cholinesterase inhibitor insecticide, is used as a pediculicide in the form of a shampoo. This product has an objectionable odor, but has some ovicidal activity. It is an effective medication available in England and some other countries but not in the United States.

7. Chlorophenothane (DDT) is not ovicidal and confers no residual protection. Body lice and head lice have become resistant. In many countries, concern about environmental contamination has restricted its use, and it is not available in the United States.

8. Topical and/or oral ivermectin have shown effectiveness in the treatment of pediculosis. Detailed studies have not been performed to date.

9. **General comments.** All pediculicides kill lice, but the dead organisms do not fall off hairs or the body spontaneously. Most patients regard the continuing presence of dead organisms as evidence of continuing infestation, and it is necessary to clearly instruct them otherwise. The only certain way to remove dead nits is with a fine-toothed comb or forceps. Pediculicides have varying ovicidal activity too, and because eggs attached to hair shafts require 7 to 10 days to hatch, a second application is needed after this interval only if living lice can be demonstrated or eggs are observed at the hair–skin junction. Combs and brushes should be soaked in 2% Lysol or a pediculicidal shampoo for approximately 1 hour or heated in water to approximately 65°C (149°F) for 5 to 10 minutes.

For pediculosis corporis, the patient needs to only wash with soap and water and apply topical antipruritic lotions. If lice get on the body, pediculicides should be used. Lice in clothing may be killed by having the clothes washed and/or dried by machine (hot cycle in each); by boiling, followed by ironing the seams; by dry-cleaning; or by applying dry heat at 140°F (60°C) for 20 minutes.

10. **Home remedies.** Parents have undertaken alternative therapies because of fear of use of pesticides and frustration with treatment failures. Products with an oil base (Vaseline, olive oil, mayonnaise, and margarine) may smother the adult lice, but have no affect on the nits. Dippity-Do styling gel applied overnight under a shower cap is water soluble and is reported to smother lice. Vinegar or formic acid has been reported to remove the glue that holds the nit firmly to the hair shaft. Detanglers, plant oils, and cream rinses will also help lubricate the hair shaft and remove nits. Alcohol, kerosene, and paint thinners have also been used but carry extreme risks.

B. SCABIES

1. Permethrin is a synthetic pyrethroid that interferes with the influx of sodium through cell membranes, leading to neurologic paralysis and death of the mite. There is minimal percutaneous absorption (<2%), which is rapidly hydrolyzed and excreted in the urine. Permethrin 5% dermal cream (Elimite) is applied for 8 to 12 hours to the entire body from the chin down and is then washed off. Burning and stinging with application have been reported especially in more severe infestations. Formaldehyde is a preservative, and there are rare reports of contact dermatitis.

   A second application is necessary 1 week later only if there is clear evidence of treatment failure. This medication has a higher cure rate and less potential toxicity than lindane. Elimite is classified as a Pregnancy Category B agent. This drug has been safely administered in children as young as 2 months of age. Cases of lindane-resistant scabies have been eradicated with this preparation; no cases of permethrin resistance have been reported to date. Patients should avoid the 1% over-the-counter permethrin (Nix), as its concentration is too low to effectively treat scabies.

2. Apply lindane (Kwell) cream or lotion to dry skin of the entire body from the neck down, with particular attention to the interdigital webs, wrists, elbows, axillae, breasts, buttocks, umbilicus, and genitalia. Mites can even take up residence under the nails, which should be trimmed, and this area should be diligently treated. Approximately 30 to 60 g, or 60 to 120 mL, is required to cover the trunk and extremities of an average adult. Medication should be applied for 8 to 12 hours and then washed off. Lindane is a CNS stimulant that produces seizures and death in the mite; it can also cause neurotoxicity in humans if the recommended dose is exceeded or if there is increased absorption through inflamed or fissured skin or a susceptible host. Because of its lipophilic properties, lindane is stored in higher concentration in fat and extensively binds to brain tissue. Lindane should be avoided in pregnant or nursing women [U.S. Food and Drug Administration (FDA) Pregnancy Category B], infants, young children, or individuals with seizure disorders or other neurologic disease. Cure rates of 90% have been reported with a single treatment of lindane but because of resistance, careful follow-up and a possible second treatment should be considered.

3. Ivermectin is a very effective antiparasitic agent that has been available in veterinary medicine for many years and as a treatment in humans for onchocerciasis ("river blindness"). A single oral dose of 200 μg/kg is generally effective in uncomplicated cases of scabies with resolution of pruritus within 48 hours. The serum half-life is 16 hours, and it is likely that a second dose in 1 week is required in many patients. This drug is not toxic to humans unless it crosses the blood–brain barrier; therefore, it should not be used in children who weigh <15 kg or in women during pregnancy or breast-feeding. Although not approved by the FDA for this indication, this may be a very promising treatment for epidemics of scabies, the infirm, or highly infested individuals. Resistance has been documented in the veterinary literature but not in humans.

4. Crotamiton (10% N-ethyl-o-crotonotoluide, Eurax) cream applied twice and left on during a 48-hour period is usually effective against scabies and has been reported to act as an antipruritic agent. Very little is known about its toxicity, and cure rates are lower than those with other therapies.

5. Precipitated sulfur 6% in a water-washable base (or in petrolatum, which is messier), applied nightly for three nights and washed off 24 hours after the last application remains a useful treatment. Patients may complain of the sulfur odor, messiness, and staining of bed linen. This treatment is often chosen for infants younger than 2 months of age and pregnant and lactating women, although sulfur, too, has produced toxicity and death in infants.

6. Benzyl benzoate in a 10% to 20% lotion is applied on three consecutive nights and may be as effective as one application of permethrin.

7. Other considerations
   a. Clothing should be thoroughly washed and/or dried by machine (hot cycle in each) or dry-cleaned and linen and towels changed; personal articles can be sealed in a plastic bag for 10 days. Transmission of scabies is unlikely after 24 hours of treatment.
   b. Persistent itching in treated scabies may be caused by continued infestation, a slowly subsiding hypersensitivity response, or irritation from medication. Four weeks is sufficient time to evaluate for healing of lesions and enough time for the eggs to have matured to an adult. If mites are present, a differentiation needs to be made between treatment failure and recurrence. Lesions should again be examined for the presence of mites. If persistent infection is present, re-treat or use the following alternative methods. Persistent pruritic nodules may remain in patients otherwise seemingly cured of scabies. These lesions are similar to prurigo (neurodermatitis) nodules and respond only to intralesional corticosteroid injection. If itching is related to sensitization, treatment with topical corticosteroid, antihistamines, or a short (7- to 10-day) tapering course of oral corticosteroids will bring relief.
   c. Family, close friends, sexual contacts, and those sharing quarters of patients with pediculosis or scabies should all be considered for treatment to prevent reinfection or a small epidemic.

C. Protection against tick infestation is best accomplished by applying repellents to clothing. The most efficient agent is diethyltoluamide (DEET). Use the recommended amount of insect repellent but avoid frequent reapplications; do not use repellents on infants; on the hands or face of young children; or on cuts, abrasions, or sunburned skin. Repellents containing >10% to 15% DEET should not be used in children; concentrations no higher than 30% to 35% should be used in adults.

D. Tick removal methods are multiple, and each has its advocates. The important consideration is that the organism not be crushed while being taken off the skin.
   1. The easiest and most efficient method entails grasping the tick near its mouth with forceps and lifting it gently upward and forward. A needle or other sharply pointed object may be inserted between the tick and skin to help pry it out. If tick mouthparts break off in the skin, they generally cause little damage. Tick removal within a few hours of attachment prevents transmission of disease.
   2. There is little objective evidence that a tick may be induced to loosen its grasp by touching it with a hot object, such as a match head that has just been extinguished

or a hot nail or by applying a few drops of a solvent such as chloroform or gasoline.
- **E.** Treatment recommendation for Lyme Borreliosis
  - **1.** Early Lyme disease (without neurologic, cardiac, or joint involvement)
    - **a.** Amoxicillin 500 mg three times daily for 21 days.
    - **b.** Doxycycline 100 mg two times/day for 21 days.
    - **c.** Cefuroxime axetil 500 mg daily for 7 days.
    - **d.** Azithromycin 500 mg daily for 7 days (less effective).
  - **2.** Treatment of meningitis, arthritis, carditis, or of the pregnant or immunocompromised patient is beyond the scope of this text, and consultation should be made with an infectious disease specialist.
- **F.** A new Lyme disease vaccine has been approved by the FDA and is manufactured by Smith Kline Beecham. The vaccine should be considered for individuals over the age of 18 who are at moderate or high risk for acquiring Lyme disease.

    This vaccine is 70% to 80% effective in individuals who have received the three doses of the vaccine (initial dose, followed by second dose 1 month later, and the final booster dose at 12 months). This vaccine offers no protection against other tick-borne diseases.

Suggested Readings

Burgess I. Head lice. *Clin Evid* 2004;11:2168–2173.

Burgess IF. Pediculosis. *J Am Acad Dermatol* 2004;50:1–12.

Elston DM. Drugs used in the treatment of pediculosis. *J Drugs Dermatol* 2005;4:207–211.

Frankowski BL. American Academy of Pediatrics guidelines for the prevention and treatment of head lice infestation. *Am J Manag Care* 2004;10:S269–S272.

Grabowski G, Kanhai A, Grabowski R, et al. Norwegian scabies in the immunocompromised patient. *J Am Podiatr Med Assoc* 2004;94:583–586.

Huynh TH, Norman RA. Scabies and pediculosis. *Dermatol Clin* 2004;22:7–11.

Karthikeyan K. Treatment of scabies: newer perspectives. *Postgrad Med J* 2005;81:7–11.

Ko CJ, Elston DM. Pediculosis. *J Am Acad Dermatol* 2004;50:1–12.

Rash EM. Arthropod bites and stings. Recognition and treatment. *Adv Nurse Pract* 2003;11:87–102.

Robinson D, Leo N, Prociv P, et al. Potential role of head lice, Pediculus humanus capitis, as vectors of Rickettsia prowazekii. *Parasitol Res* 2003;90:209–211.

Romanelli F. Treatment-resistant scabies and lice infections. *JAAPA* 2002;15:51–54.

Schoessler SZ. Treating and managing head lice: the school nurse perspective. *Am J Manag Care* 2004;10:S273–S276.

Stanek G, Strle F. Lyme borreliosis. *Lancet* 2003;362:1639–1647.

Steen CJ, Carbonaro PA, Schwartz RA. Arthropods in dermatology. *J Am Acad Dermatol* 2004;50:819–842.

Torres M, Carey V. Review of public health advice about ticks. *N S W Public Health Bull* 2004;15:212–215.

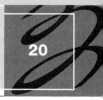

I. DEFINITION AND PATHOPHYSIOLOGY. Intertrigo is a nonspecific inflammatory dermatosis involving the opposing skin of body folds. It is most common in obese individuals during hot weather and is found principally in the inframammary, axillary, inguinal, and gluteal folds, but it may also affect other similar areas (folds of the neck creases, antecubital fossae, and umbilical and interdigital areas). As many as 11% of adult female elderly or institutionalized patients may have discomfort beneath the breasts. Patients with diabetes mellitus are also prone to developing intertrigo. As a result of skin constantly rubbing on skin, the heat, moisture, and friction lead to maceration, inflammation, and often secondary bacterial or *Candida albicans* infection. In topical regions, the genitocrural and perianal areas may be colonized with *Trichosporon beigelii.*

Incontinence may contribute to intertrigo in several ways: excessive moisture, irritant chemicals present in urine and feces, microbial contamination, and altering skin surface pH. Intertrigo is one form of diaper dermatitis in infants and is characterized by erythema only in skin folds, without pustules; it is most likely a primary irritant reaction with possible low-grade infection. Other eruptions that localize in the body folds and must therefore be differentiated from simple intertrigo include seborrheic dermatitis, psoriasis (inverse type), dermatophyte infections, erythrasma, irritant dermatitis, and miliaria.

II. SUBJECTIVE DATA. Mild or early involvement is associated with soreness or itching.

III. OBJECTIVE DATA. Mild erythema is seen initially; the red well-demarcated plaques oppose each other on each side of the skin fold, almost in a mirror image. This may then progress to more intense inflammation with erosions, oozing, exudation, and crusting. Painful fissures may develop within these erythematous plaques. Finally, vegetative changes, overt purulence, and surrounding cellulitis may arise in these areas.

Intense erythema with satellite papules and pustules is suggestive of infection with *C. albicans*; sharply marginated plaques suggest an inflammatory, noninfectious dermatosis. Macerated skin may become colonized with bacteria and then become malodorous. Incontinent patients with diaper dermatitis may develop nodules in the perianal, suprapubic, buttock, and crural fold areas.

IV. ASSESSMENT
- **A.** Examine pustule contents or scales microscopically with potassium hydroxide (KOH) preparation and by culture for evidence of bacterial, *Candida*, or dermatophyte infection.
- **B.** Examine the skin using a Wood's lamp for evidence of coral-red fluorescence suggestive of erythrasma.
- **C.** Initiate investigation for and treatment of associated medical conditions such as diabetes, obesity, and incontinence.

V. THERAPY
- **A.** Environmental changes to promote drying, aerate the body folds, and prevent skin-on-skin friction are essential.
  - **1.** The living and working areas should be cool and dry. Air-conditioning or fans will help. Have the patient disrobe for at least 30 minutes b.i.d. and expose the involved folds to a hair dryer or fan to promote drying.
  - **2.** Clothing should be light, nonconstricting, and absorbent, avoiding wool, nylon, and synthetic fibers. Bras should provide good support. Prolonged sitting and driving are obviously harmful.

3. Wash, rinse, and dry intertriginous areas at least twice daily, preferably with a mild antibacterial or low pH cleanser (pH 5.5 to 7) and liberally apply a talc-containing powder. Tucks or Wet Ones are disposable cleansing wipes useful for intertrigo and anogenital pruritus.
4. Occlusive, oily, or irritant ointments or cosmetics do more harm than good and should be avoided. In certain instances of incontinence, the benefit from a protective ointment may outweigh the potential harm. Lotions, sprays, powders, creams, or gels may be useful.
5. Careful and prompt attention to soiling by incontinent patients is mandatory.
6. Weight loss should be encouraged.

B. Specific measures
1. Apply cooling tap water or Burow's solution (aluminum acetate) compresses or soaks t.i.d. to q.i.d. to exudative areas.
2. Separate folds with absorbent material, for example, cotton sheeting well dusted with drying powders. Cornstarch should not be used, since it may encourage bacterial and fungal overgrowth. Zeasorb powder with or without miconazole (Zeasorb-AF) absorbs excess moisture and decreases friction in skin folds.
3. Initially, corticosteroid or steroid-antibiotic lotions, creams, or gels, such as triamcinolone mixed with silver sulfadiazine, should be applied b.i.d. to t.i.d. for up to 2 weeks. Prolonged use of these topical medications should be avoided, because continued application of fluorinated steroids may lead to intertriginous striae and cutaneous atrophy. Over-the-counter hydrocortisone (1%) will usually be effective, and its use reduces concern about corticosteroid side effects.
4. Bland lotions (calamine) are soothing and drying.
5. Some physicians apply drying antiseptic dye preparations to these areas and instruct patients to use them once daily thereafter. One-half- or full-strength Castellani's paint (fuchsin, phenol, and resorcinol; see Chap. 40, Antiinfective Agents, see sec. **II.C.2**) or 0.5% to 1.0% gentian violet solution may be used. These dyes are very effective but messy and may sting or burn on application.
6. Specific treatment for *C. albicans* (see Chap. 14, Candidiasis, see sec. V), dermatophytes, or bacteria may be helpful in cases where the organism has been demonstrated.

Suggested Readings
Garcia H. Dermatological complications of obesity. *Am J Clin Dermatol* 2002;3:497–506.
Guitart J, Woodley D. Intertrigo: a practical approach. *Compr Ther* 1994;20:402–409.
Mistiaen P, Poot E, Hickox S, et al. Preventing and treating intertrigo in the large skin folds of adults: a literature overview. *Dermatol Nurs* 2004;16:43–46, 49–57.

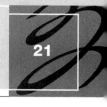

I. **DEFINITION AND PATHOPHYSIOLOGY.** Keloids and hypertrophic scars (HS) represent an excessive and aberrant healing response to cutaneous injuries, such as acne, trauma, surgery, and piercing. Both are seen in all races, especially in individuals with dark skin. Common anatomic sites for both HS and keloids include the earlobes, chest, lower legs, and upper back. Clinically, HS and keloids have many similar features and are often very difficult to distinguish. In general, HS remain in the area and shape of original injury and resolve spontaneously or with treatment (usually within several months). In comparison, keloids expand beyond the site of initial trauma and are recalcitrant to treatment.

The pathogenesis of HS and keloids are unclear. Fibroblasts from HS and keloids demonstrate excessive proliferative and low apoptosis properties. In addition to the increasing production of collagen, fibroblasts from HS and keloids also produce an increased amount of elastin, fibronectin, and hyaluronic acid. Tumor growth factor β (TGF-β) appears to play a central role in the pathogenesis process. Both TGF-β 1 and 2 stimulate the fibroblasts in keloids. *In vitro* study has demonstrated that the addition of TGF-β 1 leads to proliferation and synthesis of procollagen ribonucleic acid (RNA). Furthermore, TGF-β 1 upregulates the production of tissue inhibitor metalloproteinase and plasminogen activator inhibitor (PAI); these inhibitors protect the degradation of collagen.

II. **SUBJECTIVE DATA.** Keloids are usually asymptomatic, although some are pruritic and others may be quite painful and tender.

III. **OBJECTIVE DATA**
   A. HS appear as scars that are more elevated, wider, or thicker than expected. They are confined within the size and shape of the inciting injury.
   B. Keloids start as pink or red, firm, well-defined, telangiectatic, rubbery plaques that remain as such for several months and may be difficult to distinguish from HS. Later, uncontrolled overgrowth causes extension beyond the site of the original wound, and the tumor becomes smoother, irregularly shaped, hyperpigmented, harder, and more symptomatic. The tendency to send out claw-like prolongations is typical of keloids.

IV. **ASSESSMENT.** Keloid formation can be associated with other dermatologic diseases. These conditions, if present, should be investigated and treated aggressively. They include the Rubinstein–Taybi syndrome, dissecting cellulitis of the scalp, acne vulgaris, acne conglobata, hidradenitis suppurativa, pilonidal cysts, foreign-body reactions, and local infections with herpesvirus or vaccinia virus.

V. **THERAPY**
   A. HS usually require no treatment and often resolve spontaneously in 6 to 12 months. Intralesional corticosteroid injection is an effective treatment, and excision is another viable option because most HS do not recur. Pulsed dye laser (585 to 595 nm) surgery is also another effective modality; the laser treatment decreases redness and scar mass and improves subjective symptoms. Some clinicians feel that the combination of intralesional steroid and pulsed dye laser is more effective than either used alone.
   B. Keloids are much more difficult to treat because they are not only recalcitrant to various therapeutic modalities but also have a high rate of recurrence.
      1. **Prophylactic considerations** are of paramount importance. Optional elective surgical procedures must be avoided in individuals prone to keloid formation. When surgery is necessary for cosmetic reasons, early childhood is the best time. Scalpel surgery with strict aseptic technique and avoidance of wound tension is

mandatory. Electrosurgery and chemosurgery should be avoided; cryosurgical procedures are usually not followed by keloid formation. Surgical procedures should be avoided in patients who have been treated with isotretinoin within the past 6 to 12 months because of an increased risk of keloid and HS formation.

2. **Intralesional corticosteroid injection** often brings excellent results and is the first-line treatment. In skin fibroblast culture, glucocorticoids specifically decrease collagen synthesis in comparison with total protein synthesis. In addition, glucocorticoids may enhance collagen breakdown in keloids.

   a. Depending on the anatomic location, the use of high concentrations of medication (triamcinolone acetonide or diacetate, 10, 25, or 40 mg/mL) injected undiluted at 4- to 6-week intervals is warranted. Multiple injections directly into the bulk of the mass over several months (to years) may be necessary. Overtreatment may lead to atrophy.

   b. Initially, it may be difficult to force much medication into the tough collagenous mass. As the lesion softens and flattens, injection is accomplished more easily. Freezing the keloid with liquid nitrogen by spray or cotton swab application before injection causes the lesion to become edematous and less dense during thawing and allows the corticosteroid to be injected more easily and accurately. In addition, the freezing itself can have a therapeutic effect equal to that of the injected corticosteroids. Treatment with the pulsed dye laser before injection may be additive or synergistic in bringing about improvement from each approach.

   c. Injections at more frequent intervals may result in a depressed, atrophic lesion.

   d. Perilesional and perilymphatic atrophy around draining vessels may be seen but will resolve over the subsequent 3 to 12 months.

   e. Injection with a combination of 5-fluorouracil (5-FU) with triamcinolone acetonide, for a final concentration of 5 mg/mL 5-FU (9:1 dilution of 50 mg/mL 5-FU to a 10-mg/mL triamcinolone) has met with success in the management of keloids. This combination is more painful on injection than corticosteroids alone. Inject one to two times a week initially and then decrease to monthly intervals.

3. **Silicone gel or occlusive sheeting** applied for 12 to 24 hours daily for 8 to 12 weeks or longer, without pressure, to HS or keloids, has led to moderate success rates in small lesions. The mechanism of the treatment is unclear. Sheets (Topigel, Sil-K, Band-Aid Brand Scar Healing Strips, Curad Scar Therapy, Scarguard) are cut to size and held in place with paper tape or other adhesive and can be reused for up to 2 weeks. The dressings are removed q12h and the skin is washed. This treatment has very few side effects, and it is one of the few treatments that patients can actively self-administer in between office-based treatments such as intralesional steroid or cryotherapy. Compression or pressure devices are alternatives for home treatment. Often, a minimum of 4 to 6 months of treatment is needed to see some benefit.

4. **Cryosurgery** at monthly intervals may be effective for treating small lesions. Theoretically, cryotherapy causes ischemia that lead to subsequent necrosis and flattening of the tissue. Treat with two to three freeze-thaw cycles of 30 seconds each. Local anesthesia may be necessary. Complications include pain, edema, hypoesthesia, and hypopigmentation. The latter complication makes cryotherapy a less favorable treatment option for patients with dark skin colors.

5. **Surgical excision** is perhaps the only effective modality in converting broad-based keloid scars into narrow and cosmetically acceptable scars. However, excision alone leads to 50% to 100% recurrence. Hence, adjunctive treatments, such as intralesional steroid, radiation, or even topical imiquimod, after surgical debulkment is always needed to reduce the recurrence rate. The common **x-ray radiation** regimen is 900 cGy or greater given in fraction within 10 days of surgery. The combination of radiation with surgery can prevent recurrence in approximately 75% of patients at 1-year follow-up.

6. Both interferon-γ (IFN-γ) and IFN-α-2b suppress the synthesis of collagen both *in vivo* and *in vitro*. Intralesional IFN-α-2b injection may be used alone or in

combination with excision to reduce the size and collagen synthesis in keloids. However, most controlled trials demonstrated little evidence for the long-term efficacy of interferon treatment.

7. Pilot trials using topical imiquimod to keloids after excision is effective in reducing recurrence. The rational for imiquimod treatment is related to the drug's capability to induce local interferon at the site of application. Imiquimod is applied daily starting on the day of the surgery and continued for a total of 8 weeks.

8. Laser surgery utilizing the **CO₂ or Nd:Yag** lasers have not shown any consistent advantages over "cold steel" debulking surgery. In a number of controlled trials, **pulsed dye laser (585 nm)** has been shown to improve subjective symptoms and reduce erythema and height of keloidal scars.

9. Application of 0.05% **retinoic acid** b.i.d. for 3 months resulted in a favorable result in 77% of 28 intractable cases. *In vitro* evidence that retinoic acid reduces keloidal fibroblast collagen production lends experimental validity to this report.

10. **Ultraviolet A1** (340 to 400 nm) radiation has shown to lead softening and flattening of keloids in two case studies.

11. **Intralesional bleomycin** has been reported to achieve significant flattening in one study. The bleomycin is dripped onto the keloidal skin, and a 25 gauge needle is used to puncture the skin to facilitate the penetration of bleomycin into the dermis.

Suggested Readings

Alster TS, Lewis AB, Rosenbach A. Laser scar revision: comparison of CO₂ laser vaporization with and without simultaneous pulsed dye laser treatment. *Dermatol Surg* 1998;24:1299–1302.

Alster TS, Nanni CA. Pulsed dye laser treatment of hypertrophic burn scars. *Plast Reconstr Surg* 1998;102:2190–2195.

Alster TS, Williams CM. Treatment of keloids sternotomy scars with 585 nm flashlamp-pumped pulsed-dye laser. *Lancet* 1995;345:1198–1200.

Berman B, Flores F. Recurrence rates of excised keloids treated with postoperative triamcinolone acetonide injections or interferon alfa-2b injections. *J Am Acad Dermatol* 1997;37:755.

Berman B, Kaufman J. Pilot study of the effect of postoperative imiquimod 5% cream on the recurrence rate of excised keloids. *J Am Acad Dermatol* 2002;47(4 Suppl):S209–S211.

Dierickx C, Goldman MP, Fitzpatrick RE. Laser treatment of erythematous/hypertrophic and pigmented scars in 26 patients. *Plast Reconstr Surg* 1995;95:84–90.

Fitzpatrick RE. Treatment of inflamed hypertrophic scars using intralesional 5-FU. *Dermatol Surg* 1999;25:224–232.

Gold MH, Foster TD, Adair MA, et al. Prevention of hypertrophic scars and keloids by the prophylactic use of topical silicone gel sheets following a surgical procedure in an office setting. *Dermatol Surg* 2001;27(7):641–644.

Manuskiatti W, Fitzpatrick RE. Treatment response of keloidal and hypertrophic sternotomy scars: comparison among intralesional corticosteroid, 5-fluorouracil, and 585-nm flashlamp-pumped pulsed-dye laser treatments. *Arch Dermatol* 2002;138(9):1149–1155.

Nanda S, Reddy BS. Intralesional 5-fluorouracil as a treatment modality of keloids. *Dermatol Surg* 2004;30(1):54–56; discussion 56–57.

Niessen FB, Spauwen PH, Robinson PH, et al. The use of silicone occlusive sheeting (Sil-K) and silicone occlusive gel (Epiderm) in the prevention of hypertrophic scar formation. *Plast Reconstr Surg* 1998;102(6):1962–1972.

Norris JE. Superficial x-ray therapy in keloid management: a retrospective study of 24 cases and literature review. *Plast Reconstr Surg* 1995;95(6):1051–1055; Review.

Phillips TJ, Gerstein AD, Lordan V. A randomized controlled trial of hydrocolloid dressing in the treatment of hypertrophic scars and keloids. *Dermatol Surg* 1996;22:775–778.

Ricketts CH, Martin L, Faria DT, et al. Cytokine mRNA changes during the treatment of hypertrophic scars with silicone and nonsilicone gel dressings. *Dermatol Surg* 1996;22:955–959.

Sclafani AP. Prevention of earlobe keloid recurrence with postoperative corticosteroid injections versus radiation therapy. *Dermatol Surg* 1996;22:569–574.

Shaffer JJ, Taylor SC, Cook-Bolden F. Keloidal scars: a review with a critical look at therapeutic options. *J Am Acad Dermatol* 2002;46(2 Suppl Understanding):S63–S97; Review.

Wittenberg GP, Fabian BG, Bogomilsky JL, et al. Prospective, single-blind, randomized, controlled study to assess the efficacy of the 585 nm flashlamp-pumped pulsed-dye laser and silicone gel sheeting in hypertrophic scar treatment. *Arch Dermatol* 1999;135:1049–1055.

Zouboulis CC, Blume U, Buttner P, et al. Outcomes of cryosurgery in keloids and hypertrophic scars. *Arch Dermatol* 1993;129:1146–1151.

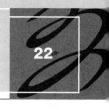

I. DEFINITION AND PATHOPHYSIOLOGY

A. Seborrheic keratoses are benign, noninvasive, hyperplastic epidermal lesions found most commonly on the face, shoulders, chest, and back; a genetic (polygenic) predisposition exists to develop seborrheic keratoses. They are the most common skin tumor in the middle-aged and elderly population and are termed **seborrheic** only in relation to their greasy appearance and their location in areas that have many sebaceous glands. Seborrheic keratoses from the genital region may contain human papillomavirus deoxyribonucleic acid (DNA). There is no known relationship to sebaceous gland function, seborrhea, or seborrheic dermatitis; the cause of seborrheic keratoses is unknown. In mature seborrheic keratoses, DNA synthesis is decreased, whereas ribonucleic acid (RNA) and protein synthesis are increased. Concern about these lesions is primarily cosmetic; occasionally, they cause anxiety because their dark color raises the question of melanoma. Rarely, malignant lesions (i.e., Bowen's disease) can arise from seborrheic keratoses, especially the reticulated type on sun-damaged skin.

B. Actinic keratoses are cutaneous neoplasms displaying chromosomal abnormalities caused by the cumulative effects of solar radiation on the skin and are commonly located on exposed surfaces such as the face, ears, scalp, dorsal forearms, and hands. They may be seen in fair-skinned individuals in their twenties and thirties but are most common after age 50. Men are more commonly affected than women, as are individuals who live in the Sunbelt latitudes and have outdoor jobs and/or hobbies. One in six white Americans will develop at least one actinic keratosis in their lifetime. Immunosuppressed individuals (organ transplant, lymphoma, and PUVA patients) are at an increased risk of developing actinic keratoses and squamous cell carcinoma (SCC); these patients also have an increased incidence of metastases. Other causes of actinic keratoses include ultraviolet (UV) light from artificial sources, x-ray irradiation, and exposure to aromatic polycyclic hydrocarbons. Actinic cheilitis is extensive involvement of the lower lip with actinic keratoses; the vermilion border is usually indistinct.

Lymphocytes and skin fibroblasts cultured from some patients with actinic keratosis show a defect in DNA repair synthesis after UV irradiation. Also, autoradiographic labeling indices have been shown to average 5.4% in non–sun-exposed buttock skin but were elevated to 11.2% in paralesional skin and 17.4% in actinic keratoses. These findings suggest that actinic keratoses develop in epidermis that is itself abnormal and that there may be a gradual progression of sun-damaged epidermis from the clinically obvious keratosis to skin cancer, and UV-induced immune suppression may contribute to tumor formation. P53 is the most commonly mutated tumor suppressor gene, and 90% of SCCs have a p53 chromosomal mutation. These changes are also present in actinic keratoses. UV light serves as both the initiator and promoter, leading to a mutation that causes the cell cycle to lose control. Activated *ras* genes have been identified in some cases of actinic keratoses.

The annual incidence of malignant transformation to SCC varies from <0.25% to 20% per year for an individual lesion. Lesions at particular high risk of malignant conversion are hyperkeratotic actinic keratoses of the dorsal hands and forearms. A white man has a 9% to 14% chance of developing a SCC in his lifetime. Progression to very aggressive lesions accompanied by metastasis occurs rarely.

Most dermatopathologists consider actinic keratoses an incipient intraepidermal SCC or keratinocyte intraepidermal neoplasia involving varying degrees of the epidermis. This change in nomenclature suggests that this lesion is neoplastic from the beginning and has implications for coverage of treatment of actinic keratoses by insurance carriers.

II. SUBJECTIVE DATA

A. Seborrheic keratoses are generally asymptomatic. Irritated lesions or those in intertriginous areas may itch intensely.

B. Actinic keratoses are usually asymptomatic but may be tender to the touch.

III. OBJECTIVE DATA (See color insert.)

A. Seborrheic keratoses start as small, multiple, flesh-colored, yellow, or tan, waxy papules and slowly grow to become dark brown or black, greasy, verrucous lesions with a distinct border. The rough scale may sometimes flake or be rubbed off but will always regrow. The keratoses appear to be "stuck on" the skin, and the surface often shows pronounced keratotic plugging. Stucco keratoses refer to light-colored, small keratotic papules on the dorsa of the hands and feet and lower legs; these are considered a variant of seborrheic keratoses. A variant of seborrheic keratoses known as **dermatosis papulosa nigra** is seen primarily on the cheeks in blacks or other dark skinned individuals with a familial predisposition.

B. Actinic keratoses first appear as flesh-colored to pink, flat or slightly raised, well-defined, scaly lesions that usually occur on the scalp, neck, ears, and dorsum of the hands. They feel rough on palpation and usually arise from obviously sun-damaged skin (dry, wrinkled, atrophic, and telangiectatic). Whereas parts of seborrheic keratoses can be scraped off easily with the fingernail or a tongue blade, this is not at all true of actinic lesions. A horny, keratotic, conical protuberance, called a **cutaneous horn**, may develop from an actinic keratosis. (Cutaneous horns may also form on verrucous epidermal nevi, warts, seborrheic keratoses, and SCCs.) Systemic chemotherapy may inflame actinic keratoses, resembling a drug rash in sun-exposed areas. Oral photosensitizing drugs such as thiazide diuretics and many others may be a risk factor for the development of actinic keratoses; further studies are needed to prove this association.

IV. ASSESSMENT.

Any doubts concerning the exact diagnosis of the keratosis may be resolved by pathologic examination of a small punch biopsy, shave biopsy, or curettage specimen. The base of all cutaneous horns should be submitted for histologic diagnosis. Shave biopsies or curettage specimens are often not sufficient for definitive histologic diagnosis.

The development of multiple seborrheic keratoses has been attributed to estrogen therapy, preexisting inflammatory dermatoses, acromegaly, and various internal malignancies. The latter association (Leser-Trélat sign), although somewhat controversial, should at least arouse one's suspicion when multiple pruritic seborrheic keratoses arise rapidly from previously normal skin.

V. THERAPY

A. Seborrheic keratoses are benign lesions, and therapy should therefore be as simple, rapid, and cosmetically acceptable as possible. After treatment, a small area of hypopigmentation may be left at the site of the keratosis. If there is any doubt regarding the diagnosis, especially in darkly pigmented individuals, a biopsy should be performed.

1. Application of liquid nitrogen (15 to 20 seconds) will result in removal of lesions without a subsequent cicatrix and is generally the simplest method. Multiple areas can be treated easily without anesthesia.

2. Simple curettage, with or without anesthesia, leaves an excellent cosmetic result. Lesions lightly frozen with a refrigerant, CO_2, or liquid nitrogen may sometimes be scraped off more easily. Monsel's solution (ferric subsulfate), ferric chloride, aluminum chloride, Gelfoam, weak acids (30% trichloroacetic), or pressure may be used for hemostasis. Light electrodesiccation will accomplish the same end but may induce a small scar. Lesions should remain uncovered or have only a light, nonocclusive dressing.

3. Very thick seborrheic keratoses may be best removed with a superficial shave excision.
4. Lesions of dermatosis papulosa nigra are best treated by simple curettage but may also be treated by Gradle scissor excision, light electrosurgery, laser surgery, or cryosurgery; it is particularly important not to treat too aggressively so as to avoid posttreatment hypopigmentation.
5. Ammonium lactate 12% lotion (Lac-Hydrin) applied b.i.d. for 1 to 2 months may reduce the height of seborrheic keratoses but will not change the length or color of the lesions.

B. Actinic keratoses

1. **Prophylactic measures.** Patients must first be told that these lesions are a result of damage from the sun and should be instructed to avoid further damage from solar radiation (see Chap. 40, Pigmenting and Depigmenting Agents, Sunscreens). The regular use of high–sun protection factor sunscreen can prevent the formation of new actinic keratoses.
2. Single or isolated lesions may be treated by any of the following methods:
   a. Cryotherapy with liquid nitrogen (10 to 20 seconds).
   b. Curettage and electrodesiccation under local anesthesia. This is a simple and rapid procedure, and the wound heals quickly; in addition, this method provides tissue for histologic diagnosis. Mild acids (30% to 50% trichloroacetic acid), Monsel's solution (ferric subsulfate), or aluminum chloride may be used for hemostasis.
   c. Shave excision (scalpel skimming) followed by electrosurgery or chemosurgery (acids). Although this may be excessive, it allows for histologic diagnosis.
   d. Excision and primary closure are almost always more extensive than the lesion warrants.
3. Multiple and/or extensive lesions are best treated with methods that allow a field effect with treatment of subclinical lesions as well as clinically obvious actinic keratoses. There are several approaches that accomplish these goals: topical 5-fluorouracil (5-FU), topical imiquimod, and aminolevulinic acid-photodynamic therapy (ALA-PDT).
   a. 5-FU is available as 1% (Fluoroplex), 2% (Efudex), and 5% (Efudex) solutions in propylene glycol and 0.5% (Carac), 1% (Fluoroplex), and 5% (Efudex) creams (see Chap. 40, Keratolytic, Cytotoxic, and Destructive Agents). The primary disadvantage is the brisk inflammatory response that accompanies successful therapy. A small number of treated patients develop an allergic contact sensitivity. Higher concentrations induce a more severe inflammatory response but may be followed by slightly more complete involution of lesions and a lower recurrence rate. The higher concentration should always be used on areas other than the head and neck. The 0.5% cream is used once daily for up to few weeks. On the face, the 1% or 2% solution or 0.5% or 1% cream is often sufficient. Medication should be applied twice daily until the inflammatory response peaks at the ulceration stage, usually 2 to 4 weeks. At this point, 5-FU may be stopped and a topical corticosteroid cream may be applied to hasten involution of the inflammation. Complete healing will be evident within 1 to 2 months. Weekly pulse dosing of topical 5-FU (1 to 2 consecutive days/week for 6 weeks) causes significantly less irritation but also a decreased level of efficacy. On resistant areas such as the forearms and trunk, the effectiveness of the medication may be increased by applying both 5% 5-FU and 0.05% retinoic acid solution (tretinoin) together b.i.d. until lesions exacerbate and then continuing with 5-FU for another 2 to 3 weeks. The tretinoin may act to increase percutaneous penetration but may also possibly have a direct effect on keratoses. An alternative regimen is to combine 5% Efudex b.i.d. and 20 mg of daily oral isotretinoin.
   b. Imiquimod 5% cream (Aldara, 3M Pharmaceuticals, St. Paul, MN) acts as a local immune response modifier with potent antiviral and antitumor activity. Imiquimod induces migration and activation of antigen-presenting cells in the skin, as well as the production of local cytokines such as interferon-α

(IFN-α), tumor necrosis factor-α (TNF-α), interleukin 1α (IL-1α), and IL-12, resulting in an enhanced innate immune response. The cream can be used in patients with normal immune systems to treat both clinical and subclinical actinic keratoses. The standard application is once a day 2 days a week with a total course of 16 weeks. However, a more rigorous dosing of thrice weekly application for 4 weeks on, 4 weeks off, and 4 weeks on has also shown successful clearance of actinic keratoses. Recent protocols call for application during weekdays only and breaks during weekends for 6 to 16 weeks. Severe skin irritation including redness, crusting, itching, and burning similar to that of Efudex may occur. An additional benefit of imiquimod cream is that it may have an effect on immunologic memory, decreasing the development of future actinic keratoses.

   c. PDT with 20% ALA may be used for the treatment of actinic keratoses. The product is marketed as Levulan Kerastick (DUSA Pharmaceuticals, Valhalla, New York). The ALA is applied diffusely over the field with an applicator; the patient returns 1 to 3 hours later and is exposed to an activating light source. Once exposed to the light, ALA produces singlet oxygen, which damages the cell membrane. Sixty-six percent of patients had total clearing of lesions at 8 weeks using blue light exposure for 15 minutes. Patients experience a burning pain but heal with an excellent cosmetic result. Photosensitivity lasts for 24 hours. An optional regimen is to apply ALA only to visible actinic keratoses; however, this method will not treat subclinical lesions. A variety of lasers and light sources can be used to activate the ALA, including blue light, yellow light, and broadband light; however, many details remain to be worked out, such as the optimal incubation times for the ALA when using each of the various light sources.

   d. Topical 3% diclofenac in a 2.5% hyaluronic acid gel (Solaraze Gel, Doak Dermatologics, Fairfield, NJ) applied b.i.d. for 6 months led to an 81% complete clearance of actinic keratoses.

4. CO_2 or Er : YAG laser resurfacing, dermabrasion, or chemical peels with various acids (trichloroacetic, glycolic, or pyruvic acid) are also effective for treatment of widespread facial actinic keratoses. The results of a Jessner's/35% trichloroacetic acid peel are similar to topical 5-FU therapy; both require retreatment at 12 to 32 months.

5. Actinic cheilitis is best treated by superficial CO_2 laser vaporization. It may also respond well to PDT with ALA and pulsed dye laser or other light sources. Vermilionectomy (surgical advancement of the lower lip) is an alternative treatment with increased morbidity. SCCs arising from actinic cheilitis are more aggressive than tumors arising from actinic keratoses on other body surfaces. A high index of suspicion for biopsy must be maintained.

Suggested Readings

Babilas P, Karrer S, Sideroff A, et al. Photodynamic therapy in dermatology—an update. *Photodermatol Photoimmunol Photomed* 2005;21:142–149.

Cockerell CJ. Histopathology of incipient intraepidermal squamous cell carcinoma ("actinic keratosis"). *J Am Acad Dermatol* 2000;42:S11–S17.

Jorizzo JL, Carney PS, Ko WT, et al. Fluorouracil 5% and 0.5% creams for the treatment of actinic keratosis: equivalent efficacy with a lower concentration and more convenient dosing schedule. *Cutis* 2004;74:18–23.

Korman N, Moy R, Ling M, et al. Dosing with 5% imiquimod cream 3 times per week for the treatment of actinic keratosis: results of two phase 3, randomized, double-blind, parallel-group, vehicle-controlled trials. *Arch Dermatol* 2005;141:467–473.

Leffell DJ. The scientific basis of skin cancer. *J Am Acad Dermatol* 2000;42:S18–S22.

Nelson C, Rigel D, Smith S, et al. Phase IV, open-label assessment of the treatment of actinic keratosis with 3.0% diclofenac sodium topical gel (Solaraze). *J Drugs Dermatol* 2004;3:401–407.

Silapunt S, Goldberg LH, Alam M. Topical and light-based treatments for actinic keratoses. *Semin Cutan Med Surg* 2003;22:162–170.

Stockfleth E, Christophers E, Benninghoff B, et al. Low incidence of new actinic keratoses after topical 5% imiquimod cream treatment: a long-term follow-up study. *Arch Dermatol* 2004;140:1542.

Tutrone WD, Saini R, Caglar S, et al. Topical therapy for actinic keratoses, II: Diclofenac, colchicine, and retinoids. *Cutis* 2003;71:373–379.

Tutrone WD, Saini R, Caglar S, et al. Topical therapy for actinic keratoses, I: 5-Fluorouracil and imiquimod. *Cutis* 2003;71:365–370.

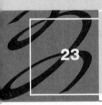

MILIA
Adrienne M. Feasel

23

I. **DEFINITION AND PATHOPHYSIOLOGY.** Milia are asymptomatic, small, subepidermal, keratinous cysts found in individuals of all ages, most often on the face. Primary milia are noninflammatory collections of lamellated keratin most frequently found within the undifferentiated sebaceous cells that surround vellus hair follicles. Milia found in infants tend to disappear spontaneously in a few months, but lesions in adults are chronic. Most arise spontaneously, but others may be localized in areas of damaged skin associated with bullous disease (porphyria cutanea tarda, bullous lupus erythematosus, epidermolysis bullosa). Milia may also arise in areas treated by dermabrasion, laser resurfacing, and, rarely, at the site of radiation therapy. These secondary milia arise predominantly from eccrine duct epithelium.

II. **SUBJECTIVE DATA.** Facial milia are of cosmetic significance only.

III. **OBJECTIVE DATA.** Milia appear as tiny (1- to 2-mm), white, raised, round lesions covered by a thinned epidermis found primarily on the cheeks and eyelids. No orifice can be seen. Some cases of idiopathic calcinosis cutis and syringomas may clinically mimic milia.

IV. **ASSESSMENT.** Enquire about previous inflammatory or blistering skin disease, trauma, use of occlusive cosmetic products, or photosensitivity. A short course of treatment with clobetasol ointment has been implicated in the formation of milia.

V. **THERAPY**
   A. Milia are easily removed without anesthesia as follows:
   1. Gently incise the thin epidermis covering the milium with a No. 11 scalpel blade.
   2. Carefully sever and tease away any connection or adhesions between the cyst and the overlying skin.
   3. Apply mild pressure with a comedo extractor, curet, tongue blade, two cotton-tipped applicators, or the dull edge of the scalpel blade. The small keratin kernel should pop out as an intact ball.
   B. Alternatively, a sterile hypodermic needle may used to enucleate the milium.
   C. Light electrodesiccation with a fine needle is also effective.
   D. Topical agents such as retinoic acid, retinol, or α-hydroxy acids may be useful adjuvant therapy to prevent formation of new milia.

MOLLUSCUM CONTAGIOSUM

Danielle M. DeHoratius

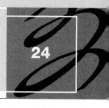

24

I. **DEFINITION AND PATHOPHYSIOLOGY.** Molluscum contagiosum (MC) is a viral tumor limited to humans and monkeys and caused by a deoxyribonucleic acid (DNA)-containing poxvirus, the largest virus known. Four subtypes exist with a high level of relatedness. The 190-kbp MC genome has been sequenced, sharing some homology with the variola virus. Although serial propagation of molluscum contagiosum virus (MCV) has been accomplished, there is no known animal model. The virus can be cultured on both human epidermis and amnion epithelium and has been transmitted experimentally to human volunteers by injections of viral filtrate into the skin. MCV is a brick-shaped particle, approximately 100 to 300 nm, which replicates in aggregates within the cytoplasm of infected cells. It may be seen in all cell layers of infected epidermis, but replication probably occurs in the more differentiated cell layers. Basal cell turnover and epidermal transit time are increased in MCV-infected epidermis, and the keratinization process is altered. Interestingly, MCV encodes an antioxidant protein named *MC066L* which functions as a scavenger of reactive oxygen metabolites and protects cells from ultraviolet (UV) or peroxide damage. However, the specific role of this protein has yet to be elucidated.

The disease is contracted from other people by direct contact or through fomites, such as bath sponges and towels, and by autoinoculation. Swimming pool outbreaks have been reported. MC has been spread locally with electrolysis. Children with atopic dermatitis may be infected more easily. Estimates of the incubation period range from 2 weeks to 2 months. Molluscum lesions were formerly found in children primarily on the face and trunk, but they are also being seen very commonly in the pubic area and genitalia of sexually active young adults. The prevalence of this viral sexually transmitted disease has increased dramatically over the past two decades. Patient visits to private physicians for MC increased 11-fold from 1966 to 1983. One Dutch study found that one in six individuals had seen a physician at least once by the time they were 15 years old for a diagnosis of MC. Antibodies to MC are the lowest in young age-groups (6 months to 2 years), and seropositivity increased with age (39% in persons older than 50 years) (1). Peak incidence is among children younger than 5 years of age with a prevalence of 25%.

MC is common in patients with acquired immunodeficiency syndrome (AIDS) as an opportunistic infection. It is often a marker for advanced disease and may exhibit multiple and disfiguring cutaneous lesions. Prevalence in human immunodeficiency virus (HIV)-positive individuals may be as high as 5% to 18%. The severity of the MC tends to be inversely proportional to the CD4 count. Widespread MC can occur in patients with atopic dermatitis, leukemia, sarcoidosis, or organ transplantation. Lesions are difficult to treat when there is any degree of immunosuppression.

MC lesions are common in the tropics and subtropics, a phenomenon attributed to increased desquamation associated with hydration. Transmission is facilitated by poor hygiene and climatic factors.

Thirty percent of individuals with perigenital MC may have concurrent sexually transmitted diseases. Many lesions are self-limited in duration (2 to 9 months), but others will last for years. Autoinoculation is common. Lesions will heal without scarring unless previously infected.

II. **SUBJECTIVE DATA.** Most lesions of molluscum are asymptomatic. Occasionally, large lesions become inflamed and can look and feel like a furuncle. Chronic conjunctivitis or keratitis may accompany lesions located on or near the eyelids. Some lesions may develop surrounding eczema, and in those patients with altered skin barrier function the molluscum may spread more rapidly in those areas. Incubation ranges from 14 to 50 days.

III. OBJECTIVE DATA (See color insert). Molluscum lesions are discrete, skin-colored or pearly white, raised, waxy-appearing, firm papules 1 to 5 mm in diameter with a central punctate umbilication. Mucosal lesions may be present, whereas involvement of the palms and soles is rare. A minority of patients may have a surrounding erythematous and scaling dermatitis. Inflamed lesions may become large, painful, and surrounded by erythema. Lesions are usually distributed on the trunk and extremities in children. In adults, lesions are found on the lower abdominal wall, inner thighs, pubic region, and genitalia.

MC in HIV-infected patients may be very atypical and difficult to treat, with either multiple small papules or giant nodular tumors up to 1.5 cm. Cutaneous cryptococcus, histoplasmosis keratoacanthoma, and basal cell carcinoma have been mistaken for molluscum in patients with AIDS. Atypical lesions should therefore be biopsied. Lesions can also occur on unusual sites such as the palms and soles and be mistaken for verruca vulgaris.

IV. ASSESSMENT. Diagnosis is usually made by clinical assessment; however, it may be confirmed by incising one of the papules, smearing the contents between two glass slides, staining (with Wright's, Giemsa's, or Gram's stain), and then viewing under low or high dry magnification. Molluscum or Henderson-Patterson bodies consisting of mature, immature, and incomplete virions and cellular debris, appear as ovoid, smooth-walled, and homogeneous up to 35 μm in diameter. The host cell can be pushed to the periphery, giving an appearance of a signet ring cell (Table 24-1). MC is self-limited and usually heals after several months. In children, lesions can resolve spontaneously and aggressive painful therapies should be avoided. Once the decision has been made to treat, certain treatments are more popular because of efficacy, ease of application, and cost-effectiveness (Table 24-2). Treatment does help minimize autoinoculation and transmission to others. Adult sexual partners should be examined and treated to prevent reinfection; evaluation for other sexually transmitted diseases should be considered. Follow-up for a second treatment should be done 2 to 6 weeks after treatment, which corresponds to the incubation period. Molluscum can be treated successfully by any of the following methods:

V. PHYSICAL ABLATION
  A. Cryotherapy with liquid nitrogen by spray or Q-tip application (5 to 10 seconds) or dry ice is generally the best treatment and one of the most popular. Treatment

TABLE 24-1	Therapy	
Treatment	**Advantages**	**Disadvantages**
"Watchful waiting"	Painless; no scarring	Potential for spread
Cryotherapy	Effective	Traumatic/painful; risk of blistering, scarring, infection
Curettage	Effective; immediate results	Traumatic/painful; risk of spread, scarring
Cimetidine	Well tolerated; readily available	Rarely effective; potential side effects, drug interactions
Tretinoin cream	Well tolerated; readily available	Minimally effective; risk of irritation
Cantharidin	Very effective; application of medication is painless	Risk of blistering, infection; requires thorough patient education

Source: Adapted from Silverberg NB, Sidbury R, Mancini AJ. Childhood molluscum contagiosum: experience with cantharidin therapy in 300 patients. *J Am Acad Dermatol* 2000;43:503–507.

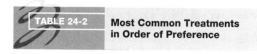

TABLE 24-2	Most Common Treatments in Order of Preference

1. Cryotherapy
2. Curettage
3. Acids; blistering agents
4. Tretinoin, imiquimod

can be repeated in 2- to 3-week intervals as needed. After this treatment, patients may experience hyper- or hypopigmentation and/or scarring.

B. Removal of the lesion by evisceration of the core of the lesion with a sharp curette, two ends of a split wooden tongue blade, or a large gauge needle. Curettage is the preferred method for eyelid lesions and can be used with or without light electrodesiccation. Anesthesia is often not necessary, but pretreatment with lidocaine and prilocaine (EMLA) or lidocaine (LMX) cream can be helpful in apprehensive children. One study showed that manual extrusion was more effective than cryotherapy (2). Some recommend touching the base of the lesion with iodine or a mild acid (30% trichloroacetic acid [TCA]).

C. Photodynamic therapy was recently used in the treatment of MC infection in six HIV-coinfected patients. There was substantial reduction in both lesional count as well as severity (3).

VI. CYTOTOXIC AGENTS

A. Podophyllin in a 10% to 25% suspension in a tincture of benzoin or alcohol can be used with success. Since this compound contains two mutagens, quercetin and kaempherol, it should used with caution in the physician's office. It should stay on for 1 to 4 hours and be applied every week for 4 to 6 weeks. Podofilox (0.05 mL of 5%) is safer than podophyllin and should be self-applied twice a day for 3 days followed by 4 rest days to complete a treatment cycle (4). Topical 0.5% podophyllotoxin cream has been used b.i.d. for 3 consecutive days for a maximum of 4 weeks with clearance in 54% of patients (5).

B. Application of a cauterizing agent causes the cornified epithelium to swell, soften, macerate, and desquamate. Within this category are chemovesicants such as cantharidin (Cantharone, Verr-Canth), an extract of Coleoptera beetles. It can be applied carefully and sparingly using a blunt wooden end of a cotton-tipped applicator to the top of the lesions once or twice a week every 3 to 4 weeks, with or without occlusion. This blistering agent can be left on for at least 4 to 4 hours. This method, though effective, may cause a severe inflammatory reaction. These agents should not be used on mucosal surfaces or on the face, especially around the eyes. Silverberg et al. showed that in a large retrospective study with this treatment, 90% of the patients experienced clearing (6). A keratolytic paint, containing 17% salicylic acid (Duofilm, Occlusal), may be used in the same fashion and will not cause as much inflammation.

C. TCA is another topical treatment that cauterizes skin and keratin and is applied in the physician's office. Concentrations vary from 25% to 50%. Scarring is rare.

D. The combination of topical sodium nitrate 5% with salicylic acid resulted in a 75% cure rate (7).

E. Silver nitrate is another cauterizing agent and coagulates cellular protein and removes granulation tissue. This should be applied everyday for approximately 5 days.

F. Topical 40% silver nitrate paste was applied after 2% lidocaine jelly, and 70% of the lesions cleared after one application. After three applications, 97.7% lesions were cleared. No scarring was reported (8).

G. 5-Fluorouracil (Efudex) is usually used topically by the patient approximately three times per week at night and washed off in the morning, for several weeks.

H. Potassium hydroxide (KOH) is a strong alkali that digests proteins and epidermal debris. In one study, 10% solution was applied b.i.d. to each lesion for 30 days with excellent clearance. The side effects included stinging of the lesion and one case of secondary infection (9). Also reported were the occurrence of a hypertrophic scar as well as some persistent or transitory hyper- and hypopigmentation. The same authors who used the 5% KOH solution completed further studies and they found it to be as effective-yet with decreased side effects (10).

I. Topical tretinoin (Retin-A) may be used in recurrent cases and should be applied twice daily. The 0.1% cream was reported to be effective by day 11 with only trace erythema in the pervious lesion sites. The 0.05% cream has also been used with decreased side effects while still achieving clearance of lesions (4).

J. Ten percent iodine solution can be placed on each papule. Upon drying, these areas can be covered with small pieces of 50% salicylic acid plaster and tape. This is repeated daily after bathing. In approximately 1 week once the lesions become erythematous, only the iodine solution should be applied. Researchers report resolution with a mean of 26 days (11).

VII. IMMUNOMODULATORY AGENTS

A. Treatment with intravenous cidofovir, a nucleotide analog of deoxycytidine monophosphate, leads to resolution of recalcitrant MC in HIV-infected patients. More recently, topical cidofovir cream 3% has been used to treat MC lesions with clearing in 2 to 6 weeks (12). Side effects include inflammation, erosion, a burning sensation, and postinflammatory hyperpigmentation (13). Also useful in immunocompromised patients are intralesional interferon-α (14) and topical injection of streptococcal antigen OK-432.

B. Topical imiquimod therapy is an immune response modifier that activates the toll-like receptor 7, perhaps mimicking a microbial antigen. It induces secretion of interferon-α as well as other cytokines thought to assist in stimulating an immunologic response to the poxvirus. It was originally approved by the U.S. Food and Drug Administration (FDA) to treat genital warts. Patients should apply imiquimod to the lesions three times per week and leave on the skin for 6 to 10 hours (15). Syed et al. reported that 80% of the patients treated with imiquimod achieved clearance of lesions (16). In one open-label study, seven children and eight adults with MC (three with HIV) self-administered 5% imiquimod cream daily, 5 days/week for 4 to 16 weeks. Eighty percent of the patients experienced either complete clearance or a >50% reduction in lesion size (17). An additional open-label study used 5% imiquimod cream daily, three times per week for a maximum of 16 weeks. Seventy-eight percent of the patients showed clearance by week 16 (18). More recently, Barba et al. reported a clearance rate of 33% in patients using imiquimod daily for 4 weeks (19).

C. Triple antiretroviral therapy has significantly decreased the frequency of MC in HIV-infected patients. Calista et al. reported three patients with recalcitrant MC lesions that cleared after 6 months of beginning highly active antiretroviral therapy (HAART) (20).

VIII. OTHER

A. Electron beam therapy and pulsed dye laser are two novel treatments reported for recalcitrant MC in immunocompromised patients. The pulsed dye laser cured almost 100% of MC lesions with one treatment in a group of nonimmunocompromised children (21). In another study, the 585-nm pulsed dye laser cleared 96.3% of the MC lesions after the first treatment and the remaining 3.7% after the second treatment (22).

B. Cimetidine (Tagamet) has been reported to be effective in some studies. Dohil and Prendiville showed clearance of the lesions in 9 of 13 patients using a dosing regimen of 40 mg/kg/day divided into twice daily dosing for 3 months. Caution is warranted because cimetidine interacts with many other systemic medications (23).

References

1. Konya J, Thompson CH. Molluscum contagiosum virus: antibody responses in persons with clinical lesions and seroepidemiology in a representative Australian population. *J Infect Dis* 1999;179:701–704.
2. White MI, Weller R, Diack P. Molluscum contagiosum in children—evidence based treatment. *Clin Exp Dermatol* 1997;22:51.
3. Moiin A. Photodynamic therapy for molluscum contagiosum infection in HIV-coinfected patients: review of 6 patients. *J Drugs Dermatol* 2003;2:637–639.
4. Valentine CL, Diven DG. Treatment modalities for molluscum contagiosum. *Dermatol Ther* 2000;13:285–289.
5. Syed TA, Ludin S, Alunad SA. Topical 0.3% and 0.5% podophyllotoxin cream for self-treatment of condylomata acuminata in women. A placebo-controlled, double-blind study. *Dermatology* 1994;189:142–145.
6. Silverberg NB, Sidbury R, Mancini AJ. Childhood molluscum contagiosum: experience with cantharidin therapy in 300 patients. *J Am Acad Dermatol* 2000;43:503–507.
7. Ormerod AD, White MI, Shah SA, et al. Molluscum contagiosum effectively treated with a topical acidified nitrate, nitric oxide liberating cream. *Br J Dermatol* 1999;141:1051–1053.
8. Niizeki K, Hashimoto K. Treatment of molluscum contagiosum with silver nitrate paste. *Pediatr Dermatol* 1999;16:395–397.
9. Romiti R, Ribeiro AP, Grinblat BM, et al. Treatment of molluscum contagiosum with potassium hydroxide: a clinical approach in 35 children. *Pediatr Dermatol* 1999;16:228–231.
10. Romiti R, Ribeiro AP, Romiti N. Evaluation of the effectiveness of 5% potassium hydroxide fir the treatment of molluscum contagiosum. *Pediatr Dermatol* 2000;17:495.
11. Ohkuma M. Molluscum contagiosum treated with iodine solution and salicylic acid plaster. *Int J Dermatol* 1990;29:443–445.
12. Zabawski EJ Jr. A review of topical and intralesional cidofovir. *Dermatol Online J* 2000;6(1):3.
13. Calista D. Topical cidofovir for severe cutaneous human papillomavirus and molluscum contagiosum infections in patients with HIV/AIDS. A pilot study. *J Eur Acad Dermatol Venerol* 2000;14:484–488.
14. Hourihane J, Hodges E, Smith J, et al. Interferon alpha treatment of molluscum contagiosum in immunodeficiency. *Arch Dis Child* 1999;80:77–79.
15. Skinner RB Jr. Imiquimod. *Dermatol Clin* 2003;21:291–300.
16. Syed TA, Goswami J, Ahmadpour OA, et al. Treatment of molluscum contagiosum in males with an analogue of imiquimod 1% cream: a placebo controlled, double-blind study. *J Dermatol* 1998;25:309–313.
17. Hengge UR, Esser S, Schultewalter T, et al. Self-administered topical 5% imiquimod for the treatment of common warts and molluscum contagiosum. *Br J Dermatol* 2000;143:1026–1031.
18. Liota E, Smith KJ, Buckley R, et al. Imiquimod therapy for molluscum contagiosum. *J Cutan Med Surg* 2000;4:76–82.
19. Barba AR, Kapoor S, Berman B. An open label safety study of topical imiquimod 5% cream in the treatment of molluscum contagiosum in children. *Dermatol Online J* 2001;7:20.
20. Calista D, Boschini A, Landi G. Resolution of disseminated molluscum contagiosum patients with highly active anti-retroviral therapy (HAART) in patients with AIDS. *Eur J Dermatol* 1999;9:211–213.
21. Hughes PS. Treatment of molluscum contagiosum with the 585-nm pulsed dye laser. *Dermatol Surg* 1998;24:229–230.
22. Michel J-L. ED2000: 585 nm collagen remodeling pulsed dye laser. *J Cosmet Laser Ther* 2003;5:201–203.
23. Dohil M, Prendiville JS. Treatment of molluscum contagiosum with oral cimetidine: clinical experience on 13 patients. *Pediatr Dermatol* 1996;13:310–312.

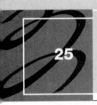

25 PITYRIASIS ROSEA
John G. Hancox and Joseph L. Jorizzo

I. **DEFINITION AND PATHOPHYSIOLOGY.** Pityriasis rosea (PR) is a mild self-limited eruption seen predominantly in adolescents and young adults during the spring and fall. Although a viral origin has often been suggested, there has not been supporting laboratory evidence. Therefore, the etiology remains unknown. Some earlier studies have suggested a role for human herpesvirus 7 (HHV-7) (1), but recent studies have failed to find serologic or tissue-based evidence for HHV-7 in patients with PR (2–4). Another study has also implicated HHV-6 as a possible cause (5). Studies have also suggested a cell-mediated immune mechanism, and some authors have postulated a relationship to the pityriasis lichenoides spectrum of disease. The eruption typically lasts 6 to 8 weeks, although in rare cases it may persist for several months. Lifelong immunity is observed in 98% of patients.

II. **SUBJECTIVE DATA.** PR may be asymptomatic, but many patients will experience pruritus, which at times can be severe (5). The onset of the eruption is sometimes coincident with mild malaise and symptoms similar to those of a viral upper respiratory tract infection or gastrointestinal symptoms (<20% of patients report some preceding viral symptoms) (6).

III. **OBJECTIVE DATA (See color insert.)**
   A. The initial lesion is frequently a 2- to 6-cm, round, erythematous, pink- to salmon-colored scaling patch or plaque, which may appear anywhere on the body but most commonly on the trunk. The collarette of scale is described as a "trailing," with the free edge pointing inward. This "herald patch" is not present, or at least not noticed, in 20% to 30% of cases.
   B. Within several days to 2 weeks, small 1- to 2-cm pale, red, round to oval macular and papular lesions with a crinkly surface and a rim of fine scales appear in crops on the trunk and proximal extremities. Minute pustules may also be seen.
   C. The face, hands, and feet are usually spared, except in children.
   D. The long axis of the lesions are oriented in the planes of cleavage running parallel to the ribs and are classically said to form a fir tree- or Christmas tree–like pattern.
   E. Lesions may be few or almost confluent, slowly enlarging by peripheral extension, and can continue to appear for 7 to 10 days.
   F. Oral lesions are unusual, but when present consist of red patches and plaques with hemorrhagic puncta or white erosions. Annular lesions have also been described in the oral mucosa.
   G. Variants of PR at times seem to appear as commonly as the classic disease.
      1. In children, the lesions are often papular, and purpuric lesions have also been described.
      2. Vesicular and bullous lesions may be seen, often with involvement of the palms and soles.
      3. Occasionally, eruptions may be limited to a small area or confined only to skin folds, which is known as *inverse PR.*
      4. Urticarial, intensely inflammatory, and very symptomatic lesions are possible.
      5. The herald patch may be absent, not noticed, or the only manifestation of the disease.
      6. In patients with Fitzpatrick skin types IV and V, individual lesions may have more of a lichenoid appearance and may show more depigmentation. The distribution may be atypical, often including the face.
   H. Either hyper- or hypopigmentation may persist after the initial eruption has resolved.

IV. ASSESSMENT

A. Except in its atypical forms, the eruption is usually easily diagnosed by its morphology and distribution.

B. A serologic test for syphilis should be considered for all patients, because secondary syphilis may closely mimic PR.

C. Other differential diagnostic considerations include guttate and acute psoriasis, nummular eczema, tinea corporis, seborrheic dermatitis, tinea versicolor, Gianotti-Crosti syndrome, pityriasis lichenoides, erythema annulare centrifugum, and scabies infestation.

D. Medications have been implicated in causing PR-like eruptions: (i) captopril or other angiotensin-converting enzyme (ACE) inhibitors, (ii) arsenicals, (iii) bismuth, (iv) tripelennamine HCl, (v) methoxypromazine, (vi) barbiturates, (vii) clonidine, (viii) nonsteroidal antiinflammatory drugs (NSAIDs), (ix) metronidazole, (x) gold, (xi) bacille Calmette-Guérin (BCG) vaccination, (xii) isotretinoin, (xiii) labetalol or other β-blockers, and (xiv) D-penicillamine.

E. PR-like eruptions have been reported with Hodgkin's disease, cutaneous T-cell lymphoma (CTCL), and solid tumors (gastric and pulmonary carcinoma, most commonly).

F. Lesions that do not resolve in 8 to 12 weeks may have pityriasis lichenoides spectrum disease (PLEVA/PLC), and a punch biopsy is indicated(7).

V. THERAPY

A. Most patients require no treatment because the disease is usually mild and self-limited.

B. Patients with pruritus may benefit from topical antipruritic lotions containing menthol or pramoxine, or even low- to medium-potency topical corticosteroids.

C. Pruritus may also be alleviated with emollients or oral nighttime antihistamines.

D. For more severe disease, one to several consecutive daily doses of erythema-producing ultraviolet B (UVB) light will decrease both the pruritus and the extent of the eruption in 50% of those treated (8). Sunlight, too, appears to have a direct beneficial effect. It has been suggested that those treated within the first week of rash will respond more readily.

E. A double-blind placebo-controlled study of 90 patients demonstrated that oral erythromycin in a dose of 250 mg four times daily in adults and 25 to 40 mg/kg in four divided doses in children (for 2 weeks) was effective in improving PR in 74% of treated patients and not in the placebo group (9).

F. Given the possible association between PR and HHV-6 and HHV-7, acyclovir may be considered. A trial using high-dose acyclovir (800 mg five times daily) cleared lesions in the treatment group in 18 days, compared with 38 days in the control group (10).

G. Rarely, a brief course of systemic corticosteroids may be required. However, caution must be used to taper the steroids slowly to avoid rebound.

References

1. Drago F, et al. Human herpesvirus 7 in patients with pityriasis rosea: electron microscopy investigations and polymerase chain reaction in mononuclear cells, plasma and skin. *Dermatology* 1997;195:374–378.
2. Kempf W, Adams V, Kleinhans M, et al. Pityriasis rosea is not associated with human herpesvirus 7. *Arch Dermatol* 1999;135:1070–1072.
3. Karabulet AA, Kocak M, Yilmaz N, et al. Detection of human herpesvirus 7 in pityriasis rosea by nested PCR. *Int J Dermatol* 2002;41:563–567.
4. Chuh AA, Chan HH, Zawar V. Is human herpesvirus 7 the causative agent of pityriasis rosea?—A critical review. *Int J Dermatol* 2004;43:870–875.
5. Broccolo F, Drago F, Careddu AM, et al. Additional evidence that pityriasis rosea is associated with reactivation of human herpesvirus-6 and -7. *J Invest Dermatol* 2005;124(6):1234–1240.
6. Tay Y, Goh CL. One-year review of pityriasis rosea at the National Skin Centre, Singapore. *Ann Acad Med Singapore* 1999;28:829–831.

7. Aiba S, Tagami H. Immunohistologic studies in pityriasis rosea: evidence for cellular immune reaction in the lesional epidermis. *Arch Dermatol* 1985;121:761–765.

8. Arndt KA, Paul BS, Stern RS, et al. Treatment of pityriasis rosea with UV radiation. *Arch Dermatol* 1983;119:381–382.

9. Sharma PK, Yadav TP, Gautam RK, et al. Erythromycin in pityriasis rosea: a double-blind, placebo controlled clinical trial. *J Am Acad Dermatol* 2000;42:241–244.

10. Drago F, Vecchio F, Rebora A. Use of high-dose acyclovir in pityriasis rosea. *Acad Dermatol* 2006;54(1):82–85.

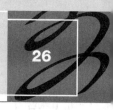

I. DEFINITION AND PATHOPHYSIOLOGY.

I. DEFINITION AND PATHOPHYSIOLOGY. Pruritus is defined as the cutaneous sensation that elicits the desire to scratch. Itching may be localized, generalized, paroxysmal, or unremitting and may be further qualified as burning, tingling, or pricking. Pruritus is almost always an unpleasant sensation and is the most common dermatologic symptom. Like pain, touch, heat, and vibratory sensation, it serves as a protective mechanism against external agents such as plants and parasites. It may be caused by a primary cutaneous disorder, but in 10% to 50% of patients, it may signal an underlying systemic disease.

The neurophysiology of pruritus is becoming better understood. Itching does not occur in an area insensitive to pain nor can it be elicited in patients with congenital absence of cutaneous pain sensation. Therefore, itching was historically believed to be a subset of pain and carried on the same unmyelinated C fibers to the dorsal root ganglia and spinothalamic tract. However, through the use of microneurography, a technique that involves the insertion of fine glass electrodes into C fibers, a subpopulation of exceptionally slow-conducting neurons has been identified. These account for only 10% to 15% of total C fibers, respond to both pruritogenic and thermal stimuli, and have extremely wide innervation territories. Interestingly, increasing temperature lowers the threshold of these receptors to pruritogenic stimuli, corresponding to the frequent patient complaint of increasing itch with higher temperature.

The specialized C fibers may be stimulated by an array of chemical mediators. Histamine is the main peripheral mediator of pruritus, but is not believed to play a significant role in most cases of pruritus secondary to systemic disease. Serotonin, which is contained in platelets, is a less potent pruritogen but can be potentiated by prostaglandin E_2. Serotonin antagonists and aspirin, which inhibits prostaglandin synthesis and aggregation, have been found to relieve the itch of polycythemia vera and uremic pruritus. Multiple neuropeptides including substance P, neurotensin, somatostatin, and melanocyte-stimulating hormone may also play a role in pruritus by mediating release of histamine. Opiates exert central regulation of itching through the central nervous system (CNS) but also act peripherally by potentiating histamine-induced itch.

Once stimulated, the specialized C fibers transmit impulses to the ipsilateral dorsal root ganglia where they synapse with itch-specific secondary neurons (1). These secondary neurons cross over and continue to the somatosensory cortex of the postcentral gyrus (2). Recent positron emission tomography (PET) scans suggest that histamine-induced itch activated both the anterior cingulate cortex, which processes the sensory and emotional aspects of itch, as well as the supplemental motor area (1). This explains the traditional observation that itch leads to an inevitable urge to scratch. Central processing of pruritus may also explain variations in the perception of itch (e.g., itching is usually worse at bedtime when there are fewer "distractions"). Psychogenic itching occurs when a psychological or psychiatric state, such as depression, causes either the itch sensation or a lowered threshold for itching (3). CNS pruritus or neurogenic itching presents with intermittent intense "seizures" of itching that cannot be ignored. This may be due to a cerebral stroke, tumor, abscess, or multiple sclerosis or be idiopathic in nature.

Seventy percent of elderly patients are affected by pruritus that may or may not be associated with a dermatologic disease. The presence of serum antibasement membrane zone antibodies has been hypothesized as one cause of senile pruritus (4). Direct and indirect immunofluorescence may be needed to exclude subclinical bullous pemphigoid in elderly patients with severe or unexplained pruritus. This testing would also exclude dermatitis herpetiformis, an autoimmune disease associated with gluten-sensitive enteropathy and characterized by deposition of immunoglobulin A (IgA) at the dermal papillae and intractable pruritus over elbows, knees, and the base of the scalp.

Itching is the cardinal symptom of most dermatologic disorders. Although scrupulous examination may be necessary to detect subtle evidence of certain pruritic dermatoses (e.g., mild atopic dermatitis, scabies, and asteatotic eczema), it is the patient who presents with itching but without rash who can pose a particularly challenging diagnostic and therapeutic dilemma. The remainder of this chapter will be devoted to such cases.

II. **GENERAL CONSIDERATIONS.** Pruritus accompanied by no visible skin alterations, other than those produced by scratching, may be a manifestation of numerous systemic disorders (Table 26-1). The evaluation of such patients must be open-minded yet orderly. A detailed history and physical examination, with particular attention to features such as pallor, icterus, adenopathy, or organomegaly, are crucial. Those diseases in which pruritus is a particularly common complaint will be discussed individually.

A. **Uremic pruritus.** Chronic renal failure is currently the most prevalent of all systemic diseases associated with pruritus. One fourth to one third of uremic patients treated without dialysis exhibit pruritus, and with maintenance hemodialysis this number increases to 70% to 80%. Many patients find that their itching is most severe during or immediately after dialysis treatments, and recent evidence suggests that this may be due to an accumulation of pruritogenic metabolites rather than a hypersensitivity reaction to the products from the dialysis equipment (2).

The etiology of uremic pruritus is unclear but is likely multifactorial, including xerosis, secondary hyperparathyroidism, abnormal mast cell proliferation, changes in endogenous opioid production, abnormal cutaneous innervation, and increased histamine concentrations.

TABLE 26-1	Systemic Disorders Associated with Pruritus

Drug reactions or drug effects (e.g., opiates)

Endocrine
      Carcinoid syndrome
      Hyperthyroidism
      Hypothyroidism
      Diabetes mellitus

Hepatitis C

HIV infection

Hypereosinophilic syndrome

Iron deficiency

Mastocytosis

Myeloproliferative disorders (e.g., polycythemia vera, Hodgkin's disease, myelodysplastic syndrome)

Neurologic disorders (e.g., brain abscess, multiple sclerosis, brain infarct, tumor)

Obstructive biliary disease (e.g., primary biliary cirrhosis)

Paraproteinemia/myeloma

Parasitic infections

Pregnancy

Uremia

Visceral malignancies

HIV, human immunodeficiency virus.

Increased levels of magnesium and vitamin A within the skin have also been postulated to contribute to itching.

B. Hepatogenic pruritus occurs in 20% to 25% of patients with jaundice, but is rare in those lacking cholestasis. Only 4% of patients with Hepatitis C without jaundice exhibit pruritus, although 100% of patients with primary biliary cirrhosis suffer from pruritus and it is the initial symptom in almost half the patients presenting with this disease. Although purified bile salts applied to the skin are pruritogenic and lowering the serum bile concentration usually ameliorates cholestatic pruritus, no convincing evidence has been found that total or individual levels of bile salts, either circulating or within the skin, correlate with the presence or absence of itching. Additional theories propose a role for an accumulated pruritogenic intermediary in bile salt synthesis, bile salt toxicity to hepatic membranes with release of a pruritogen, mast cell activation with histamine release, and centrally acting endogenous opioids accumulating as a result of hepatic failure.

C. Hematologic disorders. Between 30% and 50% of patients with polycythemia vera have pruritus, which often has a prickling sensation and may be evoked by a sudden decrease in temperature, such as when a person gets out of a hot shower. The pruritus may precede the development of the disease by several years, and successful treatment of the disease usually relieves pruritus. Although elevated plasma and urine histamine levels, correlating with an increased number of basophils, have been found in two thirds of patients with polycythemia vera, antihistamines are usually ineffective in controlling their pruritus. Iron deficiency, with or without anemia, may also be associated with pruritus, and in some patients with controlled polycythemia vera and iron deficiency, iron replacement has been shown to abolish the pruritus. However, the risks of iron therapy in polycythemia vera are significant and, in general, preclude its use.

Pruritus is seen in approximately 30% of patients with Hodgkin's disease, often many years before the correct diagnosis is evident. It is frequently most severe at night, starting with the legs and later involving the whole body. In localized disease, pruritus may localize to areas of lymphatic drainage from diseased areas, whereas generalized pruritus is seen more often in the nodular sclerosis type of Hodgkin's disease with mediastinal mass. Severe, generalized pruritus may indicate a worse prognosis.

D. Aquagenic pruritus occurs 1 to 5 minutes after water contact, regardless of temperature, and may last as long as 2 hours. Patients experience itching, tingling, or stinging sensations. No visible skin changes are seen. Polycythemia rubra vera and other myeloproliferative disorders must be excluded. Elevated acetylcholinesterase levels have been detected after water exposure in these patients.

E. Notalgia paresthetica is a sensory neuropathy in which patients present with localized pruritus of the back occasionally accompanied by pain or paresthesia in the T2-T6 distribution. Although the exact pathogenesis of the disease is not known, there is a striking correlation of nostalgia paresthetica with degenerative changes of the spine, suggesting that spinal nerve impingement may play a role (5).

F. Brachioradial pruritus is a condition with localized, intense pruritus over the distribution of the brachioradial nerve on the lateral forearm(s). The primary etiology is presumed to be a solar dermopathy as most patients have a history of excessive ultraviolet exposure, although nerve root impingement has also been hypothesized (6).

G. Scalp dysesthesia or pruritus is characterized by debilitating scalp pain and/or pruritus. Most of these patients are women, and there is no evidence of scalp disease except possibly mild erythema. The symptoms usually intensify with psychological stress, and a subset of these patients will have an associated psychiatric disorder.

H. Pruritus occurs frequently in patients with HIV and may be the presenting sign of acquired immunodeficiency syndrome (AIDS). With advancing HIV disease, there is a switch from Th1 to Th2 cytokines and an associated immune dysregulation (7). Basophils and mast cells from patients infected with HIV demonstrate enhanced degranulation. Additionally, peripheral neuropathy may also contribute to pruritus in this population.

III. SUBJECTIVE DATA. The history should include the nature, onset, and duration of the pruritus. A thorough history of medication use should be taken including prescription, over-the-counter, and alternative therapies. A detailed review of systems should be undertaken to try to establish any underlying medical problems. Occasionally, one may obtain clues to a particular underlying illness by features such as the relationship to temperature change noted previously for polycythemia vera. More extraordinary are those cases in which the discrete localization of the pruritus suggests the cause (e.g., nasal pruritus as a manifestation of a brain tumor or atypical angina). Psychogenic pruritus does not usually disturb sleep.

IV. OBJECTIVE DATA. A thorough physical examination should be undertaken, including evaluation of the liver, spleen, thyroid gland, and lymph nodes. Primary and secondary lesions, morphology, distribution, and the presence of lichenification are all important clues. In evaluating the upper back, look for sparing of this area ("butterfly sign"), indicating that the pruritus is not related to an underlying dermatologic disease.

In the case of generalized, persistent pruritus of unknown etiology, two levels of screening laboratory tests are recommended:

1. Initial screening (2)
   a. Complete blood count (CBC) with differential
   b. Chemistry profile including liver and renal function
   c. Hepatitis C screen
   d. Thyroid panel
   e. Urinalysis
   f. Occult blood in stool for patients over 40 years
   g. HIV testing
   h. Chest x-ray
   i. Referral to their primary care physician for complete physical examination to detect any possible underlying malignancy/disease not detected with the above measures
   j. Consider skin biopsy for routine histology and special stains for mast cells and a second specimen for immunofluorescence.

2. Second-level screening (8)
   a. Serum protein electrophoresis
   b. Ferritin level
   c. Ova and parasite evaluation of stool
   d. 5-Hydroxyindoleacetic acid and mast cell metabolites in the urine
   e. Additional radiologic studies as necessary.

V. THERAPY
   A. Specific measures
      1. Uremic pruritus
         a. Naltrexone (50 mg PO daily), an opiate antagonist, has been effective in relieving the pruritus associated with hemodialysis, supporting the role of opioids in renal itch. It has shown short-term benefits with few side effects (9).
         b. Activated charcoal (6 g daily) has been found in two controlled trials to be effective in some patients on dialysis (9). Charcoal may nonspecifically bind other oral drugs that patients are receiving. It is cost-effective and has a favorable side-effect profile.
         c. Ultraviolet B (UVB) phototherapy has shown effectiveness in double-blind trials, but similar effects are not seen with UVA (9). The potential carcinogenic risk in a group of patients who may later receive transplants should not be overlooked. Additionally, the psychological effects of becoming dependent on another machine should not be underestimated.
         d. Ondansetron (4 mg twice daily), a potent and selective serotonin antagonist has been reported to be effective in patients on continuous ambulatory peritoneal dialysis (9). In these patients, ondansetron reduced the plasma levels of both histamine and serotonin.
         e. Topical capsaicin 0.025% cream application has improved localized pruritus related to hemodialysis.

f. Parathyroidectomy may result in a dramatic relief from itching within 24 to 48 hours in patients with secondary hyperparathyroidism. The response is not invariable, and if patients become hypercalcemic postoperatively, the pruritus can recur.

g. Cholestyramine has been tried with some success, but often has varied results.

h. Erythropoietin therapy lowers plasma histamine levels and can reduce the symptoms of pruritus in patients with uremia on hemodialysis.

2. Cholestatic pruritus

a. Cholestyramine (4 g one to three times daily), an anion exchange resin, is frequently effective, although, as mentioned earlier, its antipruritic effect seems separate from its ability to normalize bile salt levels. Cholestyramine is a powder that is mixed with water or another fluid before ingesting. Colestipol (Colestid) is another ion exchange resin that may be substituted in patients who find cholestyramine too constipating. Like charcoal, ion exchange resins may bind other orally administered drugs. Oral vitamin K supplements (10 mg/week) should be given concurrently.

b. Phenobarbital (3 to 4 mg/kg/day PO) can reduce cholestatic pruritus, possibly by enhancing hepatic microsomal function (1). Phenobarbital is sedating and may interfere with the metabolism of many drugs.

c. Phototherapy using UVB or continuous-spectrum fluorescent bulbs (Daylite, 360 to 700 nm) may be helpful in individual patients, although seemingly not as often as for uremic pruritus.

d. Rifampin (300 to 450 mg daily) is very effective in relieving the pruritus of primary biliary cirrhosis, by inhibiting hepatic bile uptake and stimulating mixed-function oxidases. Liver enzymes should be monitored to detect drug-induced hepatitis. Children with pruritus and cholestatic liver disease have also been reported to improve with this drug.

e. Plasma perfusion through a column of charcoal-coated beads was effective in relieving pruritus in a study of eight patients. The duration of response ranged from 1 day to 5 months (1).

f. Naltrexone (50 mg daily), an oral opioid antagonist, has demonstrated effectiveness with fewer side effects than the parenterally administered nalmefene.

g. Danazol, a synthetic androgen, has been used to treat the pruritus of primary biliary cirrhosis, urticaria, and also idiopathic pruritus.

3. Hematologic diseases

a. Cimetidine, an H_2 blocker (see Chap. 40, Antihistamines), and cyproheptadine, an antihistamine and antiserotonin agent (see Chap. 40, Antihistamines), have been anecdotally reported to be effective in reducing the pruritus caused by polycythemia vera, as well as Hodgkin's disease (1).

b. Pizotifen (0.5 mg three times daily), a potent antihistamine and antiserotonin agent usually prescribed for migraine prophylaxis, has had reported success in patients with polycythemia vera (1).

c. Interferon-α-2b and psoralens plus ultraviolet A (PUVA) have both been used successfully in treating the pruritus of polycythemia vera.

d. Danazol has been used for treatment of pruritus associated with polycythemia vera and systemic lupus erythematosus. The exact mechanism of action is unknown.

e. Iron replacement will abolish pruritus due to iron deficiency, often before any measurable change occurs in the hematologic status. However, care should be taken in patients with polycythemia vera, whose underlying disease can be exacerbated by iron supplementation.

B. General measures

1. Oral antihistamines are usually ineffective for pruritus caused by systemic illness. Agents such as hydroxyzine, diphenhydramine, and cyproheptadine and may be helpful because of their sedative effect, not their primary antihistamine properties. Doxepin, a tricyclic antidepressant with antihistamine activity, is highly recommended both for its antipruritic and sedating qualities as well as mild antidepressant effects.

2. Topical antihistamines have been shown effective in decreasing pruritus in various types of dermatitis (atopic, lichen simplex chronicus) and may be helpful in other pruritic conditions. A risk for contact sensitization exists with topical antihistamines. Doxepin (Zonalon) cream is applied twice daily to localized areas or "hot spots"; there is systemic absorption, precluding its application to large body surface areas. Drowsiness may be a problem if applied to >10% of the body surface. Topical pramoxine, a topical anesthetic and antihistamine, can be useful in pruritus with low risk of contact sensitization, but with a short duration of action.

3. Coexisting conditions that may aggravate the pruritus, particularly xerosis, as is frequently observed in chronic renal failure, should be managed appropriately. Discontinuation of antistatic sheets in the dryer is sometimes helpful. The use of too many blankets or keeping the temperature of the house too high should be discouraged.

4. Dietary manipulation occasionally may be helpful—low-protein diets have been successful for uremic pruritus, whereas diets rich in polyunsaturated fatty acids may help cholestatic pruritus.

5. Topical lidocaine or topical capsaicin (Zostrix) can be effective for localized pruritus such as notalgia paraesthetica. Patients should be warned about the burning sensation associated with application of capsaicin.

6. Phototherapy with PUVA or UVB can be helpful in pruritus in general. In HIV-associated pruritus, there is theoretical evidence that ultraviolet radiation can be associated with viral activation, although no consistent alteration in CD4-positive cell counts or viral load have been determined (10).

7. Naltrexone, an oral opiate receptor antagonist, has been found to be helpful in patients with a variety of skin disorders, with a single daily dose of 50 mg. Further double-blind studies are necessary, and the issue of tolerance and withdrawal symptoms with this group of drugs needs to be taken into account.

8. Transcutaneous electronic nerve stimulation (TENS) and cutaneous field stimulation (CFS) may be helpful in generalized and localized pruritus (11,12).

9. Herbal remedies such as oatmeal baths, chamomile compresses, and aloe vera cream may provide relief with few side effects (13).

10. Occasionally, a referral to a neurologist may be helpful in detecting an underlying neurologic disorder.

References

1. Etter L, Myers SA. Pruritus in systemic disease: mechanisms and management. *Dermatol Clin* 2002;20:459–472.
2. Krajnik M, Zylicz Z. Understanding pruritus in systemic disease. *J Pain Symptom Manage* 2001;21:151–168.
3. Gupta MA, Gupta AK. Depression modulates pruritus perception: a study of pruritus in psoriasis, atopic dermatitis, and chronic idiopathic urticaria. *Psych Med* 1994;56:36–40.
4. Hachisuka H, Kurose K, Karashima T, et al. Serum from normal elderly individuals contains anti-basement membrane zone antibodies. *Arch Dermatol* 1996;132:1201–1205.
5. Savk E, Savk O, Bolukbasi O, Notalgia paresthetica: a study on pathogenesis. *Int J Derm* 2000;39:754–659.
6. Wallengren J. Brachioradial pruritus: a recent solar dermopathy. *J Am Acad Dermatol* 1998;39:803–806.
7. Smith KJ, Skelton HG, Yeager J, et al. Pruritus in HIV-1 disease: therapy with drugs which may modulate the pattern of immune dysregulation. *Dermatology* 1997;195:353–358.
8. Woodall TG. Pruritus. *Curr Probl Dermatol* 112:2000;P14–P16.
9. Murphy M, Carmichael AJ. Renal itch. *Clin Exp Dermatol* 2000;25:103–106.

10. Lim HW, Vallurupalli S, Meola T, et al. UVB phototherapy is an effective treatment for pruritus in patients infected with HIV. *J Am Acad Dermatol* 1997;37:414–417.
11. Monk BE. Transcutaneous electronic nerve stimulation in the treatment of generalized pruritus. *Clin Exp Dermatol* 1993;18:67–68.
12. Nilsson H, Levinsson A, Schouenborg J. Cutaneous field stimulation (CFS): a powerful new method to combat itch. *Pain* 1997;71:49–55.
13. Millikan LE. Alternative therapy in pruritus. *Dermatol Ther* 2003;16:175–180.

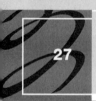

PSORIASIS
Jeffrey M. Sobell and David E. Geist

27

I. **DEFINITION AND PATHOPHYSIOLOGY.** Psoriasis is a chronic proliferative epidermal disease that affects 2 to 8 million people in the United States and 1% to 3% of the world's population. Its typical age of onset is in the third decade, although it may develop at any time from birth onward. A family history of psoriasis is found in 30% of patients; a multifactorial mode of inheritance is most likely. If one parent is affected, the incidence in the offspring is 8.1%; if both parents are affected, then 41% of the offspring may have the disease. The concordance rate in monozygotic twins is 65%; it is 30% for dizygotic twins. The histocompatibility antigen HLA-Cw6 is most strongly associated with psoriasis (relative risk is 24), and the coexistence of HLA-B17 or -B27 portends more severe skin disease or associated psoriatic arthritis. However, there does appear to be considerable genetic heterogeneity.

The pathogenesis of psoriasis involves T-cell–mediated inflammation. The clinical signs of psoriasis, epidermal hyperplasia, and vascular changes result from chronic T-cell–mediated inflammation within the psoriatic plaque. Still, the cause of psoriasis is unknown, and there is no cure. Understanding the development and maintenance of the psoriatic plaque requires an understanding of the cytokines and intercellular signaling molecules present in this disease. T-cell activation is likely triggered through typical pathways of adaptive immunity. Antigen-presenting cells (APCs) are activated in the skin, although the antigen is not known, and migrate to the lymph node. In the lymph node, APCs in turn activate T cells and program these T cells to home back to the skin. In psoriasis, APCs elaborate interleukin 12 (IL-12) and interferon-γ (IFN-γ), cytokines which direct T-cell differentiation into type 1 cells, specifically CD4$^+$ helper T cells, which predominate in the dermis, and CD8$^+$ cytotoxic T cells, which predominate in the epidermis. Once resident in the skin, activated type 1 T cells along with activated APCs and keratinocytes produce inflammatory cytokines including IL-2, IL-12, tumor necrosis factor-α (TNF-α), and IFN-γ which help sustain the T-cell response. In addition, APCs are abundant in psoriasis plaques. They may form a lymph node–like environment in the skin, which leads to continuous T-cell activation and maintenance of the psoriatic plaque (1).

In this activated T-cell milieu, psoriatic keratinocytes behave pathologically. In the presence of TNF-α and IFN-γ produced by T cells, they express increased levels of major histocompatibility complex (MHC)-II, intercellular adhesion molecule (ICAM)-1, and CD40. In addition, levels of keratin 6 and 16 (found in hyperproliferative skin) are upregulated, whereas keratin 1 and 10 (involved in terminal differentiation) are downregulated. Psoriatic keratinocytes travel from the basal cell layer to the surface in 3 to 4 days, much more rapidly than the normal 26 to 28 days. This is due to a higher proportion of basal layer keratinocytes that enter the active cell cycle. Decreased keratinocyte transit time does not allow for normal maturation and keratinization. This is reflected clinically by scaling, a thickened epidermis with increased mitotic activity, and by the presence of immature nucleated cells in the stratum corneum.

Effective and sustained T-cell activation in psoriasis requires multiple levels of intercellular signaling between T cells and both APCs and keratinocytes. The primary activation signal is delivered through the T-cell receptor (TCR)/antigen-MHC molecule interaction. Another primary signal necessary for T-cell activation is the interaction of LFA-1 on the T cell with ICAM-1 on the APC or keratinocyte. Costimulatory signals are also necessary to initiate and maintain T-cell activation and include CD28/B7 (CD80 and CD86) interactions, CD2/LFA3 interactions, and CD40Ligand/CD40 interactions. Proliferation and differentiation of T cells is driven by the cytokines IL-2 and IL-12 (and

IL-23). These essential molecular interactions, along with the cytokine TNF-α, provide the targets for several recently U.S. Food and Drug Administration (FDA)-approved psoriasis therapies.

Recently, a role for the transcription activator molecule Stat3 has been proposed. Stat3 participates in keratinocyte proliferation, survival and migration, and in wound healing. In mice, activated Stat3 in the presence of activated T cells can produce a psoriatic plaque *de novo*, which resolves when Stat3 is blocked. It is hypothesized that sensitivity of the Stat3 pathway may predispose to psoriasis (2). As such, Stat3 may be a potential future therapeutic target in psoriasis.

The course of psoriasis is prolonged but unpredictable. In most patients, the disease remains as discrete localized plaques. However, extensive or even generalized involvement may develop, and in some its severity is incompatible with a productive, happy life. Spontaneous clearing is quite rare, but unexplained exacerbation or improvement is common. Stress and anxiety frequently precede flare-ups of the disease; alcohol and smoking may also contribute to worsening of psoriasis. Psoriasis, psoriatic arthritis, and Reiter's syndrome have all been associated with human immunodeficiency virus (HIV) infection, often in a period very close to the development of acquired immunodeficiency syndrome (AIDS). Exacerbated or difficult-to-control psoriasis in an at-risk individual warrants inquiry regarding the HIV status.

II. SUBJECTIVE DATA
A. Most lesions are asymptomatic.

B. Pruritus may be noted in 20% of patients.

C. Those with generalized disease may demonstrate all the signs and symptoms of an exfoliative dermatitis (loss of thermoregulation with findings of warm skin, a feeling of chilliness and shivering, increased protein catabolism, and cardiovascular stress).

D. Oligoarticular or polyarticular pain, tenderness, and morning stiffness, especially in the small joints of the hands and feet, are the early manifestations of psoriatic arthritis. Intense pain in larger joints and the cervical and/or lumbosacral spine may also be present.

E. Alcoholism may aggravate psoriasis. A small subset of patients with psoriasis will have worsening of their clinical condition with sun exposure.

III. OBJECTIVE DATA (See color insert.)
A. The psoriatic lesion is an erythematous, sharply circumscribed plaque covered by loosely adherent, silvery scales. Acute lesions tend to be small and guttate (drop shaped). There is strong evidence that acute guttate psoriasis is induced by superantigen stimulation of T cells.

B. Inapparent scaling can be made noticeable by scratching the surface of a psoriatic lesion.

C. Any body area may be involved, but lesions tend to occur most often on the elbows and knees, scalp, genitalia, and intergluteal cleft.

D. Lesions of active psoriasis often appear in areas of epidermal injury (Koebner reaction). Scratch marks, surgical wounds, or a sunburn may heal with psoriatic lesions in their place.

E. Fifty percent of patients with psoriasis will have some degree of nail involvement. The nails may show punctate pitting or profuse collections of subungual keratotic material, clinically reflecting psoriatic involvement of the nail matrix or nail bed, respectively. A yellow-brown subungual discoloration (oil spot) is characteristic. Patients with distal interphalangeal joint involvement or arthritis mutilans usually have adjacent nail involvement.

F. Exfoliative psoriasis is clinically indistinguishable from other exfoliative dermatoses. It may occur spontaneously, follow a systemic illness or drug reaction, or occur as a reaction to some drugs or to steroid withdrawal.

G. Ten percent of patients with psoriasis may have either migratory stomatitis or glossitis.

H. Pustular psoriasis occurs in several forms: acute (von Zumbusch), subacute annular, and chronic acral. Sterile pustules are present, covering thin psoriatic plaques—the process may be generalized. The average age of onset is 50 years; flare-ups may be precipitated by infection or recent use of systemic corticosteroids. These patients require hospitalization, most necessitating systemic therapy. Impetigo herpetiformis is a rare form of pustular psoriasis during pregnancy.

  I. In acute psoriatic arthritis, one or several joints are erythematous and swollen—the distal phalanx classically has a "sausage" appearance. Long-standing or rapidly progressive disease may lead to severe bone destruction. Almost 50% to 55% of patients with psoriatic arthritis have asymmetric oligoarticular arthritis, 25% have symmetric arthritis, and another 25% have spondyloarthritis with or without peripheral arthritis; 5% of patients show a destructive polyarthritis. Most patients with asymmetric arthritis have a mild or moderately progressive course, but approximately 50% with symmetric arthritis suffer from a progressive, slowly destructive arthritis.

IV. ASSESSMENT

  A. The medical history may reveal a cause for the onset or exacerbation of psoriatic lesions. For example, acute psoriasis or a flare-up in chronic lesions may follow streptococcal pharyngitis by 7 to 10 days. T cells specific for group A streptococcal antigens can be consistently isolated from guttate psoriatic lesions. Psoriasis may be precipitated or exacerbated in patients ingesting lithium carbonate. β-Blockers, nonsteroidal antiinflammatory agents, antimalarials, gemfibrozil, chlorthalidone, and progesterone have also been implicated in aggravating psoriasis.

  B. Other causes of exfoliative dermatitis (exfoliative erythroderma) include generalized eczematous dermatitis (e.g., atopic, contact, allergic), drug reactions, lymphoma, leukemia, and several rather uncommon skin diseases; 8% to 10% of cases are idiopathic.

  C. Biopsy of lesions will reveal a psoriasiform epidermal thickening, but the histologic picture is often not diagnostic.

  D. Hyperuricemia is proportional to the amount of cutaneous involvement and is related to the increased nucleic acid degradation associated with accelerated epidermopoiesis. It rarely causes symptoms or requires therapy.

  E. Patients with psoriatic arthritis will typically have an elevated erythrocyte sedimentation rate (ESR) and, by definition, will have negative tests for rheumatoid factor. X-ray films of the hands may show characteristic subcortical cystic changes with relative sparing of the articular cartilage.

V. THERAPY

  A. It is important to emphasize that psoriasis is a treatable disease. Optimism and encouragement are justified and make it easier for the patient to conscientiously apply sometimes awkward and messy treatments. Pharmacologic data concerning the mode of action of most of these medications are limited.

  B. Treatment for mild to moderate cutaneous involvement (For scalp and nail care, see sec. V. D and E.)

    1. Topical therapies

      a. Potent topical corticosteroids applied b.i.d. to localized lesions are quite useful, especially in reducing scaling and thickness. Overnight or 24-hour occlusive therapy with these medications will initiate involution in most lesions. Hydrocolloid dermatologic patches (Actiderm, DuoDerm Extra Thin) can be applied over steroids on localized psoriatic plaques for 2 to 7 days. The patches may be worn while bathing. Corticosteroids exert their beneficial effects in this setting as inhibitors of mitoses and lymphokines and through depletion of Langerhans cells.

      Patients should apply corticosteroids to lesions without occlusion during the day, apply medication to plaques in the evening, immediately after bath or shower, and occlude with plastic wrap for 4 hours or overnight. As lesions subside, decrease the use of occlusion and increase the use of a bland emollient (e.g., Eucerin, Aquaphor, and Vaseline). After lesions have flattened, apply corticosteroids in bursts (e.g., several days on, several days off).

      If superpotent agents are used, they should be applied to limited areas only, and after achieving the desired result, they should be switched to an intermittent or staggered regimen. As little as 2 g/day of topical clobetasol propionate can suppress the hypothalamic pituitary axis (HPA).

Injection of intralesional corticosteroids beneath isolated chronic plaques will cause involution within 7 to 10 days (triamcinolone acetonide, diluted to 2.5 to 5.0 mg/mL), which lasts 2 to 4 months.

b. Topical vitamin D analogs, both calcitriol and calcipotriol (calcipotriene [Dovonex]), have shown clinical effectiveness comparable with that of topical steroids or anthralin. Vitamin D analogs bind to Vitamin D$_3$ receptors on keratinocytes and regulate keratinocyte proliferation and differentiation and also inhibit T-cell activation.

Calcipotriene (Dovonex) ointment, cream, or solution is applied b.i.d.; dosages should not exceed 100 g/week as the risk of kidney stones and hypercalcemia increases. Calcipotriene (Dovonex) may irritate facial skin (diluting Calcipotriene [Dovonex] with petrolatum may decrease this irritation). Intertriginous and genital psoriasis can be effectively treated with surprisingly minimal irritation. Any dermatitis is most likely secondary to irritancy and not allergic contact dermatitis.

A 2-week regimen of calcipotriene and halobetasol ointments daily was superior to monotherapy with halobetasol two times per day. Calcipotriol scalp solution is effective for mild to moderate scalp psoriasis but is inferior to midpotency steroids; a combination rotational therapy between the two products is recommended.

Calcipotriene (Dovonex) enhances the effectiveness of ultraviolet B (UVB) but also increases photosensitivity in UVB-treated patients. Ultraviolet light, 6% salicylic acid, 12% lactic acid, hydrocortisone valerate 0.2% ointment, and tazarotene (Tazorac) gel degrade calcipotriene (Dovonex). Halobetasol ointment and 5% tar gel are compatible with Calcipotriene (Dovonex). A British study found calcipotriene (Dovonex) to be safe and effective in a pediatric population over the age of 3, although it is not approved by the FDA.

Several new vitamin D analogs are currently involved in clinical trials.

c. Topical tazarotene gel and cream tazarotene (Tazorac 0.05% and 0.1%) are topical retinoids that modulate abnormal epidermal differentiation and proliferation; there is an upregulation of K10 terminal differentiation. Systemic absorption is minimal, but this is categorized as a category X drug, and special warnings should be provided to women of childbearing potential. Like most retinoids, this topical drug can be inherently irritating. Methods that are helpful in minimizing this irritation are as follows: (i) Apply tazarotene (Tazorac) to affected skin only at bedtime, protect normal skin with Vaseline, (ii) apply a mid-to-high–potency topical steroid in the morning, and (iii) start with a low dose (0.05%) and increase as tolerated. The 0.1% gel is slightly more effective but also more irritating than the 0.05% gel. Tazarotene is not inactivated by ultraviolet light although it will lower the erythema threshold. Tazarotene combined with UVB phototherapy is more effective than phototherapy alone.

d. Coal tar therapy may be combined or alternated with topical corticosteroids. Tars such as T/Derm, which are nearly colorless, or 1 to 5% crude coal tar ointment, which is very messy but may be more effective, are applied overnight. Tars inhibit deoxyribonucleic acid (DNA) synthesis and have an atrophogenic effect on skin, as well as sensitize the skin to long-wave ultraviolet light (UVA). Although they do not offer any advantage over lubricants such as petrolatum when used with an aggressive UVB treatment protocol, tars may provide a beneficial "light-sparing" effect when used with less aggressive UVB regimens. Tars may aggravate acne and cause folliculitis.

As directed in the instructions for corticosteroids, but on alternate nights, the patient should apply a tar formulation overnight and be exposed to ultraviolet light (UVL) the following morning or apply a corticosteroid cream with or without occlusion during the day, tar overnight, and UVL exposure in the morning.

e. Other topical agents
   i. Salicylic acid 2% to 10% formulations help remove scales and crusts and may be used along with corticosteroid or anthralin therapy. Formulations

commonly used include 3% to 10% salicylic acid cream or 3% to 6% sulfur and salicylic acid ointment.

ii. Anthralin (dithranol) is effective for treatment of discrete lesions consisting primarily of thick plaques (see Chap. 40, Keratolytic, Cytotoxic, and Destructive Agents, sec. II). This drug is derived from chrysarobin (active ingredient of Goa powder from the bark of South American Araroba Tree). This drug inhibits keratinocyte proliferation and granulocyte function and exerts an immunosuppressive effect. Anthralin's disadvantages are that it may be a primary irritant, it stains clothing and skin, and it can be difficult to apply.

Anthralin paste or cream can be used on an outpatient or inpatient basis and will clear up the lesions on most patients within 2 to 3 weeks. In short-contact therapy, start with 0.1% anthralin applied for 20 to 30 minutes and then washed off. Check for irritation at 48 hours. According to tolerance, the potency can be increased (to 0.3%, 0.5%, or 1.0%) and the contact time shortened or, for resistant plaques, increased. Use daily for clearing and then once or twice weekly for maintenance therapy.

Micanol is a temperature-sensitive formulation of anthralin that releases the anthralin product only when in contact with skin temperature. There is minimal or no staining of skin or fabrics.

iii. Topical tacrolimus or pimecrolimus does not appear effective in typical plaque psoriasis but may be helpful in intertriginous and facial psoriasis where there is better absorption.

2. Repeated exposure to sunlight or middle-wavelength, sunburn-spectrum, ultraviolet light (UVB) from artificial sources to the point of mild erythema will induce flattening or clearing of many lesions. A standardized three times weekly UVB protocol will induce complete clearing in an average of 23 treatments. While various treatment centers continue to refine its optimal parameters, UVB phototherapy remains perhaps the most rapid and effective means of inducing remission in mild to severe disease. UVB inhibits epidermal mitosis and presumably acts by this mechanism.

A new form of phototherapy is available that utilizes a narrowband wavelength of 311 nm, the wavelength determined to be the most effective in psoriasis. This limited spectrum of UVB may be less carcinogenic than traditional UVB. Widespread use of narrowband UVB treatments is limited by the expense of the units (traditional UVB units cannot be easily converted to accommodate these new bulbs).

An excimer laser with intense 308-nm UVB radiation can clear a plaque of psoriasis with as little as one treatment, although usually four to eight treatments are required. Remissions of 3 to 4 months are possible. This laser is capable of rapidly delivering multiples of the minimal erythema dose (MED) to lesions without the use of anesthesia, making it an attractive treatment option for localized and limited cutaneous areas. Pulsed dye laser treatment improves limited psoriatic plaques with some chance for pigmentary changes and scarring; the target is the enlarged and dilated blood vessels (3).

C. Treatment for more severe or widespread involvement. The management of severe or extensive psoriasis is a problem that can be best handled by a dermatologist.

1. Phototherapy

a. Aggressive UVB phototherapy is the most rapid and effective single-agent regimen for clearing psoriasis. It may be used by specific protocols three times a week, five times a week, or daily. The latter will clear most patients in 18 treatments. All protocols involve application of lubricants to psoriatic plaques before phototherapy. The 311-nm narrowband phototherapy can be used in place of broadband sources. An initial MED must be performed with narrowband UVB. Long-term studies of safety and efficacy for the 311-nm wavelength are in progress.

b. Tar and UVL therapy (Goeckerman regimen), which was once the standard of care, is little used today. It is best an inpatient or day-care facility treatment, because tars are messy to apply and potent or fluorescent lights are needed. Tars and middle-wavelength UV light (UVB) act as separate antipsoriatic agents.

c. Photochemotherapy will bring about marked improvement when used for widespread, severe psoriasis. A photoactive drug (a psoralen) is administered orally, followed 2 hours later by exposure to long-wave UVL (UVA). Psoralens form photoadducts with DNA in the presence of UVA and in this way probably reduce the increased epidermal turnover characteristic of psoriasis. Long-term side effects include increased risk of squamous cell carcinoma (SCC) (especially involving the male genitalia), malignant melanoma, atypical pigmentation, and accelerated skin aging. A long latency period (15 years or longer) and a large number of treatments (>250 J/cm^2 or >100 exposures) are required to induce the melanoma and nonmelanoma skin cancers.

Psoralen plus ultraviolet A (PUVA) is one of the most efficacious treatments for psoriasis. Repeated PUVA exposure causes disappearance of lesions in almost all patients after 10 to 20 treatments over 4 to 8 weeks. Psoriasis often recurs weeks to months after PUVA ceases, and twice-monthly treatment is necessary to keep most patients free of their disease. Scalp, body folds, and other areas not exposed to UVA respond poorly to the therapy. Topical PUVA is helpful in palmar and plantar psoriasis. Outdoor use of PUVA using natural sunlight is also possible, although hazardous (4).

d. Combined therapies appear to be most effective in clearing recalcitrant widespread and severe psoriasis. These include PUVA-UVB, retinoid-PUVA, retinoid-UVB, methotrexate-PUVA, and methotrexate-UVB (5). The latter, for example, combines thrice-weekly UVB treatments with once-weekly methotrexate administration for 8 weeks. This regimen cleared all 26 cases of disabling psoriasis in one half the number of UVB treatments (6) required without methotrexate and utilized relatively low amounts of each agent, thereby reducing cumulative methotrexate and UVL toxicity.

Six of seven studies failed to demonstrate an advantage to the addition of topical corticosteroids to UVB phototherapy. In contrast to PUVA, topical steroids appear to show a more rapid rate of clearing and a smaller total UVA dose when used in combination.

2. Oral systemic agents

a. Acitretin (Soriatane), a synthetic derivative of vitamin A, is a major metabolite of etretinate with a similar efficacy and side effect profile. Acitretin is less lipophilic than etretinate, with a significant difference in half-life (60 hours vs. 120 days). This agent is helpful in pustular, guttate, and erythrodermic psoriasis; its efficacy is less dramatic in chronic plaque psoriasis unless it is combined with some form of phototherapy, methotrexate, or cyclosporine. Care should be taken to decrease the dose of UVA and UVB by 50% when combined with acitretin.

Side effects are dose dependent and include elevation of triglycerides, hepatitis, hair loss, thinning of the nails, cheilitis, xerosis, and stickiness of the skin. Gemfibrozil (300 mg b.i.d.) corrects elevated lipid levels on this therapy.

The usual starting dose of acitretin is 10 to 20 mg/day with maximum dose of 50 mg/day. Etretinate has been identified in plasma samples of some patients treated with acitretin and is converted by ingestion of alcohol. This drug is not recommended for women of childbearing potential; if it is used, pregnancy should be avoided for 3 years after the last dose.

b. Antimetabolite therapy with agents that inhibit DNA synthesis (methotrexate, hydroxyurea) is reserved for those patients unresponsive to other approaches.

Methotrexate is given orally or by IM administration. Doses begin at 7.5 mg weekly with incremental increases of 2.5 mg/week as tolerated. Typical maximum doses reach 12.5 to 15 mg/week. Side effects include nausea, bone marrow suppression, and liver toxicity. The addition of folic acid 1 to 5 mg/day helps reduce nausea and counteract the macrocytic anemia. Complete blood count (CBC) and liver function tests should be carefully followed and a liver biopsy obtained after every 1.5 g of cumulative exposure.

Hydroxyurea dosing starts at 500 mg/day with weekly monitoring of CBC and platelets. This drug has a very narrow window between toxicity and efficacy; as many as 50% of patients will develop neutropenia at doses of 2 g/day.

c. Cyclosporine A (CSA) administration (3 to 6 mg/kg) causes dramatic clearing of widespread psoriasis. A new microemulsion formula of cyclosporine (Neoral) is better absorbed and the suggested range of dosing is 2.5 to 4 mg/kg. This drug selectively inhibits T-helper cell production of IL-2 while allowing increase of suppressor T-cell populations. Cyclosporine has no direct effect on keratinocytes and is not a mitotic inhibitor. Cyclosporine inhibits cytokine release, which results in a decreased recruitment of APCs into the epidermis and decreases immunoreactivity of lesions.

Potential long-term side effects preclude cyclosporine's use in all but very severe and recalcitrant psoriasis. Cyclosporine can be combined with low-dose methotrexate. Cyclosporine's main side effects, even at low doses, are hypertension and nephrotoxicity. Age, baseline blood pressure, and baseline creatinine levels are predictors of higher risks of side effects. Glomerular filtration rate (GFR) is a more sensitive test than creatinine for evaluating renal function, and a baseline is recommended in any high-risk patient. Long-term treatment with CSA may induce interstitial fibrosis and glomerular sclerosis, with more pronounced changes directly associated with duration of therapy. Discontinuation after 2 years at most is recommended (7). It should be administered only by dermatologists experienced in its use.

d. Treatment schedules are advocated that rotate therapies to try and minimize the adverse effects of each. One recommended schedule is as follows: UVB < PUVA, methotrexate, acitretin, and cyclosporine (8).

e. Other oral agents
   i. Mycophenolate mofetil (CellCept), an inhibitor of synthesis of the nucleotide guanosine, is administered at a dose of 500 mg four times a day to a maximum of 4 g/day. The main side effects include an increased incidence of herpes zoster, neutropenia, gastrointestinal symptoms, and opportunistic infections. In the transplant literature, 1% to 2% of patients will develop a lymphoproliferative malignancy at the doses recommended for psoriasis. This is a teratogen and should be avoided in women of childbearing age.
   ii. Fumaric acid esters have been available for a decade and have a high level of efficacy in psoriasis; the mechanism is unknown but researchers theorize that psoriasis is a disorder of defective citric acid metabolism. Side effects include flushing, gastrointestinal side effects, eosinophilia, and reports of acute renal failure.
   iii. Oral calcitriol is effective but can increase serum and urinary calcium and result in alteration of creatinine clearance.

3. **Biologic therapies**
   a. Alefacept (Amevive) is a fully human lymphocyte function–associated antigen 3/immunoglobulin 1 (LFA-3/IgG1) fusion protein. It binds to CD2 on T cells, inhibiting T-cell activation and producing selective T-cell apoptosis. Alefacept is FDA approved as a 12-week course of 15 mg weekly intramuscular injections. Long remissions can be seen in responders. Peripheral CD4 counts should be followed and doses withheld if counts drop below 250 cells/μL. Therapy should be discontinued if the CD4 count remains below 250 cells/μL for >4 weeks. A second course lengthens the period of remission without additional toxicities (9).
   b. Efalizumab (Raptiva) is a humanized monoclonal antibody that binds to the CD11a subunit of LFA-1. It blocks the interaction of LFA-1 with ICAM-1, thereby interfering with T-cell activation and trafficking. Efalizumab is FDA

approved at 1.0 mg/kg/week by subcutaneous injection. Common side effects include mild headache, fever, chills, nausea, or myalgia within the first 48 hours of injection in the first 2 to 3 weeks of therapy. Immune-mediated thrombocytopenia is rare. Worsening of psoriasis may occur after discontinuation of therapy or in unresponsive patients during therapy. Transitioning patients to alternative therapies may minimize this risk (10).

  c. Etanercept (Enbrel) is a soluble TNF receptor fusion protein. It is FDA approved for moderate to severe psoriasis at a dose of 50 mg twice weekly by subcutaneous injection for the initial 12 weeks, followed by a step-down to 50 mg weekly for maintenance. The most common side effect is injection site reactions. Rare cases of serious infection, demyelinating disease, and congestive heart failure have been reported by postmarketing surveillance (11).

  d. Infliximab (Remicade), a chimeric anti-TNF monoclonal antibody, and adalimumab (Humira), a fully humanized anti-TNF monoclonal antibody, are both promising therapies under investigation for psoriasis.

D. Scalp care

  1. Mild involvement may be treated by the patient with a tar shampoo (10% liquor carbonis detergens in tincture of green soap, Pentrax, Polytar, Sebutone, T-gel, Zetar) and steroid lotion or solution b.i.d. (betamethasone, halcinonide, Diprolene, Temovate). Steroid-containing shampoos are also available (Capex, Clobex).

  2. More severe involvement should be treated as follows:

  a. If scaling is thick, it is necessary to first remove the scales and then apply something to inhibit their reformation. Apply a keratolytic gel to a hydrated scalp and then cover it with an occlusive plastic shower cap for several hours or overnight. This will effectively loosen the scales, after which a steroid lotion or solution (Derma-Smoothe/FS, Lidex, Synalar, Valisone) should be applied under a shower cap for the rest of the night or without occlusion during the day. A betamethasone valerate mousse (Luxiq) and a clobetasol propionate mousse (Olux) were recently approved by the FDA for the treatment of scalp psoriasis. The foam distributes easily on the scalp as it liquefies at body temperature and leaves minimal residue on the hair. In warm weather, the can should be stored in the refrigerator to restore the foam to a proper consistency.

  b. Alternatively, chronic thick plaques may be treated by the patient as follows:

  i. Apply anthralin (Dritho-Scalp), or phenol/saline lotion (P&S liquid), or, in severe cases, 20% oil of cade, 10% sulfur, 5% salicylic acid (20-10-5 ointment) in hydrophilic ointment on the scalp, leaving it overnight.

  ii. Use tar shampoo (e.g., T/Gel) in the morning.

  iii. Reapply the preparation as for overnight during the day until scaling is decreased. At that point, substitute a steroid lotion or solution.

  c. Intralesional corticosteroid injections will clear isolated plaques.

E. Nail care. There is no consistently effective therapy for psoriatic involvement of the nails. The nails will often improve coincidentally with remission of cutaneous lesions and will almost always improve after systemic antimetabolite or immunomodulator therapy.

  1. Removal of subungual debris and application of corticosteroids under occlusion may offer some benefit.

  2. Injection of small amounts of triamcinolone (0.1 mL of 3 mg/mL) into the nail bed at 2- to 3-week intervals will result in cure or improvement in approximately 75% of treated nails, but it is painful and time consuming. There will be approximately 50% recurrence rate when treatment is stopped.

  Another regimen is 0.1 mL of 10 mg/mL at 3-month intervals utilizing a ring block to minimize pain. Onycholysis and pitting of the nails respond least well. Postprocedure paresthesias, hematomas, and pain of the distal tip can occur. Steroid benefit could be maintained for 9 months (12).

3. Urea 40% ointment may be useful in removing hypertrophic or dystrophic psoriatic nails. Subsequent topical therapy to the denuded nail bed and proximal nail fold may result in regrowth of "normal" nails in half of those treated.
4. A 1% 5-fluorouracil solution (Fluoroplex) applied twice daily to nail margins has been reported to decrease the severity of involvement by 75% in two thirds of patients within 3 to 6 months.
5. Subungual hyperkeratosis of a solitary nail should be further evaluated for the possibility of a wart or SCC.
6. More than 25% of patients with psoriatic nails will have an associated dermatophyte infection; oral antifungal therapy may help improve the overall condition of the nails although patients should be advised that they have two problems affecting the appearance of the nails.
7. Calcipotriol ointment and/or tazarotene (Tazorac) gel applied b.i.d. to nail beds may have some modest benefits on subungual hyperkeratosis (6).

F. Psoriatic arthritis may respond to a variety of pharmacologic agents. In general, when the disease is mild to moderate, it should be treated with either aspirin or a nonsteroidal antiinflammatory drug; if unresponsive or more severe, with hydroxychloroquine, sulfasalazine, methotrexate, etanercept (Enbrel), or infliximab; and if relentless, with gold or other immunosuppressive agents. Splinting and local heat should also be used.

1. Aspirin must be taken to near toxicity to be effective.
2. Nonsteroidal antiinflammatory agents are very effective in early psoriatic arthritis, and there is some opinion that they may be more useful than aspirin. Indomethacin is given in doses of 75 to 100 mg/day. It is essential that these drugs be administered in amounts sufficient to exert their antiinflammatory effects. Ibuprofen (Motrin) dosage should be 2,400 mg/day, or naproxen (Naprosyn), 500 to 750 mg/day. All these medications are gastrointestinal irritants and are contraindicated in patients with ulcer disease. They also affect platelets in a manner similar to aspirin and, if given to patients already on anticoagulants, may result in bleeding and clotting problems. There is no clear evidence that any one of the nonsalicylate nonsteroidal antiinflammatory agents is more effective than any other in controlling the inflammation of psoriatic arthritis.
3. Hydroxychloroquine (Plaquenil) has been shown to induce a beneficial response in 75% of 100 patients with psoriatic arthritis. The use of this antimalarial drug was not accompanied by an exacerbation in psoriasis, contrary to previous beliefs (13).
4. Sulfasalazine (3.0 g daily). Side effects include drug rash and nausea; severe side effects are minimal, making this a safe alternative to more toxic oral therapies. This can be administered with methotrexate.
5. Gold or folic acid antagonists, particularly methotrexate, are very useful in intractable cases unresponsive to the more conventional therapies. 6-Mercaptopurine may be more effective against the arthritis component but is less useful for the cutaneous lesions. Gold or immunosuppressive drugs may put psoriatic arthritis into remission.
6. TNF blockers (Enbrel and Remicade) are approved for the treatment of psoriatic arthritis. Both agents improve the signs and symptoms of arthritis and prevent the progression of joint destruction. Humira is under investigation and will likely be beneficial as well.
7. Spondylitis associated with psoriatic arthritis is treated with the same medications as spondylitis of other causes. The nonsteroidal antiinflammatory drugs described earlier are the initial agents of choice, and the disease usually responds well. Alternatively, the TNF blockers are effective.

G. Acute psoriasis should be treated gently with just emollients or topical steroids. Avoid tars, salicylic acid, and aggressive UVL therapy, because they may be irritating and lead to a more widespread eruption and chronic course.

H. HIV-associated psoriasis can be extensive and difficult to treat. Therapy with acitretin as monotherapy or in combination with UVB is recommended. Methotrexate therapy is controversial because of its immunosuppressive effects (14).

References

1. Krueger JG. The immunologic basis for the treatment of psoriasis with new biologic agents. *J Am Acad Dermatol* 2002;46:1–23.
2. Sano S, Chan KS, Carbajal S, et al. Stat 3 links activated keratinocytes and immunocytes required for development of psoriasis in a novel transgenic mouse model. *Nat Med* 2005;11:43–49.
3. Ros A-M, Garden JM, Bakus AD, et al. Psoriasis response to the pulsed dye laser. *Lasers Surg Med* 1996;19:331–335.
4. Parrish JA, White AD, Kingsbury T, et al. Photochemotherapy of psoriasis using methoxsalen and sunlight: a controlled study. *Arch Dermatol* 1977;113:1529–1532.
5. Paul BS, Momtaz K, Stern RS, et al. Combined methotrexate-ultraviolet B therapy in the treatment of psoriasis. *J Am Acad Dermatol* 1982;7:758–762.
6. Tosti A, Piraccini BM, Cameli N, et al. Calcipotriol ointment in nail psoriasis: a controlled double-blind comparison with betamethasone dipropionate and salicylic acid. *Br J Dermatol* 1998;139:655–659.
7. Zachariae H, Kragballe K, Hansen HE, et al. Renal biopsy findings in long-term cyclosporin treatment of psoriasis. *Br J Dermatol* 1997;136:531–535.
8. Spuls PI, Bossuyt PM, van Everdingen JJ, et al. The development of practice guidelines for the treatment of severe plaque form psoriasis. *Arch Dermatol* 1998;134:1591–1596.
9. Lebwohl M, Christophers E, Langley R, et al. An international, randomized, double-blind, placebo-controlled phase 3 trial of intramuscular alefacept in patients with chronic plaque psoriasis. *Arch Dermatol* 2003;139:719–727.
10. Menter A, Gordon K, Carey W, et al. Efficacy and safety observed during 24 weeks of efalizumab therapy in patients with moderate to severe plaque psoriasis. *Arch Dermatol* 2005;141:31–38.
11. Leonardi CL, Powers JL, Matheson RT, et al. Etanercept as monotherapy in patients with psoriasis. *N Engl J Med* 2003;349:2014–1022.
12. De Berker DAR, Lawrence CM. A simplified protocol of steroid injection for psoriatic nail dystrophy. *Br J Dermatol* 1998;138:90–95.
13. Schur PH, Kammer GM, Soter NA. Clinical, immunologic and genetic study of 100 patients with psoriatic arthritis. *Arthritis Rheum* 1979;22:656.
14. Buccheri L, Katchen BR, Karter AJ, et al. Acitretin therapy is effective for psoriasis associated with human immunodeficiency virus infection. *Arch Dermatol* 1997;133:711–715.

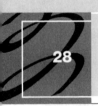

28 ROSACEA AND PERIORAL (PERIORIFICIAL) DERMATITIS

Peter C. Schalock

I. DEFINITION AND PATHOPHYSIOLOGY

A. Rosacea is a chronic disorder of unknown etiology that affects the central face and neck. At least 13 million people are affected by this noncurable disorder. It is characterized by two clinical components: a vascular change consisting of intermittent or persistent erythema and flushing and an acneiform eruption with papules, pustules, cysts, and sebaceous hyperplasia. There is no correlation between the sebum excretion rate and the severity of rosacea. Lesional blood flow as measured by laser Doppler is three to four times that of controls. Onset is most often between the ages of 30 and 50; pediatric cases have also been reported. Although women are affected three times as frequently as men, the disease may become more severe in men. Rosacea is much more common in light-skinned, fair-complexioned individuals but may also occur in darker skin types. It is estimated that 10% of individuals in Sweden have rosacea.

There is speculation that a defect in the trigeminal afferent nerve pathway contributes to a predisposition to facial flushing. Over time, after repeated bouts of flushing, the vessels become ectatic and there is permanent vasodilatation. Hot liquids are thought to promote erythema and flushing when they heat up the tissues of the oral mucosa, leading to a countercurrent heat exchange with the carotid artery. A further signal from the carotid body is then relayed to the hypothalamus (the body's thermostat), which signals the body to dissipate heat through flushing and vasodilatation because of the perceived increase in core body temperature.

The diagnosis of rosacea is made by fulfilling one of several primary and one of many secondary criteria. Primary criteria for rosacea include transient erythema/flushing, persistent facial redness, papules and pustules, and increased facial telangiectasias. Secondary criteria include burning/stinging, elevated red facial plaques with or without scale, dry/scaly skin, persistent facial edema (subtypes of solid facial or soft facial type), phymatous changes, and ocular manifestations such as burning/itching, conjunctival hyperemia, lid inflammation, styes, chalazia, and corneal damage.

There are four subtypes and one variant of rosacea that have been defined by the National Rosacea Society committee on the classification and staging of rosacea: (i) erythematotelangiectatic, (ii) papulopustular, (iii) phymatous, and (iv) ocular. Erythematotelangiectatic rosacea is characterized by flushing and persistent central facial erythema with or without telangiectasia. The papulopustular type has persistent central facial edema and transient papules, pustules, or both. Phymatous rosacea occurs most often on the nose (rhinophyma) and is characterized by thick skin with an irregular surface, nodularities, and bulbous enlargement. Careful evaluation of a nose with the changes of rhinophyma should be undertaken because basal cell carcinomas may be present, as well as less common tumors. Lastly, the ocular type of rosacea has many symptoms, which will be discussed below. Granulomatous rosacea is a variant characterized by noninflammatory, hard, brown, yellow, or red papules/nodules of the central face. It is of note that rosacea fulminans (pyoderma faciale), steroid-induced acneiform eruption, and perioral dermatitis are not considered rosacea variants but separate entities (1).

Ocular changes (blepharitis, conjunctivitis, and keratitis) and sebaceous hyperplasia of the nose (rhinophyma) may be associated with ocular rosacea. Differential diagnostic considerations include (i) acne vulgaris, which is characterized by a wider distribution of lesions and the presence of comedones, (ii) periorificial dermatitis, (iii) seborrheic dermatitis, (iv) malignant carcinoid syndrome, (v) lupus erythematosus, and (vi) photodermatoses. Ocular rosacea has been theorized to be secondary to increased local levels of interferon-1α that is proinflammatory and leads to lid irritation and erythema. Lipid breakdown in the tears releases fatty acids that are also irritating. Some studies have also shown a more alkaline pH of tears in patients with rosacea.

Helicobacter pylori, a microaerophilic gram-negative bacteria implicated in gastric ulcer disease, has been theorized to be the inciting organism in rosacea on the basis of an increased incidence of dyspepsia in this population and the responsiveness of rosacea to metronidazole. Fifty percent of the world's population and 25% of the US population may have antibodies to this organism. Colonization is associated with increased levels of serum gastrin, which can cause flushing. Also, *H. pylori* infection can increase levels of histamine, prostaglandins, leukotrienes, and various other cytokines. Therapy to eradicate this organism usually consists of a combination of oral metronidazole, amoxicillin, and omeprazole. Conflicting studies regarding this association with rosacea have recently been in the literature. In general, it is felt that strong support for a link between *H. pylori* infection and rosacea is lacking (2). Large case control studies would be needed to prove this association because of the high baseline incidence of this exposure.

Infection with *Demodex* mites is common, with infection approaching 100% in sensitive tests of healthy adults. Some have hypothesized that infection with *Demodex* is a cause of rosacea. There is controversy within the literature whether this is the case. In one study, there was a link between higher mite counts and papulopustular but not erythematotelangiectatic rosacea (2). It is unclear whether *Demodex* is pathologic or just normal skin flora.

B. Perioral (periorificial) dermatitis is a distinct clinical entity that can easily be confused with rosacea, seborrheic dermatitis, eczematous dermatitis, or acne. It primarily affects young women, is usually found around the mouth but occasionally around the nose or eyes, and is of unknown cause; *Candida, Demodex,* fluorinated toothpastes, chapping, irritation, and oral contraceptives have been implicated. Stinging/burning is usually a more significant complaint than pruritus. Pediatric cases tend to involve more boys and have periocular and perinasal papules. As with rosacea, prolonged use of potent topical corticosteroids can cause an eruption with similar features and can perpetuate preexisting disease.

Perioral (periorificial) dermatitis is found at a significantly increased rate in atopic individuals. Compared with patients with rosacea, those with perioral dermatitis have significantly increased transepidermal water loss (TEWL) and atopic diathesis (3).

II. SUBJECTIVE DATA

A. The facial lesions of rosacea and perioral (periorificial) dermatitis often cause justifiable concern about personal appearance. There may be a family history of easy flushing and blushing, as well as of a red, ruddy complexion.

B. Rosacea papules and cysts can be painful; perioral (periorificial) dermatitis papules may itch or cause a burning sensation.

C. Patients with rosacea may complain of feelings of facial heat and congestion as well as dry eyes. Other ocular complaints include stinging, photophobia, burning, tearing, scratchiness, and a sense of a foreign body being in the eye. The frequency of ocular symptoms increases as rosacea progresses. Many of these patients have also experienced multiple styes in the past. Individuals who work at video display terminals (VDTs) have complained of symptoms of facial burning and have been found to have a possible increased risk of rosacea.

III. OBJECTIVE DATA

A. Rosacea (See color insert.)

1. Recurrent erythema, located in the middle third of the face (mid-forehead, nose, malar areas, and chin), may later lead to a persistent flush and telangiectasias. Symmetric involvement of the eyelids may be the only presentation. Lupoid or granulomatous rosacea consists of uniform brown-red papules or nodules in the typical rosacea distribution. Fifteen percent of cases of granulomatous rosacea have extrafacial lesions. "Rosacea fulminans" or pyoderma faciale is a separate condition and not a variant or subtype of rosacea, according to the most recent classifications. It usually occurs in women from the age of 15 to 46 with a prior history of seborrhea. It is characterized by rapid onset, giant coalescent nodules on the face without evidence of comedones, telangiectasias, erythema, and remission with little or no scarring.

2. The lesions of rosacea may be seen in the beard region, neck, scalp, shoulders, and upper back.

3. Acneiform papules, pustules, and cysts may be present; comedones are not.

4. Central facial edema of the forehead, eyelids, nose, and cheeks with subsequent enlargement of the soft tissues may be seen.

5. Rosacea may have an associated dermatitis of the central face and cheeks. The differential diagnosis includes seborrheic dermatitis or irritant dermatitis. Often, these patients will decrease the use of soaps to minimize irritation. The surface microbes and lipids are altered, and gentle daily cleansing helps normalize this.

6. Rhinophyma, which predominantly affects men, is associated with follicular dilatation, irregular thickening of the skin, and hypertrophic soft masses centered about the tip of the nose. Pseudorhinophyma can be seen when heavy eyeglasses obstruct the lymphatic and venous drainage from the nose.

7. Fifty percent of patients will have ocular findings including blepharitis, conjunctivitis, iritis, and/or keratitis. The severity of the eye involvement does not correlate with the severity of facial involvement. Hyperplasia and plugging of the meibomian gland, a modified sebaceous gland, likely leads to the symptoms of ocular rosacea. The lid margin may show early hyperemia of the eyelids, conjunctivitis, blepharitis, and, in later stages, granules and yellow papules on the conjunctiva. Features of greater concern requiring referral to an ophthalmologist include keratitis, corneal vascularization, and severe conjunctivitis. Ocular rosacea is a rare cause of blindness.

8. Drugs associated with flushing include vasodilators, calcium channel blockers, cholinergic agents, opiates, cyclosporin, nicotinic acid, tamoxifen, and rifampin. Topical sorbic acid, a common component of cosmetics and corticosteroids, can cause facial redness and itching.

B. Perioral (periorificial) dermatitis

1. Discrete 1- to 3-mm erythematous or flesh-colored papules and pustules, often with a fine scale, are seen singly, in clusters, or in plaques around the mouth, sparing the vermillion border. Lesions may occasionally occur around the nose and on the malar areas below and lateral to the eyes. In 10% to 20% of patients, the disease will extend to the glabella and the periocular region.

2. There is often a persistent erythema of the nasolabial folds that may extend around the mouth and onto the chin.

3. Long-standing lesions show a flatter, more confluent eruption, with superimposed dry scaling.

4. The differential diagnosis includes seborrheic dermatitis, rosacea, contact or irritant dermatitis, nutritional deficiencies, or the rare glucagonoma syndrome.

IV. THERAPY

A. Rosacea

1. Precipitating factors. Patients who flush easily should avoid hot food and drinks and activities that induce this change. These may include tea, coffee, sunlight, extremes of heat and cold, and emotional stress. It has been demonstrated that the flushing caused by coffee is induced by a temperature of $60°C$ and above, but not by cold coffee or caffeine alone. A printed handout with trigger factors is helpful for the individual patient to identify any causative agents for worsening of their rosacea symptoms. If flushing is not caused by these factors, there is no evidence that avoidance will result in improvement of the disease. Vasodilator drugs that affect peripheral blood vessels will also exacerbate rosacea flushing. The vascular reactivity of rosacea flushing may be confused with menopausal flushing and carcinoid flushing.

2. Systemic therapy

a. The most effective treatment for rosacea is the administration of systemic antibiotics, particularly those in the tetracycline family. The literature supports initial therapy with tetracycline, but doxycycline or minocycline are also quite effective for initial treatment. For tetracycline, therapy should be initiated at 250 mg q.i.d. until symptoms subside, after which the dosage can be decreased slowly or discontinued. Nausea/gastrointestinal upset is a significant side effect of tetracycline therapy. Occasionally, it is necessary to use larger doses (1.5 to 2.0 g daily) for short periods of time to induce remission. Long-term administration is usually needed. Tetracycline is most effective in decreasing the acneiform component and clearing the keratitis but may also diminish erythema. Dosing of minocycline or doxycycline should be initiated at 100 mg b.i.d. and tapered as described earlier.

After discontinuing tetracycline therapy, 25% of patients can be expected to relapse within a few days; approximately 60% will have a relapse within 6 months. Keratitis always seems to recur quickly and may require continual treatment.

Ocular rosacea responds to oral tetracyclines or erythromycin. Higher doses may be required initially and then as little as 250 mg q.d. or q.o.d. of either antibiotic may be sufficient. Long-term remissions may occur, requiring episodic oral therapy.

b. If tetracycline is ineffective, minocycline, doxycycline, or erythromycin should be tried. Doxycycline monohydrate has a pH of 7.0, which decreases the chance of gastrointestinal upset, although it is more expensive.

c. Metronidazole (Flagyl) (200 mg b.i.d.) has been shown to be as effective as tetracycline for papulopustular rosacea. Patients must be forewarned of its disulfiram (Antabuse)-like side effects if alcohol is consumed during treatment, as well as an associated peripheral neuropathy with prolonged use.

d. Ampicillin (250 mg b.i.d. to t.i.d.) has also been shown to be useful.

e. Trimethoprim/sulfamethoxazole on a daily basis has a rapid onset of action but has rare associated side effects of bone marrow suppression and toxic epidermal necrolysis (TEN).

f. Clarithromycin (Biaxin) in a dose of 250 mg b.i.d. for 4 weeks and then 250 mg q.d. for 4 weeks is another oral alternative for treatment-resistant patients.

g. Menopause-related flushing or intractable flushing might respond to low doses of clonidine (Catapres), an α-adrenergic agonist, at a dose of 0.05 mg PO b.i.d. or through a transdermal patch. It is otherwise apparently ineffective in rosacea.

h. Isotretinoin (0.5 mg/kg/day for 20 weeks) can be highly effective in patients with severe refractory papulopustular rosacea. There is improvement in edema, erythema, and telangiectasias and a decrease in sebaceous gland hyperplasia, rhinophyma, and oily skin. Ocular side effects of therapy occur more frequently than with acne. One study showed efficacy with as little as 10 mg/day of isotretinoin for 16 weeks. Other dosing regimens include 10 mg two to three times per week or 20 mg two times per week. Remission rates remain to be determined, but some patients note prolonged disappearance of disease. Patients with rosacea are generally older than those with acne, and even more care concerning adverse effects is necessary when using retinoid drugs.

i. Oral spironolactone at 50 mg/day for 4 weeks improved rosacea in 11 of the 13 patients studied. The improvement was hypothesized to be secondary to changes in the metabolism of sex steroid hormones.

j. Rosacea-like demodecidosis can be treated with oral ivermectin and/or topical permethrin cream.

3. Topical therapy for the lesions is similar to that for acne vulgaris

a. Topical 1% metronidazole (MetroGel, MetroCream, and MetroLotion) applied once daily has been shown to decrease inflammatory lesions by 77%

over a 15-week period (4). This medication is a good alternative to oral antibiotic use in some patients and can help decrease flares if use is continued after discontinuing oral therapy. The gel formulation has a higher rate of penetration *in vitro*, but may cause stinging. Paresthesias have been reported with topical metronidazole.

   b. Topical erythromycin or clindamycin lotions may be used b.i.d., as in the treatment of acne vulgaris.

   c. Preparations containing benzoyl peroxide, sulfur in concentrations of up to 15%, or both benzoyl peroxide and sulfur (Sulfoxyl) can be useful.

   Sulfacetamide-containing antibiotics are available as Sulfacet-R, Plexion cleanser, Plexion TS, Novacet, and Klaron. Sulfacet-R, Plexion, and Novacet are also sulfa based. Sulfa is a good choice in some patients if *Demodex* are thought to be playing a role. Patients with sulfa allergies should avoid these preparations.

   d. Fifteen percent of azelaic acid (Finacea) applied b.i.d. is an alternative or adjunctive therapy in rosacea patients with a low side effect profile. Some stinging can be noted with application. Use of azelaic acid 15% gel twice daily decreased inflammatory rosacea lesions by 80%. In one study, erythema was completely resolved after 15 weeks of therapy in 17.9% of patients (4).

   e. Ultraviolet light (UVL) therapy is of no benefit and may worsen symptoms.

   f. Topical corticosteroids are occasionally used to decrease erythema and inflammation. The high-potency steroid preparations should never be used, because they might induce more widespread and irreversible telangiectasias. Use of 1% hydrocortisone cream is acceptable.

   g. Photodynamic therapy (PDT) has given "excellent" results in one case report. The patient had six sessions of PDT with 5-aminolevulinic acid (5-ALA) (5).

4. Telangiectatic vessels may be destroyed by multiple vascular lasers such as the long pulsed-dye laser (585 to 600 nm), the KTP laser (532 nm) or an intense pulsed light source. Several treatments may be required with each system. Pinpoint electrosurgery using the epilating needle is also an option but carries an increased risk of scarring when compared with current laser options. In one study, the pulsed-dye laser also reduced the number of papules and pustules by 60%; the intense pulsed light source is also being used to treat both the inflammatory and vascular components of rosacea.

5. Ocular rosacea with associated blepharitis can be treated with topical antibiotic bacitracin/polymyxin B. The lid margins can be gently scrubbed with baby shampoo on a cotton-tipped applicator, commercially available lid scrubs, or a nonabrasive gauze pad impregnated with a surfactant cleanser. Warm compresses q.i.d. are helpful in removing adherent crusts. If significant inflammation is present, a topical steroid ointment can be applied to the eyelid margins on only a short-term basis.

6. Surgical reduction of the soft tissue enlargement in rhinophyma may be accomplished by CO_2 laser surgery, a surgical shave, dermabrasion, or electrosurgery.

7. Cosmetic lotions and foundations with a green tint help to camouflage the redness and telangiectasias of rosacea. Estée Lauder, Origins, and Prescriptives have a broad choice of these green-based cosmetics.

8. Use of mild nonsoap cleansers as well as a SPF 15 sunscreen that protects against ultraviolet A (UVA) and UVB are recommended on a daily basis. To minimize irritation, 30 minutes should elapse after washing before applying topical products. Cool compresses, gel masks, sucking of ice chips, central facial massage, biofeedback, and flaxseed oil are all nonstudied alternative therapies.

9. A list of multiple foods is available to determine what items may be trigger factors for rosacea. The National Rosacea Society is an excellent general resource for both patients and providers at 1-888-662-5874 or www.rosacea.org.

B. Perioral (periorificial) dermatitis

   1. Systemic antibiotics used as described for rosacea are the only reliable therapy. Perioral (periorificial) dermatitis usually clears within 3 to 8 weeks, and it is then often possible to taper off antibiotics. There is moderate support in the literature for the efficacy of tetracycline use in treatment of perioral dermatitis. Dosing is the same as that used for rosacea. Some patients need longer-term maintenance therapy.

2. Isotretinoin has been successful in treating granulomatous perioral dermatitis.

3. Topical therapy can be helpful.

   a. Topical therapy with the antibiotics previously described, including metronidazole, may be helpful. One study found topical MetroGel to be an effective topical therapy in children with perioral dermatitis (6).

   b. Fluorinated corticosteroids must be avoided assiduously. Hydrocortisone 1% or other nonfluorinated corticosteroid cream may be of symptomatic benefit and can be helpful in the transition from higher potency topical steroid abuse to topical or oral antibiotic therapy but will not cure the eruption.

   c. PDT with 5-ALA and blue light activation was shown to have a 92% clearance of perioral dermatitis versus topical clindamycin (81% clearance) in a split face study of 14 individuals (7).

   d. Azelaic acid 20% cream applied twice daily has been helpful in clearing perioral dermatitis. In one series, ten patients applied the cream b.i.d. Response was seen within 2 to 6 weeks, with complete clearance of the perioral dermatitis in all patients. There was no observed recurrence after 10 months (8).

References

1. Wilkin J, Dahl M, Detmar M, et al. Standard classification of rosacea: Report of the National Rosacea Society Expert Committee on the classification and staging of rosacea. *J Am Acad Dermatol* 2002;46:584–587.

2. Crawford GH, Pelle MT, James WD. Rosacea: I. etiology, pathogenesis, and subtype classification. *J Am Acad Dermatol* 2004;51:327–341.

3. Dirschka T, Szliska C, Jackowski J, et al. Impaired skin barrier and atopic diathesis in perioral dermatitis. *J Dtsch Dermatol Ges* 2003;1:199–203.

4. Wolf JE, Kerrouche N, Arsonnaud S. Efficacy and safety of once-daily Metronidazole 1% gel compared with twice-daily azelaic acid 15% gel in the treatment of rosacea. *Cutis* 2006;77:3–11.

5. Katz B, Patel V. Photodynamic therapy for the treatment of erythema, papules, pustules, and severe flushing consistent with rosacea. *J Drugs Dermatol* 2006;5:6–8.

6. Miller SR, Shalita AR. Topical metronidazole gel (0.75%) for the treatment of perioral dermatitis in children. *J Am Acad Dermatol* 1994;31:847–848.

7. Richey DF, Hopson B. Photodynamic therapy for perioral dermatitis. *J Drugs Dermatol* 2006;5(2 Suppl):12–16.

8. Jansen T. Azelaic acid as a new treatment for perioral dermatitis: results from an open study. *Br J Dermatol* 2004;151:933–934.

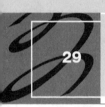

SEBORRHEIC DERMATITIS AND DANDRUFF

29

Penpun Wattanakrai

I. DEFINITION AND PATHOPHYSIOLOGY. Seborrheic dermatitis and dandruff both cause a scaling on the scalp that is often associated with itching. There are, however, distinctions between the two disorders. Dandruff is a noninflammatory form of seborrheic dermatitis with increased scaling on the scalp that represents the more active end of the spectrum of physiologic desquamation. On a normal scalp, approximately 487,000 cells/sq cm can be found after a detergent scrub; scalps affected with dandruff and seborrheic dermatitis liberate up to 800,000 cells/sq cm. Therefore, we will consider seborrheic dermatitis and dandruff to be manifestations of different severities of a similar origin.

Seborrheic dermatitis is an inflammatory, erythematous, and scaling eruption that occurs primarily in "seborrheic" areas, that is, those with a high number and activity of sebaceous glands, such as the scalp, face, and upper trunk. Although seborrheic dermatitis occurs in neonatal and postpubertal life—times during which sebaceous glands are most active—no direct relationship between the amount or composition of sebum and the presence of dermatitis has been documented. This disease is one of accelerated epidermal growth resulting in retention of nuclei in stratum corneum cells that have not had sufficient time to completely mature. On a normal scalp, there are approximately 3,700 nucleated cells/sq cm; on scalps with dandruff, there are 25,000; and on those with seborrheic dermatitis, the count is 76,000.

The etiologic agents involved in seborrheic dermatitis are multifactorial including the presence of sebum, the *Malassezia* (previously *Pityrosporum*) yeast, lipase activity, immune function, atmospheric humidity, and stress (1). Although seborrheic dermatitis occurs in skin areas with active sebaceous glands, the amount of sebum production does not directly correlate with the presence or severity of seborrheic dermatitis. Patients produce no more sebum on their scalps than controls, and reducing sebum excretion affects neither dandruff nor seborrheic dermatitis. The severity may be related to the composition of the sebum lipids or the lipase enzyme activity of *Malassezia* and/or *Propionibacterium acnes*. These lipase enzymes may split triglycerides into irritating fatty acids or release arachidonic acid, which may cause cutaneous inflammation.

The genus *Malassezia*, a lipophilic yeast, is currently classified into nine known species. Seven of the *Malassezia* yeasts, which are normal inhabitants of the skin, have been hypothesized to be the etiologic agents in seborrheic dermatitis. Although the absolute level of yeasts does not correlate with seborrheic dermatitis, its reduction in individuals with the disease does improve the symptoms. High yeast densities can also be present without symptoms. Different *Malassezia* subtypes may be more pathogenic. *Malassezia globosa* (originally described as *Pityrosporum orbiculare*) and *Malassezia restricta* (visually resembling *Pityrosporum ovale*) are most commonly found to be associated with seborrheic dermatitis (2). However, other investigators have also found *Malassezia furfur, Malassezia sympodialis, Malassezia obtuse,* and *Malassezia slooffiae,* depending on the population and geographic area studied (3). *Malassezia* has been cultured in 73% of infants with seborrheic dermatitis; the yeast may be cultured from the scalp, face, and presternal or inguinal region. Despite the many variable data found when measuring fungal load, more direct support comes from the many reports that demonstrate the response of seborrheic dermatitis to oral and topical antifungals that effectively decrease the number of *Malassezia* yeasts.

Abnormal immune response or inflammatory reaction to *Malassezia* may also be an important etiologic factor in seborrheic dermatitis. Interleukin 2 (IL-2) and interferon-γ (IFN-γ) production by lymphocytes are decreased, and there is an associated increase in production of IL-10 and immunoglobulin E (IgE) synthesis. T-cell function may be depressed and there may be an increase in the number of natural killer cells, or level of serum IgA and IgG (4). *Malassezia* antigens have been demonstrated to sensitize some patients, resulting in increased IgG levels, whereas others show conflicting results that elevated IgG titers are not related to *Malassezia* (5,6). Most adult patients with atopic dermatitis of the scalp and facial region are prick test positive to *P. ovale* (7). Strong inflammatory reactions may also be involved in seborrheic dermatitis. *Malassezia* can activate complement by both the classic and the alternative pathway and can also induce human keratinocyte cytokine production (8). The inflammation in seborrheic dermatitis may be irritant or nonimmunogenic caused by the composition of the sebum lipids or by the lipase enzyme activity or by the toxic metabolites produced by *Malassezia*.

There is a significantly increased incidence, often with extensive and severe seborrheic-like dermatitis, in human immunodeficiency virus (HIV)-positive patients and patients with acquired immunodeficiency syndrome (AIDS), ranging from 30% to 83% (9–11). Also noted is the increased incidence of seborrheic dermatitis in Parkinson's disease (idiopathic and drug induced) and other neurologic disorders. It has been theorized that there is an increased rate of sebum excretion secondary to either overactivity of the parasympathetic nervous system or action of androgens or melanocyte-stimulating hormone (MSH) (12). Other diseases associated with seborrheic dermatitis are depression, mood disorders, and pityriasis versicolor. Areas of increased skin temperature on facial skin, as documented by a sensitive thermal imager, are sites that are predisposed to seborrheic dermatitis (13). The condition is more common in male patients than in female patients and occurs most frequently in adolescents and young adults and again in adults older than 50 years. A familial tendency toward seborrheic dermatitis and an increased incidence of allergy within the family are usually present.

II. **SUBJECTIVE DATA.** The lesions of seborrheic dermatitis and dandruff are often asymptomatic with a mild clinical course. Episodic variation in intensity is common, often being precipitated by tiredness, stress, or cold weather. Pruritus is not uncommon and may be intense at times.

III. **OBJECTIVE DATA**
   A. Dandruff appears simply as noninflammatory, diffuse white or greasy scaling on the scalp usually without significant erythema or inflammation.
   B. In seborrheic dermatitis of the scalp, there is more pruritus and inflammation. The vertex and parietal regions are commonly affected. The borders of erythema and scaling are sharply demarcated and may be seen at or beyond the frontal hairline called the **corona seborrheica**.
   C. With facial seborrheic dermatitis, there is erythema, scaling, and at times exudation; the borders may be well defined. Mild erythema and fine, dry scaling may also be found on the eyebrows, eyelids, nasolabial and postauricular folds, moustache, beard, and presternal areas. The intertriginous areas, the inframammary folds, groin, gluteal crease, and umbilicus are also affected. Lesions may become thick, semiconfluent, yellow, and greasy. Secondary impetiginization and folliculitis may occur. Seborrheic dermatitis may be a cause of a generalized exfoliative erythroderma.
   D. Seborrheic marginal blepharitis, which consists of erythema and scaling of eyelid margins and cilia, is often associated with mild granular conjunctivitis or ocular irritation. Seborrheic dermatitis in other sites is often not present. Seborrheic dermatitis may also be associated with ocular rosacea.
   E. Infantile seborrheic dermatitis is self-limited and confined to the first 3 months of life. It usually starts approximately 1 week after birth and is characterized by erythema and scaling plaques involving the scalp, diaper region, or flexural surfaces; when the vertex of the scalp is involved, the condition is known as **cradle cap.** Generalized seborrheic dermatitis–like exfoliative dermatitis in an infant accompanied with systemic signs and symptoms such as fever, anemia, diarrhea, weight loss, failure to thrive, and infections is referred to as **Leiner's syndrome.** Originally reported as a disorder due to dysfunctional C5, it may be a clinical manifestation of various immunodeficiency disorders including defective phagocytic function, defect

in the third component of complement system, severe combined immunodeficiency, hypogammaglobulinemia, and hyperimmunoglobulinemia E (14).

F. Drug eruptions from gold, methyldopa, chlorpromazine or cimetidine therapy, or vitamin B deficiency may mimic seborrheic dermatitis.

G. In chronic cases, nonscarring alopecia can be noted secondary to the inflammation and the secondary effects of scratching. This should be reversible with treatment.

IV. THERAPY. Treatment modalities in seborrheic dermatitis mainly target the three important etiologic factors implicated in the disease and include keratolytic agents and antiinflammatory and antifungal preparations.

A. Agents effective in eliminating the scaling of dandruff and seborrheic dermatitis appear to act by varying mechanisms. Selenium sulfide and tars inhibit mitotic activity, and selenium kills yeasts as well. Zinc pyrithione is directly cytotoxic and has antimicrobial effects, and salicylic acid disrupts the bonds that cause stratum corneum cells to stick together. There are no studies comparing the efficacy of antiseborrheic shampoos. The following agents are listed in rough approximation of usefulness:

1. Ketoconazole is available as a 2% cream, a 2% shampoo, an oil-in-water emulsion, and a foaming gel. The 2% ketoconazole (Nizoral) shampoo is used at least twice weekly for 2 to 4 weeks, leaving the product on for 5 minutes. Placing the suds on areas of facial involvement is also helpful. Once the dermatitis is under control, treatment once a week helps prevent relapse. A 1% preparation is now available over the counter. Topical ketoconazole has been studied in children and shown to be effective and well tolerated. Its efficacy is approximately equivalent to that of 1% hydrocortisone cream. Oral ketoconazole has many potential adverse reactions and its use is warranted in only unresponsive cases.

2. A shampoo containing 0.1% triamcinolone applied on a daily basis for 2 weeks can significantly reduce scaling and itching. A maintenance regimen or an alternating schedule with another antidandruff shampoo can then be undertaken.

3. Shampoos containing 2.5% selenium sulfide (Selsun) should be applied two to three times weekly for 5 to 10 minutes each time. Studies have shown no significant difference between the efficacy of selenium sulfide shampoos and ketoconazole shampoo (15).

4. Preparations containing 1% to 2% zinc pyrithione (Danex, DHS Zinc, Head & Shoulders, Zincon) work almost as well. They are also available in a cream formulation.

5. Bifonazole 1% shampoo is a safe and effective treatment for seborrheic dermatitis of the scalp in infants and children (16).

6. Salicylic acid-sulfur shampoos (Ionil, Sebulex) are less effective.

7. Tar shampoos (DHS-T, Ionil T, Pentrax, Sebutone, T/Gel, Zetar) inhibit epidermal proliferation through cytostatic effects after an initial burst of transient hyperplasia.

8. Chloroxine (Capitrol) shampoo contains a synthetic antibacterial compound similar to the hydroxyquinoline compounds used in dermatology for many years. Comparative efficacy studies with this shampoo are unavailable.

9. Any nonmedicinal shampoo, particularly those containing surfactants and detergents, will remove scales and lead to subjective clinical improvement and decreased desquamation for approximately 4 days. These agents should be used every 2 days to control dandruff.

10. Alcohol-based preparations and hair tonics should be avoided.

B. If the lesions are extensive or very inflammatory, the patient may apply a topical corticosteroid solution, lotion, or spray (betamethasone valerate or dipropionate lotion is generally effective; other corticosteroid lotions are also useful). Alternatively, a 10% sodium sulfacetamide lotion b.i.d. to t.i.d. may be used. Topical steroid mousse formulations betamethasone valerate (Luxiq) and clobetasol (Olux) are helpful adjuncts for scalp seborrheic dermatitis because the foam melts at skin surface temperature, leaving minimal residue and with no affect on hair styling.

C. Thick crusts may be removed more easily by overnight applications of a keratolytic gel, for example, salicylic acid (Keralyt), with or without plastic cap occlusion;

3% sulfur, 3% salicylic acid, 4% cetyl alcohol-coal tar distillate (Pragmatar) cream; Baker's P&S liquid) or a 30-minute compress with warm mineral oil before shampooing.

D. Seborrheic dermatitis lesions on other areas respond rapidly to a corticosteroid cream such as 1% hydrocortisone applied one to three times a day. Aerosols or lotions are easier to apply to hairy areas. Prolonged application of high-potency fluorinated corticosteroids may lead to disfiguring telangiectasia and atrophy. Other useful topical agents for glabrous skin include sulfur-containing medications such as 10% sulfacetamide lotion; formulations such as precipitated sulfur 3% to 10%, salicylic acid 1% to 5%, and tar 2% in an ointment base; or 1% to 3% sulfur in calamine lotion.

E. A new class of topical immunomodulators, the calcineurin inhibitors, are being used with some success for treating seborrheic dermatitis (17,18). Tacrolimus ointment and pimecrolimus cream lack the side effects associated with steroid use and have been demonstrated to have *in vitro* antifungal effects against *Malassezia furfur* (19).

F. Aside from the topical azoles, which have fungistatic properties, including ketoconazole, fluconazole, miconazole, other topicals such as topical terbinafine, ciclopirox, and metronidazole has also been shown to benefit in seborrheic dermatitis.

G. A 15% propylene glycol solution applied to the scalp reduced the number of yeasts and improved seborrheic dermatitis in 90% of those treated (20).

H. For widespread or unresponsive cases, short courses of oral antifungal treatment have been shown to be effective. These include oral ketoconazole (200 mg/day for 2 to 4 weeks) (21), oral itraconazole (100 mg/day up to 21 days; 200 mg/day for 1 week) (22), and oral terbinafine at 250 mg/day for 4 to 6 weeks (23,24).

I. Oral isotretinoin reduces sebaceous gland size up to 90% by decreasing proliferation of the basal sebocytes. Sebum lipid synthesis is reduced by as much as 75% after 4 weeks of isotretinoin at a dose as low as 0.1 mg/kg/day. Patients may experience a relapse in their seborrhea for months to years (25).

J. Seborrheic blepharitis is treated one to three times a day with sulfacetamide alone or a 10% sulfacetamide, 0.2% prednisolone, 0.12% phenylephrine suspension (Blephamide, Vasocidin), or similar preparations (Cetapred, Metimyd, Optimyd). It is essential to monitor intraocular tension concurrent with intermittent or chronic steroid therapy in or around the eye. Therefore, it may be more prudent to use either topical tacrolimus or pimecrolimus as alternatives to topical steroids for treatment around the eyes as both have antiinflammatory activity without the side effects associated with long-term corticosteroid use.

K. Ultraviolet light (both UVA and UVB) is inhibitory to the growth of *Malassezia*. Many individuals note improvement of seborrheic dermatitis during the summer months (26). However, it has also been reported that some patients develop seborrheic dermatitis subsequent to psoralen plus UVA therapy (27).

References

1. Bergbrant IM. Seborrhoeic dermatitis and Pityrosporum yeasts. *Curr Top Med Mycol* 1995;6:95–112.
2. Gupta AK, Bluhm R, Cooper EA, et al. Seborrheic dermatitis. *Dermatol Clin* 2003;21:401–412.
3. Nakabayashi A, Sei Y, Guillot J. Identification of Malassezia species isolated from patients with seborrheic dermatitis, atopic dermatitis, pityriasis versicolor and normal subjects. *Med Mycol* 2000;38:337–341.
4. Bergbrant IM, Johansson S, Robbins D, et al. An immunological study in patients with seborrhoeic dermatitis. *Clin Exp Dermatol* 1991;16:331–338.
5. Silva V, Fischman O, de Camargo ZP. Humoral immune response to Malassezia furfur in patients with pityriasis versicolor and seborrheic dermatitis. *Mycopathologia* 1997;139:79–85.
6. Parry ME, Sharpe GR. Seborrhoeic dermatitis is not caused by altered immune response to Malassezia yeast. *Br J Dermatol* 1998;139:254–263.
7. Faergemann J. Pityrosporum yeasts—what's new. *Mycoses* 1997;40(Suppl 1):29–32.
8. Watanabe S, Kano R, Sato H, et al. The effects of Malassezia yeasts on cytokine production by human keratinocytes. *J Invest Dermatol* 2001;116:769–773.

9. Smith KJ, Skelton HG, Yeager J, et al. Cutaneous findings in HIV-1 positive patients: a 42-month prospective study. *J Am Acad Dermatol* 1994;31:746–754.
10. Groisser D, Bottone EJ, Lebwohl M. Association of Pityrosporum orbiculare (Malassezia furfur) with seborrheic dermatitis in patients with acquired immunodeficiency syndrome (AIDS). *J Am Acad Dermatol* 1989;20:770–773.
11. Marino CT, McDonald E, Romano JF. Seborrheic dermatitis in acquired immunodeficiency syndrome. *Cutis* 1991;48:217–218.
12. Martignoni E, Godi L, Pacchetti C, et al. Is seborrhea a sign of autonomic impairment in Parkinson's disease? *J Neural Transm* 1997;104:1295–1304.
13. Hale EK, Bystryn JC. Relation between skin temperature and location of facial lesions in seborrheic dermatitis. *Arch Dermatol* 2000;136:559–560.
14. Glover M, Atherton DJ, Levinsky RJ. Syndrome of erythroderma, failure to thrive, and diarrhea in infancy: a manifestation of immunodeficiency. *Pediatrics* 1988;81:66.
15. Danby FW, Maddin WS, Margesson LJ, et al. A randomized, double-blind, placebo-controlled trial of ketoconazole 2% shampoo versus selenium sulfide 2.5% shampoo in the treatment of moderate to severe dandruff. *J Am Acad Dermatol* 1993;29:1008–1012.
16. Zeharia A, Mimouni M, Fogel A. Treatment with bifonazole shampoo for scalp seborrhea in infants and young children. *Pediatr Dermatol* 1996;13:151–153.
17. Rigopoulos D, Ioannides D, Kalogeromitros D, et al. Katsambas A pimecrolimus cream 1% vs. betamethasone 17-valerate 0.1% cream in the treatment of seborrhoeic dermatitis. A randomized open-label clinical trial. *Br J Dermatol* 2004;151(5):1071–1075.
18. Braza TJ, DiCarlo JB, Soon SL, et al. Tacrolimus 0.1% ointment for seborrhoeic dermatitis: an open-label pilot study. *Br J Dermatol* 2003;148(6):1242–1244.
19. Nakawa H, Etoh T, Yokota Y, et al. Tacrolimus has antifungal activities against Malassezia furfur isolated from healthy adults and patients with atopic dermatitis. *Clin Drug Invest* 1996;12:245–250.
20. Faergemann J. Propylene glycol in the treatment of seborrheic dermatitis of the scalp: a double-blind study. *Cutis* 1988;42:69–71.
21. Ford GP, Farr PM, Ive FA, et al. The response of seborrheic dermatitis to ketoconazole. *Br J Dermatol* 1984;111:603–609.
22. Kose O, Erbil H, Gur AR. Oral itraconazole for the treatment of seborrheic dermatitis: an open, noncomparative trial. *J Eur Acad Dermatol Venereol* 2005;19(2):172–175.
23. Scapparo E, Quadri G, Virno G, et al. Evaluation of the efficacy and tolerability of oral terbinafine in patients with seborrheic dermatitis: a multicentre, randomized, investigator-blinded, placebo-controlled trial. *Br J Dermatol* 2001;144:854–857.
24. Vena GA, Micali G, Santoianni P, et al. Oral terbinafine in the treatment of multi-site seborrheic dermatitis: a multicenter, double-blind placebo-controlled study. *Int J Immunopathol Pharmacol* 2005;18(4):745–753.
25. Orfanos CE, Zouboulis CC. Oral retinoids in the treatment of seborrhoea and acne. *Dermatology* 1998;196:140–147.
26. Berg M. Epidemiological studies of the influence of sunlight on the skin. *Photodermatology* 1989;6:80–84.
27. Yegner E. Seborrheic dermatitis of the face induced by PUVA treatment. *Acta Derm Venereol* 1983;63:335–339.

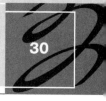

SEXUALLY TRANSMITTED DISEASES

Brian Poligone and Wanla Kulwichit

30

In the United States, more than 19 million sexually transmitted infections occur each year. Nearly half of these infections occur in people aged 15 to 24. The economic toll of these infections is estimated to be over $13 billion annually. Although there is good surveillance data regarding diseases such as syphilis, gonorrhea, and chlamydia, which are reportable infections, many other sexually transmitted diseases (STDs) are unreported. There are now >30 known infections that can be transmitted through sex. This chapter will discuss the most important of these infections.

Ulcerative and nonulcerative STDs are being implicated increasingly as risk factors in the transmission of human immunodeficiency virus (HIV) infection. Antimicrobial resistance, lack of single agents with a broad spectrum of activity against multiple genital pathogens, and poor compliance has increased the challenge of STD treatment. The therapy recommendations in this chapter reflect the recommendations of the 2002 Centers for Disease Control (CDC) Guidelines for treatment of STDs.

 GENITAL ULCER DISEASE

In the United States, a patient with a genital ulcer, especially a young and sexually active one, needs to be evaluated for herpes simplex, syphilis, and chancroid. Workup for a genital ulcer should include a culture or direct fluorescent antibody test (DFA) for herpes, serology and dark-field examination or direct immunofluorescence test for syphilis, culture for *Hemophilus ducreyi*, in addition to HIV, due to the increased risk of HIV infection associated with these other infections. Rarely, lymphogranuloma venereum (LGV) or granuloma inguinale is the cause of genital ulcers in the United States.

 HERPES SIMPLEX

Herpes simplex is the most common cause of genital ulceration in developed countries (currently 50 million cases in the United States). Although herpes simplex virus type 2 (HSV-2) is more commonly associated with genital herpes, up to 30% of first-time genital herpes is due to HSV-1 infection. Most cases of recurrent herpes are due to HSV-2. Many cases of genital herpes are transmitted when the infected individual is asymptomatic or unaware that they are infected.

 SYPHILIS

I. **DEFINITION AND PATHOPHYSIOLOGY.** Syphilis is caused by a delicate organism, *Treponema pallidum*, characterized by the closeness and regularity of its 6 to 14 thin corkscrew-like spirals. These spirochetes, 6- to 15-μm long and 0.25-μm thick, pass through intact mucous membranes or abraded skin and are disseminated by the bloodstream throughout the body within hours. Approximately 3 weeks later (9 to 90 days), the primary lesion appears at the site of infection. This chancre persists for 1 to 5 weeks and then disappears spontaneously. Fifty percent of these individuals will go on to develop secondary syphilis (bacteremia), and 50% will go into a latency period. Secondary syphilis can affect all organ systems.

Six weeks later (2 weeks to 6 months, average 9 weeks after inoculation), the signs and symptoms of secondary syphilis appear; they disappear without therapy within a

185

month. Overall, the highest rate of infectivity for the patient is during the first 1 to 2 years of infection, and infectivity decreases over time. If primary and secondary syphilis are left untreated, the clinical disease will disappear, and serologic tests will revert to nonreactive in approximately 33% of patients. Thirty-three percent will continue to have positive serologic tests for syphilis but enjoy good health, and 33% will develop signs of late syphilis afterward. Late (tertiary) syphilis is not commonly seen now. Of the latter, approximately 25% can be expected to die primarily as a result of the disease; 80% of these deaths are related to cardiovascular problems.

The incidence of primary and secondary syphilis peaked in 1990 and then declined by almost 90% until 2000. The low rate at the end of the century led to the National Plan to Eliminate Syphilis from the United States. However, the rate has increased, primarily among men, every year since 2000.

Despite the recent increase in syphilis rates, rates of congenital syphilis have decreased each year. The main clinical findings include bone involvement, hepatosplenomegaly, skin lesions, and jaundice.

II. SUBJECTIVE DATA
  A. The genital lesions of primary syphilis are either painless or much less discomforting than would be expected. Extragenital lesions may hurt.
  B. Secondary syphilis is often pruritic (40%). Patients often note flu-like syndrome with headache, malaise, sore throat, and arthralgias.

III. OBJECTIVE DATA (See color insert.)
  A. The primary chancre is usually a single, firm, indurated erosion, or ulcer covered with a crust. The base is nonpurulent and clean with a yellow-gray exudate. Thirty percent of patients have multiple chancres present and 5% of chancres are extragenital. Nontender, firm regional lymphadenopathy may be noted. In some individuals (depending on location of exposure), the primary chancre may appear as a painful anal fissure with induration of bilateral lymph nodes.
  B. The secondary rash consists of generalized, faint, red to brown ("copper colored") macules, papules, or even nodules. Syphilis has been called the **great imitator** because of the variety of clinical presentations. The maculopapular rash is, however, seen in 70% of secondary syphilis. The lesions usually start on the trunk and spread to the shoulders and extremities. Rarely, lesions can become necrotic, a condition known as **lues maligna.**
   1. The palms and soles are characteristically involved (50%).
   2. Lesions on mucous membranes appear as raised gray-white "mucous patches" (21%).
   3. A generalized nontender lymphadenopathy (85%) most commonly involving the epitrochlear lymph nodes.
   4. Other findings may include patchy hair loss or smooth-surfaced yet warty intertriginous plaques termed **condylomata lata** (10%) (considered to be the most infectious lesion of syphilis because of the eroded surface and large number of spirochetes).
  C. Tertiary syphilis may be visceral, cardiovascular, neurologic, osseous, or mucocutaneous in its manifestations. Cutaneous nodules may appear that will heal with atrophic scars. A gumma is a painless subcutaneous, destructive, ulcerative nodule with caseous or gummy-like discharge and heals with scarring.
  D. Congenital syphilis, when not leading to stillbirth or neonatal death, is noted for notched molars and central incisors (Hutchinson's teeth), snuffles (a persistent nasal discharge), a saddle nose deformity, scaling plaques, bullae, desquamation, rhagades, and mucous patches. Skin and mucosal lesions contain spirochetes.

IV. ASSESSMENT
  A. Definitive diagnosis is made by viewing the causative spirochete by dark-field microscopy in specimens collected from primary and moist secondary lesions. *T. pallidum* is not stained by ordinary reagents and is so narrow that it cannot be visualized under the normal light microscope.
  B. Invasion of the human host by this spirochete leads to production of multiple antibodies of two basic types, reflected in the two kinds of serologic tests for syphilis (STS).

1. Nonspecific, nontreponemal antibodies (reagins) directed against a lipoidal antigen that results from interaction of host and parasite are measured by flocculation tests (Venereal Disease Research Laboratories [VDRL] and rapid plasma reagin [RPR]). These tests are sensitive and easy to perform and are the screening tests of choice. They will usually be reactive within 1 to 4 weeks of the development of the chancre. The tests should reduce fourfold over the course of 6 to 12 months and become undetectable after several years. In secondary syphilis, all serologies should be reactive, whereas in late syphilis the nontreponemal tests may be negative. Titers will not decrease with tertiary syphilis. False positives can be found with collagen vascular diseases, narcotic drug use, liver disease, HIV, tuberculosis, and age.

2. The specific treponemal tests measure antibody directed against the treponemal organism and this test should be obtained after the screening test RPR/VDRL.

   a. The fluorescent treponemal antibody absorption (FTA-ABS), the reference test at present, employs the Nichol-strain treponemes on the slide as antigen to which the patient's serum is added. This test is generally positive earlier than the RPR or VDRL. However, the FTA-ABS has problems with specificity and should always be done in combination with a nontreponemal antibody test. This is because 1% of the general population will have a positive FTA-ABS. An alternative treponemal test is the microhemagglutination assay for antibody to *T. pallidum* (MHA-TP); however, it has lower specificity than FTA-ABS.

   b. These tests are needed to confirm the presence or absence of true treponemal infection in those with a positive nontreponemal test but no history or knowledge of syphilis or other treponemal disease.

3. HIV-infected patients may have abnormal serologic test results, either very high, very low, or with unusual fluctuating titers. For these patients, skin biopsy should be considered.

V. THERAPY

A. Early syphilis: primary, secondary, latent syphilis of <1 year duration

   1. Benzathine penicillin G 2.4 million units IM once. In many states and in the military, individuals are given a second dose in 1 week. Penicillin-allergic patients should take doxycycline 100 mg b.i.d. for 14 days or tetracycline 500 mg q.i.d. for 14 days. Other therapies include ceftriaxone and azithromycin. Although earlier studies had shown effectiveness of an oral, single dose of 2 g of azithromycin in treatment of early syphilis, recent data demonstrate growing resistance and treatment failure in big cities in the United States, mostly in homosexual men.

B. Syphilis of >1 year duration, cardiovascular, late benign syphilis

   1. Benzathine penicillin G 2.4 million units IM weekly for 3 weeks.
      Penicillin-allergic patients should take doxycycline 100 mg b.i.d. or tetracycline 2 g daily for 2 weeks if the duration of infection is known to have been <1 year, otherwise, 4 weeks.

   2. Cerebrospinal fluid examination should be performed if any of the following are present: neurologic or ophthalmic signs, aortitis, gumma, iritis, treatment failure, HIV infection, or serum nontreponemal titer of 1:32 or greater, unless duration of the infection is known to be <1 year.

      a. Symptomatic or asymptomatic neurosyphilis may be treated with one of the following:

         i. Aqueous penicillin G 18 to 24 million units per day IV for 10 to 14 days (administered as 3 to 4 million units IV every 4 hours), followed by benzathine penicillin G 2.4 million units IM weekly for 3 weeks.

         ii. Procaine penicillin G 2.4 million units daily, plus probenecid 2 g daily, both for 10 to 14 days.

         iii. Benzathine penicillin G 2.4 million units IM weekly for 3 weeks. (iv) Penicillin-allergic patients may take ceftriaxone 2 g daily IM or IV for 10 to 14 days. The use of tetracycline has not been well studied. Desensitization to penicillin/ceftriaxone may be appropriate.

C. Pregnant patients should be treated with penicillin. For those allergic to penicillin, desensitization should be attempted first, without switching to alternatives immediately. Tetracycline, doxycycline, and erythromycin should not be used in pregnancy. Data are insufficient to recommend ceftriaxone or azithromycin.

D. The Jarisch-Herxheimer reaction is an endotoxemia caused by the release of lipopolysaccharides from degenerating treponemes. This reaction occurs within 24 hours of treatment in 65% to 90% of patients treated for infectious syphilis. Fever, chills, malaise, myalgia, arthralgia, headache, and nausea begin several hours after therapy is initiated and usually subside within 12 to 24 hours. Antipyretics with or without corticosteroids may help alleviate symptoms and severity. Antibodies to tumor necrosis factor-α have been shown to prevent this reaction in some patients with relapsing fever, another type of spirochetal infection. The Jarisch-Herxheimer reaction may cause early labor or fetal distress; concern regarding this reaction should not delay therapy, however.

E. Retreatment. The serologies generally decrease fourfold at 3 months and eightfold at 6 months and return to normal within 6 to 12 months of treatment of primary syphilis or within 12 to 18 months of treatment of secondary syphilis. Retreatment (same treatment as for syphilis of >1 year duration) should be considered in the following cases:

   1. Clinical disease continues or recurs.

   2. The quantitative serologic titer measured at 3-month intervals does not decrease at least fourfold (two tube dilutions) within 1 year.

   3. The quantitative serologic titer increases fourfold (two tube dilutions), representing either relapse or reinfection.

F. Penicillin, ampicillin, and tetracycline treatment of gonorrhea is curative for incubating syphilis.

G. All patients with syphilis should be tested for HIV infection. In areas with a high prevalence of HIV infection, patients with primary syphilis should be retested for HIV infection after 3 months.

H. HIV-infected patients with early syphilis are at increased risk of neurosyphilis and have higher rates of treatment failure with standard regimens. Some experts recommend multiple doses of benzathine penicillin G, as suggested for late syphilis. Patients should be evaluated clinically and serologically at 3 months and then at 6, 9, 12, and 24 months after therapy.

 CHANCROID

I. DEFINITION AND PATHOPHYSIOLOGY. Chancroid, seen 20 times more commonly in men than in women, is an autoinoculable, localized STD caused by the gram-positive, facultative anaerobic coccobacillus, *H. ducreyi.* Reported cases of chancroid declined steadily from 4,986 in 1987 to 143 in 1999 and 30 in 2004. This figure may be falsely low as the organism is difficult to grow and therefore diagnose. The incubation period is only 24 to 72 hours; some lesions may heal within a few days. Chancroid is endemic in Africa, the Caribbean basin, and Southeast Asia. In central Africa, chancroid is considered the most common cause of genital ulceration. Chancroid is a cofactor for HIV infection in heterosexual men, which is particularly important for the spread of HIV in Africa. In the United States, prostitutes and crack cocaine addicts are the usual reservoir. Uncircumcised men appear to be more susceptible. Extensive drug resistance has made previous antibiotic regimens ineffective.

II. SUBJECTIVE DATA. Severe pain from both the genital lesion and involved lymph nodes is typical and helps differentiate the disease from syphilis. A foul odor may suggest chancroid even before evaluation.

III. OBJECTIVE DATA

A. The primary lesions consist of single or multiple (in approximately 50% of cases), round to oval, superficial and shallow ulcers with irregular outlines, ragged and undetermined borders, and a purulent base. The lesion is soft to palpation and is surrounded by an erythematous halo. The lesion may be 3 to 20 mm.

B. Balanitis, phimosis, and paraphimosis are frequent.

C. Inguinal lymphadenitis, present in approximately 50% of cases, develops 1 to 3 weeks after the primary lesion, is most often unilateral, and resembles an abscess (bubo). Suppuration, breakdown, and sinus tract formation can occur and are almost pathognomonic of the disease. Autoinoculation may develop with opposing ulcerations called **kissing lesions**.

IV. ASSESSMENT

A. Diagnosis is suggested by viewing this small organism on Wright's, Giemsa's, or Gram's stain under the microscope. Tissue should be taken from under the undermined borders or from material aspirated from an unruptured lymph node. Diagnosis based on morphology alone has an accuracy of 30% to 50%.

   1. *H. ducreyi* is a short, gram-negative rod with rounded ends, usually found outside the cells and in bands in parallel rows ("school of fish") and may be seen on Gram's stain.

   2. Under the best of conditions, smears are positive in <50% of cases.

B. The diagnosis is best made by isolation of the organism on enriched gonococcal agar base and enriched Mueller-Hinton agar in a biplate fashion. Polymerase chain reaction (PCR) testing has a sensitivity of 95%.

C. Up to 10% of these patients may also be simultaneously infected with syphilis or herpes simplex virus and have a "mixed chancre."

V. THERAPY

A. Azithromycin 1 g PO in a single dose. Azithromycin is class B during pregnancy.

B. Erythromycin base 500 mg PO t.i.d. for 7 days.

C. Ceftriaxone 250 mg IM.

D. Ciprofloxacin 500 mg PO b.i.d. for 3 days. Ciprofloxacin should not be used during pregnancy unless the benefit justifies potential risk.

E. Ulcers are usually symptomatically better within 3 days of initiation of therapy and objectively improved by 7 days. Fluctuant nodes can be aspirated through healthy skin; incision and drainage is a more complicated procedure.

F. Patients should be tested for HIV infection at the time of diagnosis. Retesting 3 months later for HIV infection and syphilis should be done if initial testing is negative. Healing may be slower among HIV-infected individuals, and treatment failures occur. Some experts suggest using the erythromycin 7-day regimen with these patients.

 LYMPHOGRANULOMA VENEREUM

I. DEFINITION AND PATHOPHYSIOLOGY.
Lymphogranuloma venereum, a rare disease in the United States, may account for 2% to 10% of genital ulcer disease in areas of India and Africa. Transmission is attributed to asymptomatic female carriers. This is a systemic disease caused by the obligate-intracellular parasite *Chlamydia trachomatis* immunotypes L_1, L_2, and L_3. These specific subtypes are more virulent than the other *Chlamydia* serotypes and infect macrophages. A 7- to 12-day incubation period is followed by an evanescent primary lesion and then inflammatory lymphangitis and potentially serious late sequelae.

II. SUBJECTIVE DATA

A. The primary stage lesion is a painless ulcer.

B. The secondary stage usually consists of painful inguinal lymphangitis and is accompanied by malaise, arthralgia, and fever.

C. A tertiary stage is termed the **genitoanorectal syndrome** and involves proctocolitis.

III. OBJECTIVE DATA

A. After an incubation period of 3 to 30 days, the primary lesion (which most often goes unnoticed) may be a transient papule, vesicle, or, rarely, ulceration. This lesion usually heals within a week without scarring. Mucopurulent discharge may be seen in the urethra or cervix.

B. Inguinal adenitis (the most common presenting symptom in heterosexual males) presents 2 to 6 weeks after the primary lesion and 3 to 6 weeks after inoculation;

is unilateral in 66% of cases; and initially discrete and movable and later firm, oval, and elongated. Rupture of these buboes occurs in one third of patients. The overlying skin is adherent, edematous, and violaceous in color and may form grooves between the matted nodes; suppuration and chronic sinus formation may occur. Most women do not develop the characteristic lymphadenopathy as the deep iliac and perirectal nodes are involved; they may have symptoms of rectal or back pain.

During the inguinal stage of the disease, low-grade fever, malaise, myalgias, and arthralgias may occur. Systemic spread of the organism may rarely cause arthritis, pneumonitis, or hepatitis.

C. Primary anorectal infection, most common in homosexual men and women, presents as a severe acute proctitis that may mimic Crohn's disease of the rectum. Hyperplasia of the perirectal lymphatics occurs with formation of "lymphorrhoids." Chronic involvement can lead to local destruction of tissue. (The non-LGV immunotypes cause a mild proctitis with or without symptoms.)

D. Erythema nodosum is seen in 2% to 10% of cases.

E. Late changes of chronic disease may include proctitis, rectal stricture, perirectal abscesses and fistulas, and severe genital swelling. Malignant transformation can occur.

IV. ASSESSMENT

A. The complement-fixation test becomes positive within 2 to 4 weeks of the onset of infection in 80% to 90% of patients. If only convalescent serum is available, a titer of 1:64 or greater suggests LGV. A fourfold increase in the complement-fixation rate also supports the diagnosis of LGV. Cross-reaction can occur between serotypes that produce other chlamydial infections (non-LGV *Chlamydia* titer is 1:16).

B. The organism can be cultured only with special media; this is not a clinically useful procedure with recovery at 30%.

C. The use of fluorescein-tagged monoclonal antibodies and PCR testing is available in some areas.

V. THERAPY

A. Doxycycline 100 mg b.i.d. for 21 days.

B. Alternative (but not well-evaluated) regimen includes the following:

  1. Erythromycin 500 mg PO q.i.d. for 3 weeks.

C. Aspiration or incision of suppurating adenitis should be performed before spontaneous breakdown of tissue.

 GRANULOMA INGUINALE (DONOVANOSIS)

I. DEFINITION AND PATHOPHYSIOLOGY. This mildly contagious, chronic, granulomatous disease involves the skin and lymphatics in the anogenital area. This is an extremely rare disease in the United States, but is endemic in tropical and subtropical regions such as New Guinea, India, the Caribbean, Brazil, and South Africa. A significant increase in the incidence has been noted in Africa.

The organism, *Calymmatobacterium (Donovania) granulomatis*, is related to the *Klebsiella* species. This is a gram-negative, obligate-intracellular bacillus. The incubation period is extremely variable from 1 week to 3 months.

II. SUBJECTIVE DATA. Lesions cause no discomfort but are usually malodorous.

III. OBJECTIVE DATA

A. Although rare in the United States, it is a cause of genital ulcers. Single or multiple papules and nodules develop at the site of inoculation. There is an insidious onset of tissue breakdown with painless, irregular ulcers with a soft, beefy red, friable, exuberant growth base. Lesions may become confluent and cause extensive local tissue destruction. Autoinoculation is common with the formation of "kissing lesions." A hypertrophic form exists with dry vegetating plaques that resemble condyloma acuminata.

B. Inguinal swellings are not lymphadenitis but represent subcutaneous perilymphatic granulomata that may eventually break through the skin, causing sinus formation. Complications include elephantiasis, stricture, phimosis, and pelvic abscess. Squamous cell carcinoma has been reported in persistent cases.

C. Systemic symptoms can rarely occur with extragenital involvement of sites such as the oral cavity, the bowel, bones, and bladder.

IV. ASSESSMENT. Diagnosis is confirmed by finding the organisms (Donovan bodies) in the lesions. Isolation of the organism is difficult and impractical.

A. Remove a piece of the lesion, preferably the advancing edge of the ulcer, with a scalpel or punch.

B. Smear the undersurface of the ulceration onto slides or crush the tissue between two slides for examination (tissue crush prep).

C. Fix with alcohol, and stain with Wright's or Giemsa's stain.

D. Donovan bodies will be found within mononuclear cells; they appear as straight or slightly curved rods with more deeply staining poles, thereby creating a "safety pin" appearance. The organism is gram-negative and stains red with Giemsa's and blue or purple with Wright's stain. The capsule appears pink on Wright's stain.

E. Histopathologic examination of a biopsy specimen may be necessary if touch preps are inconclusive.

F. Atypical chancroid may resemble granuloma inguinale clinically. Only appropriate bacteriologic cultures may yield the correct diagnosis.

V. THERAPY

A. Doxycycline 100 mg PO q.i.d. for 3 weeks (tetracycline is not recommended because of drug resistance).

B. Trimethoprim-sulfamethoxazole DS 160 mg/800 mg PO b.i.d. for 2 to 5 weeks. Cotrimoxazole is also effective.

C. Ciprofloxacin 750 mg b.i.d. for 3 weeks, erythromycin 500 mg q.i.d. for 3 weeks, and azithromycin 1 g once per week for 3 weeks have also been used.

D. The usual course of treatment with the above regimens is 3 weeks or until all lesions have completely healed. Even with effective therapeutic courses, relapse can occur within 6 to 18 months.

E. A secondary bacterial infection may occur or other sexually transmitted organisms may coinfect the ulcer.

F. Fluctuant masses indicate a need for aspiration.

URETHRITIS, CERVICITIS, AND/OR VAGINITIS

Chlamydia Infections and Nongonococcal Urethritis

I. DEFINITION AND PATHOPHYSIOLOGY. Nongonococcal urethritis (NGU) is an inflammation of the urethra not caused by *Neisseria gonorrhoeae.* Seventy percent to 80% of cases are associated with *C. trachomatis* and/or *Ureaplasma urealyticum.* Rarely, one of the other venereal infections (e.g., trichomonas, candidiasis, herpes simplex) will present as NGU, though in 20% to 30% of all cases no pathogen can be identified. The incubation period is 1 to 5 weeks. *Chlamydia* infection has a prevalence at least 2.5 times that of gonorrhea with many asymptomatic carriers and is the major cause of pelvic inflammatory disease (PID) (60%). *C. trachomatis,* an obligate intercellular bacterium that is cultured like a virus, can be isolated from almost half the etiologically diagnosed cases if appropriate culture and antibody tests are available. Of the 17 immunotypes of *C. trachomatis,* types D through K are usually associated with genital and perinatal infection. The mycoplasma *U. urealyticum* causes another 20% to 40% of NGU. Postgonococcal urethritis is usually due to coexisting chlamydial infection unmasked by treatment for gonorrhea with drugs ineffective against *Chlamydia.* The major complication of NGU is epididymitis, which arises in <1% of cases. Reiter's syndrome (arthritis, urethritis, and conjunctivitis) is also associated with NGU.

Mucopurulent cervicitis is the female counterpart to NGU in men. In a study of 100 randomly selected women attending a venereal disease clinic, 40% were found to have mucopurulent cervicitis; in half of these cases *C. trachomatis* could be isolated. *Chlamydia* was isolated in only 3% of women without cervicitis. *C. trachomatis* poses numerous potential health hazards in female patients: acute PID, infertility or complicated pregnancy, and transmission to the neonate if the birth canal is infected with resultant ophthalmia or lower respiratory tract infection.

II. **SUBJECTIVE DATA.** Patients with urethritis have variable symptoms; dysuria, when present, is usually not severe.

III. **OBJECTIVE DATA.** The urethral discharge is usually scant and is white or clear in appearance.

IV. **ASSESSMENT.** The diagnosis is established by the clinical presentation and a Gram's stain of urethral discharge that shows five or more polymorphonuclear leukocytes per high-power (oil-immersion) field but no organisms. Specifically, there are no gonococci or *Candida albicans* on Gram's stain, no *Candida* on potassium hydroxide smear or Swartz-Medrik stain (SMS), no *Trichomonas* on saline wet mount, and no bacteria on methylene blue and/or Gram's stain of a spun-down midstream urine: Thayer-Martin (gonococcus), Feinberg-Wittington or Bushby (*Trichomonas*), Sabouraud's (*Candida*), and phenyl ethyl alcohol/MacConkey (urinary tract bacteria).

A. A fluorescein-conjugated monoclonal antibody immunofluorescent test (Micro-Trak) permits rapid, simple, and accurate diagnosis of chlamydial infections. The test is less sensitive than tissue culture and may identify between 60% and 90% of those infected in low-risk populations. An enzyme-linked immunoassay (Chlamydiazyme II) is also available. Both must be performed by highly trained technicians to achieve maximum accuracy.

B. The leukocyte esterase test (LET) is increasingly being used to screen urine from asymptomatic males for evidence of urethritis. The test is performed on first voided urine and is indicative of >10 white blood cells per high-power field.

C. Tissue culture of *C. trachomatis* is available in most referral centers and laboratories.

D. PCR is frequently available and the other tests listed are less frequently used compared with the PCR.

V. **THERAPY**

A. Azithromycin 1 g once.

B. Doxycycline 100 mg b.i.d. for 7 days. Most patients will be cured on initial treatment, but there is a 40% relapse rate in *Chlamydia*-negative NGU within 6 weeks. Steady sexual partners should be treated.

C. Erythromycin base 500 mg q.i.d. for 7 days or erythromycin ethylsuccinate 800 mg q.i.d. for 7 days, ofloxacin 300 mg PO b.i.d. for 7 days, or levofloxacin 500 mg q.d. for 7 days are alternative treatments. If the patient is unable to tolerate high-dose erythromycin schedules, erythromycin 250 mg q.i.d. for 14 days or erythromycin ethylsuccinate 400 mg q.i.d. for 14 days is recommended.

D. Patients with multiple recurrences should be referred to an urologist to rule out structural abnormalities.

GONORRHEA

I. **DEFINITION AND PATHOPHYSIOLOGY.** Infection with *N. gonorrhoeae* occurs most often as a mucopurulent urethritis in men and as an asymptomatic or minimally symptomatic endocervical colonization in women. Transmission of the gonococcus is almost entirely through sexual practices, except for neonatal conjunctivitis and fomite-transmitted vulvovaginitis in prepubescent girls. Gonorrhea is diagnosed more often in the male patient; however, the rate is actually higher among women than men (116 vs. 110 cases per 100,000 population respectively). At least half of all reported patients are 25 years of age or younger. There has been a 75% decline in gonorrhea cases since 1975; however, this disease remains the second most prevalent STD in the United States.

Neisseria are gram-negative, nonmotile, non-spore-forming cocci that tend to grow in pairs with the adjacent sides flattened. Humans are the only natural host of *Neisseria*. *N. gonorrhoeae* is differentiated from nonpathogenic *Neisseria* through growth on selective antibiotic-containing media (Thayer-Martin agar) and from the meningococcus by fluorescent antibody techniques.

Pathogenic gonococci have tiny proteinaceous surface projections called **pili**, which cause the organisms to stick to each other as well as to mucosal cells. Other cell-surface structures and a bacterial immunoglobulin A (IgA) protease may also be relevant to pathogenicity. The gonococcus enters the body by penetrating through columnar epithelial cells of the genitourinary tract and produces an acute inflammatory response.

II. SUBJECTIVE DATA
A. Men
1. After an incubation period of 2 to 5 days, 80% to 90% of men have the sudden onset of uncomfortable sensations along the urethra followed by frequent, painful urination.
2. After a variable period of time (10 to 14 days or longer), infection may spread to the posterior urethra, prostate, seminal vesicles, and epididymis, causing pain and a feeling of fullness in the perineum or scrotum.
B. Women
1. Seventy percent to 80% of infected women have gonococci present in the endocervical canal or urethra with no symptoms or with nonspecific symptoms such as vaginal discharge, urinary frequency, or dysuria.
2. PID (salpingitis, parametritis, and localized peritonitis) causes fever, nausea, vomiting, and abdominal pain and may follow an acute infection or may occur months later.

III. OBJECTIVE DATA
A. Men. A profuse mucopurulent discharge is present.
B. Women
1. A mild discharge may be seen.
2. Patients with PID have acute abdominal pain and fever that simulates appendicitis or other acute surgical conditions.

IV. ASSESSMENT
A. Diagnosis
1. In men, the finding of intracellular gram-negative diplococci within polymorphonuclear leukocytes in a Gram-stained smear of a urethral exudate allows the presumptive diagnosis of gonococcal urethritis to be made with at least 99% accuracy. A urethral culture should be obtained from symptomatic men to ensure that the organism is sensitive to the antibiotics given and from men suspected of asymptomatic urethral colonization or for confirmation of adequate treatment.
2. In women, a smear will show approximately 5% false-positive results and 50% false-negative results and is, therefore, of no diagnostic use. Cervical culture on Thayer-Martin media will detect 80% to 85% of those infected, and the addition of a culture of the anus will increase the yield to over 90%. Cultures of skin, blood, and joint aspirates are less likely to yield organisms.
3. Several nucleotide amplification assays (e.g., PCR) for gonorrhea are now U.S. Food and Drug Administration (FDA) approved. In addition, deoxyribonucleic acid (DNA) probe assays, used to detect gonorrhea DNA in a sample, are less expensive than PCR and offer >90% sensitivity and specificity.
B. Extragenital infections and complications
1. Pharyngeal infections, usually asymptomatic, are present in approximately 20% of patients with anogenital gonorrhea who practice fellatio.
2. Anal infections in men are usually the result of anal intercourse among homosexuals. Fifty percent of women with gonorrhea will also have anal infection, presumably because of anatomic contiguity and not necessarily from intercourse. Anal infection is almost always asymptomatic.
3. Disseminated infection (gonococcemia, arthritis-dermatitis syndrome) appears initially as a triad of fever, migratory polyarthralgias and tenosynovitis, and characteristic skin lesions with subsequent development of stationary large-joint septic arthritis. One percent to 2% of patients with gonorrhea develop a disseminated infection, usually within 2 to 3 weeks of the initial infection. Women are affected more commonly, and pregnancy and menstruation appear to predispose to dissemination. Strains of *N. gonorrhoeae* that cause dissemination usually induce little genital inflammation; these strains have become less common in the United States.
   a. The cutaneous lesions are countable in number and are usually located distally over joints. Most cases have <25 to 30 lesions. Petechiae may develop over the hands and feet.

    b. Lesions start as minute erythematous papules resembling mosquito bites and progress to become pustules or, later, hemorrhagic infarcts. They are often tender. The lesions are secondary to embolization of the organisms to the skin with the development of microabscesses.

    c. Other much less common complications include hepatitis (Fitz-Hugh-Curtis Syndrome), meningitis, endocarditis, and pericarditis.

V. THERAPY. The emergence of antibiotic-resistant gonococci and therapy for possibly coexisting chlamydial infection are two of many factors to be considered in the appropriate treatment of gonorrhea. Plasmid-mediated penicillinase-producing *N. gonorrhoeae* (PPNG) is a particular problem in endemic foci in California, New York, and Florida. Chromosomal-mediated (β-lactamase-negative) resistant *N. gonorrhoeae* (CMRNG) is not only resistant to penicillin but also to tetracycline. Cases of fluoroquinolone-resistant gonorrhea have occurred with increasing frequency. Fluoroquinolones should not be used to treat proved or suspected gonococcal infections in men having sex with men in the United States and in patients whose gonorrhea was acquired in California, Massachusetts, New York City, certain counties in Michigan, the Pacific Islands (including Hawaii), Asia, and other areas such as England and Wales. Updated antimicrobial resistance data should be consulted at http://www.cdc.gov/std/gisp.

    With the exception of male homosexuals (in whom it is rare), 45% of patients with gonorrhea may have a coexisting chlamydial infection.

A. Uncomplicated infection in adults. There are several possible regimens, each with advantages and disadvantages. Selection of a treatment regimen for *N. gonorrhoeae* infection requires consideration of the anatomic site of infection, resistance of *N. gonorrhoeae* strains to antimicrobials, the possibility of coinfection with *C. trachomatis*, and the side effects and cost of the regimen. Each should be followed by a regimen effective against possible coinfection with *C. trachomatis*, such as doxycycline 100 mg PO b.i.d. for 7 days. Lastly, the availability of antibiotics has increasingly become an issue in the United States. Oral cefixime tablets and spectinomycin are now unavailable. For the most recent updates on recommended treatment, physicians should check updates at http://www.cdc.gov/std/treatment.

    1. Ceftriaxone (a third-generation cephalosporin) 125 mg IM in a single dose. No ceftriaxone-resistant strains of gonorrhea have been reported. Ceftriaxone may also abort incubating syphilis.

    2. Ciprofloxacin 500 mg PO in a single dose. Resistance data should be viewed at http://www.cdc.gov/std/gisp before using fluoroquinolones.

    3. Ofloxacin 400 mg PO in a single dose (see warning under Ciprofloxacin).

    4. Levofloxacin 250 mg PO in a single dose (see warning under Ciprofloxacin).

    5. Cefixime 400 mg PO in a single dose. (This form is currently not available in the United States.) There is a cefixime oral suspension with limited availability in the United States that has not been adequately tested and is therefore not currently recommended.

    6. Alternative treatments include spectinomycin 2 g IM once (which is now not available in the United States), other cephalosporins, or other fluoroquinolones. Cefpodoxime 400 mg, which is recommended by the California and Washington Health Departments, has not yet been adequately evaluated.

    7. The fluoroquinolones and ceftriaxone have a cure rate of >95% in anal and genital infections. If pharyngeal infection is a concern, ceftriaxone or ciprofloxacin cures >90% of these infections. However, if pharyngeal infection has been ruled out, some of the other treatments mentioned in the preceding text may be considered.

    8. Pregnant women unable to tolerate a cephalosporin may take ciprofloxacin if the benefit justifies potential risk.

B. Treatment failures. All posttreatment isolates should be tested for antimicrobial susceptibility. Infections detected after treatment with one of the preceding regimens is usually secondary to reinfection, not treatment failure. Persistent urethritis, cervicitis, or proctitis may be caused by *C. trachomatis* or other organisms.

C. PID (ambulatory patients)
1. Cefoxitin 2.0 g IM, along with probenecid 1.0 g PO, followed by doxycycline 100 mg PO b.i.d. for 14 days.
2. Ceftriaxone 250 mg IM followed by doxycycline 100 mg PO b.i.d. for 14 days.
3. Comment: These patients should be followed in consultation with a physician experienced in the management of PID.

D. Disseminated infection
1. Hospitalization is usually indicated, especially for patients who appear to have septic arthritis or other complications, have an uncertain diagnosis, or are unreliable.
2. Recommended initial regimen: ceftriaxone 1 g IM or IV q24h. Alternative regimens are cefotaxime 1 g IV q8h or ceftizoxime 1 g IV q8h, ciprofloxacin 500 m IV q12h, ofloxacin 400 mg IV q12h, or spectinomycin 2 g IM q12h (currently not available in the United States).
3. All regimens should be continued 24 to 48 hours after improvement; therapy can then be switched to an oral regimen: cefixime 400 mg PO b.i.d. (currently not available in the United States), ciprofloxacin 500 mg PO b.i.d., or ofloxacin 400 mg b.i.d. As mentioned in the preceding text, before using a fluoroquinolone, resistance data should be viewed at http://www.cdc.gov/std/gisp.
4. For persons allergic to cephalosporins, spectinomycin 2 g IM q12h is recommended but currently not available in the United States. These patients should therefore be desensitized to cephalosporins.

E. Gonococcal infections in children. Children who weigh 100 lb (45 kg) or more should receive adult regimens.
1. For those who weigh <100 lb, uncomplicated vulvovaginitis, urethritis, proctitis, and pharyngitis should be treated with ceftriaxone 125 mg IM.

F. Neonatal gonococcal ophthalmia. Prompt diagnosis, hospitalization, and treatment are necessary, because perforation of the globe and blindness may result. Ceftriaxone 25 to 50 mg/kg IV or IM in a single dose, not to exceed 125 mg. Irrigation of the eyes may reduce the discharge, though topical antibiotics are neither necessary nor a satisfactory alternative to systemic therapy. *C. trachomatis* and nonsexually transmitted agents are the more common cause of neonatal conjunctivitis.

G. Epidemiologic treatment
1. Those known to have been exposed within 1 month to symptomatic gonorrhea should be examined and treated with the same treatment as those known to have the disease. Contacts within 2 months with asymptomatic gonorrhea or PID should be examined and those within 1 month should be treated.
2. Acceptable regimens for prophylaxis of neonatal gonococcal and chlamydial ophthalmia include either tetracycline or erythromycin ointment or drops. Single-use tubes are preferable to multiple-use tubes. Use of 1% silver nitrate solution is effective against gonococcal ophthalmia but will not prevent chlamydial ophthalmia. All infants should be administered ocular prophylaxis whether delivery is vaginal or cesarean.

 TRICHOMONIASIS

I. DEFINITION AND PATHOPHYSIOLOGY. The protozoan flagellate *Trichomonas vaginalis* is the leading cause of vaginitis and may infect as many as 10% to 20% of sexually active women. It causes an infection of the vagina and urethra that may extend to involve the adjacent skin. Transmission is by sexual intercourse as well as from contaminated material or instrumentation. Organisms can be cultured from the urethra in 80% of infected women and approximately 70% of their male sexual partners. There is evidence of a relationship between vaginal trichomoniasis and adverse pregnancy outcomes, such as preterm labor, premature rupture of the membranes, and postabortal/postcesarean infection.

II. SUBJECTIVE DATA

A. When symptoms are present, vulvar pruritus is the predominant problem.

B. Dysuria and dyspareunia may be complaints.

C. Men can have mild urethral pruritus associated with dysuria and frequency; most men are asymptomatic.

III. OBJECTIVE DATA

A. The vaginal discharge is characteristically copious, malodorous, frothy, and watery.

B. Signs of secondary irritant inflammation—edema, erythema, and excoriation of external genitalia—are often seen.

C. Men will have white blood cells in their urethral secretions.

IV. ASSESSMENT

A. Diagnosis is made by visualizing motile 10- to 20-μm trichomonads on a wet mount.

   1. Mix a drop of discharge with a drop of saline on a slide, apply a coverslip, and view at 100 to 400 magnification with the condenser down.

   2. The wet mount will be positive in only 75% to 80% of patients from whom trichomonads can be cultured.

   3. Other suggestive features include vaginal secretions with a pH >4.7 and a predominance of leukocytes.

B. Organisms may be cultured on Feinberg-Wittington or other media.

C. Monoclonal antibody staining may replace wet mounts in the office diagnosis of trichomoniasis. This test is 86% sensitive and picks up 77% of wet-mount-negative cases.

V. THERAPY

A. Metronidazole (Flagyl) 2 g PO in a single dose or 500 mg b.i.d. for 7 days for the patient and for partner(s). Intravaginal metronidazole and other intravaginal medications are ineffective and should not be used. Patients should not drink alcohol for 48 hours to avoid a disulfiram (Antabuse)-like effect. Both partners should be treated.

B. Recurrent discharge may represent relapse or reinfection with *Trichomonas*, but because metronidazole therapy alters the normal vaginal flora, *C. albicans* vaginitis must be considered. If single-dose treatment fails, then treat with metronidazole 500 mg b.i.d. for 7 days. If repeated failure occurs, the patient should be treated with a single 2-g dose of metronidazole daily for 3 to 5 days.

C. Metronidazole should not be used during the first trimester of pregnancy. Acidifying douches may give adequate relief of symptoms.

   1. Clotrimazole 100 mg intravaginal at bedtime for 7 days may improve symptoms and affect some cures.

D. Tinidazole (not available in the United States) may be effective in curing refractory cases of metronidazole resistance.

 CANDIDA ALBICANS INFECTION

C. albicans organisms may cause eruption by direct infection or through an irritant action. In order to distinguish other causes of vaginitis, a potassium hydroxide prep can be utilized.

 BACTERIAL VAGINOSIS

I. DEFINITION AND PATHOPHYSIOLOGY. This infection occurs when commensal lactobacilli bacteria are replaced by anaerobic bacteria, *Gardnerella vaginalis*, or *Mycoplasma hominis*. This is the most common cause of vaginitis.

II. SUBJECTIVE DATA

A. Symptoms are similar to trichomonas vaginitis.

III. OBJECTIVE DATA

A. Objective findings are similar to trichomonas vaginitis.

IV. ASSESSMENT

A. Bacterial vaginosis can be distinguished from the other causes of vaginitis on clinical grounds. Demonstration of three of the following four criteria indicates the presence of the disease:

1. Homogenous white, noninflammatory smooth discharge.

2. Presence of clue cells.

3. Vaginal fluid pH >4.5.

4. Fishy odor with addition of potassium hydroxide to the wet prep (a.k.a. Whiff test). Clue cells are epithelial cells that have bacteria adhered to the surface. The epithelial cell wall is ill-defined because of being peppered with bacteria.

B. Gram's stain can be performed to examine the overall change in flora. Gram-positive rods (lactobacillus) make up the normal flora and coccobacilli are found in bacterial vaginosis.

C. Commercially available tests can be used which assess pH and presence of amine (present in the Whiff test).

V. THERAPY

A. Metronidazole (Flagyl) 2 g PO in a single dose. Unlike trichomoniasis, partners do not need to be treated. Patients should not drink alcohol for 48 hours to avoid a disulfiram (Antabuse)-like effect.

B. Metronidazole gel 0.75% one full applicator (5 g) intravaginally once a day for 5 days.

C. Metronidazole should not be used during the first trimester of pregnancy. Acidifying douches may give adequate relief of symptoms.

D. Clindamycin cream 2% one full applicator (5 g) intravaginally once a day for 5 days. Clindamycin is an alternative but appears to be less effective compared with the metronidazole preparations.

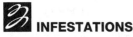 **INFESTATIONS**

Pediculosis Pubis

This disorder presents as moderate to severe pruritus in the pubic area and often elsewhere. See Chap. 19 for more discussion.

Scabies

Both scabies and pediculosis present as moderate to severe pruritus in the pubic area and often elsewhere. See Chap. 19 for more discussion.

 OTHER VIRAL INFECTIONS

Warts and Condyloma Acuminata

These slow-growing viral lesions may be found on any area of the anogenital region, and they have clearly been shown to be sexually transmitted. Referral of sexual partners for examination and obtaining Pap smears for women are essential because of the relationship of some human papilloma virus types to carcinoma of the cervix. See Chap. 36 for more discussion.

Molluscum Contagiosum

Many adult patients with molluscum have lesions in the anogenital region. See Chap. 24 for more discussion.

Other Diseases

Other infections that may be sexually transmitted include those caused by cytomegalovirus, hepatitis B virus, and HIV.

Suggested Readings

Centers for Disease Control and Prevention. Sexually transmitted diseases treatment guidelines. *MMWR Recomm Rep* 2002;51(RR-6):1–78, Available at http://www.cdc.gov/std/treatment/.

Centers for Disease Control and Prevention. *Oral alternatives to cefixime for the treatment of uncomplicated neisseria gonorrhoeae urogenital infections.* Updated 30 April 2004, Available at http://www.cdc.gov/std/treatment/Cefixime.htm.

Centers for Disease Control and Prevention. Increases in fluoroquinolone-resistant Neisseria gonorrhoeae among men who have sex with men—United States, 2003, and revised recommendations for gonorrhea treatment, 2004. *MMWR Morb Mortal Wkly Rep* 2004;53:335–338.

Centers for Disease Control and Prevention. *Sexually transmitted disease surveillance 2004 supplement: gonococcal isolate surveillance project (GISP) annual report—2004.* Atlanta, Georgia: U.S. Department of Health and Human Services, December 2005, Available at http://www.cdc.gov/std/treatment/.

Centers for Disease Control and Prevention. Notice to readers: discontinuation of spectinomycin. *MMWR Morb Mortal Wkly Rep* 2006;55:370.

Fekade D, Knox K, Hussein K, et al. Prevention of Jarisch-Herxheimer reactions by treatment with antibodies against tumor necrosis factor alpha. *N Engl J Med* 1996;335: 311–315.

Galadari I, Galadari H. Nonspecific urethritis and reactive arthritis. *Clin Derm* 2004;22: 469–475.

Ghosn SH, Kibbi A. Cutaneous gonococcal infections. *Clin Derm* 2004;22:476–480.

LaFond RE, Lukehart SA. Biological basis for syphilis. *Clin Microbiol Rev* 2006;19(1): 29–49.

Lukehart SA, Godornes C, Molini BJ, et al. Macrolide resistance in Treponema pallidum in the United States and Ireland. *N Engl J Med* 2004;351:154–158.

Miller KE, Ruiz DE, Graves JC. Update on the prevention and treatment of sexually transmitted diseases. *Am Fam Physician* 2003;67:9.

Mitchell SJ, Engelman J, Kent CK, et al. Azithromycin-resistant syphilis infection: San Francisco, California, 2000–2004. *Clin Infect Dis* 2006;42:337–345.

Morrison RP. New insights into a persistent problem: chlamydial infections. *J Clin Invest* 2003;111:1647–1649.

Peipert JF. Genital chlamydial infections. *N Engl J Med* 2003;349:2424–2430.

Rosen T Update on genital lesions. *JAMA* 2003;290:8.

Sehgal VN, Srivastava G. Chancroid: contemporary appraisal. *Int J Dermatol* 2003;42: 182–190.

SKIN CANCER

Khosrow M. Mehrany and Ken K. Lee

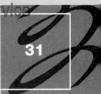

31

I. DEFINITION AND PATHOPHYSIOLOGY. Over 1.2 million new cases of nonmelanoma skin cancer are diagnosed every year in the United States. This large number of newly diagnosed skin cancers is greater than all other cancers combined. The continued increase in the incidence of skin cancer is especially concerning as it is occurring at a time when most other cancers are either decreasing or stabilizing in rate. Basal cell carcinomas (BCCs) make up most skin cancers at 75% to 80%, squamous cell carcinomas (SCCs) total 10% to 25%. Overall, BCC is three to five times more common than SCC in white populations. The expected lifetime risk for a BCC is approximately 30% and the risk for an SCC is 9%. Melanomas are the remainder (47,700 invasive cases per year, with an additional 20,000 to 40,000 cases of melanoma *in situ* per year) (1).

With changes in the ozone layer, some predict a sharp increase in the future incidence of skin cancer. The World Health Organization estimates that ozone depletion peaked in 1998 to 1999, but it will take 50 years to return to pre-1970 levels.

The etiologies of skin cancer are multiple and interrelated. Exogenous and endogenous factors interact in complex and synergistic manners, leading to carcinogenesis. This multistage process includes tumor initiation, promotion, and premalignant progression, leading to malignant conversion of normal cells into skin cancers.

Endogenous factors include (i) skin type, (ii) immunosuppression associated with effects of organ transplant medications, (iii) genetic predisposition at a cellular level, and (iv) immunosuppression secondary to leukemia, lymphoma, or human immunodeficiency virus (HIV) infection.

The most important exogenous factor is ultraviolet (UV) radiation from sunlight. Ultraviolet A (UVA) and ultraviolet B (UVB) both play a role. UVB rays promote immunosuppression, photoaging, mutations, chromosome damage, and generate reactive oxygen species. The role of UVA has only recently been established and only in recent times has sunscreen protection against UVA rays been advised. However, UVA can significantly contribute to photoaging, immunosuppression, chromosome damage, production of reactive oxygen species, and carcinogenesis.

Other exogenous factors include (i) ionizing radiation, (ii) chemical carcinogens that include hydrocarbons and industrial oils (e.g., petroleum products, coal), (iii) human papilloma virus (HPV), (iv) hyperthermia, and (v) chronic irritation.

Exogenous factors stress one's endogenous susceptibility by affecting immune function, deoxyribonucleic acid (DNA) stability and replication, enzymatic activity, cell membrane function, and overall cellular activity.

Individuals with a nonmelanoma skin cancer have a 20% chance of developing a second skin cancer in 18 months and a 36% chance in the next 5 years (2).

Organ transplant recipients are at increased risk for developing skin cancers. It is estimated that 40% to 70% of transplantation patients may eventually develop skin cancer. The ratio of SCC to BCC is 4:1 in transplantation patients, which is reversed as compared with the general population. This is due to the transplantation patients' 65-fold increased risk for SCC. SCC also behaves more aggressively in this group with higher rates of metastasis and death (3).

A. BCCs arise from a pluripotential cell in the basal layer of the epidermis or appendages. These tumors tend to grow very slowly, over months to years, with an extremely low rate of metastasis (estimated at <0.025%). Rapid destructive growth is rare; 85% of both BCCs and SCCs occur on the head and neck region.

199

Men have a higher incidence than women. There are three major subtypes of BCC: noduloulcerative, sclerosing or morpheaform, and superficial (4).

B. SCCs arise from atypical epidermal keratinocytes, usually in the setting of moderate to severe, chronic photodamage in the presence of actinic keratoses. SCCs tend to grow more rapidly than BCCs and may extend along nerves with a metastatic potential of 0.1% to 3%. Lesions on the ear, lip, penis, and dorsum of the hand have a higher metastatic rate of 10% to 15%. SCC is strongly associated with malignant melanoma (MM) and cancers of major salivary glands (5).

C. MM is the fastest growing cancer in the United States; the incidence is doubling every 10 years. Currently, 1 in 74 individuals will develop an MM. Melanoma is the most common cancer in women aged 25 to 29 and the second most common in women aged 30 to 35. The mortality rate for melanoma has increased 2% per year since 1960. It is estimated in the year 2000 that approximately 7,700 individuals will die from melanoma. Survival is directly related to early detection (6).

Melanoma is unusual in children before puberty, although the incidence in children has recently increased. Large number of nevi, an inability to tan, and a family history are strong determinants of risk (7). Blacks and Asians have 1/12th the risk of melanoma as whites; more darkly pigmented individuals have more melanomas on their hands, feet, mucous membranes, and eyes. Fair skin, prolonged sun exposure, a prior history of psoralen plus ultraviolet A (PUVA) therapy, blistering sunburns before the age of 15, family or personal history of melanoma, and the presence of atypical (dysplastic) nevi or numerous normal-appearing nevi increase the risk of developing melanoma. Fair skin, blond or red hair, blue or green eyes, freckles, and an inability to tan are all associated with an increased risk of melanoma. A prior personal history of melanoma increases the risk of a second melanoma to 3.4% (a 25-fold increased risk), but with no worse prognosis. The risk of a second melanoma is greatest in the first year, with a progressive decline thereafter (8). The *p16/CDKN2A* is an important determinant of melanoma risk in families or patients with multiple melanomas (9).

The highest risk group for melanoma is older men; women with melanoma generally have a better prognosis. Melanoma may arise *de novo* or in a preexisting lesion such as a congenital nevus, atypical nevus, or lentigo maligna. Atypical nevi are a marker for an increased risk of MM at any cutaneous site and are themselves a potential precursor lesion. Individuals with leukemia, lymphoma, and renal transplants also have an increased risk of developing melanoma (6).

D. Syndromes associated with skin cancers

1. Basal cell nevus syndrome is an autosomal dominant disorder in which individuals begin to develop multiple BCCs in childhood. The main pathology lies in mutation of the tumor suppressor *PATCHED* (*PTCH*) gene affecting cell growth control.

2. Xeroderma pigmentosum (XP) is an autosomal recessive disorder; the biochemical defect consists of defects in excision repair of UV light–induced pyrimidine DNA dimers or a defect in the synthesis of DNA after UV irradiation. These children develop multiple cutaneous neoplasms (BCC, SCC, and melanoma) before the age of 10, with devastating results.

3. Basex syndrome is a rare disorder that is both autosomal dominant and X-linked dominant in inheritance. Individuals develop BCCs between the ages of 15 and 25. These patients also exhibit follicular atrophoderma and localized anhidrosis.

4. Epidermodysplasia verruciformis is a rare autosomal recessive disorder in which HPV subtypes, most commonly type 5, induce wart-like growths in childhood that may subsequently develop an invasive SCC. A genetic defect in cellular immunity has been hypothesized.

5. Rombo syndrome is an autosomal dominant disorder featuring multiple BCCs. The gene for this disorder has not been identified yet (10).

II. SUBJECTIVE DATA

A. BCC. These tumors in their early stage are usually not painful. The patient may notice a lesion that tends to bleed and does not heal, "a pimple that wouldn't go away."

B. SCC. These tumors may be tender to the touch owing to their rapid growth and inflammatory reaction. In their later stages, they may ulcerate and invade nerves with subsequent pain and dysesthesia.

C. MM. Often the patient or a concerned individual will report a change in a nevus, a new pigmented lesion, or a change in a preexisting mole. Itching, burning, crusting, bleeding, or pain in a mole should arouse suspicion of malignant changes. Most patients with melanoma have no discomfort (11).

III. OBJECTIVE DATA

A. BCC

1. Noduloulcerative BCC

a. The BCC has rolled, easily defined borders, arises from normal or sun-damaged skin, and is found most commonly on the face.

b. The surface has a slightly translucent or pearly quality, often with a central crust or depression and surface telangiectasias.

c. Other secondary changes that may occur include ulceration, scaling and crusting, pigmentation, cyst formation, and scarring.

2. Superficial or multicentric BCC

a. Superficial BCCs appear as erythematous plaques with fine scale, often on the trunk and extremities, and may be multiple.

b. The border is well demarcated with an irregular, thread-like, elevated edge, and variable telangiectasias.

c. Lesions may resemble plaques of psoriasis or nummular eczema but are usually found in association with actinic keratoses, elastosis, lentigines, freckles, telangiectasias, wrinkles, and arcus senilis.

3. Sclerosing, morpheaform, or infiltrating BCC

a. This type of BCC is a yellow-white, flat or depressed, sclerotic papule or plaque and resembles a scar with indistinct borders and variable telangiectasias.

4. Rodent ulcer is an aggressively invasive BCC with prominent ulceration, which is found in the embryonic fusion planes of the face (nasolabial fold, anterior and posterior folds of the ear, ear canal, periorbital region, and the glabella).

B. SCC

1. An SCC presents as an enlarging, scaling, dome-shaped nodule with poorly defined borders arising from an actinic keratosis or area of dysplasia, most commonly in men.

2. SCC tumors on the lips or in a burn scar, a chronic radiation site, or sinus tract tend to be more aggressive and have a higher metastatic potential.

3. An overlying hyperkeratotic crust may produce scale with the appearance of a wart or cutaneous horn.

4. The regional lymph nodes near a suspected SCC should be evaluated for evidence of metastases.

5. Variants of SCC

a. SCC *in situ* appears as a poorly demarcated inflammatory, scaling papule or plaque in the background of actinic damage; individuals may have a history of arsenic ingestion.

b. Bowen's disease is a unique type of SCC *in situ* that is characterized by the presence of a well-demarcated macule or scaling plaque with an irregular outline, fine scale, and gray-brown pigmentation. It does not arise in skin with actinic damage. Bowen's disease does not appear to be associated with an increased risk of internal malignancy.

c. Bowenoid papulosis appears as single or multiple verrucous papules on the genitalia with histologic atypia similar to Bowen's disease. These papules are usually induced by the HPV type 16 and have malignant potential.

d. Erythroplasia of Queyrat is an asymptomatic, well-demarcated, red plaque on the penis of an uncircumcised male with the histology of an SCC *in situ*.

e. Carcinoma cuniculatum is a verrucous, slowly growing plaque on the sole of the foot, often treated for years as a recalcitrant wart. A deep incisional biopsy is required to demonstrate the invading tumor at the base of this lesion.

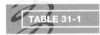

TABLE 31-1   Factors Associated with Increased Risk of Melanoma

Factor	Relative risk (%)[a]
Changing or persistently changed mole, age >15 years	Very high
One or several irregularly pigmented lesions	88
Atypical (dysplastic) mole(s) or familial melanoma (see Color Plate 44)	148
Atypical (dysplastic) mole(s) but no familial melanoma (see Color Plate 45)	17–64
Lentigo maligna (see Color Plate 46)	10
Congenital mole	17–21
White race (compared with blacks)	12
Previous melanoma	5–9
Melanoma in parents, children, or siblings	2–8
Immunosuppression — leukemia, lymphoma, renal transplantation	2–3
Sun sensitivity, tans poorly, burns easily, had multiple or severe sunburns	2–3
Excessive sun exposure, particularly during childhood	3–5
No increased risk	1

[a]Degree of increased risk for persons with the risk factor compared with persons without the risk factor. Relative risk of 1.0 implies no increased risk.
Source: Adapted from Rhodes AR, Weinstock MA, Fitzpatrick TB, et al. Risk factors for cutaneous melanoma. A practical method of recognizing predisposed individuals. *JAMA* 1987;258:3146–3154.

    f. Keratoacanthoma is a rapidly growing, well-demarcated nodule with a rolled border and cup-shaped center filled with keratinous material. A classic keratoacanthoma regresses with the formation of a scar. Although often described as a self-healing SCC, subsequent metastases have been documented from classic keratoacanthomas.

C. MM (Table 31-1 and color plate) can be found on any surface of the skin, including the mucous membranes and the retina. The physical examination should include assessment of the liver, spleen, and lymph nodes.

    1. Superficial spreading melanoma (up to 70% of MM)
        a. This lesion appears as a flat to slightly raised, pigmented papule or plaque with irregular features, most commonly found on the backs of men and the lower legs of women.
        b. The color is varied, often black and/or dark brown, with an erythematous border. Gray or white coloration represents tumor regression.
        c. The pigmented lesion may have changed with enlargement radially before deep invasion occurs.

    2. Lentigo maligna melanoma (LMM) (4% to 10% of MM)
        a. LMM occurs on sun-exposed areas, especially the face of elderly individuals.
        b. Lesions initially appear as a lentigo maligna, or Hutchinson's freckle, an irregularly pigmented macule with jagged or notched border found most often on the cheeks; 30% to 50% transform to MM.
        c. The onset of nodular growth and MM usually occurs 10 to 15 years after the initial development of the precursor lentigo maligna.

    3. Nodular melanoma (15% to 30% of MM)
        a. The tumor is located most commonly on the head, neck, and trunk (in men) and is characterized by rapid nodular growth without a radial growth phase.
        b. The pigment may be brown, black, or blue; however, amelanotic forms occur that appear as pink or red papules without pigment.

    4. Acral-lentiginous melanoma (2% to 8% of MM)

      a. This form of MM, often difficult to diagnose and occurring on palms, soles, fingers, and toes, is the most common form of melanoma in blacks.

      b. A pigmented streak in a nail may represent acral-lentiginous MM; pigmentation of the cuticle is diagnostic (Hutchinson's sign) (6,12).

D. Syndromes associated with skin cancer

    1. Basal cell nevus syndrome

      a. BCCs occur in sun-exposed and non–sun-exposed areas beginning in childhood and become more aggressive after puberty.

      b. Multiple pits occur on the palms and soles.

      c. Other signs include calcification of the falx cerebri, jaw cysts, splayed or bifid ribs, epidermal cysts, lipomas, hypertelorism, and lateral displacement of the medial canthus of the eye. Cardiac fibromas, medulloblastomas, meningiomas, and rhabdomyomas may also be found.

      d. Individuals with BCC nevus syndrome are extremely sensitive to radiation.

    2. XP

      a. The hallmarks of XP are photosensitivity, photophobia, and conjunctivitis.

      b. Multiple skin cancers develop, including BCC, SCC, and melanoma, and are often first seen before the age of 10.

      c. Some forms of XP are associated with microcephaly, progressive mental retardation, and sensorineural deficits.

    3. Basex syndrome

      a. This syndrome consists of multiple BCCs developing between the ages of 15 and 25, follicular atrophoderma of the dorsal hands and elbows, and localized areas of anhidrosis; some patients may have hypotrichosis.

    4. Epidermodysplasia verruciformis

      a. Widespread, polymorphic, verrucous plaques arise in childhood; some resemble tinea versicolor.

      b. SCCs may develop in the warty plaques.

    5. Rombo syndrome

      a. Multiple BCCs associated with trichoepitheliomas, hypotrichosis, milia, and cyanosis of hands and feet.

      b. Associated vermicular atrophoderma produces course, grainy skin texture (10).

IV. ASSESSMENT. All suspected skin cancers should be biopsied. This can be done by a shave or 3- to 4-mm punch biopsy, curettage, or incisional or excisional biopsy, depending on the diagnosis and location of the tumor. Curettage results in tissue fragments only, which can be used only to confirm a diagnosis of a BCC.

A. BCC

    1. Most BCCs can be biopsied with a simple shave biopsy.

    2. If a sclerotic BCC is suspected, a punch or incisional/excisional biopsy is preferable.

B. SCC

    1. A deep disk shave or punch biopsy may be able to demonstrate the base of the lesion, especially if the tumor resembles a keratoacanthoma clinically. The base of the lesion needs to be well visualized by the pathologist in order to rule out an invasive SCC. Lesions at high risk of metastasis include those on the lip, ear, and temple; fast growing lesions; or those with any evidence of perineural spread.

C. Melanoma. If the lesion suggests an MM and is small enough to be excised, it should be removed, full thickness, with 1- to 2-mm margins. Initial wide excisional margins are not recommended because numerous clinically suspicious tumors turn out to be non-MMs. Larger lesions, such as an LMM, can be biopsied in the most darkly pigmented, nodular area by either an incisional or a punch biopsy. Curettage or shave biopsy will not provide sufficient tissue. The following guidelines are used to establish the patient's prognosis:

    1. Melanoma staging. The stage groupings for melanoma are based on the tumor node metastasis (TNM) system which uses tumor size, nodal, and metastatic status. The T classification uses Breslow thickness, ulceration, and Clark level to differentiate the tumor (13).

   a. Breslow thickness: distance from the granular layer to the deepest tumor cell, measured in millimeters, in the primary lesion.
   b. Clark level: only used to further characterize thin melanomas (<1 mm)
      i. Level I. Tumor cells in the epidermis only (melanoma *in situ*).
      ii. Level II. Tumor cells in the papillary dermis.
      iii. Level III. Tumor cells fill the papillary dermis and extend but do not invade the reticular dermis.
      iv. Level IV. Tumor cells invade the reticular dermis.
      v. Level V. Tumor cells invade the subcutaneous fat.
      The parameters for T classification:
      Tis: *In situ* melanoma
      T1: ≤1 mm Breslow thickness
         a. Without ulceration—Clark level II/III
         b. With ulceration or Clark level IV/V
      T2: 1.01 to 2.0 mm
         a. Without ulceration
         b. With ulceration
      T3: 2.01 to 4.0 mm
         a. Without ulceration
         b. With ulceration
      T4: >4 mm
         a. Without ulceration
         b. With ulceration
      The parameters for N classification:
      N0: No regional node metastasis
      N1: Metastasis in one regional node
      N1a: Micrometastasis
      N1b: Macrometastasis
      N2: Metastasis in 2 to 3 regional nodes
      N2a: Micrometastasis
      N2b: Macrometastasis
      N2c: In-transit or satellite metastasis without nodal metastasis
      N3: Metastasis in ≥4 regional nodes, matted nodes, or in-transit or satellite metastasis with positive metastatic nodes.
      The parameters for M classification:
      M0: No distant metastasis
      M1a: Distant skin, subcutaneous, or lymph node metastasis with normal lactate dehydrogenase (LDH)
      M1b: Lung metastasis with normal LDH
      M1c: All other distant metastasis or any distant site with elevated LDH.
      When the TNM classification is used, important data on staging and survival rates can be determined (Table 31-2) (13).
   D. Sentinel lymph node biopsy (SLNB) is a sensitive detection technique to find occult metastatic lymph node foci without performing a total lymph node dissection. A sample of the first node (sentinel node) in the drainage chain is obtained after it is detected by a combination of blue dye mapping and radiolymphoscintigraphy. Detection of a positive sentinel lymph node is predictive of regional node metastases and an indication for elective lymph node dissection and/or adjuvant therapy. Polymerase chain reaction (PCR) assays for detection of submicroscopic metastases may play an increasingly important role in the future evaluation of lymph nodes. There are no current data to suggest whether SLNB or use of PCR affects ultimate prognosis/survival. The question remains whether treatment with high-dose interferon for 1 year can improve survival in patients with positive sentinel nodes (14).
   1. The most common sites of distant metastases are skin, distant lymph nodes, lung, liver, brain, and bone.

TABLE 31-2 Survival Rates for Melanoma Tumor Node Metastasis and Staging Categories

Path stage	TNM	Thickness (mm)	Ulceration	No. + Nodes	Nodal size	Distant metastasis	No. of patients	Survival 1 y	±SE 2 y	5 y	10 y
IA	T1a	≤1	No	0	—	—	4,510	99.7 ± 0.1	99.0 ± 0.2	95.3 ± 0.4	87.9 ± 1.0
IB	T1a	≤1	Yes or level IV, V	0	—	—	1,380	99.8 ± 0.1	98.7 ± 0.3	90.9 ± 1.0	83.1 ± 1.5
	T2a	1.01–2.0	No	0	—	—	3,285	99.5 ± 0.1	97.3 ± 0.3	89.0 ± 0.7	79.2 ± 1.1
IIA	T2b	1.01–2.0	Yes	0	—	—	958	98.2 ± 0.5	92.9 ± 0.9	77.4 ± 1.7	64.4 ± 2.2
	T3a	2.01–4.0	No	0	—	—	1,717	98.7 ± 0.3	94.3 ± 0.6	78.7 ± 1.2	63.8 ± 1.7
IIB	T3b	2.01–4.0	Yes	0	—	—	1,523	95.1 ± 0.6	84.8 ± 1.0	63.0 ± 1.5	50.8 ± 1.7
	T4a	>4.0	No	0	—	—	563	94.8 ± 1.0	88.6 ± 1.5	67.4 ± 2.4	53.9 ± 3.3
IIC	T4b	>4.0	Yes	0	—	—	978	89.9 ± 1.0	70.7 ± 1.6	45.1 ± 1.9	32.3 ± 2.1
IIIA	N1a	Any	No	1	Micro	—	252	95.9 ± 1.3	88.0 ± 2.3	69.5 ± 3.7	63.0 ± 4.4
	N2a	Any	No	2–3	Micro	—	130	93.0 ± 2.4	82.7 ± 3.8	63.3 ± 5.6	56.9 ± 6.8
IIIB	N1a	Any	Yes	1	Micro	—	217	93.3 ± 1.8	75.0 ± 3.2	52.8 ± 4.1	37.8 ± 4.8
	N2a	Any	Yes	2–3	Micro	—	111	92.0 ± 2.7	81.0 ± 4.1	49.6 ± 5.7	35.9 ± 7.2
	N1b	Any	No	1	Macro	—	122	88.5 ± 2.9	78.5 ± 3.7	59.1 ± 4.8	47.7 ± 5.8
	N2b	Any	No	2–3	Macro	—	93	76.8 ± 4.4	65.6 ± 5.0	46.3 ± 5.5	39.2 ± 5.8
IIIC	N1b	Any	Yes	1	Macro	—	98	77.9 ± 4.3	54.2 ± 5.2	29.0 ± 5.1	24.4 ± 5.3
	N2b	Any	Yes	2–3	Macro	—	109	74.3 ± 4.3	44.1 ± 4.9	24.0 ± 4.4	15.0 ± 3.9
	N3	Any	Any	4	Micro/macro	—	396	71.0 ± 2.4	49.8 ± 2.7	26.7 ± 2.5	18.4 ± 2.5
IV	M1a	Any	Any	Any	Any	Skin, SQ	179	59.3 ± 3.7	36.7 ± 3.6	18.8 ± 3.0	15.7 ± 2.9
	M1b	Any	Any	Any	Any	Lung	186	57.0 ± 3.7	23.1 ± 3.2	6.7 ± 2.0	2.5 ± 1.5
	M2c	Any	Any	Any	Any	Other visceral	793	40.6 ± 1.8	23.6 ± 1.5	9.5 ± 1.1	6.0 ± 0.9
Total							17,600				

TNM, tumor node metastasis.

Source: Reproduced with permission: Balch M, Buraid AC, Soong SJ, et al. Final version of the American Joint Committee on Cancer Staging for Cutaneous Melanoma. *J Clin Oncol* 2001;19:3635–3648.

2. Once a diagnosis of melanoma is established, a history and thorough physical examination should be undertaken. A baseline chest x-ray should be obtained but regular chest x-ray evaluations are not likely to detect metastases in asymptomatic individuals (15). LDH can be performed at baseline and followed, depending on the tumor thickness.

V. THERAPY. Factors such as the age of the patient, size and location of the tumor, the pathology of the tumor, the general health of the patient, cosmetic concerns of the patient, and the experience of the physician must be taken into account when planning therapy for cutaneous malignancies.

A. BCC

1. Excisional surgery with 4-mm margins is curative in 95% of small, noncomplicated BCCs. Curetting the tumor first often helps define the borders before excision.

2. **Electrodesiccation and curettage.** The tumor mass is removed by curettage, and the site is then electrodesiccated with a 1- to 2-mm margin of normal skin. This process is then repeated two more times. The crusted plaque will heal in 2 to 6 weeks with a flat, hypopigmented scar, often with a hypertrophic center. The recurrence rate is 6% to 10% for well-defined tumors located on the trunk and extremities. Recurrence rates approach 30% to 50% for tumors on the head and neck.

3. Cryotherapy by spray technique delivers liquid nitrogen to the tumor. Local anesthesia should be obtained, and then two cycles of a 30-second full freeze and a thaw of at least 90 seconds should be performed. The site will swell, become painful, and blister over 1 to 2 days. The subsequent lesion takes 2 to 6 weeks to heal and will leave a hypopigmented, slightly sclerotic scar. Side effects of this treatment may include alopecia, permanent hypopigmentation, and nerve paralysis. For tumors <2 cm, the recurrence rate is 2% to 6%.

4. Mohs' micrographic surgery is an excisional surgical technique in which horizontally oriented frozen sections are evaluated on the lateral and inferior borders of the tumor to determine where residual tumor is present. This has the advantage of sparing tissue and providing a high cure rate for difficult or recurrent tumors. Indications for Mohs' surgery are immunosuppression, location (ears, eyelids, lips, nose, temples, hands, feet, genitalia), aggressive pathology (morpheaform, micronodular, infiltrative), tumors >2 cm, those occurring on embryonic fusion planes (pre- and postauricular crease, nasofacial sulcus, nasolabial folds), recurrent tumors, poorly defined tumors, or tumors arising in scars or sites of previous radiation (16).

5. Ionizing radiation can be delivered to the tumor and its margin, often requiring multiple visits over several weeks. Acute radiation dermatitis results and heals within 4 to 6 weeks. Because of the risk of radiation-induced secondary skin cancer, this modality should generally be reserved for individuals over 70 years of age. Recurrent BCCs after radiation therapy are more difficult to eradicate because they tend to be deeper and wider.

6. Photodynamic therapy is currently in its experimental phase. Laser light treats tumors that have been rendered photosensitive after systemic or topical administration of a hematoporphyrin derivative or other photosensitizers. This technique holds promise for treatment of multiple, difficult, metastatic, or end-stage invasive tumors.

7. Medical therapies such as administration of systemic retinoids, intralesional interferon, and implantable 5-fluorouracil (5-FU) are being investigated for their antitumor properties.

   a. 5-FU is an effective agent for topical therapy of superficial or small BCCs. Apply 5% 5-FU cream or solution twice a day to the tumor until the area becomes red, crusted, and sore (usually 4 weeks on the face and 6 weeks on the extremities). Healing then takes place over the next 3 to 6 weeks, with the subsequent scar being soft, flat, and hypopigmented (17).

    b. Topical imiquimod 5% cream is an immune response modifier originally developed for the treatment of genital HPV infections. Acting through Toll-like receptor 7, it induces production of tumor necrosis factor-α, interferon-α, and numerous other cytokines. It has been indicated for the topical treatment of biopsy-confirmed, primary superficial BCCs in immunocompetent adults, with maximum diameter of 2.0 cm, located on the trunk (excluding anogenital skin), neck, or extremities (excluding feet and hands) (18).

  8. A low-fat diet may cut the risk of nonmelanoma skin cancer. Fatty acids are strong oxidants and their ability to produce free radicals is theorized to produce a cascade of cancers.

  9. Follow-up for nonmelanoma skin cancers should be on a 6- to 12-month basis. Recurrence most often develops within 3 years of treatment, usually at the periphery of the lesion. The entire cutaneous surface should be examined for the presence of a second primary. Individuals with one nonmelanoma skin cancer have a 20% frequency of another within 1 year; those with more than one have a 40% 1-year rate. The highest risk group is those with a history of three or more nonmelanoma skin cancers. All patients must be given information regarding sun protection and sunscreen use.

 10. Patients with BCC, especially those diagnosed at a young age, have an increased risk for nonmelanoma skin cancer and possible noncutaneous cancers such as testicular cancer, breast cancer, and non-Hodgkin's lymphoma (19).

B. SCC may be treated with all the preceding techniques. Because of their more aggressive growth pattern and tendency to metastasize, wider excision and Mohs' micrographic surgery are commonly preferred.

C. MM

  1. The following is a guideline for excisional margins for MM. The depth of excision should be to the level of the fascia for invasive MM (20).

    a. Melanoma *in situ* 0.5-cm margin

    b. <1-mm deep: 1-cm margin.

    c. 1 to 2 mm in depth: 1- to 2-cm margin

    d. >2 mm in depth: ≥2 cm

    e. Smaller margins are acceptable only if important surrounding structures would be sacrificed.

  2. Whereas wide local excision is widely regarded as the standard of care for MM, Mohs' micrographic surgery is indicated in certain situations. For lentigo maligna/melanoma *in situ* of the head and neck where the margins to clear the tumors are typically >0.5 cm, Mohs' micrographic surgery is valuable in more precisely determining the margins. In these cases, Mohs' micrographic surgery is usually modified by obtaining peripheral permanent paraffin sections after clearance of tumor by frozen sections or by using rapid immunohistochemical staining. Use of Mohs' micrographic surgery for invasive melanoma, though advocated by some, is controversial. In one study, this treatment modality achieved 5-year local recurrence rates, metastasis rates, and disease-specific survival rates comparable to or better than historical controls after Breslow thickness stratification (21).

  3. SLNB is now generally indicated for patients with melanomas >1 mm. SLNB is recommended for thin melanomas with ulceration and Clark level IV/V. If the SLNB is positive, an elective lymph node dissection of the involved basin is performed. However, some have cautioned against the widespread use SLNB, as it is an invasive study performed under general anesthesia with mixed data on the consequent efficacy of treatment (α-interferon) in patients with nodal disease (14,22).

  4. Regular follow-up is required to detect residual, recurrent, or metastatic disease, early primary melanomas, or precursor lesions.

    a. The entire cutaneous surface should be evaluated, including the scalp, oral mucosa, and genitalia.

    b. Annual follow-up for life is recommended for individuals who have been diagnosed with MM.

    c. A review is recommended every 3 months for the first 3 years for patients with invasive lesions, because 80% of recurrences are within this period.

After 3 years, evaluations are recommended every 6 months for the next 2 years and then annually. Most recurrences are detected by history and physical examination and not tests. All immediate family members should be evaluated for the presence of melanoma or precursor lesions (23).

5. Treatment of metastatic disease may include chemotherapy, usually a regimen with dacarbazine (DTIC). No single chemotherapeutic agent offers a response rate >25%. Adjuvant therapy and biologic response modifiers such as vaccines are being rapidly developed. Clinical trials with interleukin 2, interferon-γ, monoclonal antibodies, targeted toxins, vaccines, and gene therapy are underway.

6. Interferon α-2b is U.S. Food and Drug Administration (FDA) approved for the treatment of stage IIB and stage III disease. Treatment for 1 year resulted in a prolonged survival (2.8 years compared with 3.8 years and prolongation of disease-free survival from 1.0 to 1.7 years). The Sunbelt Melanoma Trial is under way and will attempt to answer the benefit of interferon therapy and the significance of lymph nodes that are positive only by PCR analysis.

7. Protection from UV rays is critical in the prevention of melanoma and nonmelanoma skin cancers. Currently, a regimen should include sun-protective clothing, avoidance of the midday sun, and regular use of broad-spectrum high sun protection factor sunscreens.

References

1. Eide M, Weinstock M. Epidemiology of skin cancer. In: Rigel D, Friedman R, Dzubow L, et al. eds. *Cancer of the skin*. Philadelphia, PA: Elsevier Saunders, 2005: 47–60.
2. Scheinfeld N, DeLeo V. Etiological factors in skin cancers: environmental and biological. In: Rigel D, Friedman R, Dzubow L, et al. eds. *Cancer of the skin*. Philadelphia, PA: Elsevier Saunders, 2005:61–70.
3. Berg D, Otley CC. Skin cancer in organ transplant recipients: epidemiology, pathogenesis, and management. *J Am Acad Dermatol* 2002;47(1):1–17.
4. Tilli CM, Van Steensel MA, Krekels GA, et al. Molecular aetiology and pathogenesis of basal cell carcinoma. *Br J Dermatol* 2005;152(6):1108–1124.
5. Alam M, Ratner D. Cutaneous squamous-cell carcinoma. *N Engl J Med* 2001;344(13): 975–983.
6. Tsao H, Atkins MB, Sober AJ. Management of cutaneous melanoma. *N Engl J Med* 2004;351(10):998–1012.
7. Whiteman DC, Valery P, McWhirter W, et al. Risk factors for childhood melanoma in Queensland, Australia. *Int J Cancer* 1997;70:26–31.
8. DiFronzo LA, Wanek LA, Elashoff R, et al. Increased incidence of second primary melanoma in patients with a previous cutaneous melanoma. *Ann Surg Oncol* 1999; 6:705–711.
9. Monzon J, Liu L, Brill H, et al. CDKN2A mutations in multiple primary melanomas. *N Engl J Med* 1998;338:879–887.
10. Gritsenko K, Gordon M, Lebwohl M. Genetic disorders predisposing to cutaneous malignancy. In: Rigel D, Friedman R, Dzubow L, et al. eds. *Cancer of the skin*. Philadelphia, PA: Elsevier Saunders, 2005:363–370.
11. Healsmith MF, Bourke JF, Osborne JE, et al. An evaluation of the revised seven-point checklist for the early diagnosis of cutaneous malignant melanoma. *Br J Dermatol* 1994;130:48–50.
12. Tsao H, Sober AJ. Melanoma treatment update. *Dermatol Clin* 2005;23(2):323–333.
13. Balch M, Buraid AC, Soong SJ, et al. Final version of the American Joint Committee on Cancer Staging for Cutaneous Melanoma. *J Clin Oncol* 2001;19:3635–3648.
14. Lee KK, Vetto JT, Mehrany K, et al. Sentinel lymph node biopsy. *Clin Dermatol* 2004;22(3):234–239.
15. Terhune MH, Swanson N, Johnson TM. Use of chest radiography in the initial evaluation of patients with localized melanoma. *Arch Dermatol* 1998;134:569–572.
16. Swanson NA. Mohs surgery. Technique, indications, applications, and the future. *Arch Dermatol* 1983;119(9):761–773.

17. Miller BH, Shavin JS, Cognetta A, et al. Nonsurgical treatment of basal cell carcinomas with intralesional 5-fluorouracil/epinephrine injectable gel. *J Am Acad Dermatol* 1997;36:72–77.

18. Burns CA, Brown MD. Imiquimod for the treatment of skin cancer. *Dermatol Clin* 2005;23(1):151–164, vii.

19. Frisch M, Hjalgrim H, Olsen JH, et al. Risk for subsequent cancer after diagnosis of basal-cell carcinoma. A population-based, epidemiologic study. *Ann Intern Med* 1996;125:815–821.

20. McMasters KM, Swetter SM. Current management of melanoma: benefits of surgical staging and adjuvant therapy. *J surg Oncol* 2003;82:209–216.

21. Bricca GM, Brodland DG, Ren D, et al. Cutaneous head and neck melanoma treated with Mohs micrographic surgery. *J Am Acad Dermatol* 2005;52(1):92–100.

22. Otley CC, Zitelli JA. Review of sentinel lymph node biopsy and systemic interferon for melanoma: promising but investigational modalities. *Dermatol Surg* 2000;26(3):177–180.

23. Weiss M, Loprinzi CL, Creagon ET, et al. Utility of follow-up tests for detecting recurrent disease in patients with malignant melanomas. *JAMA* 1995;274:1703–1705.

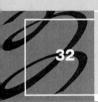

SKIN TAGS
Julie A. Neville and Gil Yosipovitch

I. **DEFINITION AND PATHOPHYSIOLOGY.** Skin tags (acrochordons) are small papillomas found commonly on the sides of the neck, axillae, upper trunk, and eyelids of middle-aged and elderly people. Obesity, pregnancy, menopause, and endocrine disorders such as acromegaly predispose to these benign epithelial hyperplastic lesions. Although controversial, it has been suggested that multiple skin tags may be a marker for diabetes mellitus or impaired carbohydrate metabolism and may indicate a significantly increased risk of colonic polyps if they occur rapidly over a short period of time. One study using polymerase chain reaction (PCR) found low but detectable levels of human papillomavirus (HPV) in 80% of the evaluated skin tags, with subtypes 6 and 11 being present 98% of the time.

II. **SUBJECTIVE DATA.** Skin tags are cosmetically bothersome but asymptomatic. Occasionally, a lesion will twist on its stalk and become painful, erythematous, and necrotic.

III. **OBJECTIVE DATA.** The lesions are single or multiple, 1 to 3 mm in diameter, soft, flesh-colored or hyperpigmented, oval or round papillomas. They are usually pedunculated.

IV. **ASSESSMENT.** Treatment of obesity or an underlying endocrinologic abnormality will decrease the likelihood of new lesion formation. Lesions may be confused with seborrheic keratoses, dermal nevi, neurofibromas, or warts. If multiple skin tags have occurred over a short period of time, referral for sigmoidoscopy or colonoscopy should be considered.

V. **THERAPY.** Treatment is easily accomplished with any of the following methods:

   A. **Excision.** Grasp the tag with forceps and sever the base with a sharp scissors (Gradle or iris scissors are excellent for this use) or a scalpel blade. Hemostasis may be secured by pressure, Monsel's solution (ferric subsulfate solution), 20% aluminum chloride, mild acids (30% trichloroacetic acid), or an electrosurgical spark, although the use of these modalities can cause stinging if the area is not anesthetized. The lesion may be anesthetized with lidocaine or ethyl chloride spray before excision, but this is rarely necessary. Never use an electrosurgical apparatus around flammable ethyl chloride spray or aluminum chloride.

   B. **Destruction.** Touch each lesion with a light electrosurgical spark or remove it with the cutting current. Administration of local anesthesia is usually unnecessary and causes as much pain as the treatment itself. Multiple lesions may be treated at one time.

   C. **Cryotherapy.** Grasp the base of the skin tag with a forceps and direct liquid nitrogen spray at the lesion until frozen. The use of the forceps helps prevent transmission of the cryogen to the skin (minimizing the chance of hyper- or hypopigmentation) and allows a deeper freeze of the individual lesion. Alternatively, dip the tip of a hemostat, forceps, or needle holder into a Styrofoam cup with liquid nitrogen for 15 seconds without allowing the hinge to freeze. Use this instrument to grasp the lesion for 10 seconds. A cotton-tipped applicator dipped in liquid nitrogen can also be used to freeze the lesion, although this can lead to damage to the surrounding tissue.

Suggested Readings

Beitler M, Eng A, Kilgour M, et al. Association between acrochordons and colonic polyps. *J Am Acad Dermatol* 1986;14:1042–1044.

Brendler SJ, Watson RD, Katon RM, et al. Skin tags are not a risk factor for colorectal polyps. *J Clin Gastroenterol* 1989;11:299–302.

Demir S, Demir Y. Acrochordon and impaired carbohydrate metabolism. *Acta Diabetol* 2002;39:27–29.

Dianzani C, Calvieri S, Pierangeli A, et al. The detection of human papillomavirus DNA in skin tags. *Br J Dermatol* 1998;138:649–651.

Goodheart HP. Surgical pearl: a rapid technique for destroying small skin tags and filiform warts. *Dermatol Online J* 2003;9:34.

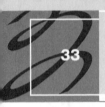

SUN REACTIONS AND SUN PROTECTION

33

Janine D'Amelio Miller

I. DEFINITION AND PATHOPHYSIOLOGY. The sun radiates a broad system of energy that may be categorized in terms of the wavelength of the electromagnetic waves. This radiation reaching the earth's surface may be broadly subdivided into (i) infrared (range 800 to 1,700 nm), felt as heat or a sensation of warmth, (ii) visible (range: 400 to 800 nm), the energy that stimulates the retina, and (iii) ultraviolet (UV) (290 to 400 nm), wavelengths shorter than the visible range.

A. Ultraviolet radiation (UVR) can be subdivided into three bands.

 1. Ultraviolet A (UVA) radiation (320 to 400 nm, long wavelength) can be further divided into UVAI (340 to 400 nm) and UVAII (320 to 340 nm). UVA causes immediate pigment darkening of preformed melanin and may play an additive role in assisting ultraviolet B (UVB) (see subsequent text) in causing sunburn or aging. In the presence of some drugs (psoralens, antibiotics such as doxycycline, sulfonamides, phenothiazides, chlorothiazides, sulfonylureas, and others), UVA may induce severe phototoxicity (sunburn and blistering). UVA can cause skin cancers in mice, induce deoxyribonucleic acid (DNA) damage through production of photoproducts, and suppress the immune system (1).

 2. UVB radiation (290 to 320 nm, middle wavelength) acutely causes erythema and edema, followed by stimulation of melanocytes to make new melanosomes, thereby causing pigment darkening and a tan. Chronic exposure induces most of the changes commonly attributed to aging and carcinogenesis.

 3. Ultraviolet C (UVC) radiation (200 to 290 nm) from sunlight is absorbed by the ozone layer in the atmosphere and does not reach the earth's surface. This radiation kills bacteria, can cause mild conjunctivitis or sunburn, and is used in operating-room germicidal lamps.

   Approximately two thirds of the total daily UVR reaches the earth between 10 a.m. and 2 p.m. Midday UVR is 10% UVB and 90% UVA, because little UVA is filtered by the atmosphere. Cloud cover can reduce the total amount of radiation by 50%. Water also reduces the penetration of ultraviolet light (UVL) by 50%. Snow and ice reflect 80% of the radiation, whereas sand reflects 20% and grass, 2.5%. A breeze will alter an individual's perception of total UV exposure as the skin is cooled. The more hydrated the skin becomes (such as after swimming), the less the reflection of UV light and, subsequently, increased absorption. Window glass blocks UV radiation below 320 nm, thereby providing protection against UVB. Tinted windows can offer increased protection against UVA (2,3).

   UVR induces genetic damage by covalent induced mutations and chromosome damage, which inactivates tumor suppressor genes such as p53. Both UVA and UVB induce DNA damage indirectly through the generation of reactive oxygen free radicals. UVB is a more potent inducer of these reactive species than UVA, although 96% of the UV spectrum is UVA. Blue light in the range of 400 to 450 nm can contribute to DNA damage. UVL also suppresses the immune system with altered response to antigens, release of immunosuppressive factors such as interleukins, and inhibition of natural killer cells.

OZONE LAYER

The ozone layer has been diminishing during the last 20 years, primarily from the release of chlorofluorocarbon compounds into the atmosphere. As a consequence, more UVB can now reach the earth's surface. In general, each degree increase in latitude corresponds to a 3% increase in UVR reaching the earth, and every 1,000 meters above sea level corresponds to a 10% increase in UVR (4,5). The impact of climate changes caused by the stratospheric ozone depletion on skin cancer incidence still remains uncertain (6). Ozone depletion might result in an increased incidence of ocular changes, leading to cataracts, the development of cutaneous melanoma, and the incidence of basal and squamous cell carcinomas (7,8).

Sunburn is usually the result of excessive exposure to UVB radiation but may be a response to excessive UVC from artificial light sources or UVA in the presence of a topical or systemic photosensitizing agent. It is seen most commonly after exposure to the sun but may also follow exposure to sunlamps or occupational light sources (welding arcs [250 to 700 nm], photoengraving [250 to 700 nm], bactericidal or cold quartz lamps [254 nm]). UVB is not screened out by thin clouds on overcast days but is fully absorbed by window glass and is partially absorbed in the smoke and smog around large cities. The epidermis reflects 10% of the UVB rays, and 20% will penetrate to the dermis. UVA penetrates deeper and has more effect on the dermis, markedly accentuating UVB damage. A great deal of UVL reaches the skin through reflection from snow, sand, or sidewalks; hats and umbrellas provide only moderate protection.

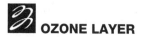 ## SKIN TYPES AND NATURAL PROTECTION

Our own natural sun-protective mechanisms include the thickness of the epidermis, natural antioxidants, melanin, urocanic acid (natural UV absorber), DNA repair mechanisms, and Fas ligand signaling. Transplantation patients are an example of what can happen in nonmelanoma skin when there is a combination of immunosuppression and prior mutations of the p53 gene. Tolerance to sunlight is based on the amount of melanin in the skin and an individual's genetic capacity to produce melanin following exposure to the sun, that is, a suntan. On the basis of the response to the first 30-minute exposure to summer sun and the tan that develops in persons with white skin, sun-reaction skin types can be classified as follows:

Skin type I: always burns easily, never tans.
Skin type II: usually burns easily, tans minimally.
Skin type III: burns moderately, tans gradually.
Skin type IV: burns minimally, tans readily.
Skin type V: rarely burns, tans profusely, and occurs in heavily pigmented individuals such as darker Mediterraneans, Mongolians, and Indians.
Skin type VI: never burns, darkly pigments, and occurs in blacks.

People with type I and II skin often have light skin color and blue eyes, may have red scalp hair, and may or may not have freckling. However, some persons with darker hair and blue or green eyes have type I and II sun reactions. People with type I and II skin will exceed their sunburn threshold tolerance in 10 to 20 minutes of noontime temperate summer sunlight. Three to eight times the minimal erythema dose (MED) will produce a moderate to severe burn.

A number of genetic (e.g., xeroderma pigmentosum), metabolic (e.g., pellagra and porphyria cutanea tarda), neoplastic (e.g., actinic keratosis, basal cell carcinoma), connective-tissue (e.g., lupus erythematosus), immunologic (e.g., solar urticaria, drug photoallergy), and idiopathic (e.g., hydroa aestivale, polymorphous light eruption) diseases may be caused or exacerbated by light exposure. In a large study that evaluated patients with photosensitive disorders, 26% had polymorphous light eruption, 17% had chronic actinic dermatitis, 8% had photoallergic contact dermatitis, 7% had systemic phototoxicity to therapeutic agents, and 4% had solar urticaria. The most frequent allergic agents were fragrances, sunscreens, and antimicrobial agents (9).

Evidence is increasing that UVL is responsible for the development of at least 10% of all cataracts and macular degeneration. Pingueculae and pterygium appear on the conjunctival surface of the eye and are more prevalent in geographic areas close to the equator. The lower eyelid, the most anatomically exposed area of the eye, is at risk for both melanoma and nonmelanoma skin cancers.

 ## ULTRAVIOLET INDEX

The UV Index is a program that informs the public about the amount of harmful UVL reaching the earth on a particular day and is a recognized part of the weather report in many cities. The SunWise program, which lists the UV Index and has developed programs for the education of the public, notably children, can be accessed on the Environmental Protection Agency (EPA) web site at www.epa.gov. The National Meteorological Center determines the index daily; a recommendation for fair-skinned individuals who burn easily and tan minimally is as follows:

1. 0 to 2: Minimal. One hour of unprotected exposure may produce UV damage in people with sun-sensitive skin.
2. 3 to 4: Low. Sunburn may occur within 30 to 60 minutes of unprotected exposure.
3. 5 to 6: Moderate. Significant risk of skin damage and sunburn in only 20 to 30 minutes of unprotected exposure.
4. 7 to 9: High. Unprotected skin may burn in 10 to 20 minutes.
5. 10 to 15: Very high. Burning will occur in <10 minutes without protection.

 ## INDOOR TANNING

The use of indoor tanning beds in the United States is a $2 billion per year industry. Dermatologists and others have expressed concern with the lack of regulation of this industry. The sunlamps (usually UVA wavelengths) in these tanning units emit 26 times more damaging UVL than the equivalent amount of sunlight. This dose can produce erythema and melanogenesis but does not provide the protection of a naturally occurring tan, because there is no thickening of the stratum corneum and the pigmentation is restricted to the basal layer.

The major concern regarding tanning beds is the carcinogenic effect of multiple doses of UVL. One systematic review of the current literature found a significantly increased risk of cutaneous melanoma subsequent to sunbed/sunlamp exposure (10). Also, a recent study evaluated the link between keratinocyte carcinomas and sunlamp usage, finding that the use of tanning devices may contribute to the incidence of nonmelanoma skin cancers (11). Additionally, polymorphous light eruption occurs in 10% to 13% of patrons. Other concerns are exacerbation of systemic lupus erythematosus, porphyria, and rosacea and the induction of phototoxic and photoallergic reactions (12).

Solar UV radiation and exposures to sun lamps and sunbeds are now listed as known human carcinogens. All sun-tanning products must now contain a package warning that says: "This product does not contain a sunscreen and does not protect against sunburn. Repeated exposure of unprotected skin while tanning may increase the risk of skin aging, skin cancer, and other harmful effects to the skin even if you do not burn."

 ## REACTIONS TO EXCESS ULTRAVIOLET EXPOSURE

I. SUBJECTIVE DATA
A. A mild sunburn will be tender to the touch and cause a hot, taut, drawn feeling. Symptoms usually peak in 16 to 24 hours.
B. Severe burns are accompanied by intense pain, inability to tolerate contact with clothing and sheets, and constitutional symptoms, including nausea, tachycardia, chills, and fever. This constellation of symptoms is what the lay public calls "sun poisoning."

II. OBJECTIVE DATA

A. The earliest sign of a burn is a pink to scarlet hue of the skin and mild edema. The more severe the burn, the earlier it will be evident. Sun exposure will cause immediate erythema, which then fades. A delayed erythema appears in 2 to 4 hours, peaks at 14 to 20 hours, and lasts 24 to 72 hours.

B. This burn may progress to a vivid erythema, intense edema, and blistering.

C. Peeling follows as a consequence of increased epidermal turnover during the repair response, usually a week or more after the burn.

D. Hyperpigmentation is seen because of UVB-induced new pigment formation and offers some protection against further sunburn. This is evident as immediate pigment darkening of preformed melanin (2 to 24 hours) and delayed tanning, reflective of new pigment formation (4 to 7 days).

E. UVA reactions follow a slower time course; erythema becomes evident as late as 48 hours, and the reaction may become more severe for several days.

F. UVC reactions are seldom severe; overexposure to short-wave UVL rarely leads to blistering but can lead to conjunctivitis and keratitis.

III. ASSESSMENT.
The patient's history will usually be adequate to explain the clinical picture. It is important to be certain that there are no predisposing or underlying factors (drug administration, topical application of photosensitizers, or systemic illnesses such as lupus or porphyria).

IV. THERAPY

MILD SUNBURN

1. Apply cool tap water or Burow's solution compresses for 20 minutes three to four times a day or more frequently.

2. A topical corticosteroid spray, lotion, cream, or gel may reduce inflammation and pain.

3. Use emollients (Eucerin, Lubriderm, Nivea, petrolatum) to soothe and relieve dryness.

4. Most proprietary over-the-counter (OTC) burn remedies contain local anesthetics (benzocaine, dibucaine, or lidocaine), antiseptics, emollients, and fragrant materials. There is little need for any of these ingredients in the care of a sunburn, and only 20% benzocaine (Americaine) has been demonstrated to be effective. The vehicles of "anesthetic" sprays, creams, and lotions may be cooling and the ointments lubricating, thereby lessening the symptoms, but this must be weighed against the hazard of becoming sensitized, especially to benzocaine. Because burns are intrinsically self-healing, it is mandatory that the therapy be less noxious than the problem.

5. Aspirin, indomethacin, and ibuprofen in usual doses can help relieve the discomfort.

SEVERE SUNBURN

1. Patients should call immediately if they are overexposed to sunlamps or to sunlight, because it is easier and more effective to abort severe inflammation than to treat an already established reaction. A short course of systemic corticosteroids may reduce potentially severe sunburn; prednisone 40 to 60 mg or its equivalent should be administered daily for 3 days and then discontinued. Some studies have been unable to confirm that prednisone suppresses sunburn, but the clinical impression still remains that it may often be useful.

2. Topical care of established severe sunburns entails almost continuous cool compresses, topical steroids and emollients, a cradle for bed linens, analgesics as needed, and careful surveillance for bacterial superinfection. Application of a class I topical steroid b.i.d. for 3 days within 48 hours of the burn can provide symptomatic relief but does not repair damage to the skin. Topical 5% indomethacin in combination with the class I steroid can provide additional benefit.

3. Some fair-skinned individuals may increase their tolerance of UVL through systemic administration of psoralen compounds. These drugs will increase the capacity of the skin to produce melanin after sun exposure and will also result in retention of melanin granules in a thickened stratum corneum. Two hours before sun exposure, trioxsalen (Trisoralen) 30 mg should be taken, and exposure during the first week should be increased gradually. Use of this medication without subsequent exposure to light will be ineffective.

PHOTOPROTECTION

Sunscreen has been shown to prevent ultraviolet-induced DNA damage, cutaneous immunosuppression, and the generation of T suppressor cells. Application of sunscreens does decrease the risk for development of nonmelanoma skin cancers and actinic keratoses; its effect on the prevention or development of melanoma is controversial.

Sun-protective topical medications are available as sunscreens, which contain multiple chemical substances and physical blockers. Chemical sunscreens, more recently termed **organic** by the U.S. Food and Drug Administration (FDA), block the penetration of UV radiation by acting as filters and by absorbing and reflecting UVL. The physical or nonchemical sunscreens scatter or reflect UV radiation. Most sunscreens are good protective agents against UVB and short-wave UVA; however, complete protection against long-wave UVA has not yet been achieved (13).

In 1997, Congress requested the FDA to create new regulations and recommendations on the prevention and treatment of sunburn. The result was the most recent FDA monograph of sunscreens containing requirements for formulation and simplified labeling (14). This new monograph listed 16 ingredients that companies can use in sunscreen products (see subsequent text). Other changes included labeling any sunscreen greater than a sun protection factor (SPF) of 30 with an "SPF 30 plus." The terms "waterproof" and "all-day protection" were dropped, replacing them with "water resistant" and "very water resistant."

SUNSCREEN ULTRAVIOLET LIGHT ABSORPTION

Most sunscreens have their peak absorption in the UVB range between 290 and 320 nm. Of the commonly used sunscreen agents, only the benzophenones and anthranilates have substantial absorption in the UVA range, from 320 to 400 nm. Newer sunscreens with padimate O and Parsol 1789 provide some increased UVA absorption but less UVB photoprotection. Parsol 1789 is a chemical with a major absorption peak at 360 nm, in the UVA range. Many photosensitizing drugs are activated at 360 nm.

SPECIFIC AGENTS

Product	Percent (%)	Absorbance
Aminobenzoic acid	Up to 15	UVB
Avobenzone	2 to 3	UVAI
Cinoxate	Up to 3	UVB
Dioxybenzone	Up to 3	UVB, UVAII
Ensulizole	Up to 4	UVB
Homosalate	Up to 15	UVB
Meradimate	Up to 5	UVAII
Octocrylene	Up to 10	UVB
Octinoxate	Up to 7.5	UVB
Octisalate	Up to 5	UVB
Oxybenzone	Up to 6	UVB, UVAII
Padimate O	Up to 8	UVB
Sulisobenzone	Up to 10	UVB, UVAII
Titanium dioxide	2 to 25	Physical
Trolamine salicylate	Up to 12	UVB
Zinc oxide	2 to 20	Physical

Physical blockers or "chemical-free" sunscreens contain small particles that scatter, reflect, or absorb in the UV and visible range. Because some of the energy is absorbed, secondary oxygen radicals can be formed. Coating the particles with silicone absorbs these free radicals and is the basis of a product called **Z-cote**. The physical blockers include the following:

a. Zinc oxide
b. Titanium dioxide
c. Iron oxide
d. Kaolin

 SUN PROTECTION FACTOR

The SPF value is defined as the dose of UVR required to produce one MED on protected skin after the application of 2 mg/cm^2 of product divided by the UVR required to produce one MED on unprotected skin. The SPF usually ranges from 2 (minimal protection) to 30+ (highest protection). SPF 2 gives 50% protection, SPF 15 produces 93% protection, and SPF 34 gives 97% protection. Some have recommended that SPF be changed to Sunburn Protection Factor, because it is a misconception that application of sunscreen will offer protection against sun-induced skin damage. The use of higher SPF sunscreens appears to increase the duration of recreational sun exposure, giving these individuals a false sense of security.

Although the general public is starting to wear sunscreen on a daily basis, studies have shown that they do not use sunscreen correctly. If a patient uses only half of the recommended amount of sunscreen, the SPF can be reduced by as much as a power of two (therefore, an SPF 15 would become an SPF 4 and an SPF 30 would become an SPF 8). The use of a higher SPF can partially compensate for underapplication. For a sunscreen to be effective, a layer of 0.5 mm should be applied. This is about a quarter of most standard-sized bottles of sunscreen when applied to the entire body. Reapplication every 20 to 90 minutes is necessary to keep most sunscreens effective, depending on the formulation and the activity level of the person (15). The American Academy of Dermatology recommends, regardless of skin type, a broad-spectrum sunscreen with an SPF of at least 15 to be worn year round.

Water-resistant labeling indicates that the SPF is maintained after two 20-minute immersions in water. Very water-resistant labeling can be used if the SPF is maintained after four 20-minute immersions. Therefore, neither of these labels translates into protection that can last for the entire afternoon at the pool with one application.

 ULTRAVIOLET PROTECTION FACTOR

The protection achieved by wearing fabrics is expressed as the "Ultraviolet Protection Factor" (UPF), which was coined in Australia in 1996 (16). Depending on material, stitch, color, moisture content, and chemical additives, clothing can provide a range of protection. Fabrics with tighter weaves, darker colors, synthetic fibers, and loose fit typically provide the greatest protection. Materials that are light in color, loosely woven, natural fibers, or material stretched tightly over the skin provide the least protection. When clothing becomes wet, it usually results in a reduction, but may result in an increase in SPF, depending on the particular fabric (17). For these reasons, clothing is usually overestimated in its protectiveness, and in one study it was estimated that 33% of summer clothing had a UPF <15, compared with the recommended UPF of >30 (18).

 METHOD OF USE

The term substantivity refers to a product's ability to remain effective under the stress of prolonged exercise, sweating, and swimming. Para-aminobenzoic acid (PABA) esters may be more effective than PABA in ethanol, and cream-based vehicles may, in some cases, be more resistant to removal than those in alcohol bases. Whatever product is used, it should be applied 15 to 30 minutes before exposure and reapplied generously several times during exposure, particularly after swimming or sweating. Application of sunscreen is variable, with one study showing that 60% of people missed an application to the posterior neck, 35% skipped the anterior neck, and 32% did not cover the ears. The average person applies only one-half or less of the recommended amount of sunscreen.

 VEHICLE

a. Lotions have low viscosity, spread easily, and are nongreasy. Lotions usually contain an SPF of 15 or less.
b. The products with a higher SPF have more sunscreen oil and have a heavier, greasy consistency. The addition of silicone liquids has decreased the greasiness and increased the water-resistant nature of the high SPF sunscreens.
c. Men, acne-prone patients, and individuals with oily skin prefer oil-free gels. Water-based gels are ideal for individuals who plan on exercising, but can only incorporate water-soluble sunscreens, therefore limiting the SPF. Hydroalcoholic gels can achieve a higher SPF, but none of these products are waterproof. It is sometimes more difficult to obtain uniform application of gel sunscreens compared with lotions.
d. Dry lotions (anhydrous) are for athletes who experience eye stinging.
e. Sticks contain lipid-soluble sunscreens and are effective for protection of limited areas such as the nose, under the eyes, and the ears. These products are the most water resistant and can be helpful in applying sunscreen to critical areas of the face in uncooperative children. They are too occlusive for general application.
f. Aerosols and sprays are a new delivery system, but problems with skip areas and uneven distribution of product decrease their level of protection.
g. Nonchemical or physical blockers and sun-protective clothing are suitable for patients with sensitive skin, individuals who are intolerant to sunscreens, and babies <6 months old.

 ADVERSE EFFECTS

PABA may stain clothing yellow, especially after exposure to the sun. Contact dermatitis develops occasionally from the use of PABA, PABA esters, benzophenones, and cinnamates; glyceryl PABA is the most common cause. Although rarely reported, allergy to a component of the sunscreen vehicle may certainly occur. Patients allergic to benzocaine, procaine, paraphenylenediamine, and sulfonamides may have allergic reactions to PABA.

GENERAL GUIDELINES FOR SUNSCREEN USE

a. Select a sunscreen with SPF 15 to 30 that has both UVA and UVB protection.
b. Apply sunscreen 15 to 30 minutes before exposure and allow to dry; reapply every 1 to 2 hours during outdoor activities.
c. Select a water-resistant sunscreen for beach or outdoor activities associated with per-spiring.
d. Reapply sunscreen after swimming or exercising.
e. All children should be protected from excessive sun exposure through avoidance of midday sun and use of sun-protective clothing and sunscreens.
f. Children <6 months of age should have sunscreen applied to the exposed areas; titanium dioxide–containing sunscreens are safe and are less likely to irritate the skin. Sun-protective clothing and avoidance are strongly recommended in this age-group.
g. To minimize eye stinging, use a sport gel formula and avoid the benzophenones.
h. For maximum eye protection, pick wrap-around sunglasses that fit close to the forehead and absorb up to 400 nm in the UVA, UVB, and blue light range. Polarizing lenses help cut the glare from reflective surfaces but do not add UV blocking properties. The Skin Cancer Foundation has a Seal of Recommendation for sunglasses that meet its criteria to block 99% of UVA and UVB.
i. Lipstick sunscreens are generally available but often overlooked as part of a sun protection program. Frequent application is also helpful in decreasing the potential for activation of herpes labialis.

Parents and children should be educated regarding the importance of sun protection. The American Academy of Pediatrics (AAP) has determined that limited sunscreen use in infants is acceptable if no other method of sun protection is available. Adverse effects of sunscreens in infants younger than 6 months of age have not been reported. The AAP still recommends that infants be kept out of direct sunlight and that they be covered with sun-protective clothing.

It has been estimated that use of sunscreen during the first 18 years of life would reduce the incidence of nonmelanoma skin cancers by 78% over one's lifetime. Chronic use of sunscreen does alter vitamin D synthesis; a normal diet should compensate for this.

 DIHYDROACETONE

Dihydroacetone (DHA), the active ingredient in skin "tanning" or "bronzing" products, produces a brown-orange staining of the stratum corneum; there is no stimulation of melanin pigmentation. There is some photoprotection against long-wave UVA and visible light. Recently, it has been shown that DHA, in addition, offers a modest SPF in humans (19). However, self-tanning creams only offer an SPF of 3 to 4, this protection is only present for several hours after application of the product, and does not last for the duration of the tan (20). Some products now include a sunscreen with SPF 15 or higher. Most products contain a concentration of 3% to 5% DHA; higher concentrations will result in a deeper color that may look unnatural. The color fades with normal epidermal desquamation over 5 to 7 days.

a. Lightly exfoliate the skin before application.
b. Apply every 2 to 3 hours until the desired skin color is achieved.
c. Different application techniques include sprays, wipes, and application by hand.
d. Wash the hands well to prevent staining.
e. Elbows, knees, and ankles take up the chemical unevenly and require less product.
f. Freckles will take up more of the color as will hair and nails.
g. Fabrics may become stained on contact with the product before drying.
h. The lotion must be applied every 3 to 5 days to maintain the color.

 FUTURE DIRECTIONS IN SUNSCREEN DEVELOPMENT

a. Experimental studies have shown that it is possible to encapsulate endonucleases into liposomes. These enzymes recognize and repair the structural defects in the DNA induced by UVL. Topical treatment with these liposomes containing T4 endonuclease V has been found to protect human skin *in vivo* from ultraviolet-induced upregulation of interleukin-10 and tumor necrosis factor-α. Therefore, correcting ultraviolet-induced skin damage with DNA repair enzymes may provide a new avenue for photoprotection.
b. 2-Furildioxime, an iron binder chelator, is capable of decreasing the free radicals formed by UVL exposure and appears to offer some degree of photoprotection.
c. The topical application of antioxidants such as vitamin C (L-ascorbic acid) and E (α-tocopherol), caffeine, isoflavones, green tea (polyphenols), ferulic acid, caffeic acid, cadmium, and cistus has been advocated, but more studies regarding efficacy and penetration of the skin are needed (21). The two most studied of these are vitamin C and vitamin E. Studies have shown that use of these agents, both orally and topically, has significantly decreased the MED from sun exposure.
d. White particulate pigments (Ciba Specialty Products), somewhat like the physical blockers, are being adapted from the clothing industry and appear to offer a broad range of photoprotection.

References

1. Nghiem DX, Kazimi N, Clydesdale G, et al. Ultraviolet a radiation suppresses an established immune response: implications for sunscreen design. *J Invest Dermatol* 2001;117(5):1193–1199.

2. Johnson JA, Fusaro RM. Broad-spectrum photoprotection: the roles of tinted auto windows, sunscreens and browning agents in the diagnosis and treatment of photosensitivity. *Dermatology* 1992;185(4):237–241.

3. Hampton PJ, Farr PM, Diffey BL, et al. Implication for photosensitive patients of ultraviolet A exposure in vehicles. *Br J Dermatol* 2004;151(4):873–876.

4. Rigel DS, Rigel EG, Rigel AC. Effects of altitude and latitude on ambient UVB radiation. *J Am Acad Dermatol* 1999;40(1):114–116.

5. Winkler P, Trepte S. Ozone decline and UV increase. *Gesundheitswesen* 2004;66(Suppl 1):S31–S36.

6. Autier P. Skin cancers and environmental factors. *Rev Med Brux* 1998;19(4):A346–A350.

7. de Gruijl FR, Longstreth J, Norval M, et al. Health effects from stratospheric ozone depletion and interactions with climate change. *Photochem Photobiol Sci* 2003;2(1):16–28.

8. Kripke ML. Impact of ozone depletion on skin cancers. *J Dermatol Surg Oncol* 1988;14(8):853–857.

9. Fotiades J, Soter NA, Lim HW. Results of evaluation of 203 patients for photosensitivity in a 7.3-year period. *J Am Acad Dermatol* 1995;33(4):597–602.

10. Gallagher RP, Spinelli JJ, Lee TK. Tanning beds, sunlamps, and risk of cutaneous malignant melanoma. *Cancer Epidemiol Biomarkers Prev* 2005;14(3):562–566.

11. Karagas MR, Stannard VA, Mott LA, et al. Use of tanning devices and risk of basal cell and squamous cell skin cancers. *J Natl Cancer Inst* 2002;94(3):224–226.

12. Spencer JM, Amonette RA. Indoor tanning: risks, benefits, and future trends. *J Am Acad Dermatol* 1995;33(2 Pt 1):288–298.

13. Pustisek N, Lipozencic J, Ljubojevic S. A review of sunscreens and their adverse reactions. *Acta Dermatovenerol Croat* 2005;13(1):28–35.

14. Sunscreen drug products for over-the-counter human use; final monograph. Food and Drug Administration, HHS. Final rule. *Fed Regist* 1999;64(98):27666–27693.

15. Diffey BL. When should sunscreen be reapplied? *J Am Acad Dermatol* 2001;45(6):882–885.

16. Georgouras KE, Stanford DG, Pailthorpe MT. Sun protective clothing in Australia and the Australian/New Zealand standard: an overview. *Australas J Dermatol* 1997;38(Suppl 1):S79–S82.

17. Gambichler T, Hatch KL, Avermaete A, et al. Influence of wetness on the ultraviolet protection factor (UPF) of textiles: *in vitro* and *in vivo* measurements. *Photodermatol Photoimmunol Photomed* 2002;18(1):29–35.

18. Gambichler T, Rotterdam S, Altmeyer P, et al. Protection against ultraviolet radiation by commercial summer clothing: need for standardised testing and labelling. *BMC Dermatol* 2001;1(1):6.

19. Faurschou A, Wulf HC. Durability of the sun protection factor provided by dihydroxyacetone. *Photodermatol Photoimmunol Photomed* 2004;20(5):239–242.

20. Draelos ZD. Self-tanning lotions: are they a healthy way to achieve a tan? *Am J Clin Dermatol* 2002;3(5):317–318.

21. Dreher F, Maibach H. Protective effects of topical antioxidants in humans. *Curr Probl Dermatol* 2001;29:157–164.

URTICARIA

Penpun Wattanakrai

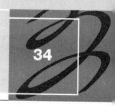

I. DEFINITION AND PATHOPHYSIOLOGY. Urticaria (hives) affects 15% to 25% of the population at some time during their lives and is more prevalent in middle-aged females (1). The same reaction taking place in deeper layers of the skin—submucosa, deep dermis, and subcutaneous and submucosal tissue—is termed **angioedema.** Angioedema may accompany urticaria but infrequently presents as angioedema alone, in which the differential diagnosis should include hereditary angioedema, acquired or paraneoplastic angioedema, idiopathic angioedema or anaphylaxis, and drug reactions especially angiotensin-converting enzyme (ACE) inhibitors or nonsteroidal antiin-flammatory drugs (NSAIDs) (2). Urticaria may be elicited by immunologic (IgE) or nonimmunologic mechanisms. The latter includes complement pathway disorders, alterations in arachidonic acid metabolism, and agents that act directly on mast cells. The resulting vasodilatation, increased vascular permeability, and extravasation of proteins and fluids seem to be mediated principally by histamine and by many other mediators such as prostaglandin D2, leukotrienes C4 and D4, platelet-activating factor, anaphylotoxins (C3a, C4a, and C5a), bradykinin, histamine-releasing factors, cytokines, and chemokines. There is also increased production of cytokines, including IL-4, IL-5, and interferon-γ (3). Although the primary effector cells in chronic urticaria are mast cells, patients with chronic urticaria do not have an increased number of mast cells (4). The inflammatory infiltrates in chronic urticaria consist of CD4+ and CD8+ T lymphocytes, eosinophils, basophils, and neutrophils (3,5). Immunoglobulin G (IgG) autoantibodies against IgE (anti-IgE) and the more common autoantibodies to the high-affinity receptor for IgE (IgG anti-FceRIa antibodies) have been described in the sera of patients with chronic urticaria. The term **autoimmune urticaria** is used to describe chronic urticaria with these functional autoantibodies that act directly on the subunit of the receptor to stimulate histamine when IgE is absent (6).

Classification of urticaria initially begins with duration and frequency of attacks. The duration of at least 6 weeks daily or nearly daily symptoms separates chronic from acute urticaria. **Acute urticaria** is most often mediated by B-lymphocyte-produced IgE and is seen in patients with anaphylaxis, serum sickness, or atopy or as a reaction to insect bites, foods, infection, or drugs. Exposure to crustaceans and ingesting NSAIDs are the most common agents to cause anaphylaxis (7). The most common foods that cause recurrent attacks of urticaria are nuts, eggs, strawberries, tomatoes, chocolate, fish, and citrus fruits. The list of infectious etiologies is long, including hepatitis B, hepatitis C, infection with *Helicobacter pylori,* gastrointestinal parasites, dermatophyte infections, sinusitis, and dental abscesses. Urticaria persisting of >6 weeks' duration, termed **chronic urticaria,** may have a multiplicity of trigger factors. Immunologic cases of chronic urticaria include reactions to drugs or, less frequently, to foods and food additives, inhalants, parasitic infestations, or Hymenoptera venom. Children have a higher incidence of acute urticaria, whereas adults, especially women, are more prone to chronic urticaria. In one retrospective study of urticaria and angioedema, 49% had both lesions, 40% had urticaria alone, and 11% had angioedema alone. The mean duration of urticaria alone is 6 months, that of angioedema alone is 1 year, and that of urticaria with angioedema is approximately 5 years. Fifty percent of patients with chronic urticaria will be in remission after 1 year; 20% of patients will have urticaria for years. The two largest subgroups of chronic urticaria are physical urticaria and autoimmune urticaria.

Physical urticarias are hives that are produced in response to a specific external physical agent (8). This subgroup is responsible for approximately 20% to 30% of

221

patients with chronic urticaria. They tend to be more persistent and less responsive to treatment than idiopathic chronic urticarias.

A. **Dermatographism or dermatographic lesions** are hives induced by trauma (stroking, scratching) or pressure (standing, tight clothing) and are present in up to 9% of the general population. Although everyone will respond to cutaneous trauma with a triple response of Lewis (erythema, flare, and wheal), in dermatographism, the response, even to minor stimuli, is excessive.

B. **Cholinergic urticaria** is a common disorder induced by an increase in body temperature and is mediated by acetylcholine, not histamine. This condition may also be caused by a neural mast cell trigger (9). The clinical presentation is distinctive with diffuse erythema and monomorphic urticarial lesions, which are usually smaller than typical urticaria. The trigger is believed to be related to the cholinergic innervations associated with the sweating reflex. It can be triggered by heat, exercise, change in temperature, and overheating even in the absence of exertion such as by spicy foods or extreme emotion (10). It has also been hypothesized that these patients have a type I allergy to their own sweat (11).

C. **Cold urticaria** is caused by immersion in cold water or exposure to cold air with lesions appearing as the skin begins to rewarm. This disorder may be due to an IgE cryoglobulin or a cold-induced skin antigen (12). Confirmatory testing for cold urticaria can be done with the cold contact stimulation test in which a cold stimulus of 0 to 4°C, such as an ice cube, can induce urticaria or angioedema after applied to the skin for several minutes.

D. **Contact urticaria** occurs after direct contact of a chemical with the skin; the mechanism may be immunologic (e.g., drug, cosmetics, natural latex rubber) or nonimmunologic (animals—caterpillars, jelly fish sting; plants—nettles; and chemicals).

E. **Pressure urticaria** is delayed dermatographism in which lesions appear 30 minutes to several hours after pressure (especially if deep and prolonged) is applied on the skin. This type of physical urticaria is uncommon and is less pruritic but more painful and prolonged. Malaise, fever, chills, and headache may also be observed, and 60% of patients have chronic idiopathic urticaria or angioedema. The diagnosis may be confirmed by hanging a weight over an arm or leg using an unpadded strap, such as hanging a 15-lb weight for 15 minutes (13).

F. **Aquagenic urticaria** is a rare water-induced urticaria. Small papules resembling the micropapular hives of cholinergic urticaria occur usually within minutes of exposure to water.

G. **Solar urticaria** a rare photosensitive disorder, produces urticarial lesions provoked minutes after sunlight exposure and disappears rapidly after sun avoidance. It is most common in young adults; females are more often affected. Phototesting is required to make the diagnosis with testing against ultraviolet A (UVA), UVB, and visible light to determine the precise action spectrum. Antihistamines, broad-spectrum sunscreens, and graded exposure to increasing amounts of light or psoralens plus ultraviolet A (PUVA) desensitization are effective treatments.

H. **Autoimmune urticarias.** At least 30% to 40% of patients with unexplained (idiopathic) chronic urticaria have clinically relevant functional autoantibodies to the high-affinity IgE receptor (FceRIa) on basophils and mast cells and, less commonly, approximately 10% have anti-IgE (14). This subgroup of patients with chronic urticaria present with highly symptomatic, severe continuous urticaria associated with systemic symptoms but without any other known cause or physical triggers.

I. **Hereditary angioedema** is a dominantly inherited disorder in which a normal serum inhibitor of the activated first component of complement C1 esterase inhibitor (C1INH) is either deficient or nonfunctional. Eighty percent of these patients will have a positive family history, and the symptoms most characteristically appear in late childhood or early adolescence. There are two types. Type I is the most common and is characterized by an insufficient production of C1INH. This affects 85% of all patients with hereditary angioedema. Patients with type 2 have normal or elevated concentrations of C1INH but the protein is functionally deficient. These patients suffer recurrent episodes of cutaneous angioedema as well as attacks of laryngeal edema and gastrointestinal involvement. Typical pruritic urticarial lesions are not seen in hereditary angioedema. Acquired C1INH deficiency is seen with lymphoproliferative and autoimmune diseases.

J. Drug-induced urticaria. As many as 5% to 8% of patients exposed to radiocontrast media (especially high-osmolar or ionic agents) or other pharmacologic mediators such as acetylcholine, opiates, curare, and certain antibiotics (notably polymyxin B, vancomycin), which directly release histamine from mast cells and basophils, will experience urticaria. Approximately 1% of individuals experience urticarial or anaphylactic reactions to aspirin. Patients with chronic urticaria related to aspirin may lose their sensitivity over time (15). Aspirin-intolerant patients also react to other nonsteroidal antiinflammatory agents such as indomethacin and ibuprofen. Up to 15% to 20% of such patients react to the ubiquitous azo dyes, notably tartrazine (U.S. Food and Drug Administration [FDA] yellow dye no. 5), and some may also be sensitive to benzoate preservatives. Although aspirin intolerance may be found in 20% to 50% of patients with chronic urticaria, it has been shown that tartrazine intolerance may be present only when the urticaria, regardless of its original cause, is in an active phase. These agents cause urticaria by altering the arachidonic acid metabolism.

K. Other types of urticaria. Acute urticaria in children <3 years of age is usually related to an underlying infection, such as benign viral illness, and antibiotic therapy or food origin. Angioedema and a cutaneous hemorrhagic pattern may be observed. Thirty percent of these children are at risk for chronic or recurrent disease (16).

Urticaria may accompany infections, collagen-vascular disease, autoimmune thyroid diseases, and malignancies. Viral infections (hepatitis B prodromal phase reaction, infectious mononucleosis, coxsackie) are believed to be a relatively common cause of urticaria. Chronic urticaria has been associated with chronic parasitic infections, chronic bacterial infections (such as sinus, dental, chest, gall bladder, urinary tract, and other infections, including *Helicobacter pylori* gastric infection, onychomycosis, and tinea pedis), and many others, although proof of these associations is lacking and these may be merely coexistent. Hives with arthralgias or arthritis may be an early sign of anicteric hepatitis or a manifestation of an underlying necrotizing vasculitis. An association between thyroid autoimmunity and chronic urticaria was first reported by Leznoff (17) and has recently been reviewed by Rumbyrt and Schocket (18), with most patients being clinically and biochemically euthyroid. ACE inhibitors and angiotensin II antagonists may cause angioedema in 1% of patients. The onset of angioedema usually occurs within hours to 1 week of starting therapy, although the angioedema may occur suddenly even after a long duration of therapy (19).

II. SUBJECTIVE DATA. Intense pruritus is the typical symptom of urticaria. Stinging and prickling sensations are also described. Pruritus is milder in angioedema because the edema occurs in deeper areas where there are fewer sensory nerve endings.

III. OBJECTIVE DATA

A. Urticarial wheals are raised, erythematous, and edematous plaques with sharply defined, serpiginous, or polycyclic borders surrounded by an erythematous halo. Intensely edematous lesions will have a blanched center. Their diameters may range from millimeters to several centimeters. Individual lesions last up to 8 to 12 hours. The clinician must entertain alternate diagnosis such as erythema multiforme or urticarial vasculitis (urticaria perstans) for lesions persisting in one location for >24 hours. The continuous spectrum of urticarial lesions, ranging from the evanescent wheal of true urticaria to the relatively fixed edema of erythema multiforme, makes precise diagnosis difficult at times.

B. Angioedema has thick, edematous plaques usually involving the face, not associated with pruritus but rather with pain and/or burning. The edema may last as long as 48 to 72 hours. Gastrointestinal or laryngeal signs may accompany the hereditary form of angioedema.

C. The lesions of cholinergic urticaria are small, monomorphic 1- to 3-mm, punctate, papular wheals (called **pencil–eraser** lesions) surrounded by a large macular erythematous flare, usually appearing on the neck and trunk, although they may spread distally. They disappear spontaneously in 30 to 60 minutes.

D. Cold urticaria may be familial or acquired. Associated symptoms include fever, arthralgias, and a leukocytosis. One third of patients have cryoproteins. Patients can develop localized or generalized pruritic urticarial wheals or angioedema. The cutaneous wheals are typically non-pseudopodic and conform to the shape of the cold stimuli.

E. Urticarial vasculitis is characterized by painful (more than pruritic), burning urticarial papules/plaques that typically last longer than 24 hours. Postinflammatory hyperpigmentation or purpura may be noted. The patient should be evaluated for signs of systemic vasculitis. One third of patients have low complement levels.

IV. ASSESSMENT. A detailed, perceptive history and thorough physical examination will often reveal the cause, physical triggers, and type of urticaria (20). It is crucial to identify all medications that are taken intermittently or regularly, including prescription, over-the-counter, oral, topical, vitamins, supplements, and herbal medications. Particular concern should be focused on the use of aspirin, NSAIDs including cyclooxygenase 2 (COX-2)-selective agents, ACE inhibitors, ACE receptor blockers, β-blockers (antihypertensive, eye drops for glaucoma) and opiate analgesics. Additionally, all products that are topically applied or contact the skin should be questioned as being possible contact or airborne allergens. After a careful and detailed history and thorough physical examination, specific lab tests and studies should be performed as specifically indicated and directed by abnormal signs and symptoms. If the history and examination is not rewarding, then other types of investigations, although usually unproductive, must nevertheless be pursued in patients with chronic urticaria, especially if persistent or difficult to control with antihistamine therapy. Pertinent tests would include a complete blood count (CBC) and differential, erythrocyte sedimentation rate (ESR), urinalysis, and liver function tests. Leukocytosis suggests chronic infection. Total eosinophil counts may implicate causes such as drugs, food, parasites, or atopy. Consider screening thyroid function tests and tests for thyroid autoimmunity (thyroid microsomal and thyroglobulin antibody titers), especially in women or in patients with a family history of thyroid disease or other autoimmune diseases. Complement (C3 and CH50) and antinuclear antibody (ANA) levels should be tested if there is suspicion of collagen-vascular disease or necrotizing vasculitis. Analysis of serum for cryoproteins or hepatitis-associated antigens and antibodies may permit specific diagnosis. Assessment of complement components C1, C4, and C1 esterase inhibitor level and functional assay may prove diagnostic for forms of C1INH deficiency. X-rays of the chest, sinuses, or teeth may be indicated in some patients with chronic urticaria. Occasionally, food diaries and a brief trial of a rigid food elimination diet are warranted, and examination of fresh stool for ova and parasites is undertaken. Skin biopsy with immunofluorescence studies of chronic urticaria lesions is indicated and will occasionally show perivascular inflammatory changes suggestive of lupus erythematosus or vasculitis. The predominant type of cellular infiltrates in the biopsy specimen may also help suggest further therapeutic approach if treatment with antihistamines alone is inadequate. Predominance of neutrophils may suggest a trial of agents such as hydroxychloroquine, sulfasalazine, or dapsone (21), whereas patients with a predominance of eosinophils may respond better to steroids (22). Skin testing is rarely of value. Dermatographism can be evaluated by firmly stroking the skin with a tongue blade or similar blunt surface. Total IgE and basophil count may implicate autoimmune urticaria. Although research centers have used immunoassays to screen sera for anti-FceRI and *in vitro* functional histamine-release assays on basophils and cutaneous mast cells to diagnose autoimmune urticaria, the simplest test for diagnosis of autoimmune urticaria is the whealing response to intradermal injection with autologous serum, known as the **autologous serum skin test (ASST)** (23).

V. THERAPY

A. Anaphylactic and acute urticarial reactions. See therapy outline in Chap. 5.

B. Chronic urticaria

    1. Identification and treatment or removal of the trigger factor is the most important and only effective long-term therapy.

a. Avoid exposures that aggravate urticaria, including overheating, stress, exposure to alcohol, opiates, NSAIDs, aspirin, and ACE inhibitors with angioedema.

b. Avoidance of food allergens such as food additives, salicylates, and as-yet-unidentified aromatic substances in tomato, white wine, and herbs may improve the condition of patients with chronic idiopathic urticaria.

2. **Local measures**

a. Cool or ice water compresses or tepid baths with colloidal oatmeal (Aveeno) may eliminate itching. Obviously, this procedure is contraindicated in cold urticaria.

b. Antipruritic lotions or emulsions may help: 0.25% menthol with or without 1% phenol in calamine lotion or petrolatum-based emollient cream (Eucerin), cooling lotions that contain menthol (Sarna lotion) and topical pramoxine and benzyl alcohol lotions (Itch-X).

3. **Systemic measures**

a. Antihistamine therapy with H1 antagonists is the therapy of choice. Hydroxyzine (Atarax, Vistaril) is often the best drug for chronic urticaria and is particularly preferred for symptomatic dermographism and cholinergic urticaria. It may be used alone or with other antihistamines, and dosage should be pushed to the limit of tolerance or to subsidence of symptoms. If hydroxyzine is ineffective, chlorpheniramine maleate (Chlor-Trimeton) or cyproheptadine hydrochloride (Periactin) should be used next, either alone or in combination. Diphenhydramine (Benadryl) may be slightly more sedating than hydroxyzine and requires t.i.d. to q.i.d. dosing. Both hydroxyzine and diphenhydramine can have a paradoxical effect in children, with central nervous stimulation rather than sedation.

Second-generation H_1 antihistamines are less sedating because of their decreased penetration of the blood–brain barrier and provide a 24-hour H_1 histamine receptor blockade. Fexofenadine (Allegra) 60 mg b.i.d. and single dose of 180 mg daily, cetirizine (Zyrtec) 10 mg q.d., and loratadine (Claritin) 10 mg q.d. are currently available. Higher doses than those suggested by the manufacturers may be required to control symptoms of urticaria.

Cetirizine is a metabolite of the first-generation H_1 antihistamine hydroxyzine. A reduced dosage (5 mg daily) is recommended in patients with chronic renal or hepatic impairment. Sedative side effects increase with dosages of cetirizine >10 mg per day.

Terfenadine and astemizole were withdrawn from the market because of drug–drug interactions and cardiac side effects. Loratadine and cetirizine have not been shown to alter cardiac repolarization described with other nonsedating antihistamines. Both have no significant drug interactions. A reduced dosage of loratadine may be required in patients with chronic liver or renal disease. A special form of loratadine (RediTabs) 10 mg rapidly disintegrates in the mouth.

Desloratadine (Clarinex) is an active metabolite of loratadine. A 5 mg daily dose has been shown to be effective. There is no evidence that it offers any advantage over loratadine.

Fexofenadine (like its parent compound terfenadine) may rarely promote cardiac arrhythmias (24). No significant difference in efficacy has been noted in the nonsedating H_1 blockers. Combinations of nonsedating antihistamines in the morning and sedating antihistamines in the evening may be more cost effective than increasing doses of the nonsedating agent.

b. **Doxepin** (Sinequan, Adapin) is a tricyclic antidepressant with potent H_1 and H_2 antagonistic effects. It also has antimuscarinic, antiserotonic, and anti-α-adrenergic activity. Use of 10 to 50 mg PO t.i.d. to q.i.d. has been shown to be effective in the treatment of primary acquired, chronic idiopathic urticaria, idiopathic cold urticaria, and for patients with anxiety or depression associated with their urticaria. Sedation and dry mouth are the most common side effects. Doxepin may interact with other drugs that are metabolized by the cytochrome P-450 system (ketoconazole, itraconazole, erythromycin, clarithromycin, etc.).

c. Because approximately 15% of histamine receptors in the skin are H_2 subtype, the combined use of an H_1 antihistamine and an H_2 antihistamine (e.g., cimetidine [Tagamet] 400 to 800 mg PO b.i.d., ranitidine [Zantac] 150 to 300 mg PO b.i.d., famotidine [Pepcid] 20 to 40 mg PO b.i.d.) may be superior to an H_1 antihistamine alone in some patients with symptomatic dermatographism, cold urticaria, or chronic urticaria. The coadministration of cimetidine and hydroxyzine significantly increased serum hydroxyzine levels with enhanced suppression of the wheal and flare reaction (25). Cimetidine may aggravate urticaria if given without an H_1 antihistamine. Compared with cimetidine, ranitidine is more potent and lacks interference with hepatic microsomal enzymes and androgen receptors.

d. Cyproheptadine (Periactin) also may be more effective than other antihistamines in the treatment of cold urticaria; the dosage is 4 mg PO t.i.d. to q.i.d.

e. Cromolyn sodium (Intal) may be considered in refractory cases of chronic urticaria. Cromolyn is administered by means of an oral nebulizer, the initial adult dosage being 1 ampoule (20 mg) q.i.d.

f. It is rarely necessary or justified to use systemic corticosteroids. However, in some refractory cases, when all diagnostic and therapeutic methods have been exhausted, a 2-week course of corticosteroids (starting at 40 to 60 mg prednisone or equivalent) will temporarily suppress the disease. Occasionally, after this treatment, the urticaria will not recur.

g. Corticosteroids are usually necessary to control urticarial vasculitis, even when not associated with another autoimmune disease. Colchicine (0.6 mg PO b.i.d. to t.i.d.) and Dapsone (up to 200 mg/day) have also been helpful in refractory cases of urticarial vasculitis.

Other medications reported to be effective are indomethacin (25 mg three times daily to 50 mg four times daily), low-dose oral methotrexate, and antimalarial drugs.

h. Prophylaxis with anabolic steroids prevents spontaneous attacks of hereditary angioedema in those patients with low levels of C1INH (26). The best drugs for prophylaxis are the attenuated androgens danazol (200 to 600 mg/day) and stanozolol (2 mg/day) (27). They need to be taken for 5 days before they become effective and are not given to pregnant women and prepubertal patients.

i. Infusions of C1INH concentrate restored normal functioning levels of C1INH and C4 in hereditary angioedema (28).

j. Low-dose cyclosporine in doses of 3 mg/kg/day can be an effective treatment for chronic idiopathic urticaria, especially as a steroid-sparing agent (29). A double-blinded, placebo-controlled trial has shown cyclosporine A to have activity in patients with anti-FceRI autoantibodies (29).

k. Ketotifen (not available in the United States) has been shown to inhibit mast cell mediators in urticaria.

l. Plasmapheresis has been effective in some cases of severe, unremitting chronic urticaria. Histamine-releasing autoantibodies have been identified in a subgroup of patients with chronic urticaria. High-dose intravenous immunoglobulin is an expensive therapeutic option in patients with recalcitrant chronic urticaria associated with histamine-releasing antibodies (30).

m. The use of many other immunosuppressive agents in the treatment of urticaria including tacrolimus, azathioprine, cyclophosphamide, mycophenolate mofetil, and intravenous immunoglobulin, interferon a (IFN-a) has been reported.

n. Thyroid autoimmunity and elevated antithyroid antibodies in euthyroid may play a role in chronic urticaria. Resolution of urticaria has been described with the use of oral thyroxine (31), although more double-blinded, placebo-controlled trials are needed to clarify which patients will respond to thyroxine. In patients with documented thyroid autoimmunity who have been unresponsive to standard therapy for chronic urticaria and/or angioedema, consider the use of levothyroxine if the patient is hypothyroid or euthyroid while monitoring the thyroid-stimulating hormone level.

o. Antileukotriene medications such as zileuton (Zyflo), a 5-lipooxygenase inhibitor, zafirlukast (Accolate 10 mg, 20 mg) and montelukast (Singulair 10 mg/day), both leukotriene receptor antagonists, have been used off-label for chronic urticaria especially in combination with antihistamines (32).

References

1. Dibbern DA, Dreskin SC. Urticaria and angioedema: an overview. *Immunol Allergy Clin North Am* 2004;24:141–162.
2. Frigas E, Nzeako UC. Angioedema: pathogenesis, differential diagnosis and treatment. *Clin Rev Allergy Immunol* 2002;23:217–231.
3. Ying S, Kikuchi Y, Meng Q, et al. TH1/TH2 cytokines and inflammatory cells in skin biopsy specimens from patients with chronic idiopathic urticaria: comparison with the allergen-induced late-phase cutaneous reaction. *J Allergy Clin Immunol* 2002;109:694–700.
4. Smith CH, Kepley C, Schwartz LB, et al. Mast cell number and phenotype in chronic idiopathic urticaria. *J Allergy Clin Immunol* 1995;96:360–364.
5. Sabroe RA, Poon E, Orchard GE, et al. Cutaneous inflammatory cell infiltrate in chronic idiopathic urticaria: comparison of patients with and without anti-FceRI or anti-IgE autoantibodies. *J Allergy Clin Immunol* 1999;103:484–493.
6. Hide M, Francis DM, Grattan CE, et al. Autoantibodies against the high-affinity IgE receptor as a cause of histamine release in chronic urticaria [see comments]. *N Engl J Med* 1993;328:1599–1604.
7. Kemp SF, Lockey RF, Wolf BL, et al. Anaphylaxis. A review of 266 cases. *Arch Intern Med* 1995;155:1749–1754.
8. Dice J. Physical urticarial. *Immunol Allergy Clin North Am* 2004;24:225–246.
9. Hirschmann JV, Lawlor F, English JS, et al. Cholinergic urticaria: a clinical and histologic study. *Arch Dermatol* 1987;123:462–467.
10. Beltrani VS. Urticaria and angioedema. *Dermatol Clin* 1996;14:171–198.
11. Adachi J, Aoki T, Yamatodani A. Demonstration of sweat allergy in cholinergic urticaria. *J Dermatol Sci* 1994;7:142–149.
12. Wanderer AA, Hoffman HM. The spectrum of acquired and familial cold-induced urticaria/urticaria-like syndromes. *Immunol Allergy Clin North Am* 2004;24:259–286.
13. Sussman GL, Harvey RP, Schocket AL. Delayed pressure urticaria. *J Allergy Clin Immunol* 1982;70:337–342.
14. Tong LJ, Balakrishnan G, Kochan JP, et al. Assessment of autoimmunity in patients with chronic urticaria. *J Allergy Clin Immunol* 1997;99:461–465.
15. Paul E, Geipel M, Moller R. Follow-up studies of patients with chronic urticaria and ASS intolerance [German]. *Hautarzt* 1994;45:12–14.
16. Mortureux P, Leaute-Labreze C, Legrain-Lifermann V, et al. Acute urticaria in infancy and early childhood: a prospective study. *Arch Dermatol* 1998;134:319–323.
17. Leznoff A, Josse RG, Denberg J, et al. Association of chronic urticaria and angioedema with thyroid autoimmunity. *Arch Dermatol* 1983;119:636–640.
18. Rumbyrt JS, Schocket AL. Chronic urticaria and thyroid disease. *Immunol Allergy Clin North Am* 2004;24:215–223.
19. Kaplan AP, Greaves MW. Angioedema. *J Am Acad Dermatol* 2005;53:373–388.
20. Kozel MMA, Mekkes JR, Bassuyt PM, et al. The effectiveness of a history-based diagnostic approach in chronic urticaria and angioedema. *Arch Dermatol* 1998;134:1575–1580.
21. Tharp MD. Chronic urticaria: pathophysiology ant treatment approaches. *Allergy Clin Immunol* 1996;98:S325–S330.
22. Zavadak D, Tharp MD. Chronic urticaria as a manifestation of the late phase reaction. *Immunol Allergy Clin North Am* 1995;15:745–759.
23. Grattan CEH. Autoimmune urticaria. *Immunol Allergy Clin North Am* 2004;24(174):163–181.

24. Pinto YM, van Gelder IL, Heeringam M, et al. QT lengthening and life-threatening arrhythmias associated with fexofenadine. *Lancet* 1994;27:343–346.

25. Simons FER, Sussman GL, Simons KJ. Effect of the H_2-antagonist cimetidine on the pharmacokinetics and pharmacodynamics of the H_1-antagonists hydroxyzine and cetirizine in patients with chronic urticaria. *J Allergy Clin Immunol* 1995;95:685–693.

26. Sheffer AL, Fearon DT, Austen KF. Clinical and biochemical effects of stanozolol therapy for hereditary angioedema. *J Allergy Clin Immunol* 1981;68:181–187.

27. Cicardi M, Bergamaschini L, Cugno M, et al. Long-term treatment of hereditary angioedema with attenuated androgens: a survey of a 13-year experience. *J Allergy Clin Immunol* 1991;87:768.

28. Waytes AT, Rosen FS, Frank MM. Treatment of hereditary angioedema with a vapor-heated C1 inhibitor concentrate. *N Engl J Med* 1996;334:1630–1634.

29. Grattan CE, O'Donnell BF, Francis DM, et al. Randomized double-blind study of cyclosporin in chronic 'idiopathic' urticaria. *Br J Dermatol* 2000;143:365–372.

30. O'Donnell BF, Barr RM, Black AK, et al. Intravenous immunoglobulin in autoimmune chronic urticaria. *Br J Dermatol* 1998;138:101–106.

31. Rumbyrt JS, Katz JL, Schocket AL. Resolution of chronic urticaria in patients with thyroid autoimmunity. *J Allergy Clin Immunol* 1995;96:901–905.

32. Ellis MH. Successful treatment of chronic urticaria with leukotriene antagonists. *J Allergy Clin Immunol* 1998;102:876–877.

VASCULAR TUMORS AND MALFORMATIONS

Ethel Ying

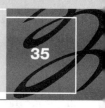

I. **DEFINITION AND PATHOPHYSIOLOGY.** Cutaneous abnormalities consisting of new vessel growths (hemangiomas) or vascular malformations and ectasias are extremely common. Vascular lesions may be most easily classified on the biologic classification described by Mullikan et al. (1).

A. **Hemangiomas**
   1. **Superficial/mixed/deep hemangiomas.** These are benign tumors of the capillary endothelium. Endothelial cell proliferation is promoted by angiogenic factors. Although considered to be a birthmark, only 1% to 3% of newborns are noted to have a lesion present at birth. Hemangiomas are characterized by a rapid proliferative phase which begins at approximately 1 to 2 months of age and continues until the infant is approximately 6 to 9 months. This is followed by the subsequent regression of the tumor. Approximately 50% of hemangiomas regress by 5 years of age and 90% by 9 years. The tumors are described on the basis of their location in the skin—superficial, mixed, and deep.

B. **Vascular malformations**
   1. **Nevus simplex/Salmon patch.** Nevus simplex is a pale red macule most commonly found on the eyelids, glabella, and the nape of the neck of infants and are present at birth. Most eyelid lesions disappear within the first year of life, whereas only half of those on the nuchal area will fade.
   2. **Nevus flammeus/Port-wine stain (PWS).** These are capillary malformations that are usually present at birth, persist, and grow in proportion with the child's growth. They can occur anywhere on the body and consist of ectatic dermal capillaries. With time, they may thicken and darken in color. Nodular lesions may also develop within them. PWSs may also be associated with other findings as in Sturge-Weber syndrome or Klippel-Trenaunay-Weber syndrome.
   3. **Venous malformations.** These result from developmental errors in vein formation and may involve the skin, subcutaneous tissues, and mucosa.

C. **Cutaneous ectasias**
   1. **Cherry angioma.** Cherry angiomas (senile angiomas) appear in early adult life and increase in number with advancing age. They are composed of mature dilated capillary vessels in the dermis with thickened walls. These asymptomatic lesions remain indefinitely.
   2. **Pyogenic granuloma.** These are believed to be caused by an abnormal healing response and are tumors composed of proliferations of endothelial tissue and contain numerous capillaries. Infection usually plays no part in the initiation or course of the lesion.
   3. **Spider angioma (nevus araneus).** Spider ectasias are seen most commonly on the face and upper trunk in women and children. Acquired lesions may appear in relation to liver disease, such as hepatitis or cirrhosis; in relation to changes in estrogen metabolism, as in pregnancy or in women on birth control pills; or as a part of hereditary hemorrhagic telangiectasia. Other causes of facial telangiectasia include actinic damage, the prolonged use of topical corticosteroids, rosacea, and postrhinoplasty "red nose" syndrome. Telangiectasias are also commonly seen on the lower extremities of women.

II. **SUBJECTIVE DATA**
   A. **Hemangiomas.** The lesions are not painful, but large lesions may erode spontaneously or become infected. Symptoms of the lesion are also dependent upon the

location of the hemangioma. Lesions at certain locations can affect vital functions such as vision, respiratory status, as well as the ability to feed.

B. Vascular malformations. There are usually no symptoms with PWSs or venous malformations.

C. Cutaneous ectasias. There are usually no symptoms. Pyogenic granulomas may be painful, but the most frequent complaint relates to their friability; these angiomas bleed easily and may become infected secondarily.

Note: Even when asymptomatic, any vascular lesion may pose a significant cosmetic problem.

III. OBJECTIVE DATA

A. Hemangiomas. The appearance of hemangiomas is dependent upon its stage of evolution, location, and depth.

  1. Superficial hemangioma (Strawberry hemangioma)
  a. Bright red papules/plaques with discrete borders.
  b. Minimally compressible.

  2. Deep hemangioma
  a. These are located deeper in the skin and present as nodules with a bluish color.

  3. Mixed hemangioma
  a. Most hemangiomas have both superficial and deep components.

B. Vascular malformations

  1. PWS
  a. Discrete pink to burgundy macules and patches of varying sizes.
  b. As the lesions age, they become darker in color and may develop blebbing and nodules. It may also lead to the overgrowth of underlying tissues.

C. Venous malformations

  1. Small to very large, ill-defined lesions that are spongy and compressible but will refill slowly.
  2. They have a distinct venous pattern which may be blue to violet in color.

D. Cutaneous ectasias

  1. Cherry angioma
  a. Discrete small bright red papules 1 to 3 mm, most commonly located on the upper trunk.
  b. Will not blanch on pressure.

  2. Pyogenic granuloma
  a. Dull red solitary papules and nodules usually located on the extremities.
  b. Bleed easily when traumatized.
  c. May be eroded, crusted, ulcerated, or infected.

  3. Spider angioma and telangiectasias
  a. Spider angiomas consist of a bright red central arteriole with radiating branches, resembling a spider.
  b. The central arteriole may be pulsating, which becomes more apparent on gentle pressure with a glass slide.
  c. More intense pressure will obliterate the lesion entirely.

IV. ASSESSMENT

A. Hemangiomas

  1. Superficial/deep/mixed. Measure and photograph the lesion to follow its evolution. Close monitoring of lesions located in critical regions.

B. Vascular malformations

  1. PWS. These may need to be further investigated with neuroimaging/ophthalmologic evaluation if located on the face to evaluate for Sturge-Weber syndrome. Bilateral facial PWSs are associated with a higher risk for Sturge-Weber syndrome. Imaging studies may also be warranted with large malformations on the extremities as this may be associated with overgrowth of the extremity.

C. Venous malformations. May require imaging studies to determine the extent of the malformation.

D. Cutaneous ectasias

  1. Cherry angiomas. May occasionally require biopsy to determine their benign nature.

  2. Venous lake. No investigation needed.

  3. Telangiectasias. History and a complete physical examination may determine the need for additional investigation to evaluate the underlying etiology of acquired telangiectasias resulting from systemic disease.

V. THERAPY

A. Hemangiomas

  1. Superficial/deep/mixed

   a. Almost all lesions will involute spontaneously. Aggressive forms of therapy may leave a significant cosmetic defect. Parents of children with hemangiomas should be educated about the nature and course of the lesions. Support and reassurance should be provided particularly in cases where treatment is not required.

   b. Lesions impinging on vital structures and in crucial locations require treatment. Systemic corticosteroids (prednisone or prednisolone) at 2 to 3 mg/kg/day is the first line therapy. Some studies recommend higher doses of up to 5 mg/kg/day. The duration of treatment is variable, depending upon the response of treatment, the age, as well as the indication for treatment. Patients should be slowly weaned off the steroids.

   c. Intralesional injection of corticosteroids (triamcinolone 3 to 5 mg/kg), which may be repeated once or twice, can also be effective in small localized lesions.

   d. Recombinant interferon-α, which inhibits angiogenesis, should be used only in patients with life-threatening hemangiomas in whom high-dose corticosteroids have failed. Side effects are common, and spastic diplegia has been reported in up to 20% of patients treated with interferon α-2a.

   e. The flash lamp–pumped pulsed-dye laser (585 to 595 nm) is effective in the treatment of superficial hemangiomas because of its limited penetration to a depth of <1 mm. This treatment is also useful for lesions that are slow in regressing in older children and for residual telangiectasia after involution. Millisecond pulsed Nd:YAG lasers (1,064 nm) may have a role for deeper vascular components. Continuous-wave lasers, such as argon and copper bromide, have been used in the past to flatten vascular nodules, but often induced nonspecific thermal damage and were associated with an increased risk of scarring.

   f. Ulcerated hemangiomas respond well to pulsed-dye laser treatments. They rapidly reepithelialize and pain decreases or is eliminated.

   g. Small superficial hemangiomas have been treated by cryotherapy but the concern of scarring has limited its use.

B. Vascular malformations

  1. PWSs

   a. Laser surgery is the treatment of choice. The pulsed-dye laser is used to treat lesions in neonates as well as in adults and is the best laser for vascular pink-red lesions. Multiple sessions are often necessary to bring about maximal fading. Continuous-wave (CW) or quasi-continuous-wave lasers (argon, CW dye, copper vapor) may be useful for more mature, darker lesions with raised, irregular surfaces but are associated with increased risk of textural change.

   b. Tattooing with flesh-colored pigments has been used on PWSs with variable success.

   c. The use of skin-colored cosmetics which can effectively cover up the lesion may be all that is necessary in some cases. Cosmetics such as Dermablend and CoverBlend are available in a variety of colors for this purpose.

  2. Cutaneous ectasias

   a. Cherry angiomas. Light electrodesiccation will readily remove these lesions. Pulsed-dye laser or millisecond pulsed 532 nm Nd:YAG laser will also destroy these lesions.

- **b. Pyogenic granulomas**
    - **i.** Excision, curettage, and electrodesiccation are the therapy of choice.
    - **ii.** Carbon dioxide and pulsed-dye lasers are also effective with minimal scarring.
    - **iii.** Cautery with silver nitrate as well as cryotherapy have also been used.
- **c. Venous lake.** Electrosurgery or laser surgery with pulsed Nd:YAG or pulsed-dye lasers is usually effective. More than one treatment may be necessary.
- **d. Telangiectasias**
    - **i.** Pulsed-dye laser surgery is an effective treatment for most lesions. The pulsed-dye laser or pulsed 532-nm laser is the instrument of choice for widespread, matted ectasias. Pulsed Nd:YAG lasers (532 nm) are preferable for treating linear vessels.
    - **ii.** Spider ectasias are easily effaced by electrosurgery or laser surgery. Electrocoagulation is more effective than electrodesiccation. If anesthesia is used, mark the "body" of the spider before injection.

Reference

1. Mullikan JB, Young AE. *Vascular birthmarks: hemangiomas and malformations.* Philadelphia, PA: WB Saunders, 1988.

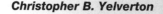
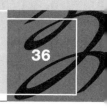

I. DEFINITION AND PATHOPHYSIOLOGY. Warts are intraepidermal tumors of the skin and mucosa caused by infection with the human papillomavirus (HPV). These papillomaviruses are host specific; there are over 100 variants known to cause disease in humans. Clinically, warts are classified by location into three main subtypes: cutaneous, anogenital/mucosal, and epidermodysplasia verruciformis (EV).

Implantation of HPV into basal keratinocytes is thought to occur primarily through mechanical disruption of the skin barrier. Because of its simple protein coat and lack of a lipid envelope, fomite and transmission through clothing may occur. The incubation period after inoculation into human volunteers varies from 1 to 12 months and averages 2 to 3 months. The virus replicates in the nucleus of the keratinocyte as it differentiates and migrates upward through the epidermis. Once the entire nuclear space is filled, virus spills into the cytoplasm; in the stratum corneum, the virus lies free within the keratin mass. Virus concentration is greatest in warts of 6 to 12 months' duration. The number of virus particles varies in warts from different locations; plantar and common warts often contain thousands of viruses, whereas condyloma acuminata and juvenile laryngeal papillomatoses contain few. HPV, a very stable virus, is shed from the superficial keratinocytes and then transmitted through hetero- or autoinoculation and even through indirect contact with contaminated articles such as swimming pool surfaces. Latent viral deoxyribonucleic acid (DNA) has been demonstrated in normal-appearing skin surrounding lesions of condyloma acuminata and laryngeal papillomatosis; latent virus clearly predisposes to posttreatment recurrences and difficulty in delineating the true extent of infection with this virus.

Although difficult to cultivate *in vitro*, *in situ* DNA hybridization, polymerase chain reaction (PCR), and molecular nucleic acid hybridization have allowed the separation and cloning of many HPV subtypes (Table 36-1). Infections by HPV subtypes show a marked preference for specific sites and are often characterized by type-specific macroscopic and microscopic features. Several HPV types are oncogenic, and there is a strong association between certain types, particularly HPV-16 and 18, and dysplasias and invasive cancers of the female lower genital tract, the penis, and the anorectal region. HPV sequences have been identified in 90% of cervical carcinomas in some studies. Recently approved HPV vaccine may help curb the incidence of related carcinomas in the future (see sec. IV.H). Recent studies have also detected the presence of β-class HPV subtypes (particularly HPV-5) within some actinic keratoses and nonmelanoma skin cancers in persons with normal immune systems (1–3). The exact significance of this association is not yet fully understood.

HPV lesions are more common in patients receiving immunosuppressive drugs and those with immune deficiency states, including lymphoma, chronic lymphocytic leukemia, Hodgkin's disease, and human immunodeficiency virus (HIV). This information, plus the increased frequency of cell-mediated responses and antibodies specific for viral antigens in patients with regression or cured warts, supports a role for immunity in the resolution of warts. Most HPV infections are latent or transient, suggesting intracellular control of viral expression; when this control is compromised, HPV-associated diseases will result. In persons with a healthy immune system, approximately 20% to 30% of all lesions will involute spontaneously within 6 months, 50% within 1 year, and 66% within 2 years. New lesions may continue to appear during this period and are seen three times more frequently in children with warts than in those without. The high rate of spontaneous involution makes it difficult to evaluate the effectiveness of hypnosis as well as the more direct methods of wart therapy.

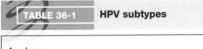

TABLE 36-1   HPV subtypes

Lesions	HPV types
Common, palmar, plantar, myrmecia, and mosaic warts	1, 2, 4
Flat warts	3, 10
Butcher's warts	2, 7
Digital squamous cell carcinoma, Bowen's disease	16
EV	3, 5, 8
EV squamous cell carcinoma	5
Condylomata acuminata	6, 11
Intraepithelial neoplasias (cervical condyloma plana, bowenoid papulosis, erythroplasia of Queyrat)	16
Buschke-Lowenstein tumor	6, 11
Recurrent respiratory papillomatosis, conjunctival papillomas	6, 11
Heck's disease	13, 32

EV, epidermodysplasia verruciformis.

II. **SUBJECTIVE DATA.** Most warts induce symptoms only when they become awkward because of their size or appearance. Although wart tissue is not inherently painful, condyloma acuminata may be discomforting for mechanical reasons; periungual lesions may develop fissures that hurt; and plantar warts can become very painful during walking or running.

III. **OBJECTIVE DATA.** There are several morphologic variants of warts such as the following:
   A. Common warts start as small, pinhead-sized, flesh-colored, translucent papules and grow over several weeks or months to larger, raised, papillary-surfaced, flesh-colored or darker, hyperkeratotic papules. Black specks of hemosiderin pigment may be seen in thrombosed capillary loops. Paring the lesion may result in punctate bleeding points. Common warts are found most often on the hands, especially in children, or on other sites often subjected to trauma. They may grow anywhere on the epidermis or mucous membranes and are spread by contact or autoinoculation. Common warts are most frequent between the ages of 12 and 16.
   B. Filiform warts are slender, soft, thin, finger-like growths seen primarily on the face and neck.
   C. Flat, plane, or juvenile warts are flesh-colored or tan, soft, 1- to 3-mm-diameter, discrete papules appearing primarily on the face, neck, extensor aspect of the forearms, and hands.
   D. Plantar or palmar warts are hyperkeratotic, firm, and elevated or flat lesions that interrupt the natural skin lines (as opposed to calluses). Red or black capillary dots may be seen. A **mosaic wart** consists of the confluence of multiple lesions into one large, usually flat lesion. As a point of contrast, corns or calluses are often more painful with direct pressure, whereas warts are more painful with lateral pressure.
   E. Warts that grow in warm, moist, intertriginous areas develop into soft, friable, vegetating clusters. These **condylomata acuminata** are found frequently on the foreskin and penis, particularly in uncircumcised men, on vaginal and labial mucosa, and in the urethral meatus and perianal area. Smaller genital warts may be hyperpigmented (resembling seborrheic keratoses or nevi). Application of a 5% acetic acid solution for 10 to 15 minutes will turn possible verrucae white. Two thirds of women and one third of men with genital warts may have accompanying genital infections that must be identified and treated.

Condyloma acuminata is the most common sexually transmitted disease and has reached epidemic proportions. The incubation period from the time of exposure is from 3 weeks to 8 months; longer latency periods up to years may occur and not everyone exposed develops lesions. Breaks in the skin likely lead to establishment of infection. Low-risk subtypes in immunocompetent individuals commonly cause external genital warts. Recent studies indicate that HPV infections are extremely common in sexually active young women, but often the infection is asymptomatic and transient.

F. EV is a chronic autosomal recessive disorder associated with chronic infection with HPV. The lesions can resemble tinea versicolor–like plaques or flat-topped papules. The lesions usually start in childhood and are often distributed on the face and extremities. During the third and fourth decades of life, one third of patients will develop actinic keratoses and nonmelanoma skin cancers in sun-exposed areas. Ultraviolet light is involved in the pathogenesis of EV through its immunosuppressive and mutagenic effects. Multiple HPV-β subtypes are involved; HPV subtypes 5 and 8 have the highest oncogenic potential. Patients with EV are immunosuppressed and might have a defect in their natural killer cell functioning.

IV. THERAPY

A. Many therapeutic modalities are available for the treatment of warts. It is important to remember that warts are benign cutaneous growths and that the therapy should also be benign. Therapy should present no hazard to the patient, no scarring should result, and side effects should be minimal. It is not difficult to cause considerable pain, as well as permanent scarring, by an overly enthusiastic approach. This curative zeal must be curbed, because it is neither necessary nor warranted to remove every wart. On the other hand, the therapist should be optimistic, because most lesions can be treated successfully with persistence.

B. A recent Cochrane review and several other similar examinations of clinical trials have shown no evidence for supremacy of any single topical wart treatment (4–6). This seems to be largely due to inadequacy of study designs and the high rate of spontaneous cure. Appropriate choice of therapy should take into consideration the number, size, and location of lesions, physician and patient preference, convenience, and cost. We suggest that most common warts can be treated effectively, safely, and conveniently with liquid nitrogen cryosurgery or salicylic acid as first-line therapy and that combination treatments may be more efficacious than monotherapy, particularly in resistant cases (7,8).

C. Common warts may be treated with the following methods:

1. Destruction by light electrodesiccation and curettage.

2. Cryosurgery with liquid nitrogen. This technique, as well as electrodesiccation, carefully executed, will remove the lesion and will usually leave no scar and little or no pigmentary change. Nonblistering therapy (10- to 20-second application) every 2 to 3 weeks until resolution is generally effective. This treatment destroys not the virus but the cells within and surrounding the lesion that contain HPV.

3. Keratolytic therapy with paints such as 5% to 20% salicylic acid and 5% to 20% lactic acid in flexible collodion may be self-administered at home and will lead to cures within 12 weeks on all but mosaic plantar warts in 60% to 80% of patients. Keratolytic agents may act by mechanical removal of infected cells and wart virus and also by providing a mild inflammatory reaction that renders the virus more available to immunologic recognition and attack. These chemicals do not reach the basal layer where the HPV DNA is present. Duofilm or Occlusal (17% salicylic acid, 17% lactic acid in flexible collodion) are commercially available preparations; patients should be instructed to use them or other keratolytic paints as follows:

a. Wash area thoroughly with soap and water.

b. Rub surface of wart gently with a mild abrasive such as an emery board, pumice stone, or callus file.

c. Apply keratolytic paint to the wart with a sharpened matchstick or orange stick.

d. Allow to dry.

  e. Keep bottle tightly closed.
  f. Repeat each night.
  g. If area becomes red or tender, discontinue therapy until this subsides and then start again. Alternatively, keratolytic paint with a lower concentration of salicylic and lactic acids may be prescribed.
  h. Do not apply paint to warts previously treated with liquid nitrogen until the inflammation has subsided.
4. Cantharidin (Cantharone), a mitochondrial poison derived from the blister beetle *Cantharis vesicatoria*, leads to changes in cell membranes, epidermal cell dyshesion, acantholysis, and blister formation and is also useful. Cantharidin can be compounded with salicylic acid and podophyllin resin; occlusion for only 2 hours is needed with this combination. Thick hyperkeratotic lesions should be pared down before painting. The lesion should then be painted with cantharidin, allowed to dry, and covered with Blenderm or other nonporous occlusive tape; 40% salicylic acid plaster may be used to achieve greater activity. The tape is left on for 24 hours or until the area begins to hurt. A blister, often hemorrhagic, will form, break, crust, and fall off in 7 to 14 days; at this time, the lesion is pared down, and any wart remnants are retreated. Because the effect of cantharidin is entirely intraepidermal, no scarring ensues. Ring-like or "donut configuration" recurrences may be seen occasionally after treatment with cantharidin or, at times, following liquid nitrogen therapy. Owing to this agent's toxicity, application by a physician is recommended. Verrusol, which contains 30% salicylic acid, 5% podophyllin, and 1% cantharidin, may be used in the same manner.
5. Podophyllum resin (podophyllin), or podofilox, a cytotoxic agent that arrests mitosis in metaphase, is used primarily for treatment of condyloma acuminata but may also be used on all other types of warts. Although now rarely available, a 25% preparation of podophyllum in compound tincture of benzoin should be applied overnight when treating common nongenital warts. A more commonly available preparation, podofilox 0.5% gel (Condylox), should be applied twice a day for 3 days, then discontinued for 4 consecutive days. The same cycle is continued until eradication of the lesions. The effectiveness as well as the irritant potential of this medication may be increased by covering with adhesive tape or plastic tape (Blenderm).
6. Occlusive tape, such as duct tape was shown to have efficacy greater than liquid nitrogen in one study (9). The treatment regimen included occlusion of the wart for 6 days, followed by warm water soaking and debridement. The following day, the tape was reapplied and the cycle repeated until resolution (up to 2 months). Eighty five percent of warts treated with duct tape were clear within 2 months, compared with 60% of those receiving up to six courses of cryotherapy (10-second freeze every 2 to 3 weeks).
7. Lesions may be painted weekly or more frequently with acids such as 50% to 80% trichloroacetic acid, saturated dichloroacetic acid, or 80% monochloroacetic acid. After a necrotic crust forms, it should be removed and the lesion should be retreated. This method is relatively painless and somewhat slow, but it may be carried out at home. Both the effectiveness and rapidity of therapy may be increased by covering the acid-treated lesion with a small pad of 40% salicylic plaster and adhesive tape for 12 to 24 hours.
8. Localized heat therapy (50°C for 30 to 60 seconds for one to four treatments) leads to an 86% regression rate (10). Other recommended treatment schedules are immersion in water baths for 30 minutes three times a week at a temperature of 45°C or 113°F. Extreme caution must be used to avoid causing a burn.
D. Filiform warts are best treated by light electrosurgery, cryosurgery, or keratolytic paints.
E. Flat warts should be treated with a short (5 to 15 seconds) application of liquid nitrogen, by "flicking" off with a sharp curette or No. 15 blade on edge, with keratolytic paint, or with tretinoin preparations. Electrosurgery may also be used, but it may leave small, hypopigmented scars. 5-Fluorouracil 5% cream applied one to two times a day has been reported to clear flat facial warts within 3 weeks.

Lesions on the male face constitute a difficult problem, because autoinoculation takes place each time the patient shaves. To avoid cosmetically damaging results, it is especially important to be conservative. Use of an electric shaver or depilatories may decrease autoinoculation. Barely visible lesions will become more prominent if lightly rubbed with liquid nitrogen on a cotton tip or sprayed with a refrigerant.

F. Plantar warts are sometimes best left untreated. Unless a wart is painful, rapidly growing, or small, it is wise to recommend no therapy or nonaggressive therapy. If treatment is necessary, the following approaches can be used:

1. Liquid nitrogen freezing may produce good results, but it does cause discomfort during application; in addition, the resultant blister makes walking uncomfortable for the next several days.

2. Enucleation by blunt dissection technique is often the therapy of choice if there is one or only a few lesions. This method of removal is also excellent for removal of verrucae vulgaris in other sites such as palms and periungual areas.

3. Intermittent flattening of the lesion with a pumice stone, callus file, or scalpel is usually enough to keep plantar lesions entirely asymptomatic.

4. Keratolytic therapy with salicylic and lactic acid paint is the most convenient and effective nontraumatic method (see sec. IV.C.3). The patient should apply medication nightly as follows:
   a. Remove the adhesive tape from the previous night's treatment.
   b. Rub the surface of the wart with an emery board, pumice stone, or callus file.
   c. Soak the foot in hot water or a bath for at least 5 minutes.
   d. Apply a drop of keratolytic paint to the wart. Allow to dry. If the wart is large, apply another drop.
   e. When dry, cover with a piece of adhesive tape. If the lesion is very thick or more aggressive treatment is desired, apply a piece of 40% salicylic acid plaster to the wart and then cover with adhesive tape.
   f. If soreness occurs, stop treatment and restart after it subsides. Use of "micropore" tape rather than adhesive tape may lead to less inflammation.

5. Weekly chemocautery with salicylic acid. Debride the wart to a point short of bleeding and apply a piece of adhesive tape with an orifice cut out in the shape of the wart. A similar shaped felt pad is then overlaid. Pack 60% salicylic acid in petrolatum (or 40% salicylic acid plaster or 35% to 50% trichloroacetic acid) onto the wart and cover caustic and surrounding tapes with more waterproof tape. Remove in 1 week, cut or curette away necrotic material, and repeat.

6. Bimonthly debridement and treatment with cantharidin is also effective but may be painful.

7. Podofilox (Condylox) is a commercially available purified preparation of podophyllin and is well tolerated when applied to common warts. Alternatively, the warts may be painted with 10% formalin and covered with 40% salicylic acid plaster for 3 to 4 days. The lesions are then debrided by the patient or physician and the formalin and dressing are reapplied. This painless therapy may be continued for weeks until the lesion is gone. Glutaraldehyde 10% in an aqueous ethanol solution can be applied for 15 minutes/day with moderate results.

8. Destructive electrosurgery, sharp scalpel excision, and radiotherapy should be avoided, because although they may remove the lesion, the resulting scar often becomes a more difficult and less easily treated problem than the wart itself.

9. **Laser therapy.** CO_2 laser surgery will frequently clear recalcitrant, chronic lesions, although the high recurrence rate and possibility for scarring limit this modality. The pulsed dye laser (PDL) has been used with triple pulse, high-power settings to target the vascular component of verruca; multiple treatments are required. One study demonstrated a 74% resolution in one treatment and a 93% clearance after 2.5 treatments (periungual and plantar warts had the lowest rate of clearance) (11). PDL treatment is better tolerated than cryotherapy, especially with pretreatment with topical lidocaine cream (EMLA cream). The long-pulse Alexandrite laser, 755 nm, has recently been used because it allows deeper penetration of the skin, heating the wart, and causing coagulation of blood vessels.

10. Studies regarding the use of topical imiquimod (Aldara) for common warts show varied results and the exact role of this drug for this type of HPV is yet to be determined. The degree of keratinization affects the efficacy of imiquimod. With common warts, application is increased to daily or b.i.d. with or without occlusion, depending on the body site. Combinations with keratolytic agents such as salicylic acid or tazarotene gel have been advocated. Specific subtypes of lesions such as flat warts and periungual warts may be most amenable to this immunomodulatory agent.

11. It is important to correct orthopaedic defects and prescribe correct footwear. Plantar warts most often occur in areas of pressure and callus, and unless the incorrect weight-bearing condition can be alleviated, it is often difficult to either cure the wart or make the patient comfortable.

G. Condylomata acuminata

1. A patient self-administration of 0.5% podofilox (Condylox) b.i.d. for 3 days for 4 weeks is convenient, cost effective, and yields good results. This has the advantage of using known amounts of active ingredients and thereby limiting potential toxicity. Side effects include pain, burning, erosions, and itching. Weekly painting of the lesion with 25% podophyllum resin in compound tincture of benzoin is also an effective therapy, although it is now used rarely. Medication should be kept off uninvolved surrounding skin; this may be accomplished by applying a thin covering of petrolatum around the lesion before therapy. After the application dries, the area should be liberally powdered to prevent undue maceration and inadvertent transfer of podophyllin from the lesions to apposing normal skin. At the start of therapy, the medication should be left on for only 1 hour and then washed off, particularly in the vulvar area and the area under the foreskin. As therapy progresses, podophyllin should be left in place 4 to 6 hours before it is removed. Treated lesions may become inflamed and painful during the following 2 to 3 days. It is wise to treat only parts of a large condyloma to prevent disabling pain, but it is important to repeat treatment every 7 to 10 days until all lesions are gone. If the lesions are very verrucous or bulky, remove the mass of the wart first by curettage, and after healing, start podophyllum therapy. A topical anesthetic preparation is often useful during the period of pain.

Podophyllin can cause severe irritation and, if absorbed in large quantities, may produce systemic toxic effects. It is inadvisable to apply it in large amounts to mucous membranes, and it is unwise to use it in pregnant women because of its possible cytotoxic action on the fetus.

2. Liquid nitrogen cryosurgery is also excellent for condylomata acuminata. The amount and intensity of therapy and the delineation of treatment margins can be better controlled than with podophyllin. Repeat the application every 1 to 3 weeks until the lesions clear.

3. Topical imiquimod (Aldara) is an immune response modifier that has antiviral and antitumor activities. This drug activates dendritic cells and keratinocytes to produce interferon, tumor necrosis factor, and interleukin-12. The cytokine production promotes migration of Langerhans cells to lymph nodes, and virus-specific T cells are generated. A dramatic decrease in the quantity of HPV DNA and messenger ribonucleic acid (RNA) occurs. The treatment regimen includes application to the wart and some surrounding skin three times a week for a maximum of 16 weeks. Irritation and erythema are expected side effects and indicate an activation of the immune system; no systemic side effects have been observed. Clearance rates are 30% on the shaft of the penis, 60% under the foreskin, and 80% on the vulva; the difference likely reflects the degree of keratinization of these sites. Imiquimod is probably at least partially effective even in those with compromised immune systems (12,13).

4. Occasionally, it is necessary and useful to approach such lesions with electrosurgery and curettage or with CO_2 laser surgery. This is particularly true when there are large masses of warty tissue, which may then be removed in one procedure, or when treatment with other methods appears to lose its effectiveness.

5. Proctoscopy and treatment of rectal lesions with podophyllin or liquid nitrogen are necessary in all patients with perianal condylomata.

6. Intraurethral and meatal condylomata may be treated conservatively with podophyllin or liquid nitrogen. The upstream proximal urethra is very rarely involved; the most commonly involved distal urethra can be visualized with a small nasal speculum. Alternatively, 1% to 5% 5-fluorouracil solution or suppositories may also be effective. Therapy must not be overaggressive if urethral stricture is to be avoided.

H. HPV vaccination

1. A quadrivalent HPV (types 6, 11, 16, 18) recombinant vaccine (Gardasil, Merck & Co., Inc.) has been approved in the United States for prevention of HPV-associated genital diseases in females between 9 and 26 years (14). This vaccine is given as three doses at 0, 2, and 6 months. Another bivalent (types 16, 18) vaccine (Cevarix, GlaxoSmithKline) is also expected to be available soon. If administered before the first sexual activity, these vaccines could potentially reduce the incidence of cervical cancer and anogenital warts considerably.

I. Special comments

1. Women with genital warts require a Pap smear for detection of cervical warts or other cytologic abnormalities. Colposcopy should be considered owing to the high false-negative rate of cervical cytology. Only a minority of women exposed to genital HPV will develop persistent infection, and very few will ever develop actual invasive carcinoma. Most external genital warts are caused by HPV types 6 and 11, which are not oncogenic. The risk of an infant developing juvenile laryngeal papillomatosis from HPV-infected women is 4%; the presence of warts does not mandate a cesarean birth.

2. If warts are recalcitrant to treatment, immunotherapy may be effective.

a. Contact immunotherapy has been advocated as a method to enhance cell-mediated destruction of warts. The agents described in the literature include squaric acid dibutyl ester, diphenylcyclopropenone, and dinitrochlorobenzene (DNCB). The individual is first topically sensitized to the agent over several weeks and then the warts are painted with the chemical, inducing a localized acute contact dermatitis. In some studies, both the treated and untreated warts resolved. Cure rates of 70% to 80% have been reported. Lack of availability and safety data limit the usefulness of these chemicals; DNCB is a known topical carcinogen, so standard recommendation of its use is extremely unlikely.

b. Systemic or intralesional injection of interferon-α or interferon-γ has been reported to clear nongenital warts and condyloma acuminata. Distant noninjected warts also disappear sometimes. Because of the expense, need to administer interferon by injection, and 60% incidence of adverse systemic effects, interferon has not gained popularity.

3. Intralesional bleomycin, a cytotoxic drug that inhibits DNA synthesis, is effective for all varieties of recalcitrant warts. Various concentrations of the drug have been used, although the total dose must be carefully tracked over time to avoid potential systemic toxicity. Administration with a bifurcated needle and multiple punctures resulted in elimination of 92% of 258 treated warts (15). Local side effects that have been described are moderate to severe pain; nail dystrophy, and persistent Raynaud's phenomenon. The area needs to be anesthetized; full-strength bleomycin should be used; small amounts (0.025 to 0.1 mL/3 mm^2) should be injected into the upper dermis, not exceeding a total of 1 mL per session. A dark hemorrhagic crust develops that should be pared after 3 weeks.

4. Injection of 0.1 mL of 1:1,000 candida antigen into the base of each wart led to 85% clearance of common warts compared with 25% of controls. The candida antigen is available from many pharmaceutical laboratories but is not approved by the U.S. Food and Drug Administration (FDA).

5. Therapy for children should be gentle and nonaggressive. Keratolytic solutions and applications of acids are useful and nonpainful. Cantharidin is effective and does not cause pain during application. Electrosurgery and cryosurgical procedures are often traumatic to all involved. In this age-group, hypnosis appears to work well at times (16). Pretreatment with topical EMLA cream and analgesics may be helpful.

6. Cimetidine, an H_2 receptor antagonist with some immunomodulatory effects at high doses (30 to 40 mg/kg/day), had been reported to be successful in treatment of warts in children and adults. The proposed mechanism is an enhanced delayed-type hypersensitivity reaction that blocks the H_2 receptor stimulation of T cells. However, the largest placebo-controlled double-blind study to date failed to show any advantage of cimetidine over placebo (17). There is still some feeling that this drug may be more effective in children than in adults. Cimetidine at a dose of 25 to 40 mg/kg/day is divided into three to four doses per day for 8 to 12 weeks. Side effects include diarrhea and headache; there are multiple potential drug interactions including those with phenytoin and theophylline.

7. A clinical trial of etretinate (1 mg/kg/day) in 20 children led to complete regression of extensive warts in 80%, with 2-year follow-up (18).

8. Treatment with keratolytic paints, liquid nitrogen, or cantharidin generally produces the best cosmetic results. Acids and electrosurgery have a greater potential for scarring.

9. Periungual lesions are best treated with liquid nitrogen, cantharidin, or blunt dissection.

10. Over-the-counter (OTC) wart remedies such as Compound W and WartAway are liquids that contain 13% to 14% salicylic acid (a keratolytic) and acetic acid (a caustic). The OTC corn and callus remedies are usually salicylic acid compounds. A dimethyl-ether-propane cryogenic spray (Freeze Away, Dr Scholl's) is also available over the counter. This $-59°C$ compound has shown efficacy at removing warts, similar to that of liquid nitrogen in one single-blinded study (19).

11. CO_2 laser surgery is useful for recalcitrant or very bulky warts. It is particularly helpful in clearing difficult palmoplantar, anogenital, and periungual lesions. Surgical small-pore masks should be used during electrocoagulation or CO_2 laser destruction of warts because the plume contains HPV DNA. Postoperative pain, prolonged healing time, and scarring add to the morbidity of this form of treatment. Infrared coagulation has been used effectively in the treatment of warts and has the advantage of not producing a plume and being much less expensive than a CO_2 laser (20).

12. There are multiple reports of chronic periungual warts developing squamous cell carcinomas with an association of HPV-16. An atypical wart that is unresponsive to therapy in the periungual distribution should be considered for biopsy. HPV may be involved in nonmelanoma skin cancer occurring in immunocompromised patients. Warts that are resistant to therapy, have atypical features, and/or are present in an immunocompromised patient should be biopsied to rule out an associated squamous cell carcinoma.

13. The risk of genital warts increases with any amount of smoking. Counseling regarding smoking cessation may help impact the resolution of HPV infections.

References

1. Karagas MR, Nelson HH, Sehr P, et al. Human papillomavirus infection and incidence of squamous cell and basal cell carcinomas of the skin. *J Natl Cancer Inst* 2006; 98(6):389–395.

2. Pfister H, Fuchs PG, Majewski S, et al. High prevalence of epidermodysplasia verruciformis-associated human papillomavirus DNA in actinic keratoses of the immunocompetent population. *Arch Dermatol Res* 2003;295(7):273–279.

3. Weissenborn SJ, Nindl I, Purdie K, et al. Human papillomavirus-DNA loads in actinic keratoses exceed those in non-melanoma skin cancers. *J Invest Dermatol* 2005;125(1): 93–97.

4. Gibbs S, Harvey I, Sterling JC, et al. Local treatments for cutaneous warts. *Cochrane Database Syst Rev* 2003;(3):CD001781.

5. Bacelieri R, Johnson SM. Cutaneous warts: an evidence-based approach to therapy. *Am Fam Physician* 2005;72:647–652.

6. Scheinfeld N, Lehman DS. An evidence-based review of medical and surgical treatments of genital warts. *Dermatol Online J* 2006;12(3):5.

7. van Brederode RL, Engel ED. Combined cryotherapy/70% salicylic acid treatment for plantar verrucae. *J Foot Ankle Surg* 2001;40(1):36−41.

8. Housman TS, Jorizzo JL. Anecdotal reports of 3 cases illustrating a spectrum of resistant common warts treated with cryotherapy followed by topical imiquimod and salicylic acid. *J Am Acad Dermatol* 2002;47(4 Suppl):S217−S220.

9. Focht DR III, Spicer C, Fairchok MP. The efficacy of duct tape vs cryotherapy in the treatment of verruca vulgaris (the common wart). *Arch Pediatr Adolesc Med* 2002; 156(10):971−974.

10. Stern P, Levine N. Controlled localized heat therapy in cutaneous warts. *Arch Dermatol* 1992;128:945−948.

11. Kauvar AN, McDaniel DH, Geronemus RG. Pulsed dye laser treatment of warts. *Arch Fam Med* 1995;4:1035−1040.

12. Harwood CA, Perrett CM, Brown VL, et al. Imiquimod cream 5% for recalcitrant cutaneous warts in immunosuppressed individuals. *Br J Dermatol* 2005;152(1):122−129.

13. Kreuter A, Brockmeyer NH, Weissenborn SJ, et al. German Competence Network HIV/AIDS. 5% imiquimod suppositories decrease the DNA load of intra-anal HPV types 6 and 11 in HIV-infected men after surgical ablation of condylomata acuminata. *Arch Dermatol.* 2006;142(2):243−244.

14. *Quadrivalent Human papillomavirus (Types 6, 11, 16, 18) recombinant vaccine. FDA Product Approval Information—Licensing Action.* 2006; Jun 8. available at: http://www.fda.gov/Cber/products/hpvmer060806.htm. Accessed 06/13/2006.

15. Shelley WB, Shelley ED. Intralesional bleomycin sulfate therapy for warts. A novel bifurcated needle puncture technique. *Arch Dermatol* 1991;127:234−236.

16. Ewin DM. Hypnotherapy for warts (verruca vulgaris): 41 consecutive cases with 33 cures. *Am J Clin Hypn* 1992;35:1−10.

17. Yilmaz E, Alpsoy E, Basaran E. Cimetidine therapy for warts: a placebo-controlled, double-blind study. *Am Acad Dermatol* 1996;34:1005−1007.

18. Gelmetti C, Carri D, Schiuma AA, et al. Treatment of extensive warts in children with etretinate: a clinical trial in 20 children. *Pediatr Dermatol* 1987;4:254−258.

19. Caballero Martinez F, Plaza Nohales C, Perez Canal C, et al. Cutaneous cryosurgery in family medicine: dimethyl ether-propane spray versus liquid nitrogen. *Aten Primaria* 1996;18(5):211−216.

20. Halasz CL. Treatment of common warts using infared coagulator. *J Dermatol Surg Oncol* 1994;20:252−256.

Procedures and Techniques

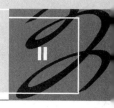

II

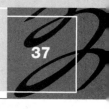
Skin is uniquely available for diagnostic procedures as well as for the direct application of therapeutic agents. This ease of access allows multiple procedures to be performed in a short period with little discomfort to the patient. Most techniques are easily learned and require only simple equipment.

BIOPSY

I. PROCEDURES

  A. The punch biopsy is an extremely simple procedure that, in all but a very few circumstances, removes sufficient tissue for histopathologic study. The information derived from this procedure is important not only for diagnostic purposes but also to clarify a disease process and to assess the extent of tissue involved, because full-thickness tissue is usually obtained.

    1. It is generally best to select a mature, well-developed, untreated lesion for biopsy. However, if blisters are present, choose the earliest lesion available, and take care to keep the roof intact; this is one of the few instances when one should intentionally include adjacent normal skin. Several biopsies should be obtained from evolving eruptions or those with various types of lesions (in this instance, too, biopsy of early lesions may be of higher diagnostic yield). Lesions altered by trauma or prior treatment or old, "burned-out" areas will not yield useful information. It should be noted that biopsies on the legs and feet heal more slowly than proximal biopsies, especially if the circulation is poor; if possible, choose a lesion above the knees. Choose a site entirely within the lesion; avoid including normal skin in the biopsy unless specifically desired, in which case the pathologist should be informed of its inclusion and how the specimen is oriented.

    2. Clean the area gently with alcohol, taking care to leave scales, crusts, and vesicles intact. It is often useful to outline small lesions before the injection of local anesthetic, because the effect of epinephrine distorts and blanches the site.

    3. Anesthetize the area by injecting into the deep dermis 0.2 to 0.5 mL of 0.5% to 2.0% lidocaine or 1% to 2% lidocaine with 1:100,000 epinephrine. Addition of sodium bicarbonate to the lidocaine (approximately one part of 8.4% sodium bicarbonate to nine parts of 2% lidocaine) will attenuate the sting on infiltration. Patients allergic to local anesthetic ether compounds (procaine, tetracaine) can tolerate amide compounds (lidocaine, bupivacaine) without difficulty (i.e., procaine [Novocaine] and lidocaine [Xylocaine] do not cross-react). Other alternatives for delivering local anesthesia include antihistamines such as diphenhydramine HCl or normal saline with preservative. The local vasoconstriction produced by epinephrine will diminish bleeding and prolong the duration of anesthesia, thereby making the procedure much easier to perform. (For maximal vasoconstriction, 15 to 20 minutes is required.) Epinephrine-containing solutions should not be used when anesthetizing acral areas such as the penis, earlobes, or distal fingers or toes or when vasoconstriction might interfere with the significant histopathologic finds, as in vascular lesions. It is probably preferable to ring block an area with anesthesia, although intradermal injection directly into or below a lesion appears to cause little or no perceptible microscopic alteration. For larger excisions, patients with severe diabetic angiopathy or Raynaud's disease or those receiving monoamine oxidase inhibitors or β-blockers should also not receive vasoconstrictors.

    a. To inject with the least trauma for both the physician and the patient, a 30- or 32-gauge needle should be used.

    b. A topical anesthetic cream may be used to dull the pain of injection in children or for larger excisions. However, it must be applied at least 1 hour before the procedure for maximal effects. Use of occlusion may enhance the effects.

4. Biopsy punches, circular instruments with a cylindrical sharp cutting tip and a handle, are available in sizes ranging from 1 to 8 mm in diameter; the 4-mm punch is generally the most useful. Six-millimeter to 8-mm punch biopsies tend to leave excess cones of tissue ("dog ears") at the edges during subsequent wound repair. Removal of a specimen <4 mm in diameter may allow the histologic confirmation of a tumor, but is often inadequate for diagnosis of inflammatory processes.

    The skin surrounding the lesion should be stretched taut perpendicular to the wrinkle (relaxed skin tension) lines before the circular punch is inserted vertically, as demonstrated in Fig. 37-1. See figures on the inside front and back covers for a guide to the most common configuration of the relaxed skin tension lines. When the punch is removed, an ellipsoidal defect will be left (Fig. 37-1, *insets*). The biopsy punch is pressed firmly downward into the lesion with a rotary cutting motion until it is well into the subcutaneous tissue (Fig. 37-1). If the incision is made only to mid-dermis, the tissue will be more difficult to remove and the wound will heal less rapidly and with a less satisfactory cosmetic result. Care should be taken to avoid underlying structures when visible (e.g., visible vessel, tendons, etc.), especially in areas with thinner skin.

5. The biopsied skin plug will either pop up or lie free within its circular margin. The specimen must be grasped gently and lifted out with a forceps without applying undue pressure, the base must be severed with a scissors or scalpel blade as deep into the fat as possible, and the tissue placed in 10% neutral buffered formalin. The amount of formalin should be at least 20 times that of the

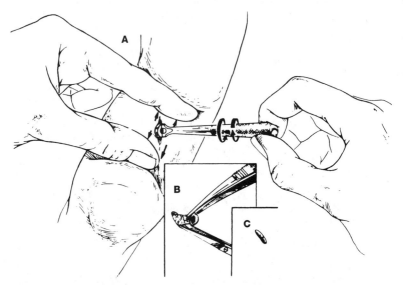

Figure 37-1. Punch biopsy technique. (*A*) Stretch the skin taut perpendicular to the relaxed skin tension lines before biopsy. (*B*) Gently grasp the skin plug with tissue forceps and sever as deep into the fat as possible. (*C*) An oval defect is left, which should be sutured.

specimen by volume. To avoid an artificial split in the skin, grasp the specimen close to the base with the forceps.

6. Simple pressure is generally adequate for hemostasis. Rarely, 20% aluminum in ethyl alcohol (e.g., Drysol), ferric subsulfate (Monsel's solution), absorbable gelatin (Gel foam), or electrodesiccation may be needed. Ferric subsulfate may occasionally result in pigmented tattoos and may destroy more tissue than other methods. Lesions heal more rapidly and with a linear scar, rather than a round defect, if either a 4-0 or 5-0 nylon or silk suture is put in place (left for 3 to 7 days on the face or 7 to 14 days on the trunk) or adhesive strips are applied across the defect (left for 14 to 21 days). If the patient cannot return for suture removal, an absorbable suture can be used to close the punch biopsy site.

7. The histologic interpretation of cutaneous reaction patterns requires a great deal of judgment and experience. It is wise to seek the help of a dermatopathologist. A clinical pathologic correlation should be made and follow-up consultation or a second opinion requested if there are questions regarding the diagnosis, especially of a pigmented lesion.

B. A shave biopsy removes that portion of skin elevated above the plane of surrounding tissue and is useful for biopsying or removing many exophytic benign epidermal growths, including keratoses and viral tumors. It allows the easy removal of epidermal and papillary dermal tissue for histopathologic inspection. It is also a convenient procedure for obtaining a tissue diagnosis of malignant lesions such as basal cell carcinomas before initiating therapy. This procedure is quickly and easily performed, heals rapidly, yields a good cosmetic result, and leaves the lower levels of the dermis intact if further procedures such as curettage, electrosurgery, or cryosurgery are necessary. The decision to perform a shave biopsy requires some judgment and, in particular, a reasonably good impression of the preoperative diagnosis. A shave biopsy may fail to distinguish, for example, between an actinic keratosis and an invasive squamous cell carcinoma if the shave is too superficial. Also, suspected melanomas or inflammatory lesions should not be biopsied by means of a shave.

1. Clean and anesthetize the area.

2. If a substantial margin of tissue surrounding and below the lesion is needed, the shave should take place immediately after injection of anesthesia, when the tissue is still elevated from the injection fluid (Fig. 37-2, *inset, right*). Tissue is removed with a lateral (horizontal) "sawing" motion of a No. 15 scalpel blade, a halved Gillette Super Blue Blade, a Persona Blade, or DermaBlade on the level of the surrounding skin (Fig. 37-2). The last three blades have the potential advantages of being thinner, sharper, and more flexible. When handheld, they can be used flat or bent to the precise arc desired to conform to the shape of the lesion and the depth of the biopsy. Presuming the elevated lesion alone is being removed, it is necessary before proceeding to wait a few minutes until any sublesional swelling subsides (Fig. 37-2, *inset, left*). Tissue may then be put into formalin and submitted for pathologic examination.

   a. Biopsy of a flat or depressed lesion may be performed by a saucerization technique, although this procedure requires even greater clinical judgment and technical expertise. It is used to obtain both superficial and deep tissues down to subcutaneous fat.

   b. Pedunculated lesions may be easily removed by use of scissor biopsy.

3. Pressure, ferric subsulfate (Monsel's solution), 20% aluminum chloride in ethyl alcohol, or electrodesiccation may be used for hemostasis.

C. Surgical excision biopsy should be considered when (i) there are lesions with active expanding borders; (ii) the junction of lesion and normal skin is important to survey; (iii) the lesions are atrophic, sclerotic, or bullous; (iv) it is important to acquire adequate full-thickness skin, for example, in panniculitis such as erythema nodosum; and (v) the lesion may be melanoma.

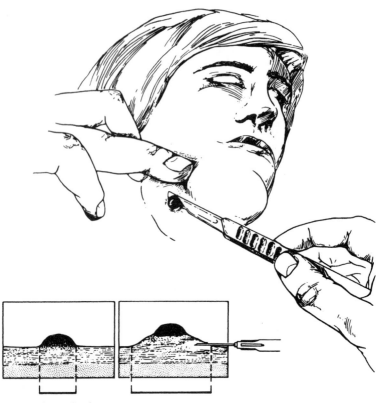

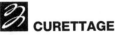

Areas to be excised

Figure 37-2. Shave biopsy technique.

CURETTAGE

I. DISCUSSION. Curettage is a simple and useful technique for removing benign cutaneous lesions such as warts, molluscum, milia, and keratoses; combined with electrodesiccation, it is also effective for treating basal and squamous cell carcinomas. Curettage before excision or Mohs' micrographic surgery allows the surgeon to define the margins of the tumor better. The curette, a cutting instrument with a circular or oval, loop-shaped cutting edge and a handle, is available in varying sizes. Large curettes will remove masses of tissue more quickly, whereas smaller ones are needed to probe for small extensions of lesions into subjacent dermis; the curette 4 mm in diameter appears to be the most generally useful one. The more friable the tissue, the easier it is to curette. Curettage is difficult to perform on normal skin or on lesions covered with a full thickness of intact skin. The curette is neither sharp enough nor does it have sufficient strength for this purpose, and the resulting tissue is usually too fragmented and distorted for pathologic examination.

II. PROCEDURE

A. Clean the area with alcohol.

B. Anesthesia is not always necessary. The process of anesthetizing can be more painful than the surgical procedure in removal of lesions such as seborrheic keratoses,

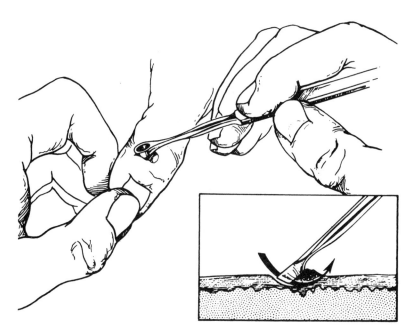

Figure 37-3. Curettage technique.

molluscum, and milia. If anesthesia is used, wait until any swelling has diminished or subsided, because it is difficult to scrape the spongy tissue.

C. Apply the cutting edge of the curette to the lesions, and remove the tissue with a firm, quick, downward scoop (Fig. 37-3). The first tissue removed will come off relatively intact and should be submitted for pathologic examination if indicated. Scrape the base and margins of the lesion well. Normal dermis is resilient and feels rough and scratchy when scraped, whereas most lesions are of softer composition.

D. Hemostasis is secured by pressure, hemostatic agents (ferric subsulfate [Monsel's solution], 20% aluminum chloride in ethyl alcohol [Drysol]), or electrodesiccation. Use of pressure alone yields the best cosmetic result.

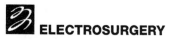 **ELECTROSURGERY**

I. DISCUSSION. The small electrosurgical units found most often in physicians' offices and in hospital clinics are versatile and useful tools. They deliver a high-frequency alternating current, producing an electrical field about the tip of the treatment electrode. The high resistance of tissue to this electric current generates heat. The electrode tip delivers the current but does not become hot.

The principal uses of electrosurgery are (i) the destruction of benign superficial lesions such as warts, keratoses, and skin tags; (ii) hemostasis and the ablation of vascular growths and (iii) the destruction of some malignant tumors of the skin. Special precautions should be taken when using these instruments on patients with indwelling cardiac pacemakers (especially the spontaneous, demand type) or implanted cardiac defibrillators. There is considerable risk of spread of hepatitis B or other viral-associated infections such as acquired immunodeficiency syndrome (AIDS) from patient to patient with the use of reusable, nonsterilized electrosurgical electrode tips. Transmission of hepatitis B virus by such electrodes has been demonstrated during simulated use with electrodesiccation and has been documented with reusable needles such as those for ear piercing, tattoo procedures, or acupuncture. Sterile disposable needle electrodes should be used for the procedure. If only reusable needle electrodes are available, gas or steam sterilization is recommended after each use.

A. Electrodesiccation and electrofulguration produce superficial destruction by dehydrating cells. Both types of electrosurgery are monoterminal, markedly damped, high-voltage (2,000 V or more), low-amperage (100 to 1,000 mA) operations where the patient is not incorporated into the circuit. The needle is either held in contact with the tissue (electrodesiccation) or kept a short distance away (electrofulguration) and the current is transmitted through a spark. The tissue is dehydrated by the heat produced through the resistance to the electric current generated at the tissue.

B. Electrocoagulation produces a deeper, more severe destruction, primarily by heat and secondarily by disruptive mechanical forces. This operation is a biterminal, relatively low-voltage (under 200 V), low-frequency, high-amperage (2,500 to 4,000 mA) procedure in which the patient is grounded by being placed in contact with a large "indifferent" electrode. The treatment needle, placed in or on the tissue, delivers an intensely hot current and literally "boils" and coagulates the lesion. Electrocoagulation is used primarily for large lesions that require extensive destruction, some neoplasms, or very vascular tumors such as pyogenic granulomas. It produces wider and deeper damage, more scarring, and better hemostasis. However, too vigorous electrocoagulation may produce delayed hemorrhage.

C. Electrocautery uses a red-hot wire heated by a low-voltage (5 V), high-amperage (15 A) current produced by a step-down transformer with a variable reactor. In this instance, the wire is hot, is not an electrode, and no current flows into the patient. Disposable battery-operated units are available in high- and low-temperature varieties. Electrocautery is an excellent alternative when hemostasis is required in patients with indwelling cardiac pacemakers or defibrillators. The extent of tissue destruction of lesions is readily apparent and sharply localized about the cautery tip.

II. PROCEDURE

A. Clean the skin with alcohol and let dry. Alcohol and some anesthetic gases are flammable. Strict asepsis is unnecessary because the procedure is itself antiseptic.

B. Infiltrate with lidocaine containing epinephrine. Treatment of some lesions, such as telangiectatic vessels, is so rapid that anesthesia is not required.

C. When tissue is needed for histologic examination, first curette the lesion, removing all the accessible pathologic tissue. The difference in texture between abnormal and normal tissue becomes difficult to "feel" after a lesion has been altered by electrosurgery. Continue the curettage until the base and borders of the lesion are firm and clean and all pockets of abnormal material have been scraped away. If there is a diagnostic question, shave excision is a better method for obtaining intact tissue specimens for histologic study. It may be followed by curettage and electrosurgery or by electrosurgery alone.

D. Apply the electrodesiccating current onto or into the tissue and deliver recurrent bursts of electricity (Fig. 37-4). It is not necessary to deliver a large spark, because this chars tissue, leads to greater tissue destruction, and offers no added therapeutic advantage. The area being treated should be as dry as possible.

   1. Use as little current as will do the job when treating spider and other angiomas and seborrheic keratoses or when ensuring hemostasis of the base of a lesion.

   2. Warts, actinic keratoses, molluscum contagiosum, and skin tags should be treated with slightly more current. The best technique for treating warts is to insert the needle electrode into the lesion and deliver current until the lesion "bubbles." The gelatinous charred tissue is removed with a curette, and a spark of less intensity is used to desiccate the base lightly. Deeper destruction will not increase the cure rate and will result in a more prolonged healing time and excessive scarring. More precise localization of destruction may be accomplished by inserting a 30-gauge needle (attached to a plastic syringe) into the lesion and then touching the active electrode to the needle shaft.

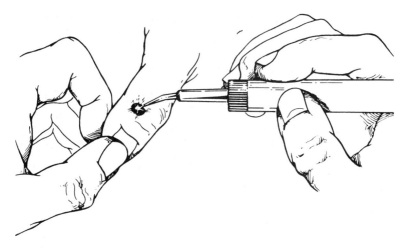

Figure 37-4. Electrosurgical technique.

3. Repeated curettage and a wider margin are needed when removing malignant cutaneous neoplasms.

E. The wound produced by electrosurgery is best treated with a topical bland or antibiotic ointment and dressing. Reepithelialization takes place from the base and sides of the lesion and is complete in 1 to 6 weeks, depending on the size of the lesion, its location, and the amount and depth of tissue destruction.

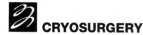 **CRYOSURGERY**

I. DISCUSSION. The application of graded degrees of cold to the skin may be used to treat a wide spectrum of skin conditions, including preneoplastic and neoplastic processes. In addition, benign problems such as seborrheic keratoses, viral warts, lentigines, keloids, and myxoid cysts, as well as other conditions, may be treated with cryosurgery. Cryogenic agents are easy to apply, usually require no anesthesia, and cause epidermal–dermal separation above the basement membrane, thereby leaving no scarring after reepithelialization. The lower the boiling point of the agent, the more efficient its freezing capabilities. The boiling point of Freon 11 is $+23.8°C$; that of ethyl chloride, $+13.1°C$; that of Freon 114, $+3.6°C$; that of dichlorotetrafluoroethane (Frigiderm), $+3.6°C$; that of Freon 12, $-29.8°C$; that of solid CO_2, $-78.5°C$; that of liquid nitrous oxide, $-89.5°C$; and that of liquid nitrogen, $-195.6°C$. Liquid nitrogen, which is readily available from medical and industrial sources, is inexpensive, noncombustible, and has become a standard therapeutic agent.

Skin is relatively resistant to freezing because of its rich vascular supply and because frozen tissue itself acts as a good insulator. Although skin freezes at 0 to $-2°C$, it is necessary to cool tissue to -18 to $-30°C$ for destruction to occur. Application of liquid nitrogen to the skin with a cotton-tipped applicator stick four times within 60 seconds will lower the temperature 2 mm below the cutaneous surface to $-18°C$. Direct spray of liquid nitrogen for an equal period will cool the tissue to $-90°C$ and, after 120 seconds, to $-125°C$ at 2 mm and $-70°C$ at 5 mm below the skin's surface. Such temperatures are needed only for cryosurgery of skin cancer. The degree of injury is roughly proportional to the intensity of freezing. Repeated freeze thawing is more damaging than a single freeze. Rapid cooling and slow thawing produce the most damage.

The exact mechanism of injury is unclear, but the following changes, all of which take place in frozen tissue, may be operative at any time: (i) mechanical damage to cells by intracellular and extracellular ice formation, (ii) osmotic changes related to dehydration of cells and increased concentration of electrolytes as a result of water withdrawal during ice crystal formation, (iii) thermal shock, a term used to denote a precipitous fall in the temperature of living cells to subnormal temperatures above 0°C, (iv) denaturation of lipid–protein complexes within the cell membrane, and (v) vascular stasis due to freezing of feeding vessels with resulting necrosis of tissue.

Freezing with liquid nitrogen is accompanied by a stinging, burning pain that peaks during thawing approximately 2 minutes after treatment is over. It is usually unnecessary to use local anesthesia. Pressure, which increases both the rate and depth of freezing, should be applied only to lesions over thick, hyperkeratotic sites such as the feet. Freezing of lesions on the hands, feet, lips, ears, and eyelids is more painful

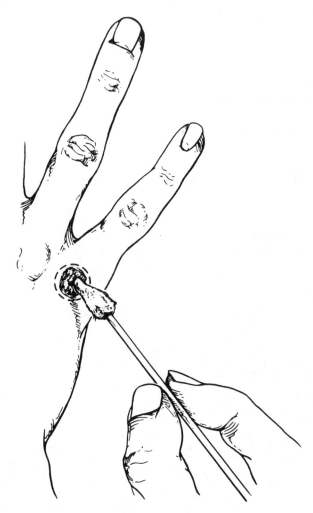

Figure 37-5. Cryosurgical technique. Liquid nitrogen is delivered to the lesion on a loosely wrapped cotton-tipped applicator stick (or larger cotton swab). The nitrogen should be repeatedly applied until the freezing front extends 1 to 3 mm around the lesion (*dotted line*).

than elsewhere. Within minutes of thawing, a triple response with redness, wheal, and surrounding flare will develop. Intense edema or a blister at the dermoepidermal junction forms 3 to 6 hours later, flattens in 2 to 3 days, and sloughs off in 2 to 4 weeks. Reepithelialization is under way within 72 hours of superficial freezing, and superinfection is rare. Melanocytes, which begin to die in the range of -3 to $-14°C$, are more susceptible to cold injury than keratinocytes; mild hypopigmentation is sometimes seen in areas previously frozen with liquid nitrogen. Cryosurgery may also produce nerve damage, and extra care should be taken when treating areas in which nerves lie superficially (e.g., the sides of the fingers). Because the nerve sheath is relatively resistant to cold injury, sensory loss is almost always temporary, though a year or more may pass before full recovery of normal sensation.

II. PROCEDURE

A. Liquid nitrogen is best kept in specially made vacuum flasks and may be poured into an insulated plastic cup or spray apparatus for immediate use. Liquid nitrogen can rarely cause normal thermos bottles to explode. An air vent must always be present in all storage apparatus.

B. When using the application tip method, dip a loosely wrapped cotton-tipped applicator into the nitrogen and place it promptly onto the cutaneous lesion (Fig. 37-5). Large fluffy swabs such as those used for sigmoidoscopy or gynecologic examination will hold greater amounts of nitrogen. When these are used, the cotton tip should be shaped into a point slightly smaller than the lesion under treatment. Do not apply pressure routinely. Thick lesions should be surgically pared first and may be treated with moderate pressure. Small lesions are treated most successfully by interrupting contact between the applicator and skin frequently, preventing the zone of freezing from extending to a greater depth and width than necessary. Large lesions can be treated by rolling the applicator over the surface.

C. A 5- to 30-second application is adequate for small, superficial lesions, such as lentigines, especially when located on thin skin. Most other benign growths, such as warts, keratoses, and molluscum contagiosum, require a 10- to 60-second application. Within seconds, the lesion begins to turn white. Nitrogen is applied repeatedly until the white freezing front extends 1 to 3 mm onto the surrounding normal skin (Fig. 37-5). The zone of frozen tissue reaches a depth of 1.5 to 2.0 mm within 1 minute of the initiation of nitrogen application and does not advance significantly farther. If using spray technique, apply for shorter times, because freezing occurs more rapidly at greater depth.

D. The posttreatment lesion usually requires no dressings. If a topical anesthetic cream such as 4% to 5% lidocaine is applied to lesions in the immediate posttreatment period, pain will be sharply diminished. If a blister forms, it may be large or hemorrhagic. If it is uncomfortable or awkward, it may be decompressed with a sterile blade or pin, leaving the roof intact. Patients with warts should be seen in 2 to 4 weeks, at which time the lesions are debrided and any remaining wart tissue is either refrozen or treated with caustics or electrodesiccation.

Suggested Readings

Boughton RS, Spenser SK. Electrosurgical fundamentals. *J Am Acad Dermatol* 1987;16: 862–867.

Graham GF. Cryosurgery. *Clin Plast Surg* 1993;20:131.

Heidenheim M, Jemice GBE. Side effects of cryotherapy. *J Am Acad Dermatol* 1991;24:653.

Johnson TM, Tromovitch TA, Swanson NA. Combined curettage and excision: a treatment method for primary basal cell carcinoma. *J Am Acad Dermatol* 1991;24:613–617.

Kuflik EG, Gage AA. The five-year cure rate achieved by cryosurgery for skin cancer. *J Am Acad Dermatol* 1991;24:1002–1004.

Kuflik EG. Cryosurgery for cutaneous malignancy. *Dermatol Surg* 1997;23:1081–1087.

Morganroth GS, Leffel DJ. Nonexcisional treatment of benign and premalignant cutaneous lesions. *Clin Plast Surg* 1993;20:91–104.

Sebben JE. Electrosurgery and cardiac pacemakers. *J Am Acad Dermatol* 1983;9:457–463.

Sebben JE. Electrosurgery: high frequency modalities. *J Dermatol Surg Oncol* 1988;14:367–371.

Sebben JE. Electrosurgery principles: cutting current and cutaneous surgery, part I. *J Dermatol Surg Oncol* 1988;14:29–31.

Sebben JE. Electrosurgery principles: cutting current and cutaneous surgery, part II. *J Dermatol Surg Oncol* 1988;14:147–150.

Sebben JE. Monopolar and bipolar treatment. *J Dermatol Surg Oncol* 1989;15:364–366.

Stewart JH, Chinn SE, Cole GW, et al. Neutralized lidocaine with epinephrine for local anesthesia, part II. *J Dermatol Surg Oncol* 1990;16:842–845.

Younis I, Bhutiani RP. Taking the 'ouch' out—effect of buffering commercial xylocaine on infiltration and procedure pain—a prospective, randomised, double-blind, controlled trial. *Ann R Coll Surg Engl* 2004;86(3):213–217.

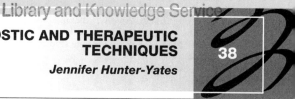

DIAGNOSTIC AND THERAPEUTIC TECHNIQUES

38

Jennifer Hunter-Yates

CYTOLOGIC SMEARS

I. DISCUSSION. Cytologic techniques in dermatology are useful in the diagnosis of bullous diseases, vesicular viral eruptions, and molluscum contagiosum. Examination of the smear is not a substitute for a biopsy, but it does enable multiple lesions to be tested on repeated occasions and allows immediate confirmation of some disease processes.

II. TECHNIQUE

A. Select an early lesion that shows no signs of trauma or infection.

B. Separate or remove the blister top with a scalpel or sharp scissors. Absorb excess fluid with a gauze pad.

C. Gently remove the blister contents and scrape the floor of the vesicle with a No. 10 or No. 15 scalpel blade or curette. Do not provoke bleeding.

D. Make a thin smear on a clean glass slide. With solid lesions such as molluscum, squeeze the material between two slides.

E. Air-dry. If the following reagents are available, fix tissue by dipping it four to five times in 95% ethanol or methanol or immerse the slide in these solutions for 1 to 2 minutes.

F. Stain with Wright, Giemsa (one-half dilution with tap water for 30 to 40 seconds), or hematoxylin and eosin stain.

G. Microscopic appearance. Examine first with a low-power objective to gain an impression of cell size and depth of stain relationships, then examine with $45\times$ or oil objective for the morphologic details.

  1. The Tzanck smear can identify an infection as herpetic in origin but cannot distinguish between herpes simplex virus and varicella-zoster virus. Between 60% and 70% of Tzanck smears show the characteristic changes of herpesvirus infection, including large, bizarre, epidermal mononucleate and multinucleate giant cells, and "ballooning degeneration." The giant cells contain eight to ten nuclei, which are often molded and may vary in size and shape. Occasionally, intranuclear inclusion bodies may be identified. For more specific identification of the causative virus, direct immunofluorescent antibody staining provides a rapid and useful laboratory aid.

  2. Molluscum contagiosum bodies appear as multiple, large, oval to round, smooth-bordered masses up to 25 μm in diameter.

  3. In most bullous eruptions, the smear will show only inflammatory cells. In pemphigus vulgaris, benign familial pemphigus, and staphylococcal scalded-skin syndrome, numerous rounded acantholytic epidermal cells with large nuclei and condensed cytoplasm are found.

FUNGAL SCRAPING AND CULTURE

I. DISCUSSION. Two techniques are available for diagnostic confirmation of a fungal infection: direct microscopy and fungal cultures. Immediate confirmation of the presence of a fungal infection may be accomplished easily by microscopic identification of organisms. Fungal culture will identify the causative organism specifically. This is therapeutically important because some nondermatophytic molds [*Hendersonula toruloidea*

(*Nattrassia mangiferae*) and *Scytalidium hyalinum*], as well as *Candida* "species," may mimic dermatophytes on potassium hydroxide (KOH) examination but are often resistant to conventional dermatophyte therapy. All scaling lesions from the scalp, angles of the mouth, axillae, groin, inframammary area, and feet, as well as blisters on the hands and feet, should be considered for both studies.

II. TECHNIQUE

A. Scraping examination

  1. Skin

    a. If lesions are soiled or macerated, clean the skin well with alcohol and let dry.

    b. Scrape with a scalpel or edge of a microscope slide at the active border of a lesion and collect scales on a glass slide. With blistering eruptions, the fungus is in the roof of the vesicle, which can be (i) gently dissected off with sharp scissors or scalpel or (ii) reflected back and the underside scraped with a No. 15 scalpel blade.

    c. When obtaining culture specimens from anxious or uncooperative patients, vigorous rubbing of the lesion with a moistened sterile cotton swab provides an effective atraumatic alternative to actual scraping (1).

    d. Small, thin fragments of tissue may be examined directly. Large pieces should be minced with a scalpel blade. Thick pieces should be discarded.

    e. Gather scrapings together in the center of the slide.

    f. Cover with Swartz–Lamkins stain (SLS) or 10% to 20% KOH and a coverslip and heat gently, but not to boiling, for 15 to 30 seconds. Note that two types of KOH are available: one in water and the other in dimethyl sulfoxide (DMSO). The KOH in DMSO does not require heating.

    g. SLS preparations can be examined immediately. Let KOH slides cool for 10 minutes (during which time the tissue is hydrolyzed and rendered clear), and then press the coverslip gently to flatten the tissue and push out air bubbles.

    h. Examine under a scanning lens or high-dry magnification. It is very important to avoid getting KOH on the microscope objective, because it will etch the lens. The diaphragm should be closed down and the condenser lowered as far as possible. The ease of identification of hyphae varies inversely with the intensity of light passing through the slide.

    i. With SLS, hyphae and spores appear blue against the unstained background of cells. The fungal stain consists of a dye, a surfactant to clear the tissues quickly, and less KOH (2%) than will etch glass and ruin microscope lenses. Because the hyphae stain selectively and are seen more easily with SLS, slides may be scanned more quickly at a lower power.

      In KOH preparations, hyphae and spores will stand out as refractile tubes and oval bodies against the background of cells and debris. It is not possible to make a species identification from tissue scrapings.

  2. Hair and nails

    a. Examine the scalp with a Wood's lamp. If individual lesions fluoresce, pull out 10 to 15 hairs for examination. Otherwise, examine scales and 10 to 15 random hairs from the involved site. Fungus invades the hair in two ways: ectothrix involvement, where the hair shaft is surrounded by tiny spores, and endothrix infection, where the spores are found inside the hair shaft. Ectothrix fungi include *Microsporum* species as well as *Trichophyton mentagrophytes* and *Trichophyton verrucosum*. Endothrix infections are seen with *Trichophyton tonsurans, Trichophyton violaceum,* and *Trichophyton schoenleinii*. Altered, dystrophic, hypertrophic, or pigmented nails should be snipped off and minced on a slide. Subungual debris is less suitable for examination.

    b. Heat the specimen on a slide or in a test tube with 10% to 40% KOH and let cool for 15 to 30 minutes. Tissue may then be stained with SLS or examined directly.

B. **Culture.** In addition to direct examination of scales, scrapings from a suspicious lesion should be cultured at room temperature on Sabouraud's glucose agar,

Sabouraud's agar with chloramphenicol and cyclohexamide (Mycobiotic, Mycosel), or dermatophyte test medium (DTM). Sabouraud's agar with chloramphenicol and cyclohexamide is more selective for dermatophytes because the chloramphenicol inhibits bacteria and the cyclohexamide inhibits contaminants. DTM contains cyclohexamide, gentamicin, and chlortetracycline, preventing growth of bacteria and saprophytic fungi. DTM contains phenol red, which turns the agar from yellow to bright red when its pH becomes alkaline from dermatophyte growth. Contaminant growth does not alter the pH of the medium. Using DTM medium, the specimen should be inoculated onto the media and the cap loosely placed, thereby providing the fungi with the air they require for growth. If no color change takes place within 2 weeks, the culture may be discarded. If the color does change, it may be presumed that a pathogenic dermatophyte or yeast is present. Microscopic examination of the culture (culture mount) should then identify the exact species.

 WOOD'S LIGHT EXAMINATION

I. **DISCUSSION.** Wood's glass, primarily barium silicate containing 9% nickel oxide, is opaque to all light except for a band extending from 320 to 400 nm. When light from a high-pressure mercury arc is passed through this filter, it is principally the 360-nm radiation that is transmitted as Wood's light. Fluorescent bulbs (black lights) that emit a similar, although slightly broader, spectrum are also available. The Wood's light was first found to have medical importance in detecting fungal infections, but it is useful for many other diagnostic tasks as well. Because ointments, exudates, tetracycline in sweat, makeup, deodorants, and soap may fluoresce, the skin should be well cleansed before examination, except if erythrasma is suspected. Wood's lamp examination may be used in the following situations:

A. **Detection and control of scalp ringworm.** Hairs infected with *Microsporum audouinii*, *Microsporum canis*, or *Microsporum distortum* fluoresce a bright blue green. Fluorescent hairs may be selected for microscopic examination and culture. Pteridine compounds have been postulated as the cause of this fluorescence. As normal hair regrows, a band of nonfluorescent hair will emerge. The emergence of *T. tonsurans*, a nonfluorescent dermatophyte, as the most common cause of tinea capitis limits the usefulness of Wood's lamp examination for screening purposes.

B. **Detection of other fungal infections.** Tinea versicolor may fluoresce a golden yellow. Although this is often imperceptible, Wood's light examination nevertheless allows the accompanying pigmentary changes to be seen more vividly.

C. Detection of bacterial infections

1. Erythrasma, an intertriginous infection caused by *Corynebacterium minutissimum*, fluoresces a brilliant coral red or pink orange. The fluorescent substance is a water-soluble porphyrin and, therefore, may not be present if the area has been washed recently.

2. *Pseudomonas aeruginosa* infections give off a yellow-green fluorescence due to pyocyanin. Fluorescence due to fluorescein is detectable before obvious purulence appears, and it is useful in screening burn patients for infections.

D. **Delineation of pigmentary disorders.** Long-wave ultraviolet light (UVL) is transmitted into the dermis, where it gives a white to blue-white fluorescent color. Melanin present in the epidermis (but not dermis) acts to absorb long-wave UVL and thereby prevents this "white" color. Under Wood's light, variations in epidermal pigmentations (freckles, melasma, vitiligo) are more apparent, and variations in dermal pigmentation (Mongolian spot, some instances of postinflammatory hyperpigmentation) are less apparent or unchanged compared with their appearance in ambient visible light. Wood's light accentuates the contrast between pigmented and nonpigmented skin, but, more importantly, it separates hypopigmented from totally amelanotic areas (the latter have true white to blue-white fluorescence). It is used for examining patients with vitiligo, albinism, leprosy, and other disorders of hypopigmentation and is also useful as a screening procedure in nurseries to look for the small, ash-leaf-shaped, white macules, indicative of tuberous sclerosis.

E. Detection of porphyrins. Acidified urine, feces, and, rarely, blister fluid from patients with porphyria cutanea tarda will fluoresce a brilliant pink orange.

F. Drug detection. Patients who ingested tetracycline in childhood during formation of their deciduous teeth may have teeth which fluoresce yellow. A pink fluorescence of the nail bed lunulae can be observed in patients on oral tetracycline therapy, whereas topical therapy will produce yellow fluorescence of the treated sites.

G. Miscellaneous. Fluorescent ingredients or markers in cosmetics, medications, or industrial compounds may be detected with Wood's lamp examination.

 PATCH TESTING

I. DISCUSSION. Patch testing is used to document and validate a diagnosis of allergic contact sensitization and to identify the causative agent. It may also be of value as a screening procedure in some patients with chronic or unexplained eczematous eruptions (e.g., hand and foot dermatoses). It is a unique means of *in vivo* reproduction of disease in diminutive proportions, because sensitization affects the whole body and may therefore be elicited at any cutaneous site. The patch test is easier and safer than a "use test" because test items can be applied in low concentrations on small areas of skin for short periods of time.

II. TECHNIQUE

A. Delay patch testing until any acute inflammation has subsided. Reexposure to the antigen may cause the eruption to flare. Neither low-dose systemic steroids nor antihistamines will influence the results.

B. Test only with potential allergens. There are no methods available for assaying primary irritants easily.

C. Be certain that the substances being tested will not irritate the skin. Cosmetics may be applied full strength, but items of unknown irritant potential should be diluted to 1% to 2% in petrolatum, mineral oil, or less preferably, water. Suitable dilution and vehicle data are available in Fisher's Contact Dermatitis (2001), other references cited at the end of this chapter, and the textbooks mentioned previously (2).

D. The True Test is a prepackaged double adhesive strip with the 24 most common allergens in the United States. This is a general screen and tests <2% of the >3,700 known allergens. The True Test identifies the cause of the allergic contact dermatitis in <80% of patients. This testing is limited and can miss some other important allergens such as newer preservatives and corticosteroids. Supplemental allergens can be purchased and applied individually.

Apply test substances to a disk of filter paper bound to plastic-coated aluminum (Al-Test) or in Finn chambers and attach to the skin with occlusive tape. The Al-Test is the standard utilized by the North American and International Contact Dermatitis groups. Alternatively, one can use a 1-in. square piece of soft cotton (Webril) and cover with occlusive tape (Scanpor) or cellophane and tape. A smaller patch, which may be slightly less effective, may be applied with a 1/4-in. piece of gauze, linen, cotton, or filter paper and covered with tape (or Dermicel for those who cannot tolerate tape). Liquids and ointments may be applied directly to the cotton or gauze. Volatile liquids should be applied directly to the skin and allowed to dry before being covered. Solids must be powdered before application. Moisten powders and fabrics with water before application. The site of application should be normal hairless skin on the back or inner arms. Pay careful attention to applying the appropriate concentration of the test substance. Too high a concentration may result in a false-positive reaction or may even sensitize the patient.

E. Leave the patches in place for 48 hours. If pain, pruritus, or irritation under a patch is noted, the patient should remove it at once. Readings should not be made until the patches have been off at least 20 to 30 minutes, because positive reactions may not be immediately apparent. Delayed reactions are not uncommon, and a final reading should be made at 4 days (96 hours).

F. The results are interpreted and noted as follows:

?+ = doubtful reaction

+ = weak (nonvesicular) reaction—erythema and/or papules

++ = strong (edematous or vesicular) reaction—erythema, papules, and/or small vesicles

+ + + = extreme reaction—all the foregoing plus large vesicles, bullae, and at times, ulceration

IR = irritant reaction

A positive patch test only proves that the patient has a contact sensitivity but not necessarily that the eliciting substance is the cause of the clinical eruption.

G. False-negative tests may be caused by the following:

1. Low concentration or insufficient amount of antigen.
2. Improper testing, including inadequate occlusion, inappropriate vehicle, wrong site, incorrect reading times, or deteriorating substances.
3. Depressed reactivity owing to the administration of high amounts of systemic steroids or recent and aggressive topical steroid application.
4. Failure to reproduce the true conditions of exposure to antigen and lack of heat, friction, or trauma.

H. False-positive tests may be related to the following:

1. Primary irritant reactions.
2. Tape reactions and pressure effects.
3. Reactions to occlusion: maceration, miliaria, and folliculitis.
4. Contamination from another site.
5. Presence of impurities in the test material.
6. Multiple concomitant positive patch tests may result in a state of hyperreactivity (excited skin syndrome or angry back syndrome). Subsequent retesting with individual allergens will reveal those that were reactive spuriously (3).

I. Once developed, positive reactions may sometimes take several weeks to subside. A topical corticosteroid may be used on test sites with active or prolonged inflammation. Patch tests positive at 2 days and negative at 3 to 2 days are often irritant in origin.

ULTRAVIOLET LIGHT THERAPY

I. DISCUSSION. UVL, the part of the electromagnetic spectrum that begins next to the violet end of the color spectrum (400 nm) and extends to the beginning of the x-ray region (200 nm), may be used in the therapy of psoriasis, vitiligo, cutaneous T-cell lymphoma (mycosis fungoides), eosinophilic pustular folliculitis, pityriasis rosea, and chronic eczematous eruptions, as well as uremic or aquagenic pruritus. It has also been used in conjunction with psoralens administration for photochemotherapy of psoriasis, vitiligo, cutaneous T-cell lymphoma, alopecia areata, chronic graft-versus-host disease, and urticaria pigmentosa. In addition to these standard therapies, it may also be used as effective prophylactic therapy for polymorphous light eruption and other photodermatoses. UVL causes many profound biologic changes, including temporary suppression of epidermal basal cell division, followed by a later increase in cell turnover, and UVL-induced immunosuppression. The UVL spectrum is subdivided into three bands: ultraviolet C [UVC (200 to 290 nm)], UVB (290 to 320 nm), and UVA (320 to 400 nm). Each region has different photobiologic characteristics and will be discussed here separately.

II. SOURCES AND TECHNIQUES

A. Sunlight is often the optimal source of UVL. It is the least expensive and most effective under most circumstances. Sun emits radiation with a continuous emission spectrum. The ozone layer in the upper atmosphere acts as a filter and absorbs virtually all UVL <290 nm. The erythema dose for a fair-skinned person is

20 minutes at latitude 41 degrees (Boston) at midday in June. The disadvantages of sunlight radiation are its variable absorption by clouds and the difficulty in controlling or monitoring its intensity.

B. UVC radiation from artificial sources is present in operating room germicidal lamps and in cold quartz lamps. These lamps (low-pressure, low-temperature mercury arcs) emit a band of radiation predominantly at 253.7 nm through a quartz envelope filter. The erythema dose is 30 seconds at 25 cm. The advantages are that (i) little or no pigmentation follows the erythema and (ii) severe burns cannot occur, because large increases in exposure time lead to only minimal increases in redness. Cold quartz radiation has been used to produce erythema and desquamation in acne patients, particularly in pigmented individuals who wish to avoid more intense melanin pigmentation. UVC radiation can cause a painful conjunctivitis after only seconds of exposure. You should not look directly into these lamps or spend much time around the lamp without adequate protection (protective clothing, glasses, and sunscreens).

C. UVB radiation is responsible for most of the therapeutic effects of sunlight and conventional artificial UVL therapy. Detailed protocols for aggressive UVB phototherapy of psoriasis have been developed and are very effective. They are administered best in hospital or office settings using UVB fluorescent bulb–lined phototherapy booths. UVB dose depends on skin type; skin type depends on constitutive color or inherent melanin content, as well as facultative color or genetic capacity to tan. Occasionally, patients may want to treat small areas of psoriasis at home. There are several sources of UVB for clinical use as follows:

1. UVB sources

a. Fluorescent sunlamp bulbs (FS40) (low-pressure, low-temperature mercury arc sources) emit a continuous spectrum with a peak at 313 nm. The radiation is filtered through calcium, zinc, and thallium phosphate phosphor in the glass envelope. The erythema dose is 90 to 120 seconds at 25 cm. These lamps are easily obtainable, relatively inexpensive, and good sources of sunburn radiation (290 to 320 nm). They are frequently used as a bank of four bulbs for home use or constructed into a light box lined by reflecting metal and many 2-, 4-, and/or 6-ft lamps for office or clinic use. Six units of 4- or 6-ft-long bulbs, which can be wall mounted or hung from door frames, are available for home phototherapy at a reasonable cost.

Narrowband UVB (311 to 312 nm) therapy using a Philips bulb model TL-01 has greater selectivity for the treatment of psoriasis. Other reports document its usefulness in vitiligo, cutaneous T-cell lymphoma, and disseminated cutaneous lichen planus. A standard minimum erythema dose (MED) must be obtained at baseline for dosimetry; treatments are typically delivered three times a week starting at 50% of the MED and then increasing by 10% to 15% increments. Narrowband UVB phototherapy has also been combined with psoralens. Long-term studies are still required to further define the efficacy and safety parameters of narrowband UVB, but it appears to confer less risk than psoralens plus ultraviolet A (PUVA) in terms of carcinogenesis.

b. Sunlamp bulbs or units are low-pressure mercury lamps that emit UVL in the sunburn spectrum.

c. Hot quartz lamps (high-pressure, high-temperature mercury arc sources) emit a discontinuous UVL spectrum with bands at 254, 265, 297, 303, 313, and 365 nm but with particular effectiveness in the erythema-producing midrange. The erythema dose is 30 to 60 seconds at 46 cm. Overexposure can lead to severe burns. These large lamps (Hanovia) are expensive and have been used primarily for hospital and office patient care. Booths containing fluorescent bulbs emitting UVB or UVA have generally supplanted use of hot quartz lamps.

D. UVA radiation from sunlight or fluorescent tubes will not, by itself, cause erythema or pigmentation except with extremely large doses. However, in the presence of a circulating photosensitizer such as psoralens, the long-wave UVL spectrum becomes an excellent therapeutic tool. This combination of light and drug is termed

photochemotherapy or **PUVA therapy.** In the doses used, neither the drug alone nor the light alone has any biologic activity. Absorption of electromagnetic energy in the UVA wave band in the presence of psoralens results in transient inhibition of deoxyribonucleic acid (DNA) synthesis as well as alterations of immune reactivity. PUVA treatment is useful in severe psoriasis and is also effective in some patients with vitiligo and mycosis fungoides. It is sometimes helpful in treating atopic dermatitis and other inflammatory dermatoses. PUVA therapy can be restricted to hand/foot exposure for limited disease. The treatment regimen is divided into a clearance phase, with more frequent therapy, and a maintenance phase after clinical response. Dosing of methoxsalen (Oxsoralen-Ultra) depends on weight (0.4 mg/kg); the pills should be taken 2 hours before light exposure. A fatty meal may enhance absorption. Topical PUVA requires application of 0.1% methoxsalen (Oxsoralen-Ultra) in Cetaphil 20 minutes before UVA.

Short-term side effects of PUVA therapy include tanning, pruritus, nausea, headache, and dizziness. Long-term side effects include cataracts, lentigines, photoaging, squamous cell carcinoma, and melanoma. An ophthalmologic examination should be done before starting PUVA. Also, an antinuclear antibody (ANA) blood test should be confirmed negative. Contraindications to PUVA include lupus erythematosus, xeroderma pigmentosum, pregnancy, and severe liver or kidney disease. PUVA should also be avoided in children and in patients with pemphigus vulgaris, bullous pemphigoid, multiple skin cancers, or a family history of melanoma.

For the treatment of psoriasis, PUVA may be combined with other modalities (methotrexate, retinoids), thereby reducing the number of PUVA treatments needed to attain remission, as well as reducing adverse effects from treatment and overall cost.

1. UVA sources
   a. Fluorescent blacklight lamps (FS40BL) (low-pressure, low-temperature mercury arcs) emit a spectrum of 320 to 450 nm filtered through the barium disilicate phosphor in their glass envelopes. The peak emissions vary dramatically, depending on the bulb manufacturer; this variability and their overall low-intensity UVA emission limit their usefulness.
   b. High-intensity UVA fluorescent bulbs were developed by GTE Sylvania, and it is these and similar bulbs that are best used in PUVA light boxes.
   c. PUVA treatment boxes are used in hospital clinics and in some dermatologists' offices. Two hours after ingestion of 8-methoxypsoralen, patients are exposed to incremental doses of UVA, starting at 1 to 5 J/cm² (approximately 2 to 10 minutes), depending on the degree of melanization and skin type determination of a minimum phototoxic dose (MPD) (see Chap. 33). The treatment protocols are complicated, should be administered only under the direction of dermatologists experienced in their use, and will not be discussed here.
   d. Sunlight-produced UVA can be used with psoralens for the treatment of vitiligo and psoriasis. This technique is potentially dangerous because it is nearly impossible to gauge UVL exposure accurately, and, hence, severe burns can result.
   e. A topical psoralens solution can be painted on the skin of the hands and feet and then exposed to UVA radiation from a hand/foot unit. This method minimizes the total ultraviolet exposure, although care must be taken to protect the normal surrounding skin.
   f. Some physicians advocate the delivery of psoralens through bath water immersion in a diluted solution of psoralens before the administration of the UVA. Studies have found equal efficacy and, more importantly, decreased total radiation requirement with this treatment option.
2. Biologic reaction to PUVA
   a. The redness caused by PUVA may be absent or minimal at 12 to 24 hours after exposure (when UVB erythema is most intense) and may peak at 48 to 72 hours or later. Severe PUVA burns can continue to intensify for up to 1 week after exposure and can be treated with prednisone.

b. PUVA pigmentation, which appears clinically and histologically similar to normal UVB-induced melanogenesis (tanning), maximizes approximately 5 to 7 days after exposure, may become very intense after repeated PUVA treatments, and lasts longer than a normal suntan, sometimes weeks to many months.

c. Repeated high-dose UVA or PUVA exposure to laboratory animals causes cataracts and skin cancer, just as UVB or sun exposure does. An increased number of basal cell carcinomas, squamous cell carcinomas, and melanoma have been found in patients with long-term PUVA psoriasis. Men being treated with PUVA therapy should always wear some form of protection for their genital skin. Patients must be observed carefully for evidence of accelerated actinic damage and melanoma and nonmelanoma skin cancers. Sunglasses with UVA-blocking properties must be worn on PUVA treatment days to decrease UVA exposure to the lens of the eye.

PHOTODYNAMIC THERAPY

I. DISCUSSION. Photodynamic therapy (PDT) is used to treat numerous skin diseases, most commonly actinic keratoses and superficial nonmelanoma skin cancers. PDT involves exposure to a photosensitizer followed by light activation and resultant cell death through the formation of singlet oxygen and other free radicals. Because the photosensitizer concentrates in epidermal cells with higher metabolic activity (i.e., rapidly growing cells found in malignancies, hair follicles, and sebaceous glands), more singlet oxygen and other free radicals accumulate in, and more damage is done to, the desired target as compared with normal skin. The light source used must emit a wavelength which falls within the absorption spectrum of the photosensitizing agent for activation to occur.

PDT has been reported in the medical literature since the early 1900s, and its use by dermatologists to treat actinic keratoses and superficial nonmelanoma skin cancers has increased recently, particularly when large body surface areas require treatment. PDT has also been reported to be effective in the treatment of actinic cheilitis, acne vulgaris, sebaceous hyperplasia, localized scleroderma, cutaneous T-cell lymphoma, Hailey-Hailey disease, psoriasis, human papillomavirus, molluscum contagiosum, and other cutaneous infections. In addition, PDT is currently being used for photorejuvenation in sun-damaged skin.

II. TECHNIQUE. Patients undergoing PDT must first be exposed to a photosensitizer. Photosensitizing agents may be either systemic [e.g., porphimer sodium (Photofrin)] or topical [e.g., 5-aminolevulinic acid (ALA)]. Topical ALA is converted to protoporphyrin IX, a potent photosensitizer. The absorption spectrum for porphyrins, including porphimer sodium and protoporphyrin IX, exhibits a maximum peak in the Soret band ranging from 360 to 400 nm and smaller peaks between 500 and 635 nm. Topical use of ALA has become more widespread because of ease of application and accumulation in desired target lesions. Typically, 20% ALA solution (with 48% ethanol) is applied to the area to be treated and left in place for several hours (14 to 18 hours per initial protocols). Newer studies suggest that shorter incubation time (15 to 60 minutes) does not decrease the effectiveness of treatment but may help minimize side effects and increase treatment convenience.

After an appropriate incubation time, the patient is exposed to a light source. Many different light sources have been used, such as incoherent sources (slide projectors, halogen lamps, xenon lamps, and fluorescent lamps), blue light (405 to 420 nm), red light (635 nm), pulsed dye lasers (585 nm), and intense pulsed light sources (500 to 1,200 nm). Depth of penetration is proportional to the wavelength of the light source. Hence, longer wavelengths may be more effective in the treatment of thicker skin lesions, whereas shorter wavelengths may be used for superficial lesions. Recommended times of exposure and light dosing vary considerably, depending on the disease and the light source used. PDT may be repeated at various intervals if needed.

Stinging, burning, itching, and localized erythema and edema at the treatment site have been reported from PDT. Pain and hyperpigmentation of the treatment site are less common side effects but have been reported, especially with the treatment of acne vulgaris. Treated lesions, which respond to PDT, often exhibit scaling and crusting followed by healing in 2 to 8 weeks. Severe reactions such as blistering and ulceration are rare and may signify overexposure to light or increased sensitivity to light (as seen in diseases such as porphyria cutanea tarda and systemic lupus erythematosus). Prolonged cutaneous photosensitivity is the major side effect encountered in patients treated with PDT. Patients receiving PDT should be counseled to avoid sunlight and excessive indoor light and to use appropriate protective measures (sunscreen and tightly woven clothing) for approximately 1 to 2 weeks after treatment.

References

1. Head ES, Henry JC, Macdonald EM. The cotton swab technique for the culture of dermatophyte infections—its efficacy and merit. *J Am Acad Dermatol* 1984;11:797–801.
2. Rietschel RL, Fowler JF, eds. *Fisher's contact dermatitis*, 5th ed. Baltimore, MD: Lippincott Williams & Wilkins, 2001.
3. Bruynzeel DP, Maibach HI. Excited skin syndrome (angry back). *Arch Dermatol* 1986; 122:323–328.

Suggested Readings

Alam M, Dover JS. Treatment of photoaging with topical aminolevulinic acid and light. *Skin Therapy Lett* 2004;9(10):7–9.

Alexiades-Armenakas MR, Geronemus RG. Laser-mediated photodynamic therapy of actinic keratoses. *Arch Dermatol* 2003;139:1313–1320.

Alster TS, Tanzi EL. Photodynamic therapy with topical aminolevulinic acid and pulsed dye laser irradiation for sebaceous hyperplasia. *J Drugs Dermatol* 2003;2(5):501–504.

Alster TS, Tanzi EL, Welsh EC. Photorejuvenation of facial skin with topical 20% 5-aminolevulinic acid and intense pulsed light treatment: a split-face comparison study. *J Drugs Dermatol* 2005;4(1):35–38.

Belsito DV. Patch testing with a standard allergen ("screening") tray: rewards and risks. *Dermatol Ther* 2004;17(3):231–239.

Cohen DE, Brancaccio R, Andersen D, et al. Utility of a standard allergen series alone in the evaluation of allergic contact dermatitis: a retrospective study of 732 patients. *J Am Acad Dermatol* 1997;36:914–918.

Coors EA, von den Driesch P. Topical photodynamic therapy for patients with therapy-resistant lesions of cutaneous T-cell lymphoma. *J Am Acad Dermatol* 2004;50:363–367.

Daniel CR III. The diagnosis of nail fungus infection revisited [editorial]. *Arch Dermatol* 2000;136:1162–1164.

Enk CD, Elad S, Vexler A, et al. Chronic graft-versus-host disease treated with UVB phototherapy. *Bone Marrow Transplant* 1998;22(12):1179–1183.

Ferguson J. The use of narrowband UV-B (tube lamp) in the management of skin disease. *Arch Dermatol* 1999;135:589–590.

Fisher AA. Special issue: the current status of contact dermatitis. *Cutis* 1993;52:237–322.

Gathers RC, Scherschun L, Malick F, et al. Narrowband UVB phototherapy for early-stage mycosis fungoides. *J Am Acad Dermatol* 2002;47(2):191–197.

Gold MH, Bradshaw VL, Boring MM, et al. Treatment of sebaceous gland hyperplasia by photodynamic therapy with 5-aminolevulinic acid and a blue light source or intense pulsed light source. *J Drugs Dermatol* 2004;3(6):S6–S9.

Gold MH, Goldman MP. 5-aminolevulinic acid photodynamic therapy: where we have been and where we are going. *Dermatol Surg* 2004;30:1077–1084.

Goossens A, Matura M, Degreef H. Reactions to corticosteroids: some new aspects regarding cross-sensitivity. *Cutis* 2000;65:43–45.

Habib F, Stoebner PE, Picot E, et al. Narrowband UVB phototherapy in the treatment of widespread lichen planus. *Ann Dermatol Venereol* 2005;132(1):17–20.

Krob HA, Fleischer AB Jr, D'Agostino R Jr, et al. Prevalence and relevance of contact dermatitis allergens: a meta-analysis of 15 years of published T.R.U.E. test data. *J Am Acad Dermatol* 2004;51(3):349–353.

Laube S, George SA. Adverse effects with PUVA and UVB phototherapy. *J Dermatolog Treat* 2001;12(2):101–105.

Lawry M, Haneke E, Strobeck K, et al. Methods for diagnosing onychomycosis. *Arch Dermatol* 2000;136:1112–1116.

Man I, Dawe RS, Ferguson J. Artificial hardening for polymorphic light eruption: practical points from ten years' experience. *Photodermatol Photoimmunol Photomed* 1999; 15:96–99.

Morison WL, Baughman RD, Day RM, et al. Consensus workshop on the toxic effects of long-term PUVA therapy. *Arch Dermatol* 1998;134:595–598.

Morison WL. Phototherapy and photochemotherapy: an update. *Semin Cutan Med Surg* 1999;18:297–306.

Nahass GT, Goldstein BA, Zhu WY, et al. Comparison of Tzanck smear, viral culture, and DNA diagnostic methods in detection of herpes simplex and varicella-zoster infection. *JAMA* 1992;18:2541–2544.

Piacquadio DJ, Chen DM, Farber HF, et al. Photodynamic therapy with aminolevulinic acid topical solution and visible blue light in the treatment of multiple actinic keratoses of the face and scalp. *Arch Dermatol* 2004;140:41–46.

Pratt MD, Belsito DV, DeLeo VA, et al. North American Contact Dermatitis Group patch-test results, 2001–2002 study period. *Dermatitis* 2004;15(4):176–183.

Rietschel RL. Experience with supplemental allergens in the diagnosis of contact dermatitis. *Cutis* 2000;65:27–30.

Ruiz-Rodriguez R, Alvarez JG, Jaen P, et al. Photodynamic therapy with 5-aminolevulinic acid for recalcitrant familial benign pemphigus (Hailey-Hailey disease). *J Am Acad Dermatol* 2002;47(5):740–742.

Ruocco V, Ruocco E. Tzanck smear, an old test for the new millennium: when and how. *Int J Dermatol* 1999;38:830–834.

Scherschun L, Kim JJ, Lim HW. Narrow-band ultraviolet B is a useful and well-tolerated treatment for vitiligo. *J Am Acad Dermatol* 2001;44(6):999–1003.

Tanew A, Radakovic-Fijan S, Schemper M, et al. Narrowband UV-B phototherapy vs. photochemotherapy in the treatment of chronic plaque-type psoriasis. *Arch Dermatol* 1999;135:519–524.

Taub AF. Photodynamic therapy for the treatment of acne: a pilot study. *J Drugs Dermatol* 2004;3(6):S10–S14.

Treatment Principles and Formulary

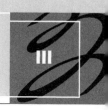

III

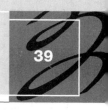

DERMATOLOGIC PRESCRIPTIONS AND DRUG COSTS

The prescribing of medications today is very different from the early 1900s, when most medications were compounded on the basis of physicians' recipes. Currently, hundreds of single-ingredient as well as multiple-ingredient products are available to the dermatologist, both in prescription and over-the-counter forms. The fixed-dose combination products can offer effective alternatives to extemporaneous products compounded by the pharmacist. A wide range of fixed-dose products are now available, many offering comparable therapeutic benefits but at different costs. A major factor to influence price is whether the product is generic or branded. A drug manufacturer has exclusive rights to a compound it develops for the first 17 years after discovery (not market entry, but creation and patenting of the chemical entity). This product will possess a commercial brand name, making it readily identifiable, and a generic chemical name. Only the brand name is available until the patent expires, unless the company signs a licensing agreement with another firm. Once patent expiration occurs, generic forms are manufactured and available to the market. In most states, once a U.S. Food and Drug Administration (FDA)-approved generic product is available, the pharmacist must dispense the less expensive version unless the physician specifically writes "no substitution" or "dispense as written" or checks the appropriate box on the prescription. In most cases, generic products are less expensive than brand-name versions, but the difference can range from as little as pennies to as much as 50% to 80%. The exception to this is insurance arrangements where patients pay a fixed amount (co-pay) per prescription. This price may be less for a generic version or could be the same for all prescriptions. Although generics have to meet FDA specifications to be marketed as equivalent, permissible variations in the vehicle or base may produce alterations in products.

Another essential component of economically prudent prescribing is package size, where larger tubes (60 g) cost less per gram than smaller (15- or 30-g) ones. Although there are books available listing the retail pharmacies' acquisition costs of medications (Drug Topics Red Book and American Druggist Blue Book), these become outdated quickly because of the twice-yearly price changes from drug manufacturers. The most accurate way to gauge patient cost is to speak to your local pharmacist. The retail marketplace for prescriptions is very competitive, with an average profit on a prescription of approximately 20% (i.e., the pharmacy acquires the drug for $20 and sells it for $24). As a rule, generic drugs cost, on average, 30% to 40% less than brand names. By working closely with neighboring pharmacies and using a consistent selection of prescription products, the pharmacist will be more likely to carry the products you prescribe, often purchasing them in volume and providing them at a lower cost to your patients. Lastly, be sure to write all prescriptions with explicit directions for use, including duration of treatment when applicable. The pharmacist will put this on the medication label, preventing any confusion or errors in patient understanding.

TYPES OF TOPICAL MEDICATIONS

It is important to note that there are two variables in topical therapy. Both the medication and the vehicle chosen must be appropriate for the condition being treated. In general, acute inflammation is treated with aqueous drying preparations, and chronic inflammation is treated with greasier, more lubricating compounds (see also Chap. 40, Dermatologic Topical Preparations and Vehicles).

I. POWDERS. Powders promote drying by increasing the effective skin surface area. They are used primarily in intertriginous areas to reduce moisture, maceration, and friction. Powders may be inert or may contain active medications. They may be nonabsorptive, making the skin slippery (talc), or absorptive (cellulose). Absorptive powders may form clumps or small aggregates after absorbing water and can act as irritants.

II. LIQUIDS. Lotions consist of suspensions of a powder in water. Tinctures are alcoholic or hydroalcoholic solutions. As lotions and tinctures evaporate, they cool and dry; lotions leave a uniform film of powder on the skin. Sprays and aerosols act in a similar manner. Active agents are often incorporated into the aqueous phase.

III. CREAMS AND GELS. Creams are semisolid emulsions of oil in water (O/W). As the proportion of oil increases and the proportion of water decreases, the preparation becomes more viscous and at some undefined ratio will no longer be considered a cream, but will enter the classification of ointments. A gel is a transparent and colorless semisolid emulsion that liquifies on contact with the skin, drying as a thin, greaseless, nonocclusive, nonstaining film. Aqueous, acetone, alcohol, or propylene glycol gels of organic polymers such as agar, gelatin, methylcellulose, pectin, and polyethylene glycol are primarily used.

IV. OINTMENTS. These consist of water droplets suspended in the continuous phase of oil (W/O) or of inert bases such as petrolatum. Ointments are of three types: those soluble in water, those that will emulsify with water, and those completely insoluble in water.

V. PASTES. These, which are rarely used today, are mixtures of a powder and an ointment.

VI. OPEN WET DRESSINGS. These types of dressings cool and dry through evaporation. They therefore cause vasoconstriction, decreasing the augmented local blood flow present in inflammation. In addition, wet dressings cleanse the skin of exudates, crusts, and debris and help maintain drainage of infected areas. They are indicated in the therapy of acute inflammatory conditions, erosions, and ulcers. Although various medicaments and antibacterial substances may be added for specific causes, water is by far the most important ingredient of wet dressings. Wet dressings covered by an impermeable cover (closed wet dressings) retain heat, prevent evaporation, and cause maceration, which may not be desirable.

VII. LUBRICANTS, BASES, AND PROTECTIVE COVERINGS. The following preparations are most often used as lubricants, bases in which to incorporate drugs, and protective coverings for the skin:

A. The oil-in-water creams, which are water washable ("vanishing cream") and cosmetically pleasing, account for most topical items prescribed.

B. Water-in-oil emulsions, which are better lubricants than oil-in-water creams, retain heat, impede water loss, increase hydration, and may thereby encourage percutaneous absorption. Because W/O preparations are occlusive, they should be avoided in oozing or infected areas. To provide smooth mixtures, dispersing and emulsifying agents, surfactants, and detergents are usually added to these emulsions.

C. Lotions and sprays are most easily applied to hirsute areas and scalp.

 AMOUNT TO DISPENSE

It will become apparent on long-term patient follow-up that when inadequate amounts of medication are dispensed, the patient will tend to apply too little, will use the drugs less frequently than prescribed, will soon run out of medication, and then may not refill the prescription. If a medication is known to be effective and is to be used on a long-term basis, dispensing large quantities will be more economical and will ensure continuous supply, resulting in better treatment.

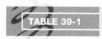

| TABLE 39-1 | | | Amount of Topical Medication Needed for Single or Multiple Application(s) | | |

Area treated	One application (g)	b.i.d. for 1 wk (g)	t.i.d. for 2 wks (g)	b.i.d. for 1 mo (g)	t.i.d. for 6 wks (g)
Hands, head, face, anogenital area	2	28	90 (3 oz)	120 (4 oz)	270 (9 oz)
One arm, anterior or posterior trunk	3	42	120 (4 oz)	180 (6 oz)	360 (12 oz)
One leg	4	56	180 (6 oz)	240 (8 oz)	540 (18 oz)
Entire body	30–60	420–840 (14–28 oz)	1.26–2.52 kg (42–84 oz; 2.5–5 lb)	1.8–3.6 kg (60–120 oz; 3.75–7.5 lb)	3.8–7.5 kg (126–252 oz; 7.5–15 lb)

One gram of cream will cover an area of skin approximately 10 cm by 10 cm, or approximately 100 sq. cm, assuming a layer 100 μm in thickness. The same amount of ointment will cover an area 5% to 10% larger. Total body self-application of different vehicles was studied in 29 adults and found to average 22 g. Subjects used twice as much medication from a large jar than from a small tube. Table 39-1 gives conservative figures for the amounts needed for a single application of an ointment or cream and for t.i.d. application for a 2-week period.

The fingertip unit (FTU) is a practical, visually simple means of explaining how much ointment is adequate to cover a specific region. One FTU is the amount of ointment expressed from a tube with a 5-mm-diameter nozzle applied from the distal skin crease to the tip of the index finger, roughly equivalent to 0.5 g. The area of involved skin covered by one flat, closed hand requires approximately 0.5 FTU, or 0.25 g, of ointment. Four hand areas require 2 FTUs, or 1 g, of ointment. Also, the number of ounces of ointment needed for one application per day equals the number of grams needed for a single application.

 GENERAL PRINCIPLES OF NORMAL SKIN CARE

Recommendations for the care of normal skin are based on principles of moderation and common sense as well as on knowledge derived from the study of skin structure and function. Routine daily care is far simpler than one may be led to believe by the profusion of astounding advertising claims. Whereas much is known about adverse reactions to cosmetics and other products for topical use, well-controlled scientific studies related to the care and maintenance of healthy skin are either so limited or so rudimentary that they preclude precise recommendations in most instances. "Normal" skin refers to skin that is not affected by any disease process. Within "normal," there is obviously a wide variation of skin textures, complexions, and appearances. The principles in this section are applicable to almost everyone within this category, whether the skin is on the "dry" or the "oily" end of the spectrum. The various systems and categorizations of skin types so readily available at cosmetic counters of department stores yield little useful information, are not based on any basic pathophysiologic principles, and are useful primarily for the cosmetic company whose products are subsequently recommended. It is not at all clear that normal skin benefits from much, if anything at all, in the way of specific care, except for protection from harsh chemical and physical agents (especially sunlight). On the other hand, many products used for skin care or cosmetic purposes can occasionally produce adverse reactions, such as allergic and irritant contact dermatitis, phototoxic and photoallergic reactions, and induction of acne (acne cosmetica). Neither price range nor brand name provides absolute assurance that a given product will be of high quality or will not cause adverse reactions. The area of skin care is beset with an amazing number of unsubstantiated claims, "secret" ingredients, and fads. It is beyond the scope of this book to address all of them.

I. PROTECTION

A. Changes induced by sunlight are the major factors in causing alterations in the skin that contribute to the appearance of aging. Sunscreens and sunblocking agents can prevent or retard these changes. The more fair the skin, the stronger the indication for a stronger sun-protective agent.

    1. A variety of topical agents can camouflage the appearance of aging or induce transient changes that make the skin look or feel "younger." For example, mild irritation caused by certain chemicals in "rubefacient" masks accomplishes this by inducing mild erythema and edema. Apart from cosmetic surgical techniques, the same generally applies to remedies for wrinkles and for sagging. Application of tretinoin, adapalene, or tazarotene cream will not prevent aging, but can alter, or "normalize," keratinization in photodamaged skin and may induce production of new dermal collagen. Wrinkles and dyspigmentation may diminish. α-Hydroxy acids (glycolic, lactic) may bring about similar changes.

B. Efforts to protect the skin from harsh chemicals (e.g., strong acids and alkalis) and physical agents (e.g., cold, wind, and extreme dryness) that may damage the skin are also sensible and desirable.

II. NUTRITION

A. The normal epidermis, hair follicles, and nail matrices receive their nutrition from the cutaneous (dermal) vasculature, and there is little evidence that any topically applied "nutrient" can enhance their performance. Except in *bona fide* nutritional disorders such as avitaminoses (e.g., pellagra), there is no convincing proof that any dietary supplement can enhance skin, hair, or nail growth.

B. Because the stratum corneum, hair, and nails consist of dead cells, there is no evidence or reason to believe that external application of "protein," "amino acids," "collagen," "elastin," ribonucleic acid ("RNA"), "nucleic acids," or the like will have anything more than a transient effect on the appearance or texture of the skin or its appendages.

III. CLEANING THE SKIN; "FACIALS"

A. Soap is not inherently harmful to the skin. Use of cleansing creams instead of soap has no benefits and may induce acneform lesions.

B. However, excessive washing with water and with soap or detergents can lead to dryness of the skin. Also, exposure to air with low relative humidity in either a warm or cold environment permits a significant degree of moisture loss from the skin.

C. The use of a "mild" soap or detergent bar, and a reduction in the number of washings per day (to once, twice, or at most three times) will minimize the drying effects of washing. Recent studies showed that the soap-like cleanser Dove was the least irritating among 18 soaps and detergent bars tested.

    1. People who are obliged to wash their hands frequently are well advised to use as little soap as possible and to apply an emollient such as petrolatum or an O/W lubricant after washing.

D. The pH of normal skin at its surface is approximately 6.8. Most soaps and shampoos are alkaline. Whereas extremes of acid or alkaline pH may be harmful to hair or skin, no skin care or cosmetic product—even inexpensive ones—achieves such extremes. For the most part, products that claim to be "pH balanced" offer no particular advantage over other products on that score alone.

E. Facial massage, saunas, mud packs, pore cleaning, "facials," and so on, may temporarily improve the appearance of the skin but have not been shown to have any long-term beneficial effects other than those that can be attributed to looking and feeling good (which may be substantial).

IV. ASTRINGENTS; FACIAL MASKS; CLARIFIERS; LARGE PORES

A. "Large pores" can be camouflaged or temporarily altered but cannot be permanently changed or prevented.

B. Astringents, also called skin bracers or after-shave lotions in products for men, contain water (as much as 50%) and alcohol or witch hazel. As the alcohol evaporates, it cools the skin, which is interpreted as feeling refreshed.

1. Astringents with aluminum salts (alum) added are called **refiners.** Alum irritates the skin and causes mild erythema and edema, which makes the face rosy and the pores look transiently smaller.

C. Clarifiers are meant to act as keratolytics. The lotions may contain resorcinol or salicylates, and the cleansers contain grains that are scrubbing agents. They are meant to thin the stratum corneum to leave the skin rosy and refreshed.

D. Masks, which may contain an absorbent clay or synthetic resin, form a film that tightens on the skin as it dries. This produces mild irritation and similar effects as noted for astringents.

V. LUBRICATING THE SKIN

A. Water is the most important plasticizer of the epidermis. Used appropriately, emollients or "moisturizers" can restore water to the skin for a short period or help the skin retain moisture when applied after bathing.

1. Emollients may make the skin look better or feel more supple transiently, but there is no evidence that aging or wrinkling can be slowed down or prevented by such measures. Furthermore, some emollients can cause or exacerbate acne.

2. The most effective lubricants are usually the least cosmetically acceptable— petrolatum, mineral and "baby" oil (Albolene or Eucerin). The next most helpful ones are O/W emulsions such as cold creams and Nivea Skin Oil, which contains oils, fatty alcohols, and waxes with emulsifiers and humectants. The least effective but most comfortable ones to use are W/O creams and "moisturizers," which are principally water along with emulsifiers, colors, fragrances, preservatives, and humectants.

B. Certain lipids and oils are thought to lubricate the skin by reducing surface friction between lamellae of the stratum corneum. "Humectants" such as lactic acid and urea may enhance the water-bearing capacity of the stratum corneum and hold water in the skin for prolonged times.

C. A variety of compounds such as aloe, jojoba oil, and vitamin E receive commercial attention as lubricants, for cosmetic use, and as home healing aids. Some have been in use as folk remedies for many years. How they will stand up to rigorous testing remains to be seen. On the other hand, cases of allergic sensitization to such substances have been reported.

VI. HAIR CARE

A. Daily shampooing of normal scalp and hair will not ordinarily cause dryness or other damage and will remove exfoliated skin and debris.

1. If hair becomes too alkaline, the cuticular cells may become rough and the hair catches and looks dull.

2. Detergents may be more alkaline than soaps. Sodium lauryl sulfate and ammonium lauryl sulfate are the strongest; laureth sulfate detergents are less alkaline; the amphoterics, which are present in some baby shampoos, are the mildest.

B. Use of electric rollers, curling irons, hot combs, and exposure to permanent waving solutions can alter and "dry out" hair and make it more brittle. This damage only affects hair that has already grown out of the follicle; hair growth is not altered.

C. Physical abuses to hair, such as some straightening techniques, and hairstyles that promote prolonged traction on hair can cause follicular scarring and permanent alopecia.

D. Acid hair rinses counteract the temporary effects of the alkaline shampoos, smooth down cuticular cells, and reduce swelling of the hair shaft so that the hair looks smooth and shiny.

1. They also change the electrical charge on the hair and remove mineral deposits left by soaps.

E. Conditioning rinses put an oily coating back on the hair to replace that removed by the shampoo. In addition to ingredients that change the electrical charge, they also contain emollients, thickeners, preservatives, humectants, fragrances, colors, and sometimes an alkali to make the hair swell so that the conditioner can penetrate.

1. These rinses are useful for hair damaged by chemical treatments, physical abuse, or excessive exposure to ultraviolet light or harsh weather.

VII. "HYPOALLERGENIC" AND "NONCOMEDOGENIC"

    A. "Hypoallergenic" cosmetics are theoretically designed to eliminate the most common and notorious allergy-producing compounds but still contain components allergenic to some individuals. The term *hypoallergenic* does not necessarily imply that there are fewer antigens present. Any product may legally call itself "hypoallergenic."

        1. Even inexpensive cosmetics are usually screened and tested quite thoroughly to eliminate potential allergens. The rate of adverse reactions to cosmetics of all types is quite low.

    B. A long history of problem-free use is no guarantee that a particular product is not the cause of an allergic reaction. It is possible for an individual to become allergic to a compound even if it has been applied to the skin for years without difficulty. Furthermore, manufacturers may change the ingredients in a preparation without concomitant labeling changes.

        1. The investigation and prevention of allergic contact dermatitis from cosmetic products may be complex and require dedication on the part of patient and physician. A single fragrance or scent may contain >200 chemicals. It is often necessary to discontinue use of all cosmetics.

    C. Persons with suspected allergies to cosmetic ingredients will often benefit from patch testing, so knowledge of sensitivity to particular compounds can help in the choice of alternative products. In some instances, it is wise for individuals with multiple sensitivities or with sensitivity to an undetermined compound to perform pre-use open patch tests.

    D. Acne cosmetica is not an allergic reaction but is caused by the inclusion of comedogenic substances that can be found in many cosmetic products, especially emollients and oil-based makeups. Hypoallergenic does not mean noncomedogenic. Some notable comedogenic compounds are sodium lauryl sulfate, isopropyl isostearate, isopropyl myristate, butyl stearate, hexadecyl alcohol, lauryl alcohol, oleic acid, lanolin, and cocoa butter.

    E. Water-based, rather than oil-based, cosmetics should be used to decrease the risk of acne cosmetica in susceptible individuals. "Oil-free" cosmetics are not necessarily noncomedogenic and may contain certain comedogenic organic oils. Some soaps also contain comedogenic materials; certain "creamy" or "moisturizing" soaps should be avoided by individuals with acne.

VIII. IT IS DIFFICULT TO RECOMMEND SPECIFIC PRODUCTS. Except for advice to be on the lookout for adverse reactions, trial and error in combination with individual preference is about the only rational way for people with normal skin to choose among most cosmetic products.

Suggested Readings

Begoun P. *Don't go to the cosmetics counter without me*, 4th ed., Tukwila, WA: Beginning Press, 1999.

Schoen LA, Lazar P. *The look you like: medical answers to 400 questions on skin and hair care*. New York: Marcel Dekker Inc, 1990.

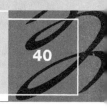
$\mathcal{T}$his chapter includes the topical and systemic medications most useful in treating cutaneous disease. Drugs are listed alphabetically in each instance. This chapter is not a complete listing of all the pharmaceutical preparations available for dermatologic use, and many useful products may have been omitted. For uniformity and ease of conversion, all package sizes are listed in metric terms (Table 40-1). Medications that require a prescription are noted by R_x.

 ACNE PREPARATIONS

I. DISCUSSION. See Chap. 1.

II. PRESCRIPTION DRUGS

A. Isotretinoin (13-*cis*-retinoic acid, Accutane, Amnesteem)

1. Structure: cis isomer of tretinoin.

2. Use: See Chap. 1. Note: Patients allergic to parabens will also react to isotretinoin, which contains these agents as preservatives. Isotretinoin also contains glycerin and ethylenediamine tetraacetic acid (EDTA) in a soybean suspension. Isotretinoin is also useful in disorders of keratinization.

3. Adverse effects: Isotretinoin is teratogenic to humans and should not be administered to pregnant women or women contemplating pregnancy. Refer to Chap. 1 for a complete list of adverse effects. Concomitant use of isotretinoin with drugs of the tetracycline class increases the incidence of *Pseudotumor cerebri*. There have been recent reports of an increased risk of depression, suicide, and suicide attempts in individuals taking isotretinoin, but the causality has not been absolutely proved. The manufacturers have formulated a new informed consent to reflect these concerns. No population-based studies have documented this risk to date. The manufacturers have also initiated risk management programs to prevent adverse outcomes. The U.S. Food and Drug Administration (FDA) approved a combined program named *iPledge*.

4. Packaging:

Isotretinoin soft gelatin capsules, 10 mg, 20 mg, 30 mg, 40 mg: packs of 10.

B. Spironolactone

1. Structure: Synthetic steroid that resembles aldosterone.

Spironolactone

TABLE 40-1	Metric Measures with Approximate Equivalents

Liquid measure	Weight	Length (exact equivalents)
4000.0 mL = 1 gal (4 qt)	1 kg = 2.20 lb (Av.)	1 m = 39.37 in. 30.48 cm = 1 ft.
1000.0 mL (1 L) = 1 qt (32 oz)	0.454 kg = 1 lb 454 g = 16 oz (lb Av.)	2.54 cm = 1 in. 1 cm = 0.39 in. 1 mm = 0.04 in.
500.0 mL = 1 pt (16 oz)	30 g = 1 oz 4 g = 60 gr (1 dr)	
250.0 mL = 8 fluid oz	1 g = 15 gr	
30.0 mL = 1 fluid oz	60 mg = 1 gr	
15.0 mL = 1 tbsp		
5.0 mL = 1 tsp		
4.0 mL = 1 dr		
0.06 mL = 1 minim, the rough equivalent of 1 drop		

Note: 1 milliliter (mL) = 1 cubic centimeter (cc): Most of these approximate dose equivalents have been approved by the U.S. Food and Drug Administration. They may be used as a convenience in prescribing, but must not be used for compounding specific pharmaceutical formulas.

> 2. **Use:** See Chap. 1. Also useful for other androgen-responsive disorders such as hirsutism. Poor tolerance in men owing to adverse endocrine side effects.
> 3. **Packaging (Searle):**
>   Spironolactone: 25-mg, 50-mg, 100-mg tablets
> C. Tretinoin (vitamin A acid, Retin-A, Retin-A Micro, Avita, Renova)
>   1. **Structure:** *trans*-Retinoic acid.

Tretinoin

> 2. **Contains:** 0.05% tretinoin (vitamin A acid) in the liquid; 0.1%, 0.05%, or 0.025% in the cream; and 0.01%, 0.025%, or 0.04% in the gel. The 0.025% cream or 0.01% gel is usually the least irritating. Tretinoin does not function as a vitamin in this therapy.
>   Retin-A Micro gel 0.1% and 0.04% contain small time-released microsponges that are designed to release the drug slowly into the upper layer of skin and, therefore, to decrease irritation. Avita cream 0.025% and gel 0.025% contain a large polymer that also releases the drug slowly.
>   Renova was formulated in a water-in-mineral oil emollient base for the mature complexion and for the indication of photoaging. This product could conceivably make acne worse because of the base.

3. **Use:** See Chap. 1. Tretinoin is a photosensitizing agent. Therapy need not be discontinued during times of increased ultraviolet (UV) exposure, but patients should be instructed in photoprotection. Tretinoin does not function as a vitamin in this therapy.
4. **Packaging (many companies):**
   Avita, 0.025% cream, 0.025% gel: 20-g, 45-g tube
   Renova, 0.02%, 0.05%, cream: 20-g, 40-g, 60-g tube
   Retin-A Micro gel, 0.1%, 0.04%: 20-g, 45-g
   Tretinoin 0.05% liquid: 28-mL bottle
   Tretinoin 0.025%, 0.05%, 0.1% cream: 20-g, 45-g tube
   Tretinoin 0.01%, 0.025% gel: 15-g, 45-g tube

D. Tazarotene (Tazorac)
1. **Structure:** Retinoid prodrug, converted to active form, the carboxylic acid of tazarotene by rapid de-esterification. This drug binds to all three retinoic acid receptors with some increased affinity for the β and γ receptors.
2. **Use:** See Chap. 1. Also useful in treatment of plaque psoriasis. Tazorac is a Pregnancy Category X drug; adequate birth control measures should be emphasized with women in their childbearing years.
3. **Packaging:**
   Tazarotene 0.05%, 0.1% gel: 30-g, 100-g tube
   Tazarotene 0.05%, 0.1% cream: 15-g, 30-g, 60-g tube

E. Adapalene (Differin)
1. **Structure:** Retinoid-like compound that binds to retinoic acid nuclear receptors, but not to cytoplasmic receptor proteins.
2. **Contains:** 0.1% solution in 30% alcohol.
3. **Use:** See Chap. 1.
4. **Packaging:**
   Adapalene 0.1% solution: 30-mL bottle
   Adapalene 0.1% cream: 45-g tube
   Adapalene 0.1% gel: 45-g tube
   Adapalene 0.1% pledgets: 60/box

F. Benzoyl peroxide preparations [also available over the counter (OTC)]
1. **Structure:** (Owing to the myriad of manufacturers and products, the following consists of only a partial list of the available preparations.)

$$O=C-O-O-C=O$$

Benzoyl peroxide

2. **Contains:** 2.5%, 3%, 4%, 5%, 6%, 8%, 9%, or 10% benzoyl peroxide, oil-base lotion alcohol gel base (PanOxyl/AQ); aqueous gel base (Benzac W, Desquam-E, Desquam-X); aqueous base cleanser with EDTA (Desquam-X Wash), glycerin base cleanser (Benzac AC Wash), aqueous base cleanser with menthol, glycolic acid, lactic acid, and zinc (Triaz).
3. **Use:** See Chap. 1.
4. **Packaging:**
   Benzagel wash, 10%: 60 g
   Benzac 5%, 10% gel: 60 g
   Benzac AC gel 2.5%, 5%, 10%: 60 g, 90 g
   Benzac AC liquid wash 2.5%, 5%, 10%: 8 oz
   Benzac W gel 2.5%, 5%, 10%: 60 g, 90 g

Benzac W liquid wash 5%, 10%: 4 oz, 8 oz
Brevoxyl gel 4%, 8%: 42.5 g, 90 g
Brevoxyl cleanser 4%, 8%: 170 g
Desquam-E gel 5%, 10%: 42.5 g
Desquam-X gel 5%, 10%: 42.5 g, 85 g
Desquam-X bar, 10%: 106 g
Pan Oxyl gel, 5%, 10%: 56.7 g, 113.4 g
Pan Oxyl AQ gel 2.5%, 5%, 10%: 56.7 g, 113.4 g
Triaz liquid 3%, 6%, 9%, 10%: 81.5 g, 170.3 g, 340.2 g
Triaz gel 3%, 6%, 9%, 10%: 42.5 g
Triaz pad 3%, 6%, 9%: 30/box

G. Topical antibiotics

1. Clindamycin phosphate (Cleocin T, Clindets, Clindagel, ClindaMax)

   a. Contains: 10 mg/mL clindamycin as phosphate in 50% isopropyl alcohol and propylene glycol solution, in methylparaben as a topical gel or lotion, or in isopropyl alcohol as pledgets.

   b. Structure: Semisynthetic derivative of lincomycin.

   c. Use: See Chap. 1. Contraindicated in patients with a history of regional enteritis, ulcerative colitis, or antibiotic-associated colitis.

   d. Packaging:

   Clindamycin phosphate 1% suspension: 30 mL, 60 mL
   Clindamycin phosphate 1% gel: 30 g, 60 g
   Clindamycin phosphate 1% lotion: 60 mL
   Clindamycin phosphate 1% pledgets: 60/box

2. Erythromycin base solution

   a. Contains: Erythromycin base in propylene glycol and alcohol solution. The alcohol content is 92% (Erygel), 77% (EryDerm), 71% (T-stat), 66% (A/T/S), and 55% (Staticin).

   b. Structure: Macrolide antibiotic derived from *Streptomyces erythreus*.

   c. Use: See Chap. 1.

   d. Packaging: The following consists of a partial list of all available preparations.

   Akne-mycin, 2% ointment: 25 g
   A/T/S, 2% gel: 30 g
   A/T/S, 2% solution: 60 mL
   Emgel, 2% gel: 27 g, 50 g
   EryDerm, 2% solution: 60 mL
   Erygel, 2% gel: 30 g, 60 g
   Staticin, 1.5% solution: 60 mL
   T-stat, 2% solution: 60 mL
   T-stat, 2% pads: 60/box

3. Metronidazole (MetroCream, MetroGel, MetroLotion, Noritate)

   a. Contains: 0.75% and 1.0% metronidazole with parabens (MetroGel), with benzyl glycol (MetroCream) or benzyl alcohol, glycerin, and mineral oil (MetroLotion); 1% metronidazole with parabens (Noritate). Patients with parabens allergies may react to formulations containing this product.

   b. Use: See Chap. 28.

   c. Packaging:

   MetroCream 0.75% cream: 45 g
   MetroGel 0.75% and 1.0% gel: 28.4 g, 45 g
   MetroLotion 0.75% lotion: 59 mL
   Noritate 1% cream: 30 g

4. Sodium sulfacetamide (Klaron, Novacet, Sulfacet-R, Vanocin, Plexion, and others)

   a. Mechanism of action: Postulated to act as a competitive inhibitor of *para*-amino benzoic acid (PABA), which is essential for bacterial growth.

   b. Contains: 10% sodium sulfacetamide with 5% sulfur [Novacet, Plexion, Vanocin), with parabens (Sulfacet-R)]. Patients with allergies to parabens may react to Sulfacet-R. Some contain tints to camouflage the erythema associated with rosacea (Avar Green).

   c. Packaging:

       Avar cleanser 10%/5%: 226.8 g
       Avar Gel 10%/5%: 45 g
       Avar Green Gel 10%/5%: 45 g
       Clenia Cream 10%/5%: 28 g
       Clenia Foam 10%/5%: 170 mg, 340 mg
       Klaron 10% lotion: 59 mL
       Nicosyn Lotion 10%/5%: 45 g
       Novacet 10% lotion/5% sulfur: 30 mL,
       Plexion 10% cleanser/5% sulfur: 170 g, 340 g
       Plexion SCT Cream 10%/5%: 120 g
       Rosanil Cleanser 10%/5%: 170 g
       Rosula Gel 10%/5%: 45 mL
       Sulfacet-R 10% lotion/5% sulfur: 25 mL
       Vanocin 10% lotion/5% sulfur: 30 g, 60 g

H. Oral antibiotics. Indicated for inflammatory papulopustular acne (see Chap. 1)

   1. Tetracycline (Sumycin)

      a. Dosage: 1 to 2 g/day divided every 6 hours. Once improvement is noted, dosage may be reduced to 125 to 500 mg/day for maintenance.

      b. Adverse effects: Photosensitivity, abdominal discomfort, oral and vaginal yeast infections, onycholysis, discoloration of the nails, gram-negative folliculitis, glossitis, and cheilitis. Medication deposits in growing teeth and bones, and hence it is contraindicated during pregnancy, lactation, and childhood (<12 years of age). It may potentiate lithium and oral anticoagulants, as well as antagonize aminoglycosides and penicillins. May decrease effectiveness of oral contraceptives. Avoid administration with milk, meals, or antacids. Adjust dosage with renal impairment. *P. cerebri* may develop and must be managed expediently.

      c. Packaging:

          Tetracycline capsules: 250 mg, 500 mg
          Tetracycline oral suspension, 125 mg/5 mL: 473 mL

   2. Doxycycline (Vibramycin, Monodox, Doryx, Periostat, Vibra-Tabs)

      a. Dosage: 50 mg b.i.d. to q.i.d.; 100 mg q.d. to b.i.d. Recent evidence suggest that sub-antimicrobial dose of 20 mg b.i.d. is also effective. No dosage adjustments needed for renal impairment.

      b. Adverse effects: Same adverse effects as tetracycline. Doxycycline is the most significant photosensitizer of all the tetracyclines and its use should be avoided during increased UV exposure. May be taken with food and/or milk products.

      c. Packaging:

          Doxycycline capsules: 20 mg, 50 mg, 75 mg, 100 mg
          Doxycycline powder for oral suspension: 25 mg/5 mL when reconstituted
          Doxycycline syrup, 50 mg/5 mL: 473 mL
          Doxycycline tablets: 50 mg, 75 mg, 100 mg

   3. Minocycline (Minocycline HCl, Dynacin, Minocin, Vectrin)

      a. Dosage: Up to 200 mg daily in divided doses.

      b. Adverse effects: Vestibular reactions including headache and vertigo, abdominal discomfort, onycholysis, blue-gray pigmentation of the oral mucosa and sites of cutaneous inflammation or trauma, as well as generalized muddy brown pigmentation in sun-exposed regions. May possibly decrease effectiveness of oral contraceptives containing estrogens. Drug-induced systemic lupus erythematosus, leukemoid reaction, serum sickness–like reaction, pulmonary edema, pulmonary infiltrates with eosinophilia, and *P. cerebri* have been described and require expedient care. Photosensitivity is less common than with other tetracyclines. May be taken with food and/or milk products.

c. Packaging:
Minocycline capsules: 50 mg, 75 mg, 100 mg
Minocycline oral suspension, 50 mg/5 mL: 60 mL
Minocycline pelleted capsules: 50 mg, 100 mg

4. Erythromycin (Erythromycin base, EES, Ery-tabs, PCE Dispertab, erythrocin stearate, E-mycin)
   a. Dosage: 1 g/day in divided doses.
   b. Adverse effects: Abdominal pain, nausea, vomiting, and diarrhea are generally dose related. Inhibits cytochrome P-450 microsomal enzyme system and thereby decreases hepatic metabolism of some drugs, including cyclosporine, theophylline, carbamazepine, lovastatin, bromocriptine, and disopyramide. Dose adjustments of these medications must be made accordingly.
   c. Packaging: Available in enteric-coated or time-release forms to reduce amount of gastrointestinal irritation.
   Erythromycin tablets: 250 mg, 333 mg, 400 mg, 500 mg

5. Trimethoprim-sulfamethoxazole [Bactrim (DS), Cotrim (DS), Septra (DS), Trimpex]
   a. Contains: 80 mg trimethoprim and 400 mg sulfamethoxazole; DS contains 160 mg trimethoprim and 800 mg sulfamethoxazole. Trimethoprim is available as a single agent in a dose of 100 or 200 mg.
   b. Dosage: One to two tablets a day. Trimethoprim is dosed at 200 mg/24 hours given either q.d. or b.i.d.
   c. Adverse effects: Nausea, vomiting, and anorexia are generally dose related. Hypersensitivity reactions (including Stevens-Johnson syndrome and hematologic reactions) occur in <5% of patients.
   d. Packaging:
   Trimethoprim-sulfamethoxazole tablets: single or double strength (DS).

I. Other topicals
   1. Benzamycin
      a. Contains: 3% erythromycin and 5% benzoyl peroxide in 16% alcohol.
      b. Use: Apply one to two times a day. Note: Refrigerate after mixing.
      c. Packaging:
      Benzamycin gel: 23 g, 46 g
   2. Azelaic acid (Azelex, Finacea)
      a. Mechanism of action: Naturally occurring dicarboxylic acid that is bacteriostatic to *Propionibacterium acnes*. It also decreases conversion of testosterone to 5{pi}ga-dihydrotestosterone (DHT) and alters keratinization of the microcomedone. It may also be beneficial in the treatment of melasma. The mechanism of action is not fully understood. Deoxyribonucleic acid (DNA) synthesis is reduced, and mitochondrial cellular energy products are inhibited in melanocytes.
      b. Use: Apply to face b.i.d.
      c. Packaging:
      Azelaic acid cream 20%: 30 g, 50 g
      Azelaic acid gel 15%: 30 g
   3. Clindamycin/benzoyl peroxide combination (BenzaClin, Duac)
      a. Contains: 1% clindamycin and 5% benzoyl peroxide in an aqueous-based gel.
      b. Use: Apply one to two times a day. This topical combination is contraindicated in individuals with a known sensitivity to lincomycin or with a history of regional enteritis, ulcerative colitis, or antibiotic-associated colitis.
      c. Packaging:
      BenzaClin gel: 25 g
      Duac gel: 45 g

III. OTC DRUGS

  A. Structure of common ingredients

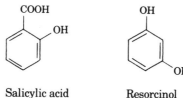

                Salicylic acid   Resorcinol

  B. Abrasive soaps

    1. Brasivol

      a. Contains: Aluminum oxide particles in a surfactant cleansing base.

      b. Use: See Chap. 1.

      c. Packaging:

           Fine, medium, or rough grain

    2. Pernox

      a. Contains: Polyethylene granules, 2% sulfur, 1.5% to 2% salicylic acid in EDTA.

      b. Use: See Chap. 1.

      c. Packaging:

           Pernox cleanser: 2 oz, 4 oz

           Pernox lotion: 4 oz

  C. Cleansers (only a few OTC products are listed in the following text)

    1. Aveeno Cleansing Bar for Acne

      a. Contains: 0.5% salicylic acid, 38% colloidal oatmeal, glycerin, and titanium dioxide. Soap-free.

      b. Use: q.d. to b.i.d.

      c. Packaging:

           Bar: 85 g

    2. Basis All Clear Bar

      a. Contains: Triclosan, tea tree oil, glycerin.

      b. Use: q.d. to b.i.d.

      c. Packaging:

           Bar: 113 g

    3. Clearasil Antibacterial Soap

      a. Contains: Triclosan

      b. Use: q.d. to b.i.d.

      c. Packaging:

           Bar: 92 g

    4. Clinique Antiacne Soap

      a. Contains: 8% sulfur, 1% resorcinol.

      b. Use: q.d. to b.i.d.

      c. Packaging:

           One bar

    5. Neutrogena Medicated Cleansing Pads

      a. Contains: 0.14% benzethonium chloride, witch hazel extract, octoxynol-9, methylparaben, menthol, peppermint, eucalyptus oil, rosemary oil, and camphor.

      b. Use: q.d. to b.i.d.

      c. Packaging:

           Individual pads: 40/box

    6. Seba-Nil Cleansing Mask

      a. Contains: SC alcohol-40, castor oil, and methylparaben.

      b. Use: p.r.n. for oily skin.

      c. Packaging:

           Mask: 105 g

7. Stri-Dex Acne Medicated Pads
  a. Contains: 0.5% salicylic acid (regular strength, sensitive skin pads) and 2% salicylic acid (maximum strength, super scrub pads).
  b. Use: q.d. to b.i.d.
  c. Packaging:
      Regular strength, jar: 55 pads
      Maximum strength, jar: 32, 55, 90 pads
      Sensitive skin pads, jar: 55, 90 pads
      Super scrub pads, jar: 55 pads
D. Other drying and antiseptic topicals. Although benzoyl peroxide, retinoic acid preparations, and topical antibiotics are the drugs of choice, a partial list of other acne medications are listed here for comparison of ingredients.
  1. Acnomel cream
    a. Contains: 8% sulfur, 2% resorcinol, and 11% alcohol in tinted vehicle.
    b. Use: Apply one to two times daily.
    c. Packaging:
        Bottle: 28 g
  2. Clearasil Adult Care
    a. Contains: 8% sulfur and 1% resorcinol.
    b. Use: Apply one to two times daily.
    c. Packaging:
        Bottle: 18 g
  3. Liquimat lotion
    a. Contains: 4% sulfur and 22% alcohol in tinted lotion in five shades.
    b. Use: Apply one to three times daily.
    c. Packaging:
        Bottle: 45 mL

 ANESTHETICS FOR TOPICAL ADMINISTRATION

See Antipruritic and External Analgesic Agents for more details.

I. DISCUSSION. Before the advent of EMLA (eutectic mixture of local anesthetics) cream, topical anesthetics had limited use because the stratum corneum provided an intact barrier through which anesthetic agents could not penetrate. In addition, although benzocaine was previously considered the most effective of the topical anesthetics, it was rarely used because of its potent sensitization capacity. EMLA represents a breakthrough in transdermal delivery of anesthesia. By combining lidocaine and prilocaine, the hydrophilic and lipophilic properties of each are enhanced, thereby allowing penetration through cornified skin. Topical anesthetics provide some relief from pain in a variety of situations, including superficial surgery, split-thickness skin grafts, venipuncture, laser surgery, epilation, and debridement of infected ulcers. Other potential uses include postherpetic neuralgia and painful ulcers. Because mucosal surfaces lack a stratum corneum, the older anesthetic agents may be used in aphthous stomatitis, primary or recurrent herpes simplex infections, or painful condyloma after treatment. Additional topical anesthetics, including LMX 4% and 5%, 4% tetracaine gel, and betacaine-LA ointment, have been developed for transdermal delivery of anesthesia. Note: With topical anesthetics, esters are potential sensitizers. It is rare for amides to induce a contact dermatitis.

Amides
      Bupivacaine
      Carticaine
      Dibucaine
      Etidocaine
      Lidocaine
      Mepivacaine
      Oxethazaine

Prilocaine
Ropivacaine
Aminobenzoate esters
Amylocaine
Benzocaine
Butacaine
Butyl aminobenzoate
Chloroprocaine
Cocaine
Isobucaine
Meprylcaine
Oxybuprocaine
Piperocaine
Procaine
Propoxycaine
Tetracaine hydrochloride
Nonamide, nonaminobenzoate esters
Benzyl alcohol
Cyclomethycaine sulfate
Diperodon
Dyclonine hydrochloride
Pramoxine hydrochloride

Local Anesthetics

Selected brand names are given, but some agents are available as generic products.

II. PRESCRIPTION DRUGS

  A. EMLA

    1. Contains: 5% eutectic mixture of 2.5% lidocaine and 2.5% prilocaine in an oil-in-water emulsion cream.

    2. Use: Application of 1/2- to 1-in. thick EMLA cream to treatment site 1 to 2 hours before a procedure, under occlusion, provides safe and effective analgesia. The duration of action depends on both the amount of cream applied and the time under occlusive dressing. There are guidelines for use of EMLA in the pediatric population.

Age and weight	Maximum dose (g)	Maximum area (cm^2)	Maximum application time (h)
Up to 3 mo or 5 kg	1	10	1
3–12 mo and 5–10 kg	2	20	4
1–6 y and 10–20 kg	10	100	4
7–12 y and <20 kg	20	200	4

    3. Adverse effects: Minimal: include transient blanching or vasodilation and erythema with longer application. One case of methemoglobinemia in a child who had prolonged application of EMLA and who had also received sulfamethoxazole has been reported.

    4. Structure

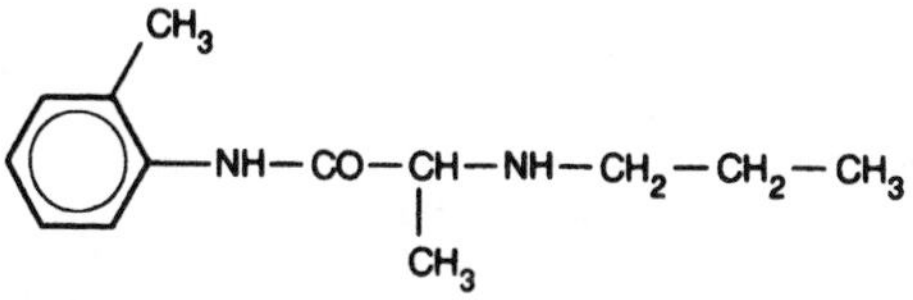

Prilocaine

    5. Packaging:
        EMLA cream: 5-g tube with Tegaderm dressing
        EMLA cream: 30-g tube without dressing (must supply own plastic wrap)

B. LMX
  1. Contains: 4% to 5% lidocaine in a liposomal vehicle
  2. Use: Apply to treatment site 15 to 45 minutes before procedure. No occlusion is required.
  3. Packaging:
      ELA-Max cream: 5-g tube box of 5, 30 g

C. Betacaine gel
  1. Contains: Lidocaine 5%. Also contains an epinephrine-like vasoconstricting agent. FDA approval pending.
  2. Use: Apply to treatment site 30 to 35 minutes before procedure. No occlusion required.
  3. Packaging:
      10- and 30-g tubes, or 100-g pump bottle

D. Dyclonine HCl
  1. Structure

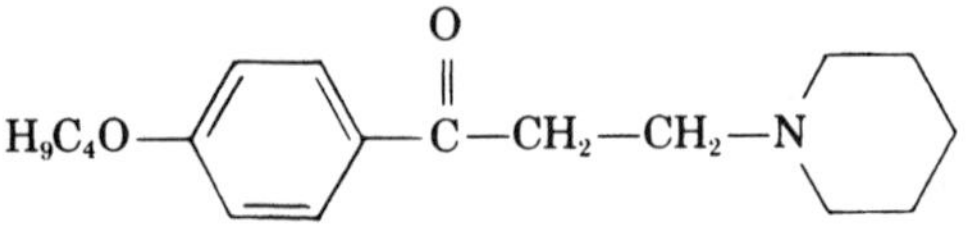

Dyclonine

  2. Contains: Synthetic organic ketone, related in structure to antihistamine.
  3. Use: Provides anesthesia of mucous membranes. Apply 5 to 10 minutes before a procedure; apply b.i.d. to t.i.d. for pain relief. Onset of action is within 2 to 10 minutes. Anesthesia lasts 30 to 60 minutes.
  4. Packaging:
      Dyclone, 0.5%, 1% solution: 1 oz

E. Dibucaine HCl is an amide-like quinoline derivative and is one of the most potent and longest acting of the commonly used local anesthetics.
  1. Structure (amide-like quinoline derivative)

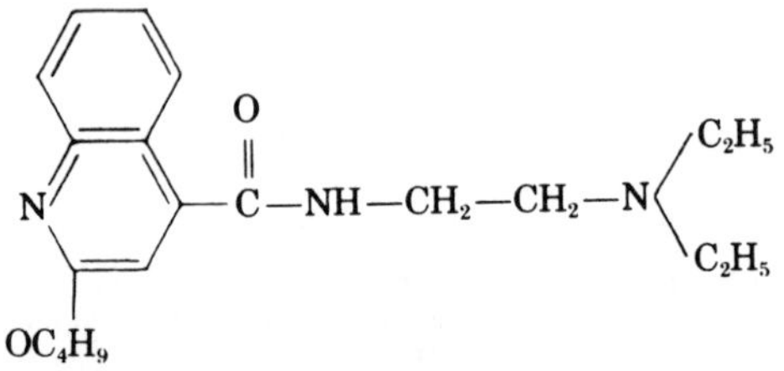

Dibucaine

  2. Contains: 0.5% cream in acetone, glycerin; 1% ointment in acetone, lanolin, mineral oil, and petrolatum.
  3. Packaging:
      Nupercainal 0.5% cream: 42.5 g
      Nupercainal, 1.0% ointment: 30 g, 60 g

F. Lidocaine HCl (Lidocaine, Xylocaine, Anestacon, Dentipatch, Zilactin-L, Solarcaine, Burn-O Jel, DermaFlex, Lidoderm)

1. **Structure:** Amine acyl amide anesthetic.

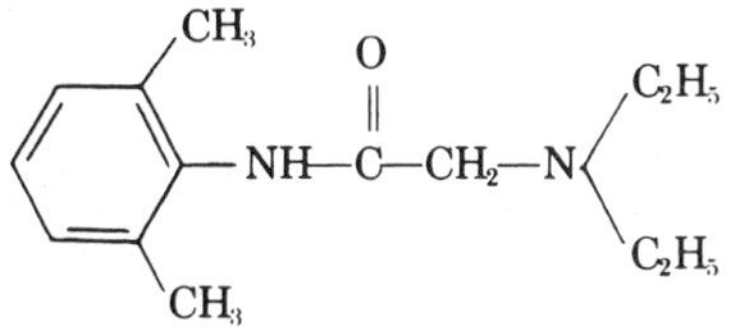

Lidocaine

2. **Contains:** 0.5% to 5% lidocaine in cream, gel, ointment, jelly, spray, patch, or solution; dental patches.
3. **Use:** Apply to affected site 5 to 10 minutes before procedure. Duration of anesthesia is relatively short (<1 hour).
4. **Packaging:**
   Lidocaine cream, 0.5%, 4%: 5 g, 30 g, 120 g
   Lidocaine gel, 0.5%, 2.5%: 15 g, 85 g, 120 g, 240 g
   Lidocaine jelly, 2%: 15 mL, 240 mL
   Lidocaine ointment, 5%: 50 g
   Lidocaine viscous solution, 2%, 4%: 20 mL, 50 mL, 100 mL, 450 mL
   Lidocaine spray, 0.5%: 135 mg
   Lidocaine liquid 2.5%: 10 mL
   Lidocaine patch 5%: cartons of 30 patches

III. NONPRESCRIPTION DRUGS

A. Benzocaine

   1. Structure: Ethyl aminobenzoate, a para-aminobenzoate derivative (PABA)

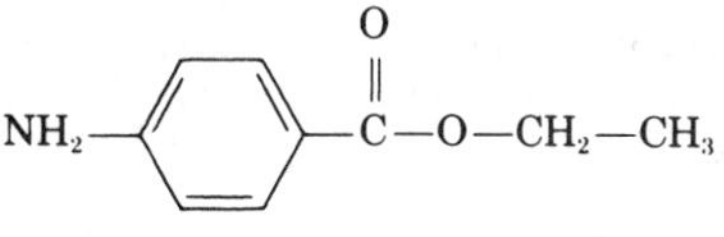

Benzocaine

   2. Contains: PABA-based anesthetic. Patients allergic to PABA may react to this medication and other anesthetics based on PABA (i.e., dibucaine, cocaine, procaine, monocaine, tetracaine, and propoxycaine). These patients may have a cross-sensitivity to products containing paraphenylenediamine, sulfonamides, hydrochlorothiazide, and PABA-containing sunscreens as well.

   3. Use: Apply to a maximum of three to four times a day to the affected area, as directed by the physician.

   4. Packaging: Numerous brands and formulations available, both OTC and by prescription. The following is an abbreviated list of these products.

      Anbesol liquid or gel, 6.3% benzocaine with 0.5% phenol, povidone-iodine, 70% alcohol, camphor, and menthol (OTC): 9 mL, 22 mL

      Benzodent ointment, 20% benzocaine with 0.4% eugenol and 0.1% hydroxyquinoline sulfate in a denture adhesive–like base (OTC): 7.5 g, 30 g

      Cetacaine aerosol, gel, liquid, ointment, 14% benzocaine, 2% tetracaine HCl, 2% butamben, and 0.5% benzalkonium chloride in a water-soluble base (R_x): 30 g, 60 g, 75 mL, 150 mL

      Dent's Extra Strength Toothache Drops and Gum (OTC): 1 g

      Lanacane Maximum Strength Creme, 20% benzocaine, glycerin in water-soluble base (OTC): 1 oz

      Orajel Mouth-Aid gel, 20% benzocaine with benzalkonium chloride and 0.1% zinc chloride and saccharin (OTC): 10 g

B. Pramoxine HCl (Prax, PrameGel, Tronothane HCl, AmLactin AP, Itch-X, Bactine)
   1. Structure: Ether-like topical anesthetic. Resembles antihistamine.

$$CH_3CH_2CH_2CH_2O-\text{(benzene ring)}-OCH_2CH_2CH_2-N\bigg\langle \text{morpholine ring with } O \text{ and } H$$

Pramoxine

   2. Contains: 1% pramoxine HCl.
   3. Use: Apply to affected area t.i.d. to q.i.d., as directed by a physician. Useful for patients sensitive to ester and/or amide anesthetics. Onset of anesthesia is within minutes. Duration of anesthesia is 2 to 4 hours.
   4. Packaging:
      Pramoxine 1% cream: 28.4 g, 30 g, 113.4 g, 140 g, 1 lb
      Pramoxine 1% lotion: 15 mL, 120 mL, 240 mL
      PrameGel, 1% gel: 35.4 g, 118 g
      Pramoxine 1% spray: 60 mL
      Pramoxine 1% wipes: in 16s

 ANTIHISTAMINES

I. DISCUSSION. These drugs bear a close structural resemblance to histamine and antagonize the pharmacologic actions of histamine by occupying histamine receptor sites, but only if histamine has not yet reached its target receptors (competitive inhibition). Antihistamines do not elicit any direct effect at the receptor sites, affect antibody production or antigen–antibody interactions, react chemically with histamine, or prevent histamine's release. They may diminish capillary permeability to substances other than histamine and may also have a mild local anesthetic effect.

$$N\text{(imidazole ring)}N-CH_2-CH_2-N\bigg\langle{}^{H}_{H}$$

Histamine

$$X-CH_2-CH_2-N\bigg\langle{}^{X}_{X}$$

Most antihistamines

There are two types of histamine receptors, H_1 and H_2, and two corresponding groups of antihistamines. Classic antihistamines (H_1 blockers) do not alter gastric acid secretion. H_2 antagonists decrease gastric acid secretion and find their greatest utility in the treatment of peptic ulcer and related diseases. Cutaneous blood vessels possess both H_1 and H_2 receptors. If histamine is experimentally injected into the skin, combined H_1 and H_2 blockade reduces the histamine response better than either agent alone. The combination of H_1 and H_2 antihistamines is effective therapy for dermatographism, cold urticaria, and the flush associated with metastatic carcinoid.

The classic H_1 antihistamines are most effective in the management of acute urticaria and seasonal rhinitis. They are also currently the drugs of choice in the therapy of chronic urticaria and other allergic cutaneous reactions, including drug reactions. They are, however, of only limited value when given systematically for the relief of nonspecific pruritus. Antihistamines have been shown to be no more effective than aspirin or a placebo for relief of non–histamine-related itching (i.e., eczematous eruptions, as opposed to urticaria), but there is an enormous placebo effect; in dealing with patients bothered by pruritus, the magnitude of this beneficial phenomenon should not be overlooked. The classes of antihistamines show only minor variations in their properties. However, individuals frequently react differently to each antihistamine class. One or several antihistamines of different classes may have to be used, occasionally in combination, before the best treatment effect is obtained. Many antihistamines have a sedating effect, which the patients must be made aware of, especially if they will be driving. These medications include hydroxyzine, diphenhydramine, chlorpheniramine maleate, and cyproheptadine. Hydroxyzine appears to be the most effective sedating antihistamine in suppressing histamine-induced pruritus. In one experimental system, cyproheptadine and placebo administration necessitated a 5-fold increase in the intra-dermal histamine dose required to produce pruritus, compared with a 10-fold increase following diphenhydramine and a 750-fold increase following hydroxyzine HCl. For general use, chlorpheniramine maleate, hydroxyzine hydrochloride, and hydroxyzine pamoate have proved consistently effective.

The development of nonsedating H_1 antagonists was a significant advance in anti-histamine therapy. These agents penetrate the blood–brain barrier minimally and have greater affinity for peripheral H_1 receptors. Thus, compliance is often better because of fewer bothersome side effects. Examples of these medications include cetirizine, fexofenadine, and loratadine.

Antihistamines are rapidly absorbed after oral or parenteral administration. Following an oral dose, symptomatic relief is noted within 15 to 30 minutes and usually lasts 3 to 6 hours. These drugs are metabolized mainly in the liver, and excretion by the kidney is nearly complete in 24 hours. Antihistamines are also incorporated into some topical antipruritic lotions. Previous concern about antihistamine-induced contact dermatitis was based on anecdotal evidence and is unwarranted. Recent studies reveal no risk of contact hypersensitivity. The most common untoward systemic effect is sedation. Gastrointestinal side effects can also be seen. Because H_1 antihistamines are structurally similar to atropine, they may all produce peripheral and central anticholinergic effects, including excitation, dry mouth, blurred vision, and urinary retention. Patients should be cautioned to avoid the use of alcoholic beverages and barbiturates during antihistamine therapy because the depressant action of these drugs is additive.

To be used most effectively, antihistamines should be increased gradually until either clinical remission occurs or side effects (most often sedation) become significant. It is unwise to start at too high a dose.

II. SPECIFIC AGENTS (all R_x except where noted)
  A. Ethanolamine derivatives are potent antihistamines. However, there is a high inci-dence of sedation, and they have an additive effect with hypnotics and sedatives. Possible hypertension, tachycardia, T-wave changes, or shortened diastole may further complicate the clinical picture.
    1. Diphenhydramine hydrochloride (Benadryl, Caladryl, Dermamycin, Dermarest, Sleepinal, Sominex, etc.)—OTC
      a. Structure

Diphenhydramine

      b. Contains: 1% to 2% diphenhydramine hydrochloride as cream, gel, injection, lotion, solution, spray, capsule, and tablet.
      c. Use: 25 to 50 mg PO q4h. Maximum daily dose is 300 mg in adults. The maximum oral dose for children is 150 mg/day. The topical agents are not as effective as antihistamine drugs.

   d. Packaging:
> Diphenhydramine capsules: 25 and 50 mg
> Diphenhydramine cream and gel, 1% to 2%: 15 g, 30 g, 180 g
> Diphenhydramine elixir (12.5 mg/5 mL): 118 mL
> Diphenhydramine injection (50 mg/mL): 1-mL ampules, 10-mL vials
> Diphenhydramine liquid 12.5 mg/5 mL: 118 mL, 236 mL, 473 mL
> Diphenhydramine oral solution: 12.5 mg/5 mL: 473 mL
> Diphenhydramine syrup 12.5 mg/5 mL: 30 mL, 118 mL, 473 mL, 3.8 L
> Diphenhydramine spray: 60 mL

  2. Other ethanolamine antihistamines include carbinoxamine maleate (Clistin), clemastine fumarate (Tavist), and dimenhydrinate (Dramamine).

B. Ethylenediamine derivatives cause less drowsiness than ethanolamine derivatives but have more gastrointestinal side effects. These antihistamines must be avoided in individuals with contact allergy to ethylenediamine. Because of structural similarities, it would also be wise to avoid piperazine and hydroxyzine antihistamines in these patients. Ethylenediamine antihistamines include methapyrilene hydrochloride (Histadyl) and pyrilamine maleate [Triaminic (OTC)].

C. Piperazine antihistamines are sedative in nature. They include hydroxyzine hydrochloride (Atarax), hydroxyzine pamoate (Vistaril), cyclizine hydrochloride (Marezine), buclizine hydrochloride (Bucladin-S), and meclizine hydrochloride (Bonine, Antivert). They are also utilized for their antiemetic, sedative, anticholinergic, analgesic, and skeletal muscle relaxant effects.

  1. Structure

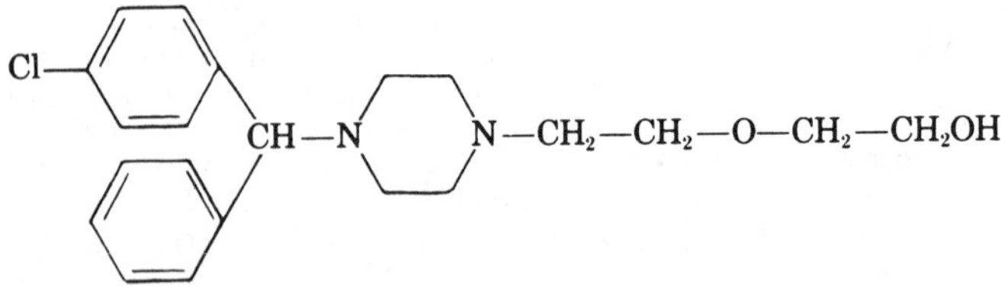

Hydroxyzine

  2. Use: Drugs of choice for the treatment of dermatographism and cholinergic urticaria. They are also effective alone or in combination with other antihistamines in the management of acute and chronic urticaria, atopic and contact dermatoses, and histamine-induced pruritus.

  3. Dosage: 25 mg, three to four times a day.

  4. Packaging:
> Hydroxyzine tablets: 10 mg, 25 mg, 50 mg, 100 mg
> Hydroxyzine injection: 25 mg/mL, 50 mg/mL
> Hydroxyzine syrup, 10 mg/5 mL: 118 mL, 473 mL
> Hydroxyzine capsule: 25 mg, 50 mg, 100 mg
> Hydroxyzine oral suspension 25 mg/5 mL: 120 mL, 473 mL

D. Alkylamine derivatives include some of the most active antihistamines effective in low dosage. There is no variation in the effectiveness of members of this antihistamine class. Emphasis should be placed on the lower cost and easy availability of these medications.

  1. Brompheniramine maleate (This drug is only available in combination with other medications: Bromfed, Dimetane, Dimetapp, Drixomed, Histatab, Nasahist). The only difference between this agent and chlorpheniramine is the substitution of a bromine for a chlorine atom in brompheniramine. The side effects of this medication are similar to other classes of sedative antihistamines. Some medications include parabens. Patients sensitive to parabens may develop a sensitivity reaction.

2. Chlorpheniramine maleate (Alka-Seltzer Plus, Allerest, Chlor-Trimeton, Comtrex, Contact, Norel Plus, Sinarest, Sinutabs, TheraFlu)

a. Structure

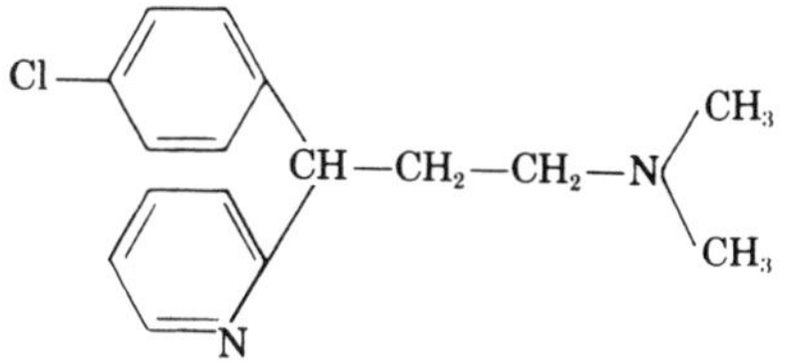

Chlorpheniramine

b. Dosage: 4 to 6 mg PO q4–6h. Maximum daily dose is 24 mg for adults and children 12 years or older. Found frequently in combination with acetaminophen and pseudoephedrine.

c. Packaging (OTC and R$_x$):

Chlorpheniramine syrup, 2 mg/5 mL: 118 mL
Chlorpheniramine tablets: 4 mg
Chlorpheniramine extended tablets: 8 mg, 12 mg, 16 mg
Chlorpheniramine chewable tablet: 2 mg
Chlorpheniramine sustained-release capsule: 8 mg, 12 mg

3. Dexchlorpheniramine maleate is the dextrorotatory isomer of chlorpheniramine.

a. Dosage: 4 or 6 mg qhs or q8–10h.

b. Packaging:

Dexchlorpheniramine extended-release tablets: 4 mg, 6 mg

E. Phenothiazine derivatives are used primarily as central nervous system (CNS) depressants or CNS stimulants but are also potent antihistamines. They also possess antiemetic, anticholinergic, and local anesthetic effects. They demonstrate side effects similar to those of other sedative antihistamines.

1. Promethazine hydrochloride (Phenergan)

a. Structure

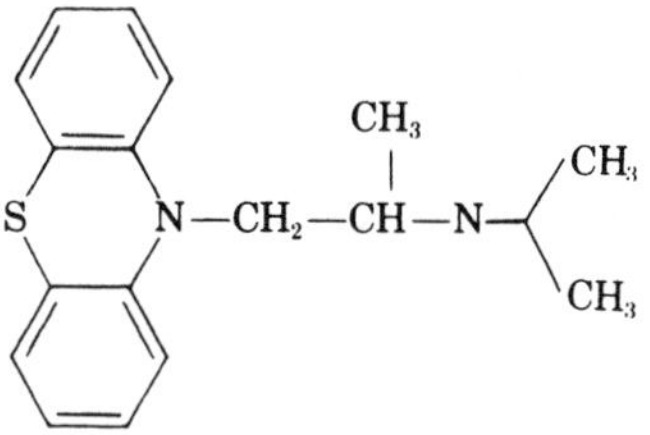

Promethazine

b. Dosage: 12.5 mg PO q.i.d.; 25 mg PO at bedtime. May contain saccharin.

c. Packaging:

Promethazine injection, 25 mg/mL, 50 mg/mL: 1-mL ampules; 10-mL multidose vials
Promethazine suppositories: 12.5 mg, 25 mg, 50 mg
Promethazine syrup: 6.25 mg/5 mL, 473 mL
Promethazine tablets: 12.5 mg, 25 mg, 50 mg

F. Piperidine derivatives

1. Cyproheptadine hydrochloride is an antihistamine in which antiserotonin activity has been demonstrated both *in vivo* and *in vitro*. As yet, however, there is no evidence that this action contributes to clinical therapeutic effects. Anticholinergic and sedative effects are observed. Cyproheptadine may be more effective than other H_1 blockers in the management of cold urticaria.

a. Structure

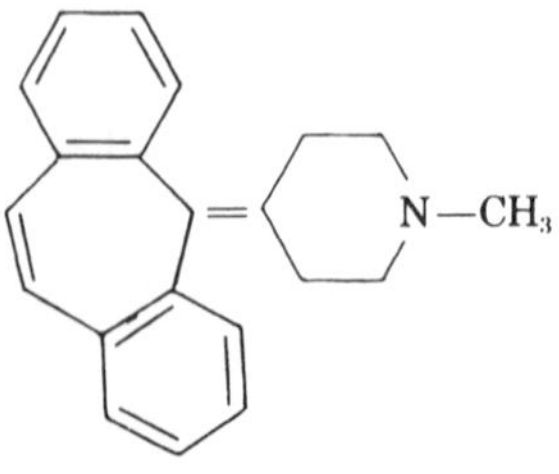

Cyproheptadine

b. Dosage: 4 mg PO t.i.d. Maximum daily dose is 0.5 mg/kg/day for adults.
c. Packaging:
  Cyproheptadine tablets: 4 mg
  Cyproheptadine syrup, 2 mg/5 mL: 473 mL
 2. Azatadine maleate (Optimine) and phenindamine (Nolahist) are other piperidine antihistamines.
G. Nonsedating H_1 antihistamines
 1. Fexofenadine HCl (Allegra) is a selective, specific H_1 antagonist that is structurally related to the butyrophenone tranquilizer haloperidol. It is the active carboxylic acid metabolite of terfenadine (no longer commercially available in the United States). It binds mainly to the peripheral H_1 receptors, with minimal crossing of the blood–brain barrier and hence minimal sedative effects. Fexofenadine lacks the cardiotoxic effects of its parent drug, terfenadine. However, it has been associated with increased QT interval, syncope, and ventricular arrhythmia in at least one susceptible patient with preexisting cardiovascular risk. To date, no significant interactions have been demonstrated with fexofenadine when administered concomitantly with azole antifungals or macrolide antibiotics. Indicated for seasonal allergic rhinitis and chronic idiopathic urticaria.
  a. Dosage: 60 mg PO b.i.d.
  b. Packaging:
    Fexofenadine capsules: 60 mg
    Fexofenadine tablets: 30 mg, 60 mg, 180 mg
 2. Loratadine (Claritin) is a long-acting, potent peripheral H_1 blocker with minimal sedative effects. It does not appear to have the same adverse cardiac effects as the other nonsedating H_1 antihistamines. It is indicated for allergic rhinitis and chronic urticaria.
  a. Dosage: 10 mg daily. Patients with liver or renal impairment should be started on a lower dose.
  b. Packaging:
    Loratadine syrup, 1 mg/mL: 480 mL
    Loratadine tablets: 10 mg
    Loratadine orally disintegrating tablet: 10 mg
 3. Cetirizine HCl (Zyrtec) is the carboxylic acid metabolite of hydroxyzine. It is a selective, peripheral H_1 receptor antagonist. It is a long-lasting antihistamine. It does not appear to have the same adverse cardiac effects as the other nonsedating H_1 antihistamines; however, additional data are required. Indicated for allergic rhinitis and chronic urticaria.
  a. Dosage: 5 to 10 mg daily.
  b. Packaging:
    Cetirizine syrup, 5 mg/5 mL: 120 mL, 473 mL
    Cetirizine tablets: 5 mg, 10 mg

H. Thioguanidine derivatives. Block H_2 histamine receptors

1. Cimetidine (Tagamet) is an H_2 histamine antagonist that contains an imidazole ring and is structurally similar to histamine. It is used primarily for the treatment of peptic ulcer disease by blocking gastric parietal cell receptors and reducing gastric acid secretion. Additionally, it has an immunomodulatory effect by inhibiting suppressor T cells, apparently by competitive blockade of their H_2 receptors. This effect has resulted in its use in various infections, including severe mucocutaneous candidiasis, resistant condyloma acuminata, and herpes simplex. Its antiandrogen side effects are due to its competitive inhibition of DHT at the receptor site; this side effect makes it useful in treating female androgenetic alopecia.

a. Structure

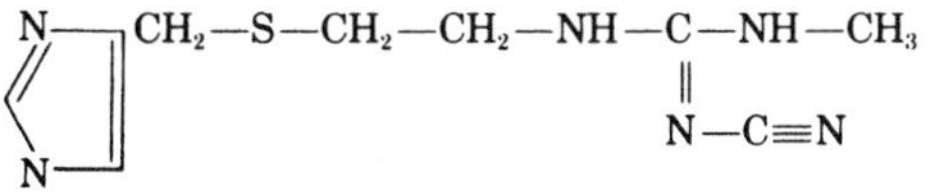

$$\text{CH}_2-\text{S}-\text{CH}_2-\text{CH}_2-\text{NH}-\overset{\displaystyle \|}{\underset{\displaystyle \text{N}-\text{C}\equiv\text{N}}{\text{C}}}-\text{NH}-\text{CH}_3$$

Cimetidine

b. Dosage: 300 mg PO q.i.d. or 800 mg at bedtime.

c. Packaging:
Cimetidine injection, 150 mg/mL: 2-mL vials; 8-mL multidose vials
Cimetidine liquid, 300 mg/5 mL: 240 mL, 470 mL
Cimetidine tablets: 200 mg, 300 mg, 400 mg, 800 mg

2. Ranitidine (Zantac) is another H_2 receptor antagonist that does not have the same antiandrogen side effects as cimetidine. Note that both cimetidine and ranitidine inhibit the cytochrome P-450 microsomal enzyme system.

a. Dosage: 150 mg b.i.d.

b. Packaging:
Ranitidine tablets: 75 mg, 150 mg, 300 mg
Ranitidine injection, 1 mg/mL, 25 mg/mL: 2-mL, 6-mL, 50-mL vials
Ranitidine syrup, 75 mg/5 mL: 10 mL, 480 mL

I. Doxepin (Sinequan, Zonalon) is a combined H_1 and H_2 receptor antagonist. It is also a tricyclic antidepressant with antianxiolytic effects. Adverse side effects include sedation and anticholinergic symptoms, in addition to tachycardia, hypotension, and prolongation of the PR and QRS intervals on electrocardiogram. A topical form of doxepin cream is available (Zonalon 5% cream) for use in patients with atopic dermatitis, lichen simplex chronicus, and other eczematous dermatoses. Side effects are usually mild and may include burning, stinging, drowsiness, and dry mouth. The incidence of side effects increases when applied to more than 10% of the body surface area or when duration of therapy exceeds 8 days. Cases of acute contact dermatitis to topical Zonalon have been reported.

1. Structure

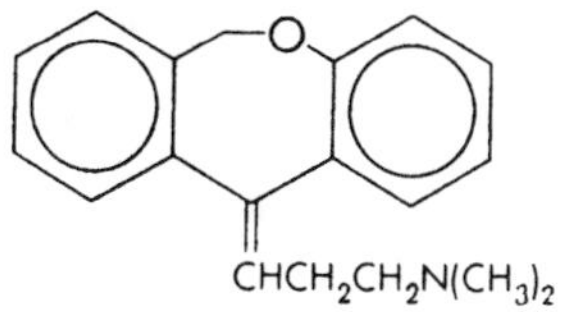

$$\text{CHCH}_2\text{CH}_2\text{N(CH}_3)_2$$

Doxepin

2. Dosage: Tablets: 10 mg PO q.i.d., may increase dose as tolerated. Zonalon cream: apply to affected areas t.i.d. to q.i.d. up to 8 days.

3. Packaging:
Doxepin cream, 5%: 30 g
Doxepin capsule: 10 mg, 25 mg, 50 mg, 75 mg, 100 mg, 150 mg
Doxepin oral solution, 10 mg/mL: 120 mL

ANTIINFECTIVE AGENTS

I. ANTIBACTERIAL AND ANTISEPTIC AGENTS, TOPICAL. Antiseptic agents are applied to tissue to destroy microorganisms or inhibit their reproduction or metabolic activity. The major uses of antiseptics are as hand scrubs, cleansers, irritants, and protective dressings. Commonly used antiseptics include ethyl and isopropyl alcohols, cationic surfactants (e.g., benzalkonium), chlorhexidine, iodine compounds, and hexachlorophene. Disinfectants are used on nonliving agents to destroy microorganisms and prevent infection. Some diluted disinfectants are used as antiseptics. The most commonly used disinfectants are the aldehydes (formaldehyde and glutaraldehyde), elemental chlorine, and cresol (a phenolic compound). Topical antibiotics have long been used to prevent or treat cutaneous bacterial infection, yet it is only recently that the effectiveness of this therapy has been evaluated critically.

Numerous antibacterial agents are available for topical use. Topical erythromycin is also effective and is the drug of choice when contact irritation or allergy occurs to the poorly absorbed agents. Use of broad-spectrum germicides or topical antibiotics, singly or as mixtures, is justified for many reasons:

1. They can treat a wide range of potential pathogens in mixed infections. Frequently, more than one pathogen is present and quick identification of organisms is difficult.
2. They are used in small amounts and therefore permit use of drugs that are relatively toxic when given systemically. There is no percutaneous absorption of these antibiotics from normal, psoriatic, or eczematous skin; therefore, the possibility of producing nephrotoxicity or ototoxicity is extremely unlikely. Neomycin is a frequent cause of allergic contact dermatitis; approximately 1% of the general population is sensitized.
3. The concentration of the topical medications is high, although the total amount used is small. This represents large multiples of the minimum effective concentration for potential pathogens.
4. Topically administered drugs are in more direct contact with organisms, so that the problems of absorption, distribution, and availability to the infected site are not involved.
5. The combined effects of bactericidal agents such as bacitracin, neomycin, and polymyxin B are predominantly synergistic, thereby increasing the rate and spectrum of bactericidal action, and *Staphylococcus aureus* is highly susceptible to the bactericidal action of mupirocin and neomycin and bacteriostatic action of tetracyclines, whereas *Streptococcus pyogenes* is particularly susceptible to bacitracin and neomycin. Neomycin is approximately 50 times more active against staphylococci than bacitracin (by weight), but bacitracin is 20 times more active against streptococci. Of gram-negative invaders, all but *Proteus* species are sensitive to polymyxin B and all but *Pseudomonas* are sensitive to neomycin. Therefore, to cover this spectrum, combinations of two or three antibiotics may be necessary.
6. Another effect of combination therapy is to retard the emergence of resistant organisms, which is true particularly with use of neomycin and gentamicin. Although outbreaks of neomycin-resistant infections have been reported in closed communities, the incidence of resistance to this antibiotic has not significantly changed during the last 20 years.

Note: The risk of combination topical antibiotic use is that if a contact dermatitis/allergic reaction were to develop while on this combination therapy, it would be difficult to ascertain which antibiotic the patient is allergic to. Further testing would be required to determine the etiology.

Local treatment of secondarily infected dermatoses may not diminish the reservoir of pathogens elsewhere on the body. Systemic antibiotics may be required for full eradication of the infection. Additionally, impetigo and other bacterial pyodermas should be treated with systemic antibiotics as discussed in previous chapters.

By reducing bacterial colony counts, topical antibiotic preparations are effective for axillary deodorization, controlling nasal carriage of staphylococci, and preventing infections in clean wounds. When used promptly, they might hasten healing and diminish the local or systemic morbidity of infected wounds. Nonetheless, some topical antibiotics and antibiotic-corticosteroid creams are classified by the FDA as lacking adequate evidence of effectiveness.

These preparations should be applied frequently (three to six times a day) after the skin is cleansed of adherent crusts and debris and should not be applied under occlusive dressings.

A. Alcohol. Both ethyl and isopropyl alcohol are used as topical antiseptics; 70% isopropyl alcohol (rubbing alcohol) is the more commonly used agent. There is a 75% reduction in surface microorganisms, specifically gram-positive bacteria, after wiping the skin with alcohol. The treated area must be allowed to dry completely for the full antiseptic effect. Spores, viruses, and fungi are resistant. Because of the short duration of action, other longer-acting antiseptics should be used for prolonged procedures. Be sure that the surface is completely dry before electrosurgery and laser surgery, for alcohol may easily be ignited.

1. Packaging:
Isopropyl alcohol, 70% USP: 500 mL
Ethyl alcohol, 60% to 70%: 500 mL
Alcare foam, 62%: 210, 330, 600 mL
Isagel gel, 60%: 120, 630, 3,840 mL
System TLC gel, 70%: 118 mL
Sebanil solution, 49%: 105, 240, 480 mL

B. Aluminum salts have strong antibacterial effects. Formulations include 1% aluminum chlorohydrate (Ostiderm), aluminum diacetate (Burow's solution, Domeboro's powder), and aluminum chloride hexahydrate (Drysol, Xerac AC). These compounds completely inhibit representative dermatophytes, yeasts, and gram-positive and gram-negative bacteria *in vitro. In vivo*, 20% aluminum chlorohydrate, 10% to 20% aluminum acetate, and 20% to 30% aluminum chloride hexahydrate have appreciable direct killing effects, with the chlorohydrate salt being most potent. The recommended use concentrations (1:20 and 1:40) of 5% aluminum diacetate exert no *in vivo* bacteriostatic or bactericidal effects. Aluminum chloride hexahydrate 20% to 30% solution is effective in treating symptomatic interdigital tinea pedis owing to its bactericidal effects as well as this salt's unique astringent (drying) properties. In the management of folliculitis, notably of the buttocks, 6.25% aluminum chloride hexahydrate (Xerac AC) has been found useful. Aluminum salts are also effective as antiperspirants.

1. Packaging (OTC):
Aluminum chloride hexahydrate, 20% solution (Drysol): 35 mL, 60 mL
Aluminum chloride hexahydrate, 20% lotion (Bromil Lotion): 120 mL
Aluminum chloride hexahydrate, 6.25% solution (Xerac AC): 35 mL
Burow's solution, tablets, and powder (Bluboro, Domeboro): 12/box, 100/box

C. Bacitracin. This polypeptide antibiotic, which is produced from *Bacillus subtilis*, interferes with bacterial cell wall growth and is bactericidal against many gram-positive organisms such as streptococci, staphylococci, and pneumococci but is inactive against most gram-negative organisms. All anaerobic cocci, *Neisseria*, and the tetanus and diphtheria bacilli are also sensitive to bacitracin. Resistance is rare, but some staphylococcal strains are inherently resistant. Hypersensitivity reactions are uncommon. Bacitracin is stable in petrolatum (but not water-miscible preparations) and is available as an ointment or as a component of antibiotic mixtures. Sensitization to bacitracin has been reported more recently, particularly in patients with leg ulcers.

1. Structure

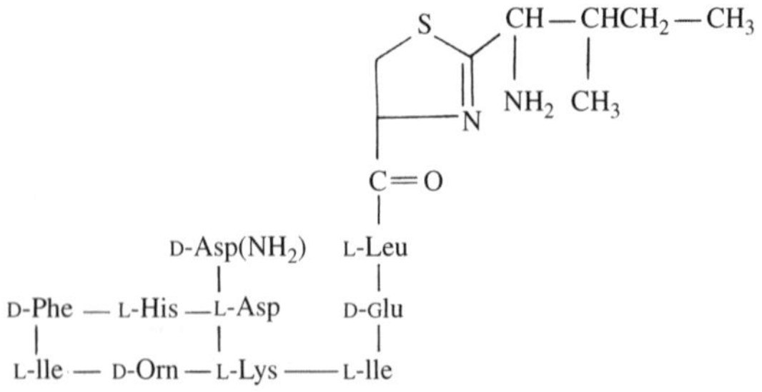

Bacitracin

2. Use: Clean wound and apply one to three times a day.

3. Packaging (OTC):
Bacitracin ointment, 500 U/g: 1-g, 15-g, 30-g tube; 1 lb

D. Benzalkonium chloride is a quaternary ammonium detergent that treats gram-positive and gram-negative organisms. Strains of *Mycobacterium* tuberculosis and *Pseudomonas aeruginosa* are often resistant. It is not effective against spore-forming organisms. It is nonirritating to mucous membranes and may be used near the eyes. Drawbacks include lack of sustained activity and ease of contamination of this antimicrobial. It is inactivated by anionic compounds such as soap. A 0.1% solution takes 7 minutes to decrease the bacterial count by 50%. All traces of soap must be removed with 70% alcohol before use.

1. Use: Must be diluted to correct concentration before use.
For unbroken skin, superficial injuries: 1:750 dilution.
For denuded skin, deep wounds: 1:2,000 to 1:10,000 dilution
For mucous membranes: 1:5,000
For mouthwash: 1:1,000
For wet dressings or irrigation: 1:5,000

2. Packaging (OTC):
Benzalkonium chloride concentrate, 17%: 500 mL, 4,000 mL
Benzalkonium chloride towelettes: 24/box
Benzalkonium chloride solution, 1:750: 60 mL, 120 mL, 240 mL
Benzalkonium chloride tincture, 1:750: 1 gal
Benzalkonium chloride topical solution 1%: 30, mL

E. Chlorhexidine. This topical antiseptic product acts rapidly but, like hexachlorophene, persists on the skin to give a cumulative, continuing antibacterial effect. Like iodophors and alcohol, it is active against gram-positive and gram-negative bacteria, including *P. aeruginosa*, as well as common yeasts and fungi. It does not lose effectiveness in the presence of whole blood. Many consider it the antiseptic of choice for skin cleansing and surgical scrubs. Contact allergy is not uncommon. Chlorhexidine should not be used near the eyes or mucosal surfaces, because it may cause irritation or even anaphylaxis.

1. Structure

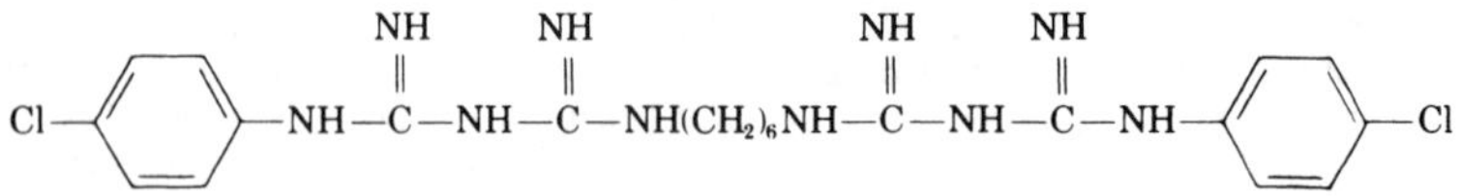

Chlorhexidine

2. Use: Apply to treatment area and swab for >2 minutes. Repeat treatment for an additional 2 minutes.

3. Packaging (OTC):

Chlorhexidine liquid, solution, 2%, 4%: 120 mL, 240 mL, 480 mL, 946 mL, 960 mL, 1 gal

Chlorhexidine towelettes, 0.5%: 50/box

Chlorhexidine 0.5% rinse: 120 mL, 240 mL,

Chlorhexidine 0.12% oral rinse: 480 mL

Chlorhexidine 4% foam: 180 mL

Chlorhexidine sponge/brush 4%: 22 mL

F. Gentamicin (Garamycin). This antibiotic is a combination of three related amino-glycoside agents obtained from cultures of *Micromonospora purpurea* and acts by interfering with the bacterial synthesis of protein. It prevents bacterial protein synthesis by irreversibly binding to 30S ribosomal subunits. Its antibiotic spectrum is similar to that of neomycin, and cross-resistance does occur. Gentamicin is active against gram-negative organisms including *Escherichia coli* and a high percent-age of strains of *Pseudomonas* species and other gram-negative bacteria. *Proteus* organisms show a variable degree of sensitivity. Some gram-positive organisms, including *S. aureus* and group A β-hemolytic streptococci, are also affected. In general, higher concentrations are needed to inhibit streptococci than those needed to inhibit staphylococci and many gram-negative bacteria. It is inactive against fungi, viruses, and most anaerobic bacteria. The most important use of gentamicin is in the treatment of systemic gram-negative infections, particularly those due to *Pseudomonas* organisms. Widespread use is unwarranted not only because equally effective drugs are available but also because of the risk of increasing the background of gentamicin-resistant organisms. Allergic reactions to gentamicin are unusual but may occur with prolonged use. Cross-reactivity with neomycin may occur.

1. Structure

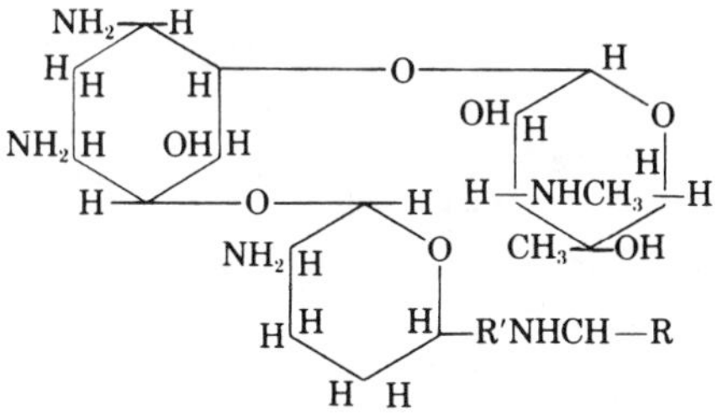

Gentamicin sulfate

2. Use: Clean lesion and apply one to three times a day.

3. Packaging:

Gentamicin 0.1% cream: 15 g

Gentamicin 0.1% ointment: 15 g

G. Hexachlorophene is a bacteriostatic antiseptic effective against gram-positive organ-isms, specifically *Staphylococcus*. It has a cumulative and sustained effect. Although it has a slow onset of action, with repeated use a film develops on the skin that has long-acting properties. It is not effective against gram-negative organisms or yeast. It is postulated to affect bacterial electron transport and membrane function. With repeated use, it penetrates through the stratum corneum. It is often used for preoperative surgical scrubbing. One retrospective study showed that it may be teratogenic if used excessively by pregnant women, although there have been no subsequent, well-controlled studies that substantiate this. It should not be used in infants, particularly those who are premature or have dermatoses. It is toxic to tissues when applied to open wounds.

1. Use: Apply to treatment area and scrub for 3 minutes. Repeat treatment for addi-tional 3 minutes. Not to be used on mucosal surfaces. Rinse thoroughly after use.

2. Packaging (R_x only):

Hexachlorophene 3% liquid: 8 mL, 150 mL, pt, gal

H. Iodophors (Acu-Dyne, Aerodine, Betadine, Iodex, Operand, Polydine). These consist of a water-soluble organic complex of iodine with a carrier that slowly liberates iodine on contact with reducing substances in body tissues. These broad-range germicidal antiseptics are effective against bacteria, fungi, viruses, protozoa, and yeast. They are water soluble, nonirritating, and nonstinging but may lose effectiveness on contact with whole blood or serum. They are often used for preoperative skin cleansing and surgical scrubbing because their sustained action provides protection even through lengthy procedures. They are also used in treating skin infections and burns. They are available in many vehicles. The solubilizing carrier substances include polyvinyl–pyrrolidone (povidone-iodine, as in Betadine products or available as generics) and poloxamer–iodine complexes. Because iodophors may be absorbed through the skin, they should be avoided in neonates or in patients with thyroid disorders. Also, extensive use for prolonged periods should be minimized. Iodine preparations may slow wound healing on actively granulating tissue.

1. Structure

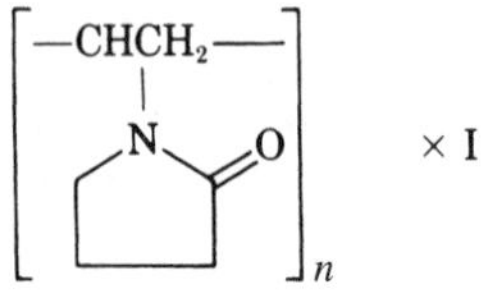

Povidone-iodine

2. Use: Apply to treatment area and scrub for 2 minutes. Repeat treatment for an additional 2 minutes.

3. Packaging (OTC): Numerous products are available; the following are some examples:

  Iodine/povidone aerosol, 5%: 909 mL
  Iodine/povidone gel, 5%: 5 g, 151 g
  Iodine/povidone ointment, solution, 10%: 30 g 1 lb
  Iodine/povidone skin cleanser/surgical scrub, 7.5%: 170 g

I. Mupirocin (Bactroban, Centany) is a topical antibiotic produced by fermented *Pseudomonas fluorescens*. It has a narrow spectrum of activity, mostly against gram-positive aerobic bacteria (including *Staphylococcus* and methicillin-resistant *Staphylococcus*) and many strains of *Streptococcus*. It is also active against some gram-negative aerobic bacteria but is inactive against anaerobes, *Chlamydia*, and fungi. It has proved equal in efficacy in the treatment of impetigo when compared with oral erythromycin, with fewer adverse side effects.

Mupirocin does not interfere with wound healing. It is active only on topical administration and is converted to an inert molecule on systemic administration. Prolonged use of mupirocin increases the risk of evolution of resistant organisms. The mechanism of action has not yet been fully classified, but it does differ from other available antiinfective agents, and there is little chance of cross-resistance developing. Also, unlike many other topical antibiotics, it rarely causes allergic sensitization.

1. Structure

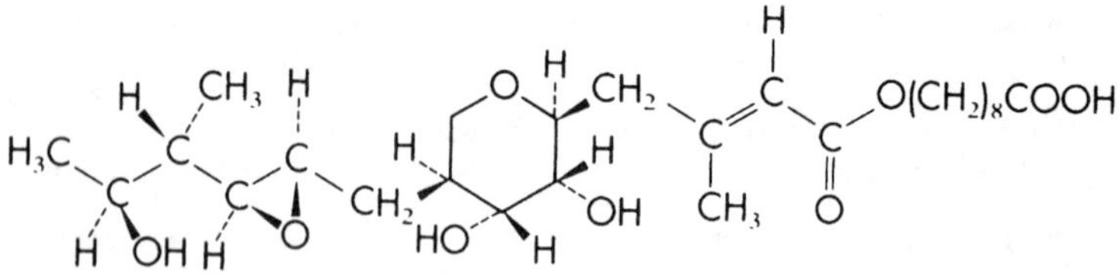

Mupirocin

2. Use: Clean lesion and apply b.i.d. to t.i.d. for 10 to 14 days.
To eradicate nasal colonization, apply b.i.d. for 14 days.

3. Packaging:
Bactroban cream and ointment, Centany ointment 2%: 15 g, 22 g, 30 g
Bactroban nasal cream, 2%: 1 g

J. Neomycin sulfate. This drug is obtained from species of the actinomycete *Streptomyces* and is an aminoglycoside antibiotic (as are streptomycin, gentamicin, and kanamycin) effective against most aerobic gram-negative organisms. Group A streptococci are relatively resistant. Neomycin acts to inhibit bacterial protein synthesis by irreversibly binding to the 30S subunit. It is responsible for a greater incidence of allergic contact sensitivity than any other topical antibiotic. This diagnosis often remains hidden, because morphologically the eruption is of a mild eczematous nature. Rarely, anaphylaxis may occur.

1. Structure

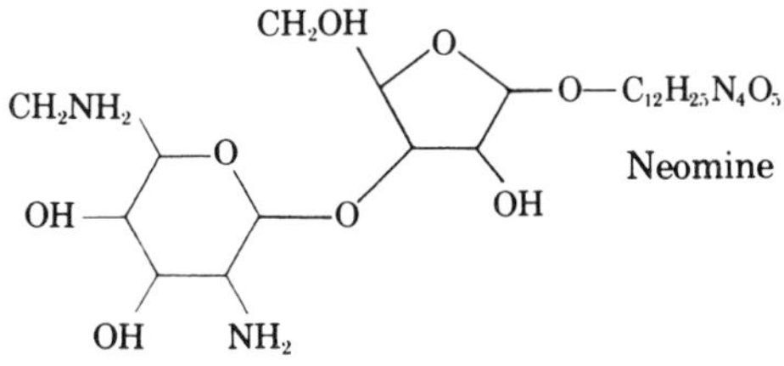

CH_2OH

CH_2NH_2

$O—C_{12}H_{23}N_4O_5$

Neomine

OH

OH

OH NH_2

Neomycin B

2. Use: Apply one to three times a day.

3. Packaging:
Neomycin cream, ointment, 0.5%: 15 g, 30 g

K. Polymyxin B. Polymyxin B is one of a group of cyclic polypeptides elaborated by *Bacillus polymyxa*. The drug is a surface-active agent. It is thought to alter the lipoprotein membrane of bacteria so that it no longer functions as an effective barrier, thereby allowing the cell contents to escape. Polymyxin B is effective against *Pseudomonas, E. coli*, and other gram-negative bacteria except the *Proteus* and *Serratia* species. It has little effect on gram-positive organisms.

1. Use: Apply to affected area one to three times a day.

2. Packaging (available in combination with other agents—see the following text):

L. Combination topical preparations

1. Neomycin/polymyxin B/bacitracin ointment (Neosporin)

   a. Contains: 5,000 units polymyxin B sulfate, 400 U bacitracin zinc, and 3.5 mg neomycin sulfate (as base) per gram.

   b. Use: Apply one to three times a day.

   c. Packaging (OTC):
   Neomycin/polymyxin B/bacitracin ointment: 0.9 g, 14 g, 15 g, 28 g, 30 g, 454 g

2. Polymyxin B/bacitracin (Polysporin) ointment

   a. Contains: 10,000 U polymyxin B sulfate with 500 U zinc bacitracin per gram.

   b. Packaging (OTC):
   Polysporin ointment: 15 g, 30 g

II. ANTIFUNGAL AGENTS

A. DISCUSSION. See Chap. 14.

B. Prescription drugs

1. Systemic therapy (Table 40-2)

   a. Fluconazole is a synthetic triazole derivative that is structurally related to the imidazole antifungals. Replacement of the imidazole ring with a triazole ring increases antifungal activity and expands the antifungal spectrum. It works to inhibit fungal cytochrome P−450 14-α-demethylase, with a resultant decrease

TABLE 40-2   **Comparison of Oral and Topical Antifungal Agents**

Drug	Route of administration	Organisms treated	Mechanism	Side effects
Allylamine				
Naftifine (Naftin)	Topical	Dermatophytes	**1.** Blocks squalene epoxidase **2.** Alters PMN chemotaxis	Rarely an irritant, burning
Terbinafine (Lamisil)	Topical	Dermatophytes	Blocks squalene epoxidase	Oral: delayed gastric emptying, hepatitis, metallic taste, and decreased white blood cells count
Butenafine				
(Mentax)	Topical	Dermatophytes and yeasts	Blocks squalene epoxidase	
Azole compounds				
Clotrimazole (Lotrimin, Mycelex)	Topical	Dermatophytes and yeasts	Inhibits ergosterol synthesis by inhibiting 14 α-demethylation of lanosterol	
Econazole (Spectazole)	Topical	Dermatophytes and yeasts		
Fluconazole (Diflucan)	Oral	Above plus systemic mycoses		Drug interactions
Itraconazole (Sporonox)	Oral	Above plus systemic mycoses		Drug interactions, congestive heart failure, rash, hepatitis
Ketoconazole (Nizoral)	Topical/oral	Dermatophytes and yeasts		Pituitary-testosterone-adrenal axis, hepatitis
Miconazole (Micitin, Monistat)	Topical	Dermatophytes and yeasts		
Oxiconazole	Topical	Dermatophytes and yeasts		
Sertaconazole (Ertaczo)	Topical	Dermatophytes and yeasts		
Sulconazole (Exelderm)	Topical	Dermatophytes and yeasts		
Polyene antibiotics				
Fungizone	Topical	Yeast (*Candida*)	Binds to cell membrane sterols (*ergosterol*) causing cell leakage and permeability changes	Nausea, vomiting, diarrhea, with oral use

(continued)

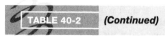 **TABLE 40-2** *(Continued)*

Drug	Route of administration	Organisms treated	Mechanism	Side effects
Nystatin (Mycostatin Nilstat)	Oral/topical	Yeast (*Candida*)		
Griseofulvin	Oral	Dermatophyte	Inhibits synthesis of fungal cell walls	Gastrointestinal side effects; headache, lupus erythematosus flares; precipitates acute intermittent porphyria; granulocytopenic

PMN, polymorphonuclear leukocyte

in ergosterol. Fluconazole is approved by the FDA for systemic candidiasis and is prescribed primarily in patients with oropharyngeal and esophageal candidiasis. It is also useful in cryptococcal, histoplasmosis, and *Blastomycetes* infections. It is ineffective against *Malassezia* and *Scopulariopsis* infections. Existing data suggest that fluconazole accumulates in the stratum corneum, where it is delivered both through sweat and direct diffusion through the dermis and epidermis. Because it concentrates in the stratum corneum and nails, it is useful for therapy of cutaneous fungal infections, although it is fungistatic. Rare side effects include hepatotoxicity, anaphylaxis, and Stevens-Johnson syndrome.

i. Structure

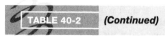

Fluconazole

ii. Use: Coadministration with other drugs metabolized by cytochrome P-450 system may result in increased concentration of the drug. Dose adjustment may be necessary. Levels of oral contraceptives decrease when used in combination with fluconazole. Hydrochlorothiazide increases fluconazole levels.

    Vaginal candidiasis: 150 mg PO single dose.

    Pityrosporum infections: 200 to 400 mg PO, single dose.

    Dermatophytosis: 150 mg/week for 4 to 6 weeks (2 additional weeks after clinical resolution of symptoms).

    Onychomycosis: 300 mg/week for 4 months (fingernails) or 8 months (toenails).

iii. Packaging:

    Fluconazole tablets: 50 mg, 100 mg, 150 mg, 200 mg

    Fluconazole injection, 2 mg/mL: 100 mL, 200 mL

    Fluconazole powder for oral suspension (when reconstituted): 10 mg/mL, 40 mg/mL

b. Flucytosine (Ancobon) is a synthetic, fluorinated pyrimidine that is structurally related to fluorouracil (FU) and floxuridine. It can be fungistatic and fungicidal. Although it is used more frequently in the treatment of systemic infections caused by *Candida* and *Cryptococcus*, dermatologic indications may include infections due to chromomycosis, sporotrichosis, *Cladosporium*, and *Sporothrix* species. It is generally ineffective against *Aspergillus* species.

  i. Structure

Flucytosine

  ii. Use: Generally administered at 50 to 150 mg/kg daily in four divided doses.

  iii. Packaging:

    Flucytosine capsule: 250 mg, 500 mg

c. Griseofulvin is an antifungal antibiotic effective against all dermatophyte fungi but not against yeast (i.e., *Candida* or *Pityrosporum*) or molds. It is derived from *Penicillium* species, but there is no structural homology or cross-reactivity with penicillin or the cephalosporins. Griseofulvin resembles colchicine structurally, and one of its major cellular effects is to inhibit fungal mitosis by interfering with microtubular proteins and thereby causing metaphase arrest. The rate of absorption and the total amount of drug absorbed are increased after a high-fat meal. Microsize griseofulvin is produced by a special process that fractures the particles into minute crystals of irregular shape that offer a greater surface for increased gastrointestinal absorption. Further processing to achieve ultramicrosize particles doubled the bioavailability; 125 mg was originally thought to be equivalent to 250 mg of microsize griseofulvin, but more recent data indicate that it takes 150 to 200 mg to achieve bioequivalent plasma levels.

    Griseofulvin enters the epidermis by diffusion forces from extracellular fluid (through transepidermal water loss) and from sweat and reaches higher concentrations in the horny layer than in serum. With excessive sweating in hot, humid climates, the amount of griseofulvin in skin is likely to be reduced, and more of the drug should be taken. The response to therapy depends on the rate of keratinization and the time necessary for desquamation of infected keratinized structures. Griseofulvin is deposited in newly formed nails but does not diffuse through the nail bed, which may account for the need for prolonged time of therapy for onychomycosis.

    Griseofulvin is metabolized by the liver, and its metabolites are excreted in the urine. It is highly protein bound and, therefore, may have high tissue levels. However, tissue levels decrease and fall as soon as griseofulvin is discontinued such that its presence is no longer detectable 2 to 3 days after cessation of therapy.

    Griseofulvin may cause a reversal of the hypoprothrombinemic effect of anticoagulants, necessitating an increase in the dose of anticoagulant to maintain a therapeutic range of anticoagulation. This effect occurs through increased synthesis of drug-metabolizing liver enzymes, leading to more rapid inactivation of anticoagulants. Phenobarbital has been postulated to decrease the gut absorption of griseofulvin, thereby decreasing blood levels and presumably decreasing antifungal action.

Griseofulvin has the following cure rates: tinea capitis, 93.1%; tinea of the glabrous skin, 64.8%; tinea of the palms and soles, 53.3%; tinea of the fingernails, 56.9%; and tinea of the toenails, 16.7%. Failure of fungal infection to respond to this therapy may occur because of inadequate dosage, poor compliance, inadequate absorption, microsomal enzyme inactivation and drug interaction, failure of griseofulvin to enter the site of infection or diminished activity within that site, or infection with an organism not sensitive to griseofulvin. The latter had long been postulated, but it has been shown that for *Trichophyton rubrum* infections of body, palms, and soles, a poor clinical response correlates with a diminished *in vitro* sensitivity to this antimycotic. Minimal inhibitory concentration determinations for griseofulvin can be used to determine the appropriateness of this therapy. Griseofulvin is contraindicated in patients with porphyria, pregnancy, and hepatocellular failure.

i. Structure

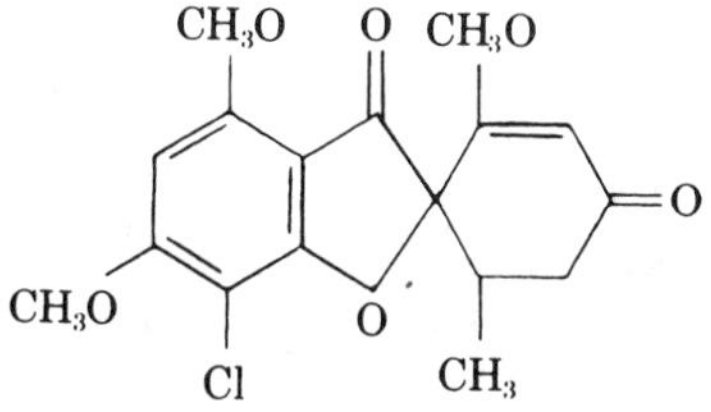

Griseofulvin

ii. Dosage: See Chap. 14.

The average treatment time for tinea capitis is 4 to 6 weeks; for tinea corporis, 2 to 4 weeks; and for tinea pedis, 4 to 8 weeks. Because of the low cure rate and length of therapy, griseofulvin is not commonly used for onychomycosis of the fingernails or toenails. Complete blood count (CBC) is monitored every 3 months during long-term therapy.

iii. Packaging:

Griseofulvin ultramicrosize: tablets, 125 mg, 165 mg, 250 mg, 330 mg

d. Itraconazole (Sporanox) is a triazole antifungal that is related to the imidazole ketoconazole. Similar to ketoconazole, it interferes with ergosterol synthesis and cell membrane integrity. It is clinically active against dimorphic fungi, yeast, dermatophytes, *Blastomycetes*, histoplasmosis, sporotrichosis, and *Aspergillus*. It is ineffective against *Scopulariopsis*. Side effects are fewer compared with ketoconazole, with reportedly less hepatotoxicity. Less than 5% of patients may have asymptomatic elevations in serum transaminase. Early investigational studies showed less effect on the pituitary-testosterone-adrenal axis in patients on low doses of itraconazole. Higher doses for prolonged duration may rarely cause hypokalemia. Itraconazole is highly lipophilic, has a high affinity for keratinous tissue, and has been shown to persist in nails. One study found evidence of the drug in nail clippings 7 to 12 months after cessation of therapy, and another study showed evidence in tissue up to 6 months after treatment was discontinued. Plasma levels, in contrast, rapidly decrease after therapy is stopped.

Itraconazole is a potent inhibitor of the cytochrome P450 3A enzyme system, which may elevate blood levels of other drugs metabolized by this system if taken concomitantly. Itraconazole levels may decrease in patients who are concurrently taking rifampin, phenobarbital, or phenytoin. Cyclosporine, felodipine, digoxin, warfarin, and oral hypoglycemic levels may increase when given in conjunction with itraconazole.

Itraconazole, like ketoconazole, is contraindicated in patients taking cisapride. Itraconazole may induce torsades de pointes, ventricular arrhythmias, and congestive heart failure.

i. Structure

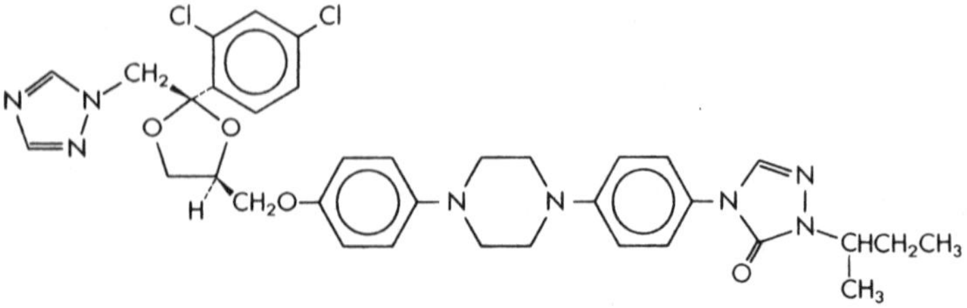

Itraconazole

ii. Use: Monitor Liver function tests (LFTs) monthly while on medication

Fingernail onychomycosis: daily dosing 200 mg q.d. ×6 weeks; pulse dosing 200 mg b.i.d. ×1 week/month for 2 months

Toenail onychomycosis: daily dosing 200 mg q.d. ×12 weeks; pulse dosing 200 mg b.i.d. ×1.week/month for 3 to 4 months

Blastomycosis, histoplasmosis, aspergillosis: 200 to 400 mg q.d.

Candidiasis: 100 mg q.d. for 2 weeks after resolution of symptoms

iii. Packaging:

Itraconazole capsules, 100 mg: pulsepak 28

Itraconazole injection, 10 mg/mL: 25-mL ampules

Itraconazole oral suspension, 10 mg/mL: 150 mL

e. Ketoconazole (Nizoral) is a water-soluble imidazole derivative with a wide spectrum of activity against pathogenic fungi at concentrations achievable with oral treatment. Unlike miconazole, it is well absorbed after oral administration, and unlike clotrimazole, it does not induce a liver enzyme that inactivates any absorbed drug. This drug, like other imidazoles, affects fungi by mechanisms involving increased membrane permeability, inhibition of uptake of precursors of ribonucleic acid (RNA) and DNA, and synthesis of oxidative and peroxidative enzymes. It is fungistatic. Ketoconazole's spectrum of activity includes *Candida* species, *Cryptococcus neoformans, Coccidioides immitis, Histoplasma capsulatum, Blastomyces dermatitidis, Paracoccidioides brasiliensis,* and pathogenic dermatophytes. It is effective in chronic dermatophyte infections, including those resistant to griseofulvin. Although it is useful in treating chronic mucocutaneous candidiasis, fluconazole has been shown to be more effective against *Candida albicans* than ketoconazole.

When used systemically, the most worrisome adverse reaction to ketoconazole is hepatotoxicity. Two percent to 5% of patients may experience asymptomatic elevations of hepatic enzymes. Acute hepatic injury resembling viral hepatitis is an apparently idiosyncratic reaction that occurs in approximately 1 patient in 10,000; fatalities have occurred. Appropriate liver function tests should be monitored in patients on ketoconazole, and if any evidence of hepatic injury develops, the drug should be discontinued. Hepatitis is twice as common in women than men and rarely occurs in patients on oral therapy <2 weeks.

Nausea, gynecomastia, infertility, decreased libido, and oligospermia have also been reported, although most frequently at doses exceeding 400 mg/day. Other side effects are uncommon. Ketoconazole is best absorbed if taken on an empty stomach. Because gastric acidity facilitates absorption, concomitant use of antacids, H_2 blockers, or anticholinergic agents should be avoided. Rifampin also prevents adequate therapeutic levels from being achieved. Ketoconazole should not be administered in patients taking cisapride because of adverse cardiac effects, including torsades de pointes, ventricular arrhythmias, and sudden death.

Ketoconazole is a potent inhibitor of the cytochrome P450 3A4 enzyme system. This may result in increased plasma concentrations of drugs metabolized by this system if given concomitantly. Ketoconazole levels may decrease in patients who are concurrently taking rifampin, phenobarbital, or phenytoin. Cyclosporine, felodipine, digoxin, and warfarin levels may increase when given in conjunction with ketoconazole.

Ketoconazole is extensively degraded by the liver, and very little active drug is excreted in either the urine or bile; the dose need not be modified for renal insufficiency. Adverse reactions to topical ketoconazole are very rare.

i. Structure

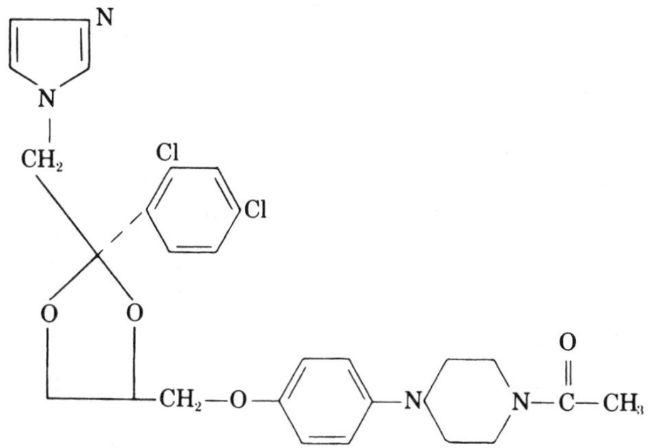

Ketoconazole

ii. Use: See Chap. 14, Dermatophyte Infections.

iii. Packaging:

        Ketoconazole tablets: 200 mg

        Ketoconazole cream, 2%: 15 g, 30 g, 60 g

        Ketoconazole shampoo, 2%: 120 mL

        Ketoconazole shampoo, 1%: 207 mL

f. Nystatin, a polyene antibiotic derived from a species of the actinomycete *Streptomyces noursei*, binds to sterols in fungal membranes, causing a change in the permeability of cell membranes and leakage of cell components. It is nontoxic and available for oral, vaginal, and topical administration. Nystatin is poorly absorbed from the gastrointestinal tract and will therefore rid the oral and gastrointestinal mucosa of *Candida* but has no effect on systemic or cutaneous lesions when given orally. Nystatin is unstable in heat, light, moisture, and air. Aqueous-alcohol suspensions are stable for 10 days under refrigeration.

i. Use: See Chap. 14, Candidiasis.

ii. Packaging:

        Nystatin cream and ointment, 100,000 U/g: 15 g, 30 g, 240 g

        Nystatin oral suspension, 100,000 U/mL: 5 mL, 60 mL, 480 mL

        Nystatin powder, 100,000 U/g: 15 g, 30 g

        Nystatin oral tablets, 500,000 U: box of 100

        Nystatin vaginal tablets, 100,000 U: 15s, 30s

g. **Terbinafine Hydrochloride (Lamisil).** A synthetic allylamine antifungal agent, structurally related to naftifine. It inhibits fungal sterol biosynthesis by inhibiting the enzyme squalene 2,3-epoxidase. The deficiency of ergosterol and concomitant accumulation of squalene within the fungal cell results in cell death. It can be fungicidal or fungistatic, depending on the concentration used, and is effective against dermatophytes, *Aspergillus*, blastomycosis, and histoplasmosis. It is only minimally effective against *Candida*.

Adverse reactions include lens and retinal disturbances (red/green visual perception), metallic taste disturbance that may last up to 4 weeks after medication discontinuation, hepatoxicity, and pancytopenia. Five percent of patients will experience delayed gastric emptying with symptoms of nausea, fullness, and/or dyspepsia. Terbinafine does not appear to have any effect on the cytochrome P-450 systems (Check baseline CBC and LFTs; repeat if taken for >6 weeks).

i. **Use:**

Fingernail onychomycosis: 250 mg/day for 6 weeks

Toenail onychomycosis: 250 mg/day for 12 weeks

ii. **Packaging:**

Terbinafine (Lamisil) tablets: 250 mg

2. **Topical therapy** (Table 40-2)

a. Amphotericin B (Fungizone) is an amphoteric polyene macrolide produced by *Streptomyces nodosus*. It exerts its antifungal activity principally by binding to sterols in the fungal cell membrane, resulting in loss of membrane-selective permeability, leakage, and subsequent cell death. It is used topically in the treatment of superficial *C. albicans* infection and is orally active against *Aspergillus, Coccidioides, Cryptococcus*, Exophilia, histoplasmosis, *Mucor, Paracoccidioides*, and *Rhodotorula*. It is also active against many strains of *Leishmania, Naegleria,* and *Acanthamoeba. Fusarium, Pseudallescheria,* and *Scedosporium* are generally resistant to amphotericin B. It is fungistatic or fungicidal, depending on the concentration used and the fungal susceptibility. It is ineffective against dermatophytes. The drug is yellow orange, odorless, and may stain skin. Adverse reactions with topical administration are limited. When administered by IV, amphotericin B may be associated with infusion reactions, nephrotoxicity, anemia, gastrointestinal distress, hepatitis, and neurologic effects.

i. **Structure**

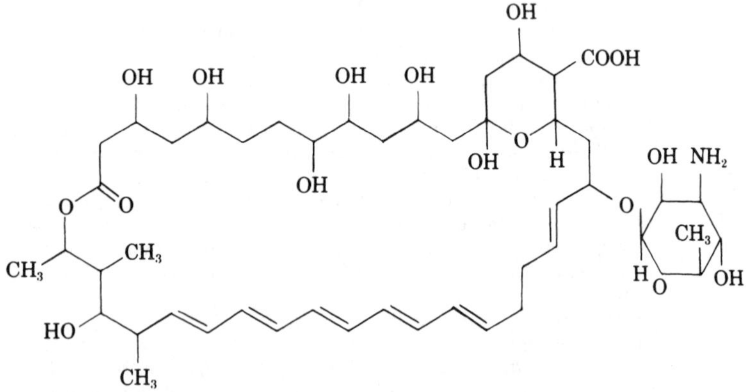

Amphotericin B

    ii. Use: Oral candidiasis: use 1 mL four times a day, applying directly to tongue, then swish and swallow.

    iii. Packaging:

        Fungisone oral suspension, 100 mg/mL: 24 mL

b. Butenafine (Mentax) is a synthetic benzylamine antifungal agent, related structurally and pharmacologically to terbinafine. It is thought to act by inhibiting the enzyme squalene 2,3-epoxidase, resulting in decreased ergosterol and corresponding increase in squalene, with subsequent cell membrane permeability alteration and cell death. It is active against dermatophytes, yeast, and *Sporothrix*.

    i. Use: Tinea corporis/cruris/pedis: apply to affected areas q.d. until fully resolved, generally 2 to 4 weeks.

    ii. Packaging:

        Butenafine (Mentax) cream, 1%: 12 g, 15 g, 24 g, 30 g

c. Ciclopirox olamine (Loprox, Penlac) is a synthetic, broad-spectrum hydroxypyridone antifungal agent. It is chemically unrelated to the imidazoles or any other antifungal agent currently available in the United States. It appears to act through intracellular depletion of substrates and/or ions principally by inhibition of transmembrane transport of these substances. It is active against dermatophytes, yeast, and *Pityrosporum orbiculare*. It also demonstrates activity against *Trichomonas vaginalis*, some mycoplasma, and some gram-positive and gram-negative bacteria.

    i. Structure

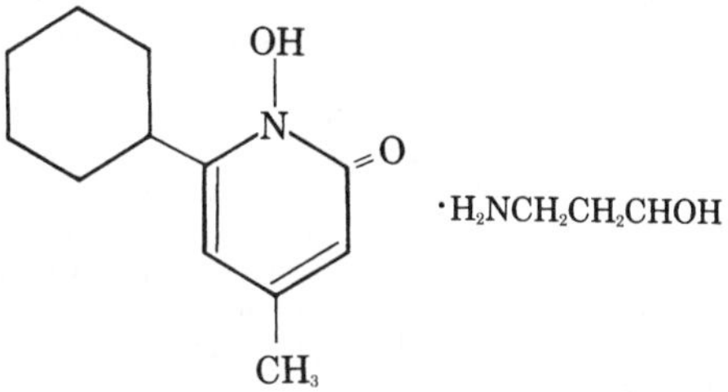

$\cdot H_2NCH_2CH_2CHOH$

Ciclopirox olamine

    ii. Use: Tinea corporis/cruris/pedis: apply to affected areas b.i.d. until complete resolution. Generally 2 to 4 weeks of treatment is necessary.

        Tinea versicolor: apply to affected areas b.i.d. × 2 weeks.

        Onychomycosis, mild to moderate: apply nail lacquer to nail plate (entire surface) and 5 mm surrounding skin q.d. Remove with alcohol every 7 days. No nail polish to be used when on treatment. Requires 6 to 12 months of use for effective treatment.

    iii. Packaging:

        Ciclopirox (Loprox) cream or gel, 0.77%: 15 g, 45 g, 30 g, 90 g, 100 g

        Ciclopirox (Loprox) topical suspension, 0.77%: 30 mL, 60 mL

        Ciclopirox (Penlac) nail lacquer, 8% topical solution: 3.3 mL with applicator, 6.6 mL

        Ciclopirox (Loprox) shampoo 1%: 120 mL

d. Econazole (Spectazole) is a synthetic imidazole. Econazole blocks C-14 demethylation of sterols, interfering with the biosynthesis of ergosterol, which results in disorganization of the fungal plasma cell membrane and increased permeability. It is active against dermatophytes, yeast, *P. orbiculare, Aspergillus, Cladosporium*, and *Sporothrix*.

i. Structure

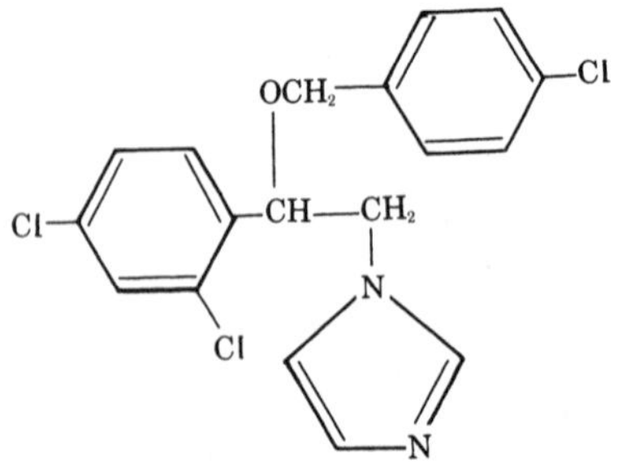

Econazole

  ii. Use: Cutaneous candidiasis: apply to affected areas b.i.d. until resolved, generally 2 to 4 weeks.

      Tinea corporis/cruris/pedis: apply to affected areas q.d. until resolved, generally 4 to 6 weeks.

      Tinea versicolor: apply to affected areas q.d. until resolved, generally 2 weeks.

iii. Packaging:

      Econazole (Sporonox) 1% cream: 15 g, 30 g, 85 g

e. Ketoconazole: see sec. 1.e.

f. Naftifine (Naftin) is a synthetic allylamine derivative topical antifungal agent that works by blocking squalene 2,3-epoxidase, resulting in increased cell membrane permeability and cell death. It is structurally and pharmacologically related to terbinafine. It also has some antiinflammatory properties that may be due to its ability to alter chemotaxis by polymorphonucleocytes. It is most effective against dermatophytes, moderately active against molds, and less active against yeasts, including C. *albicans*.

  i. Structure

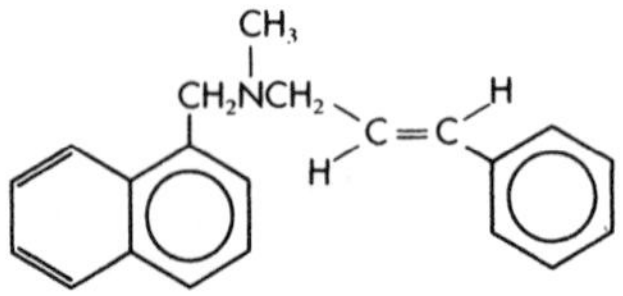

Nâftifine

  ii. Use: Tinea corporis/cruris/pedis: apply q.d. (cream) or b.i.d. (gel) to affected areas, continuing treatment for 2 weeks after symptoms have subsided.

iii. Packaging:

      Naftifine (Naftin) cream, 1%: 15 g, 30 g, 60 g

      Naftifine (Naftin) gel, 1%: 20 g, 40 g, 60 g

g. Nystatin: see sec. sec 1.f.

h. Oxiconazole (Oxistat) is a synthetic imidazole that works, in part, by inhibiting ergosterol 2,3-epoxidase synthesis and thereby disrupting cell membrane integrity.

  i. Dosage: Apply daily to affected area, continuing treatment for 2 weeks after symptoms have subsided.

ii. Packaging:
Oxiconazole (Oxistat) cream, 1%: 15 g, 30 g, 60 g
Oxiconazole (Oxistat) lotion, 1%: 30 mL

i. Sulconazole (Exelderm) is a synthetic, sulfur-substituted imidazole that is structurally related to the other imidazole antifungals (ketoconazole, econazole, and miconazole). It is postulated to inhibit 14-α-demethylase for decreased ergosterol synthesis, increased cell membrane permeability, and resultant cell death. It is active against most dermatophytes, yeast, and *P. orbiculare*. It also displays activity against some aerobic and anaerobic gram-positive bacteria. Sulconazole is a mild inducer of the cytochrome P-450 microsomal enzymes CYP1A1 and CYP2B1 and could theoretically induce the metabolism of other drugs.

i. Structure

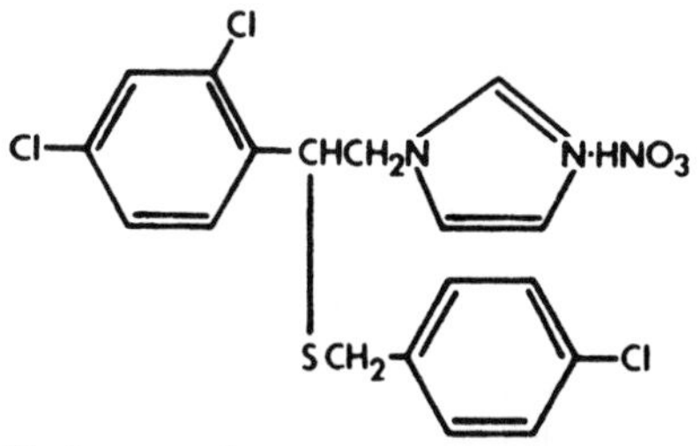

Sulconazole

ii. Use:
Tinea corporis/cruris/pedis: apply to affected areas b.i.d., continuing treatment for 2 weeks after symptoms have subsided.
Tinea versicolor: apply to affected areas b.i.d. until resolved.

iii. Packaging:
Sulconazole (Exelderm) cream 1%: 15 g, 30 g, 60 g
Sulconazole (Exelderm) solution 1%: 30 mL

j. Terbinafine (Lamisil) is a second-generation allylamine that is related to naftifine; however, it is 10 to 100 times more potent *in vitro*. It is fungicidal, whereas griseofulvin, ketoconazole, itraconazole, and other azole derivatives are all fungistatic. Because it is fungicidal, duration of therapy is shorter, and relapse rates are less than with other oral or topical therapies.

Terbinafine acts by inhibiting squalene epoxidase and thereby decreasing synthesis of ergosterol, an essential component of fungal cell membranes. It is highly lipophilic and concentrates in the stratum corneum, sebum, and hair follicles. Slightly better cure rates are attained with b.i.d. than with daily dosing.

i. Structure

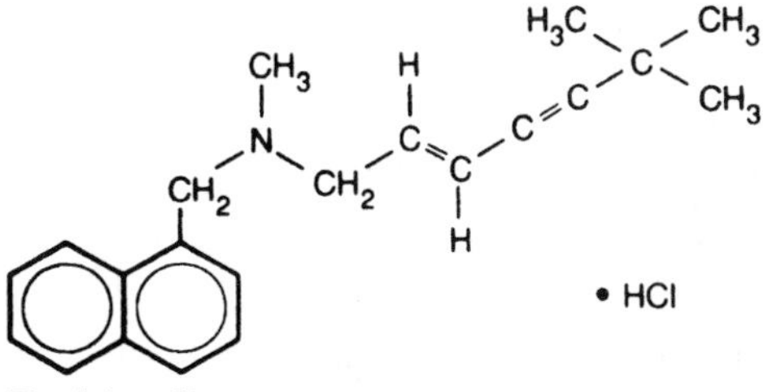

Terbinafine

    ii. Dosing: Tinea corporis/cruris/pedis: apply to affected areas b.i.d. until clinically resolved (1 to 4 weeks). Discontinue after 4 weeks.

    iii. Packaging:

        Terbinafine (Lamisil) cream, 1%: 15 g, 24 g, 30 g

        Terbinafine (Lamisil) spray 1%: 30 mL

k. Benzoic acid and salicylic acid (Whitfield's, Benzal HP) ointment is a potent keratolytic agent and is used in the treatment of dermatophyte infections (see also Chap. 14, Dermatophyte Infections). It has, however, a strong potential for causing irritant reactions.

    i. Structure

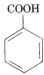

COOH

Benzoic acid

    ii. Dosage: Apply to affected areas b.i.d. to t.i.d.

    iii. Packaging:

        Benzoic acid 6%/salicylic acid 3%: 15 g, 30 g, 1 lb

l. Carbol-fuchsin solution (Castellani's paint) is an aqueous alcohol-acetone solution containing phenol (4.5 g/100 mL), resorcinol (10 g/100 mL), and basic fuschin (300 mg/100 mL). The basic fuschin appears as a dark purple liquid that appears red on the skin and can stain. It has local anesthetic, bactericidal, and fungicidal properties. It has also been reported to stimulate granulation and epithelization. It is applied topically in the treatment of subacute and chronic superficial fungal infection. It is particularly effective in intertriginous areas.

    Carbol-Fuschin is poisonous when ingested and is treated in the same manner as phenol or resorcinol poisoning.

    i. Structure

$$NH_2-\!\!\!\bigcirc\!\!\!-\!\!\!\underset{\displaystyle\quad\bigcirc-NH_2}{\overset{\displaystyle\bigcirc-NH_2}{C}}=\!\!\!\bigcirc\!\!\!=NH_2-Cl$$

Fuchsin (pararosaniline hydrochloride)

    ii. Use: Apply to affected areas one to three times a day with swab. Clean skin with soap and water before application.

    iii. Packaging (Pedinol):

        Castellani's paint, color or colorless: 30 mL, 480 mL

m. Clotrimazole (Lotrimin, Mycelex, etc.) is a synthetic imidazole agent. It acts by altering cell membrane permeability. It inhibits the growth of most dermatophyte species, yeast and *Malassezia furfur*.

i. Structure

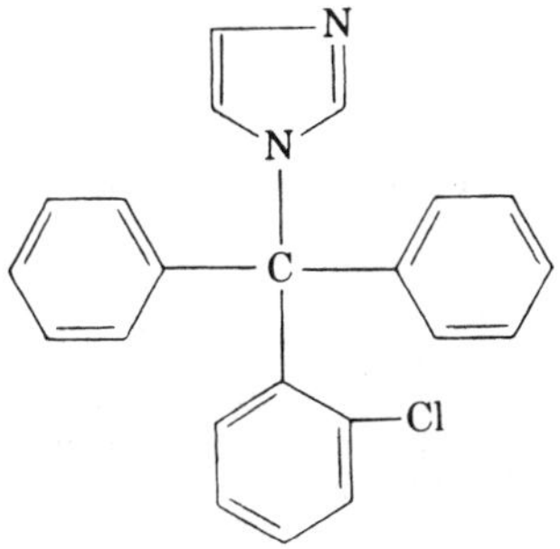

Clotrimazole

ii. **Use:** Tinea corporis/cruris/versicolor/pedis: apply b.i.d. until eruption clears, generally 2 to 4 weeks.

iii. **Packaging (R_x and OTC):**

Clotrimazole cream 1%: 12 g, 15 g, 24 g, 30 g, 45 g

Clotrimazole lotion 1%: 20 mL

Clotrimazole topical solution 1%: 10 mL, 30 mL

Clotrimazole vaginal cream 1%: 15 g, 30 g, 45 g

Clotrimazole vaginal suppositories, 100 mg, 200 mg: packs of three, packs of seven

Clotrimazole vaginal cream 2%: 21 g

n. Miconazole (Monistat-Derm, Micatin, etc.) is a synthetic imidazole antifungal compound that acts by altering cell membrane permeability. It is effective against most dermatophyte species, *P. orbiculare*, and *C. albicans*.

i. Structure

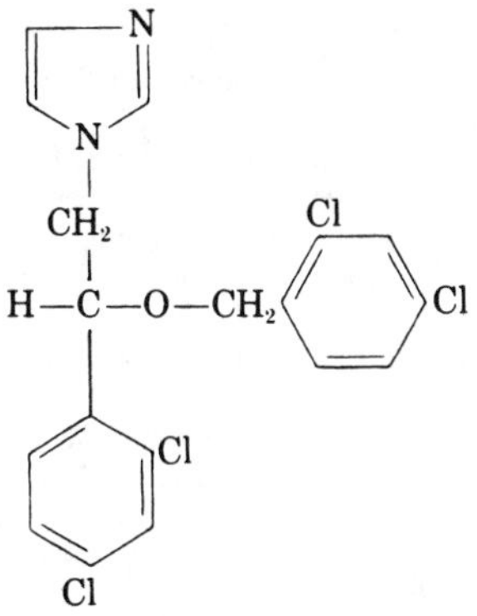

Miconazole

ii. **Use:** Apply to affected areas b.i.d. until resolution, generally 2 to 4 weeks.

iii. **Packaging (R$_x$ and OTC):**

Miconazole 2% cream: 15 g, 30 g, 90 g

Miconazole 2% ointment: 28.4 g

Miconazole 2% powder: 70 g, 90 g

Miconazole 2% spray powder: 90 mL, 85 g, 90 g, 100 g

Miconazole 2% solution: 7.39 mL, 29.57 mL

Miconazole 2% vaginal lotion, cream: 15-g, 30-g, 35-g, 45-g tube with applicator

Miconazole 200 mg vaginal suppositories: pack of three

Miconazole 100 mg vaginal suppositories: pack of seven

Miconazole 1,200 mg vaginal suppositories: pack of one

Miconazole 2% spray liquid: 105 mL, 113 mL

o. Tolnaftate (Aftate, Tinactin, etc.) is an odorless and nonstaining synthetic antifungal agent whose exact mechanism of action is unknown. It is effective against dermatophytes and *P. orbiculare* and *Pityrosporum ovale*. It is ineffective against *C. albicans* and bacteria.

i. **Structure**

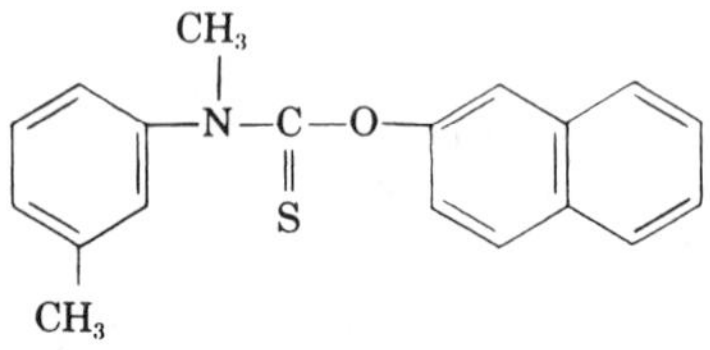

Tolnaftate

ii. **Dosage:** Apply to affected areas b.i.d. until resolved, generally 2 to 6 weeks.

iii. **Packaging:**

Tolnaftate 1% cream: 15 g, 21.3 g, 30 g

Tolnaftate 1% gel: 15 g

Tolnaftate 1% powder: 45 g, 90 g

Tolnaftate 1% solution: 10 mL

Tolnaftate 1% spray liquid: 59.2 mL, 118.3 mL, 120 mL

Tolnaftate 1% spray powder: 100 g, 105 g, 150 g

p. There are numerous OTC antifungal remedies that contain fatty acids and fatty acid salts (undecylenic acid $CH_2 = CH(CH_2)_8$ COOH, propionic acid), organic acids and their salts (benzoic acid, salicylic acid), and miscellaneous other compounds. They are all reasonably effective (see Chap. 14, Dermatophyte Infections). Some common preparations follow.

i. **Packaging:**

Cruex cream (20% total undecylenate, as undecylenic acid and zinc undecylenate): 15 g

Cruex powder (10% calcium undecylenate): 45 g, 60 g, 120 g

Desenex powder (25% total undecylenate, as undecylenic acid and zinc undecylenate): 45 g

Fungoid AF solution (25% undecylenic acid): 30 mL

III. ANTIVIRAL AGENTS

A. Oral therapy

1. Acyclovir (Zovirax) is a synthetic purine analog derived from guanine. It exerts its effects on the herpes simplex virus (HSV) and varicella-zoster virus by interfering with DNA synthesis through phosphorylation by viral thymidine kinase and subsequent inhibition of viral DNA polymerase, thereby inhibiting viral replication. It is effective against HSV-1 and 2, varicella-zoster virus, Epstein-Barr virus, herpesvirus simiae, and cytomegalovirus. Acyclovir may be administered intravenously, orally, or topically.

a. Structure

Acyclovir

b. **Use:** See Chaps 15 and 16.
c. **Packaging:**
  Acyclovir capsules: 200 mg
  Acyclovir suspension, 200 mg/5 mL: 473 mL
  Acyclovir tablets: 400 mg, 800 mg

2. Famciclovir (Famvir) a synthetic acyclic purine analog derived from guanine. It is the diacetyl ester (prodrug) of penciclovir, which exhibits no antiviral activity until hydrolyzed to penciclovir and its active metabolites. It is indicated for the management of acute herpes zoster infections. It has been shown to relieve acute symptoms as well as to shorten the duration of postherpetic neuralgia. It is also used for the treatment or suppression of recurrent episodes of genital herpes in immunocompetent patients and in the treatment of recurrent herpes simplex types 1 and 2 infections in patients with human immunodeficiency virus.

   a. **Use:** See Chaps 15 and 16.
   b. **Packaging:**
     Famciclovir (Famvir): 125-mg, 250-mg, 500-mg tablets

3. Valacyclovir (Valtrex) is the 1-valine ester (prodrug) of acyclovir that exhibits no activity until hydrolyzed in the intestinal wall or liver to acyclovir and its active metabolite. Its modified structure allows increased intestinal absorption and concomitant higher plasma levels of acyclovir. It demonstrates activity against HSV types 1 and 2, varicella-zoster virus, and cytomegalovirus. It exerts its effects by interfering with DNA synthesis through phosphorylation by viral thymidine kinase and subsequent inhibition of viral DNA polymerase, thereby inhibiting viral replication. Valtrex is indicated for the treatment of acute herpes zoster and recurrent genital herpes in immunocompetent adults. The most common side effects are headache, nausea, and vomiting.

   a. **Use:** See Chaps 15 and 16.
   b. **Packaging:**
     Valacyclovir (Valtrex): 500 mg, 1,000 mg

B. **Topical therapy.** Three agents (vidarabine, idoxuridine, and trifluridine) that act by interfering with viral DNA synthesis are currently approved for topical therapy of herpetic keratitis. These drugs are similarly effective in the treatment of uncomplicated dendritic keratitis, and patients allergic or resistant to one agent may be treated with another. Local allergic and irritant reactions have been observed with all three drugs. Treatment should be continued for 3 to 7 days beyond the time of apparent healing.

   A topical ointment containing 5% acyclovir in polyethylene glycol is useful in initial infections of herpes genitalis in promoting healing, relieving pain, and reducing viral shedding. It is less useful in recurrent episodes. Another indication for use is in limited mucocutaneous herpes simplex infections in immunocompromised patients. Penciclovir 1% cream (Denavir) is approved for the treatment of recurrent herpes labialis.

1. Acyclovir (Zovirax)
   a. Use: Apply 1/2-in. ointment/4 sq. in. six times a day for 7 days.
   b. Packaging:
   Acyclovir (Zovirax) 5% ointment: 3 g, 15 g
   Acyclovir (Zovirax) 5% cream: 2 g.
2. Penciclovir (Denavir) is a topical antiviral that inhibits HSV polymerase, thereby decreasing the replication of the virus. It is indicated for oral and facial HSV caused by HSV-1 or HSV-2.
   a. Use: For 4 days, apply to the affected area every 2 hours while awake.
   b. Packaging:
   Penciclovir (Denavir) 1% cream: 1.5 g
3. Vidarabine (Vira-A) is a purine nucleoside obtained from cultures of *Streptomyces* antibioticus. The antiviral mechanism of action has not been established, but is postulated to block viral DNA synthesis by inhibiting viral DNA polymerase.
   a. Structure

Vidarabine

   b. Use: Apply 1/2-in. thick in the lower conjunctival sac(s) five times a day for 7 days.
   c. Packaging:
   Vidarabine (Vira-A) 3% ointment: 3.5 g
4. Trifluridine (Viroptic) is a pyrimidine nucleoside structurally related to idoxuridine and thymidine. Postulated to alter viral replication by incorporation into viral DNA during replication with subsequent formation of defective proteins.
   a. Dosage: One drop every 2 hours while awake for maximum daily dosage of nine drops.
   b. Packaging:
   Trifluridine (Viroptic) 1% solution: 7.5 mL

IV. SCABICIDES AND PEDICULICIDES (For discussion, see Chap. 19)
   A. Lindane (Gamma benzene hexachloride, Kwell, Thionex) is a cyclic chlorinated hydrocarbon originally developed as an agricultural insecticide. It is absorbed through the chitinous exoskeleton and stimulates the nervous system, resulting in seizures and death of the insect. It is both a pediculicide and scabicide, with a 45% to 70% ovicidal effect. Resistance has been shown to *Pediculosis capitis* and *Sarcoptes scabiei*. Lindane can be absorbed through intact skin following topical application and has the potential for CNS toxicity. It should therefore be used with great caution in infants, children <2 years of age, elderly patients, and pregnant and lactating women. It may be irritating to the eyes or mucous membranes; hence, these areas should be avoided. Irritant dermatitis may occur with use of excessive

amounts or over prolonged periods. Toxicity, if overused, may result in nausea, vomiting, seizures, or even bone marrow suppression.

1. Structure

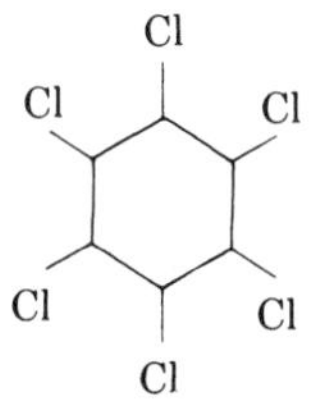

Gamma benzene hexachloride

2. Use: Scabies: apply lotion uniformly to all skin surfaces, including folds and creases from the neck to the toes. Rinse off in 8 to 12 hours. Head/pubic lice: with shampoo, apply to affected hairy areas and rinse off in 4 minutes. Remove all residual nits with nit comb or tweezers.

3. Packaging:
  Lindane lotion: 30 mL, 59 mL, pharmacy-size only pint
  Lindane shampoo: 30 mL, 59 mL, pharmacy-size only pint

B. Permethrin (Acticin, Elimite, Nix). Permethrin is a synthetic pyrethrin derivative of the flowers of the plant *Chrysanthemum cinerariifolium*. It has a broad spectrum of insecticidal activity. It acts to disrupt neuronal sodium channel repolarization and cause paralysis and eventual death of the insect. It is both a pediculicide and scabicide. It can cause breathing difficulty or an asthmatic episode in susceptible patients. It is generally nonirritating and offers a 90% cure rate after a single application. Although no resistance has been demonstrated in the United States to date, decreased susceptibilities have been shown, indicating the possible emergence of resistance. It is also effective against ticks, fleas, and other arthropods.

1. Structure

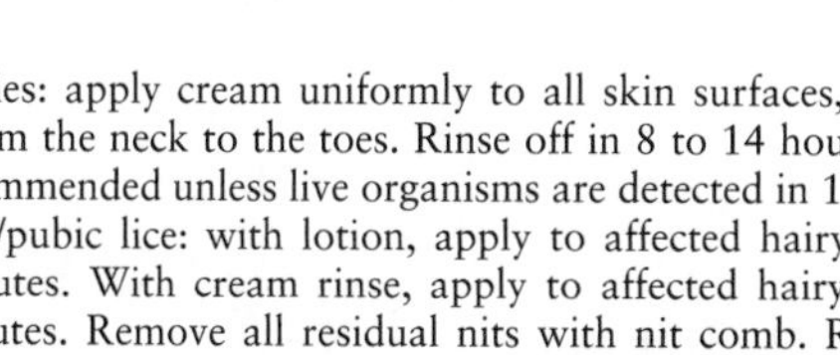

Permethrin

2. Use: Scabies: apply cream uniformly to all skin surfaces, including folds and creases from the neck to the toes. Rinse off in 8 to 14 hours. Repeat treatment is not recommended unless live organisms are detected in 1 week.

  Head/pubic lice: with lotion, apply to affected hairy areas and rinse off in 10 minutes. With cream rinse, apply to affected hairy areas and rinse off in 10 minutes. Remove all residual nits with nit comb. Repeat treatment not recommended unless live organisms are detected in 1 week.

3. Packaging:
  Permethrin 5% cream: 60 g
  Permethrin 1% liquid: 60 mL
  Permethrin 1% lotion: 60 mL

C. Pyrethrin (Licide, R&C, RID, Tisit) compounds and synthetic pyrethroids are used for the treatment of pediculosis (see Chap. 19). These are currently the drugs of choice in treating pediculosis. They demonstrate no scabicidal effect. Resistance has been shown to these compounds. They are absorbed through the chitinous exoskeleton and stimulate the nervous system, resulting in seizures and death of the insect.

1. Packaging:

> Pyrethrin 0.3% gel: 30 mL
> Pyrethrin 0.3% lotion: 59 mL, 118 mL
> Pyrethrin 0.33% mousse: 165 mL
> Pyrethrin 0.33% shampoo: 59 mL, 60 mL, 118 mL, 120 mL, 240 mL

D. Ivermectin (Stromectol) is a semisynthetic antihelminthic agent derived from *Streptomyces avirmitilis*. It acts to bind with high affinity to glutamate-gated chloride ion channels in nerve and muscle cells. Chloride ion permeability is increased, with resultant hyperpolarization, paralysis, and death of the insect. It is indicated for strongyloidiasis and onchocerciasis and for crusted scabies or scabetic infection that has failed multiple courses of topical therapies.

1. Use: 200 μg/kg as a single dose; may require to be repeated in 1 week.

2. Packaging:

> Ivermectin (Stromectol): 3 mg, 6 mg

E. Benzyl benzoate: 20% to 25%. This agent is relatively nontoxic and is widely used in developing countries to treat scabies and pediculosis capitis and pubis. Only a veterinary preparation is available in the United States. Benzyl benzoate is synthetically derived from the esterification of benzoic acid with benzyl alcohol. Its mechanism of action is unknown. It is toxic to *Sarcoptes scabei* and may be toxic to *Pediculosis capitis* and *Phthirus pubis*. No resistance has been demonstrated to date.

1. Structure

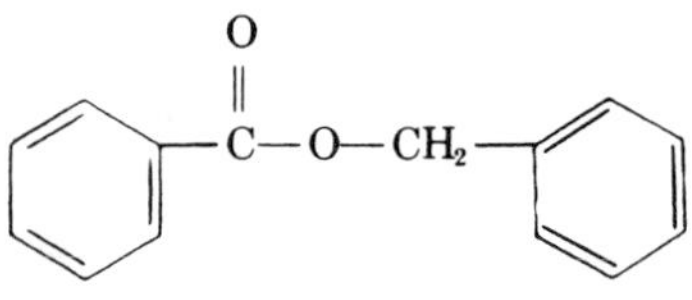

Benzyl benzoate

2. Use: Rub into affected hairy areas, avoiding eye exposure. Rinse off in 12 to 24 hours. Repeat treatment in 1 week.

3. Packaging (prepared extemporaneously):

> Benzyl benzoate 28% lotion: 500 mL

F. Crotamiton (*N*-ethyl-*o*-crotonotoluide, Eurax) is a synthetic chloroformate salt used for the prevention and treatment of scabies, although cure rates tend to be lower for the same number of applications compared with lindane and permethrin. It may have an antipruritic effect independent of its scabetic effect. Its mechanism of action is unknown. It is not effective as a pediculicide.

1. Structure

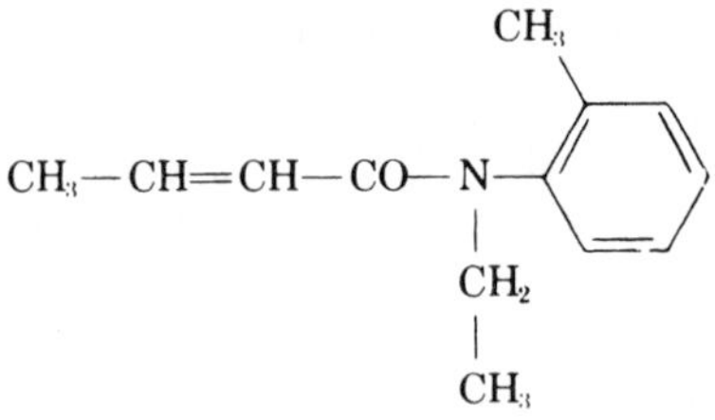

Crotamiton (*N*-ethyl-*o*-crotonotoluide)

2. Use: Apply uniformly to all skin surfaces, including folds and creases from the neck to the toes. Repeat every 24 hours for 2 days. The patient should bathe 48 hours after the last application to remove the drug.

3. Packaging:

Eurax 10% cream: 60 g

Eurax 10% lotion: 60 g, 454 g

G. Malathion (Ovide) is highly effective in the prevention and treatment of pediculosis. It displays 95% ovicidal activity and has no scabicidal activity. It works through cholinesterase inhibition.

1. Structure

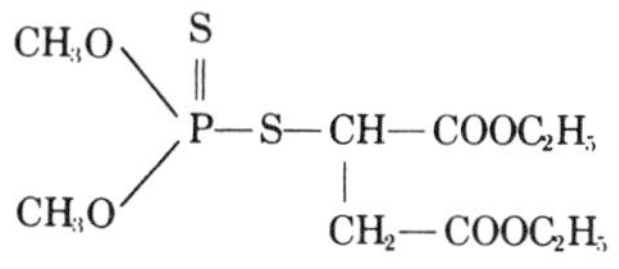

$$CH_3O\diagdown \underset{\|}{\overset{S}{P}}-S-CH-COOC_2H_5$$
$$CH_3O\diagup \qquad \quad | \qquad$$
$$\qquad\qquad CH_2-COOC_2H_5$$

Malathion

2. Use: Apply to affected hairy areas and rinse off in 8 to 12 hours. Remove all nits. Repeat treatment if live organisms are observed in 7 to 9 days.

3. Packaging:

Malathion (Ovide) 0.5% lotion: 59 mL

H. Petrolatum, physostigmine 0.025% ophthalmic ointment, and yellow oxide of mercury are useful for infestation of eyelashes with pediculosis pubis. These agents are generally thickly applied b.i.d. for 8 days with a cotton-tipped applicator.

I. Precipitated sulfur was used previously in infants and pregnant women, but with the discovery that permethrin cream 5% is equally safe, it is now prescribed less often. Although systemic effects are rare, it may stain clothing and it also has an unpleasant odor. It is applied daily for 3 days.

1. Packaging:

Must be compounded, generally as 6% (5% to 10%) sulfur in petrolatum or Cetaphil: 1 lb

V. MISCELLANEOUS AGENTS

A. Iodochlorhydroxyquin (Clioquinol), containing 40% iodine, was originally developed as a substitute for iodoform as an antiseptic dusting powder. Although its most effective use is in the treatment of amebiasis, it also has mild antibacterial and antifungal effects and may be used alone or with steroids in the treatment of eczematous and impetiginized processes and some dermatophyte, yeast, and *Trichomonas* infections. However, more specific agents are available. Because of neurotoxicity, the oral form of this drug has been withdrawn in the United States. A recent study demonstrating significant percutaneous absorption when applied to intact human skin raises concern regarding its topical use as well. The medication may stain the skin, hair, and clothing yellow and may induce contact allergy.

1. Structure

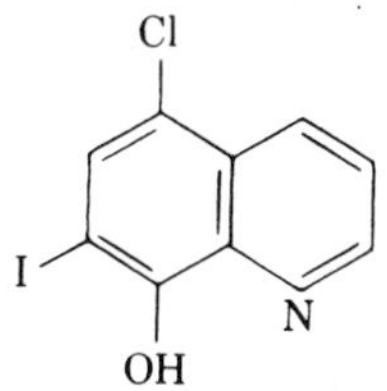

Iodochlorhydroxyquin

2. **Use:** Apply to affected areas b.i.d.
3. **Packaging:**
Clioquinol 3% and hydrocortisone 1% (Vioform): 20 g and 50 g

B. Mafenide (Sulfamylon) is a synthetic antibacterial agent related chemically, but not pharmacologically, to the sulfonamides. The drug appears to interfere with bacterial cellular metabolism and is not antagonized by PABA, pus, or serum. It is bacteriostatic against many gram-positive and gram-negative organisms, including staphylococci, streptococci, and *Pseudomonas* species. Mafenide is highly soluble and diffuses easily through an eschar. After percutaneous absorption, the drug is metabolized; it acts as a weak carbonic anhydrase inhibitor and may therefore cause systemic acidosis.

Mafenide is used primarily in the adjunctive treatment of second- and third-degree burn wounds. It may cause severe pain on application, and active allergic contact sensitivity may develop.

1. **Structure**

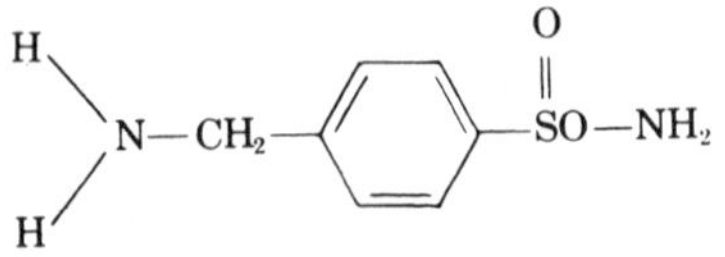

Mafenide

2. **Use:** Apply q.d. to b.i.d. with hand in a sterile glove.
3. **Packaging:**
Mafenide (Sulfamylon) cream, 85 mg/g: 37 g, 114 g, 411 g
Mafenide (Sulfamylon) solution, 5%: 50-g packets for reconstitution

C. Mercurial compounds have bacteriostatic effects, most likely mediated through inhibiting sulfhydryl enzymes, but fall far short of being ideal antibacterial compounds. Mercurial compounds may be absorbed and can sensitize; more effective and less hazardous antiseptic agents are available.

1. Insoluble mercury compounds are used as antibacterial and antiparasitic agents. Yellow mercury oxide ointment has been used for pediculosis involving the eyelashes; ammoniated mercury, containing 78% mercury, has been utilized in pyoderma and scaling processes.
2. The organic mercurial antiseptics are more bacteriostatic and less irritating and toxic than inorganic salts. Merbromin (Mercurochrome), containing 25% mercury, is not particularly active and suffers further from having its activity decrease in the presence of organic material. Thimerosal, containing 49% mercury, has the same drawbacks although is more effective although a significant contact sensitizer.

D. Nitrofurazone (Furacin), a synthetic nitrofuran derivative with a broad antibacterial spectrum. Although its exact mechanism of action is unknown, it is thought to inhibit bacterial enzymes involved in carbohydrate metabolism. It is not effective against fungal or viral organisms. It is used as adjunctive therapy in patients with second- and third-degree burns when bacterial resistance to other antiinfective agents is a potential problem. It is not effective in the treatment of minor burns or superficial bacterial infections involving wounds, cutaneous ulcers, or various pyodermas. It is rarely used by dermatologists as it carries a high risk of acquired contact sensitivity.

1. **Structure**

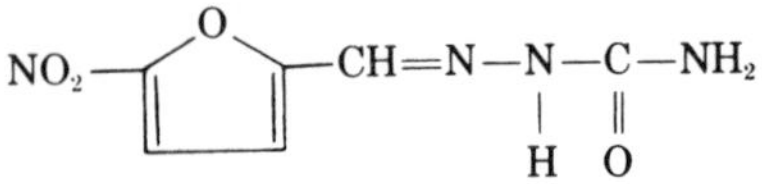

Nitrofurazone

2. Use: Apply once daily.
3. Packaging:

Nitrofurazone 0.2% cream: 28 g
Nitrofurazone 0.2% ointment: 28 g, 56 g, 454 g
Nitrofurazone 0.2% solution: 480 mL, gal

E. Silver sulfadiazine (Silvadene, SSD) is a synthetic agent that combines the beneficial properties of silver nitrate and sulfonamides. It acts upon the cell membrane and cell wall. It is used primarily as an adjunct in the prevention and treatment of wound sepsis in patients with second- and third-degree burns and for wound care of chronic ulcers. It is bactericidal against many gram-positive and gram-negative bacteria as well as *C. albicans* and is reasonably effective against *P. aeruginosa* and *S. aureus*. Bacteria susceptible to sulfadiazine but resistant to silver nitrate, as well as those sensitive to silver nitrate but resistant to sulfadiazine, have shown good response to silver sulfadiazine. It does not stain, is unlikely to produce electrolyte imbalance, and does not cause systemic acidosis. Some patients note a stinging sensation on application, and because this compound can be absorbed, systemic sulfonamide reactions similar to those caused by sulfonamides may occur.

1. Structure

$$H_2N- -SO_2N $$

AG

Silver sulfadiazine

2. Use: Apply q.d. to b.i.d. 1/16-in. thick. Dressing not required.
3. Packaging:

Silver sulfadiazine cream, 10 mg/g: 20 g, 25 g, 50 g, 85 g, 400 g, 1,000 g

 ANTIINFLAMMATORY AGENTS

Topical and Intralesional Corticosteroids

I. Corticosteroids are the most potent and effective local antiinflammatory medications available and also have a striking ability to inhibit cell division. They are the therapy of choice in most inflammatory, pruritic eruptions (e.g., dermatitis) and are also effective in hyperproliferative disorders (e.g., psoriasis) and infiltrative disorders (e.g., sarcoid and granuloma annulare). Since 1952, when these preparations first became available commercially, hundreds have been marketed. Their continuous wide usage has been ensured by their numerous desirable qualities: broad applicability in treating a wide variety of common eruptions, rapidity of action in small amounts, ease of use, absence of pain or odor, relative lack of sensitization, prolonged stability, compatibility with almost all commonly used topical medications, and rarity of untoward clinical systemic effects from percutaneous absorption. The effectiveness of a topical corticosteroid is related to the potency of the drug and its percutaneous penetration. Activity of a particular preparation is dependent on binding to a cytosol glucocorticoid receptor; the order of clinical potency of different agents parallels the binding to receptor proteins. Potency is also significantly affected by the vehicle. For example, the enhanced potency of two of the strongest preparations is caused by alteration of the corticosteroid moiety in one (Temovate) and optimization of the vehicle in the other (Diprolene).

Approximately 1% of a hydrocortisone solution will penetrate normal skin on the forearm and about twice that will penetrate through eczematous skin. There is a marked regional variation in corticosteroid penetrations; compared with the data for the forearm, hydrocortisone is absorbed 0.14 times as well through the back, 3.5 times through the scalp, 6.0 times through the forehead, 13 times through the cheeks at the jaw angle, and 42 times through scrotal skin. If the skin is completely hydrated, absorption will be increased four- or fivefold. Inflamed skin, such as that found with atopic dermatitis, allows increased percutaneous penetration; with conditions such as exfoliative psoriasis, there seems to be very little barrier to absorption. Small changes in molecular structure related to enhancing the intrinsic activity of the corticosteroid moiety, increasing lipophilicity to facilitate better skin penetration, and retarding the metabolic inactivation of the molecule result in enormous alterations in clinical effectiveness. To be active, cortisone must be reduced to cortisol (hydrocortisone), just as prednisone must be converted to prednisolone before it can be utilized. Addition of halogen atoms to the steroid nucleus may dramatically increase activity. The potency of topical corticosteroids is most often assessed *in vivo* by their ability to produce vasoconstriction on human skin, and results of this bioassay correlate well with clinical trials. Other potency assays include suppression of experimentally induced allergic contact dermatitis (e.g., to Rhus antigen) or irritant dermatitis (produced by kerosene or croton oil) or reduction in size of histamine-induced wheals. Antimitotic activity may be assessed by *in vitro* fibroblast inhibition and/or *in vivo* epidermal mitotic assay.

Systemic absorption of topical steroids depends on both the pharmacokinetic properties of the substance applied and the integrity of the stratum corneum. Suppression of the hypothalamic-pituitary-adrenal (HPA) axis has been shown to occur with medium- and high-potency agents.

In 1960, it was discovered that placing corticosteroids on the skin under occlusion with thin, pliable plastic wraps dramatically increased their efficacy (up to 100-fold); occlusion causes hydration of the stratum corneum, increases the surface of skin almost 40%, and appears to induce a reservoir of corticosteroid in the horny layer that persists for several days after application. Percutaneous absorption of steroids under wrap, particularly through altered skin, always occurs. It should be assumed that all patients under substantial occlusive therapy have temporary suppression of the HPA axis. Adults applying a potent steroid in excess of 50 to 100 g weekly (10 to 20 g in small children) for 2 or more weeks face the possibility of having HPA axis suppression. Clobetasol has been shown to suppress the HPA axis at doses as low as 2 g/day. Occlusion and application over large areas increase the risk of suppression. Patients with liver failure or children are particularly at greater risk. Suppressed HPA axis function was noted in 5 of 13 children with atopic or seborrheic dermatitis after application of 1% hydrocortisone cream. Normal function returns within days to weeks of dressings being discontinued, depending on the duration, extent, and intensity of prior therapy. Undesirable effects from occlusive therapy include infection, miliaria, folliculitis, disagreeable odor, interference with heat exchange, and an increased tendency to sunburn, atrophy, and striae.

Multiple potential adverse effects are associated with the use of topical corticosteroids. If used injudiciously even without occlusion, the more potent formulations may induce mild hypercortisolism, HPA axis suppression, or, rarely, Cushing's syndrome. Burning, itching, irritation, and dryness are the most common acute problems and are usually related to the vehicle of the steroid preparation and to the pretreatment state of the skin. The prevalence of contact allergy to topical steroids is higher than initially thought; patients with stasis dermatitis and leg ulceration are at increased risk, without regard to duration of dermatitis. Ointments are better tolerated on inflamed skin than creams or gels. Miliaria, folliculitis, and maceration may occur from excessive occlusion and plastic films. Atrophy and telangiectasia are frequent findings if potent corticosteroids have been used over prolonged periods, particularly with the use of occlusive techniques. Early atrophic changes are generally limited to the epidermis, but the dermis and subcutaneous tissue may also be affected with prolonged use. The atrophy is generally due to reduction in cell size rather than in number. Minor atrophic changes as well as telangiectasia are reversible on discontinuation of the topical steroid within 6 months. Concomitant use of 12% ammonium lactate (Lac-Hydrin Lotion) reduces the amount of epidermal and dermal atrophy without influencing the bioavailability or antiinflammatory properties of the corticosteroid. Purpura may be found in atrophic areas. Thinning with or without atrophic striae can be seen within 1 month of use on more susceptible sites such as the face and intertriginous and anogenital areas. Striae are irreversible. The more potent the corticosteroid, the more rapidly and more severe the adverse effects will be. Complications are related to potency but not restricted to halogenated corticosteroids. Less common side effects include perioral dermatitis or a rosacea-like dermatitis, acneiform lesions, hypertrichosis, hypopigmentation, contact dermatitis to the vehicle or to the actual corticosteroid, and ocular hypertension from application in or around the eyes. Topical steroids may also mask superficial infections or worsen fungal infections.

Injection of small amounts of corticosteroids (betamethasone sodium phosphate and betamethasone acetate suspension, triamcinolone acetonide, triamcinolone diacetate, triamcinolone hexacetonide) into cutaneous lesions has the advantage of achieving high local concentration with prolonged depot effects and no systemic side effects. Intralesional use is of particular value in the treatment of acne cysts, psoriatic plaques, circumscribed neurodermatitis, keloids, and occasionally, chronic plaques of nummular eczema, insect-bite reactions, alopecia areata, discoid lupus erythematosus, sarcoidosis, myxoid cysts, and nail disorders. Local adverse reactions include atrophy (especially when the concentration is too high or the steroid is injected too high in the dermis), hypopigmentation of deeply pigmented skin, growth of occasional tufts of hair in susceptible individuals, infection, and ulceration. Injection with a 1-mL tuberculin syringe using a 30-gauge needle is best. Air-powered guns can be used but are less precise, disrupt the dermis, and are associated with increased risk of pyogenic infection or transmission of hepatitis virus. Usually a dilution of the medication (i.e., to 2.5 mg/mL triamcinolone acetonide) will provide enough steroid to reduce inflammation while avoiding these problems. (See discussion of individual diseases for proper dilution.)

II. DOSAGE CONSIDERATIONS

A. Dose–response relationship. It is usually possible to observe a clear dose–response relationship in the use of topical corticosteroids. Compounds vary markedly in their potency and efficacy, and most products are available in standard and diluted concentrations; some may also be obtained in high-potency concentrations. Efficacy may also be altered by method of use (e.g., prior hydration, occlusion). The diluted concentration products may be equipotent to full-strength agents on vasoconstriction assays. Ointment vehicles generally give better biologic activity to the incorporated steroids than do cream or lotion vehicles.

In most instances, initial therapy should be with one of the most potent compounds and maintenance therapy should involve a less concentrated compound such as 1% hydrocortisone. At least 33% to 50% of patients can be managed with medium- to low-strength topical corticosteroids, which should always be tried. The less potent corticosteroid formulations (e.g., 1% hydrocortisone) should be used for the scrotum, groin, axillae, eyelids, and face.

B. Frequency of application. There is a paucity of pharmacokinetic data dealing with the optimal dose–response characteristics of topical corticosteroid use. One study of 12 patients with corticosteroid-responsive dermatoses found that six treatments per day were no more effective than three applications per day. Other studies involving patients with psoriasis or atopic dermatitis have shown no advantage of application three to four times a day compared with once daily. Overnight application of corticosteroids to hydrated skin, used with or without occlusion, should be as effective and far less costly than multiple daily applications. During the day, simple lubricants can be used. If desired, topical corticosteroids may be used b.i.d. to t.i.d. but there are no data supporting the notion that more frequent use leads to better or faster resolution of hyperplastic or inflammatory processes.

C. Tachyphylaxis. Repeated application of a potent topical steroid may result in a diminished effect. Tachyphylaxis may occur within 1 week of initial use, but the ability to respond fully returns within a week of stopping drug application. It is therefore best to treat effectively for short periods of time (days to 2 weeks) followed by corticosteroid treatment–free intervals of a week or more during which time lubricants alone are applied. This regimen also avoids the possible increased percutaneous absorption of topical corticosteroids that may occur after long-term administration.

D. Relative potency. The "perfect test" to measure the relative potency of topical steroids and the bioequivalence of generic brands has yet to be established. The vasoconstrictor assay visually measures the amount of vasoconstriction produced by a glucocorticoid. The degree of pallor produced after application of a steroid over a standard period of time increases with the concentration of the steroid. The assay is imprecise because of the variation between observers and other parameters within an individual study. Clinical models, such as psoriasis, have also been used to evaluate relative potency. Table 40-3 lists the relative potency of topical corticosteroids based on the summation of available information from bioassays, clinical models, and literature reviews.

E. Generics. Some discrepancy may exist in the efficacy of the trade name topical corticosteroids and the corresponding generics, with some generics demonstrating up to 50% less activity in vasoconstrictor assays. Several generics may exist for a particular trade name [i.e., Valisone (betamethasone valerate) has 28 generic forms]. The only way to ensure consistency is to prescribe brand name only, although this is often impractical with managed care pharmacy plan limitations.

F. Occlusive therapy. Some conditions such as psoriasis, lichen simplex chronicus, and hand eczema respond poorly, if at all, to creams alone. The use of occlusive (airtight) dressings will increase the efficacy of these preparations. Occlusion with class 1 agents is not recommended. Patients should be instructed to do the following:

1. Soak the area in water for up to 20 minutes.
2. Rub medication into lesions while the skin is still moist.
3. Cover the area with a plastic wrap (Saran Wrap, Handi Wrap), plastic gloves for hands, plastic bags for feet, bathing cap for scalp, and vinyl exercise suit for large areas of the legs or torso. Tubular plastic dressings are also useful.
4. Seal edges with tape or cover plastic with an ace bandage, a long stocking, panty hose, or any dressing that will ensure close adherence to skin. Blenderm tape will stick particularly well to skin. Paper tape may be less irritating.
5. Use for at least 6 hours. Overnight application is usually sufficient to induce clinical remission, but such a technique may also be used during the day. Occlusion for even a few hours may be very beneficial.

As noted previously, significant percutaneous absorption of steroids will occur with occlusive therapy, and patients undergoing stressful procedures (i.e., operations) should be supplemented with IV corticosteroids. The most potent preparations should be used rarely, if at all, under occlusion.

III. PACKAGING: Because topical corticosteroids are stable preparations, buying in bulk is feasible and will frequently result in significant cost savings to the patient. Some pharmacies and institutions will buy 5-lb containers and repackage, with resultant enormous decreases in unit cost. With corticosteroids, the cost of purchasing multiple small tubes is particularly high in contrast to buying one larger size. For example, the price of four 15-g tubes of fluocinonide (Lidex) is 170% that of one 60-g tube. All topical corticosteroids are available by prescription only, with the exception of 0.5% and 1% hydrocortisone. Selected agents will be discussed in more detail in the following text.

A. Betamethasone valerate (Psorion, Beta-Val, Luxiq) is a synthetic fluorinated corticosteroid.

1. Structure

Betamethasone valerate

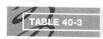

TABLE 40-3	Topical Corticosteroid Potency

1 (Most potent)	Betamethasone dipropionate cream, ointment 0.05% (optimized vehicle) (Diprolene)
	Clobetasol propionate cream, ointment 0.05% (optimized vehicle) (Clobex, Temovate)
	Diflorasone diacetate ointment 0.05% (optimized vehicle) (Apexicon, Psorcon)
	Halobetasol propionate cream, ointment 0.05% (Ultravate)
2	Amcinonide ointment 0.1% (Cyclocort)
	Desoximetasone cream, ointment 0.25% (Topicort)
	Desoximetasone gel 0.05% (Topicort)
	Diflorasone diacetate ointment 0.05% (Florone, Maxiflor)
	Fluocinonide cream, gel, ointment (0.05%) (Lidex)
	Halcinonide 0.1% cream (Halog)
	Mometasone furoate ointment 0.1% (Elocon)
	Triamcinolone acetonide ointment 0.5% (Kenalog)
3	Amcinonide cream, lotion 0.1% (Cyclocort)
	Betamethasone benzoate gel 0.025% (Benisone, Uticort)
	Betamethasone valerate ointment 0.1% (Valisone)
	Diflorasone diacetate cream 0.05% (Florone, Maxiflor)
	Fluticasone propionate ointment, 0.005% (Cutivate)
	Fluocortolone cream, 0.25% (Ultralan)
	Fluocinonide cream 0.05% (Lidex E cream)
	Halcinonide ointment 0.1% (Halog)
	Triamcinolone acetonide ointment 0.1% (Aristocort A) cream 0.5% (Aristocort-HP)
4	Betamethasone benzoate ointment 0.025% (Benisone, Uticort)
	Betamethasone valerate lotion 0.1% (Valisone)
	Desoximetasone cream 0.05% (Topicort-LP)
	Fluocinolone acetonide cream 0.2% (Synalar-HP)
	Fluocinolone acetonide ointment 0.025% (Synalar)
	Flurandrenolide ointment 0.05% (Cordran)
	Halcinonide cream 0.025% (Halog)
	Hydrocortisone valerate ointment 0.2% (Westcort)
	Mometasone furoate cream 0.1% (Elocon)
	Triamcinolone acetonide ointment 0.1% (Kenalog)
5	Betamethasone benzoate cream 0.025% (Benisone, Uticort)
	Betamethasone dipropionate lotion 0.05% (Diprosone)
	Betamethasone valerate cream 0.1% (Betatrex, Valisone)
	Clocortolone cream 0.1% (Cloderm)
	Fluocinolone acetonide cream 0.025% (Fluonid, Synalar)
	Fluocinolone acetonide oil 0.01% (Derma-Smoothe/FS)
	Flurandrenolide cream 0.05% (Cordran)

(continued)

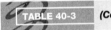

TABLE 40-3 *(Continued)*

	Fluticasone propionate cream 0.05% (Cutivate)
	Hydrocortisone butyrate cream 0.1% (Locoid)
	Hydrocortisone valerate cream 0.2% (Westcort)
	Prednicarbate 0.1% cream (Dermatop)
	Triamcinolone acetonide cream 0.1% (Kenalog)
6	Alclometasone dipropionate cream, ointment 0.05% (Aclovate)
	Betamethasone valerate lotion 0.1% (Valisone)
	Desonide cream 0.05% (DesOwen, Tridesilon)
	Fluocinolone acetonide cream, solution 0.01% (Synalar)
	Triamcinolone acetonide cream 0.1% (Aristocort)
7 (Least potent)	Dexamethasone cream 0.1% (Decadron phosphate)
	Hydrocortisone 0.5%, 1%, 2.5% (generic, Hytone, others)
	Methylprednisolone 1% (Medrol)

Source: Modified from Cornell RC, Stoughton RB. Correlation of the vasoconstriction assay and clinical activity in psoriasis. *Arch Dermatol* 1985;121(1):63–67.
Stoughton RB. Are generic formulations equivalent to trade name topical glucocorticoids? *Arch Dermatol* 1987;123(10):1312–1314. Reproduced, with permission.

2. Packaging:

Betamethasone valerate 0.05% cream: 15 g, 45 g
Betamethasone valerate 0.1% cream, ointment: 15 g, 45 g
Betamethasone valerate 0.1% lotion: 60 mL
Betamethasone valerate 1.2 mg/g foam: 100 g

B. Clobetasol propionate (Cormax, Temovate, Embeline, Olux) is one of the most potent of the currently available agents and is indicated for short-term treatment of inflammatory or hyperplastic disorders. It is a synthetic fluorinated corticosteroid. It may cause a more rapid or prolonged response than other topical corticosteroids. It is recommended that clobetasol have a maximum application of 60 g/week for no longer than 14 days without occlusion and that it should not be used in children below age 12.

1. Structure

CH_2Cl
|
$C=O$
CH_3
HO — H ---$OCOCH_2CH_3$
CH_3 CH_3
CH_3 H H
F H
$O=$

Clobetasol

2. Packaging:
Clobetasol propionate 0.05% cream or ointment: 15 g, 30 g, 45 g
Clobetasol propionate 0.05% solution: 25 mL, 50 mL
Clobetasol propionate 0.05% gel: 15 g, 30 g, 60 g
Clobetasol propionate 0.05% foam: 100 g

C. Desonide (DesOwen, Tridesilon) is a synthetic corticosteroid.

1. Structure

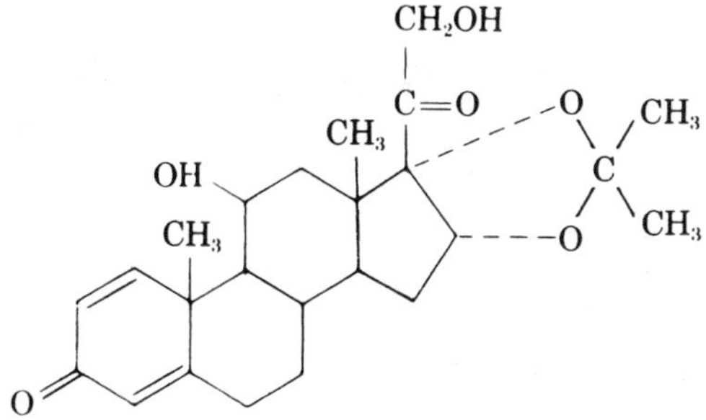

Desonide

2. Packaging:
Desonide 0.05% cream, ointment: 15 g, 60 g, 90 g
Desonide 0.05% lotion: 60 mL, 120 mL

D. Fluocinolone acetonide (Derma-Smoothe/FS, Flurosyn, Capex, Synalar) is a synthetic fluorinated corticosteroid.

1. Structure

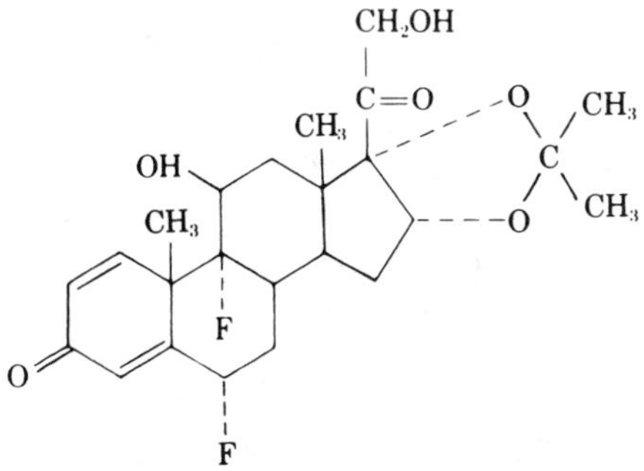

Fluocinolone acetonide

2. Packaging:
Fluocinolone acetonide 0.01% cream: 15 g, 30 g, 42.5 g, 60 g
Fluocinolone acetonide 0.2% cream: 12 g
Fluocinolone acetonide 0.025% cream, ointment: 15 g, 30 g, 60 g, 425 g
Fluocinolone acetonide 0.01% shampoo: 180 mL
Fluocinolone acetonide 0.01% solution: 20 mL, 60 mL
Fluocinolone acetonide oil 0.01%: 120 mL

E. Fluocinonide (Lidex, Lidex E, Fluonex) is a synthetic fluorinated corticosteroid.

1. **Structure**

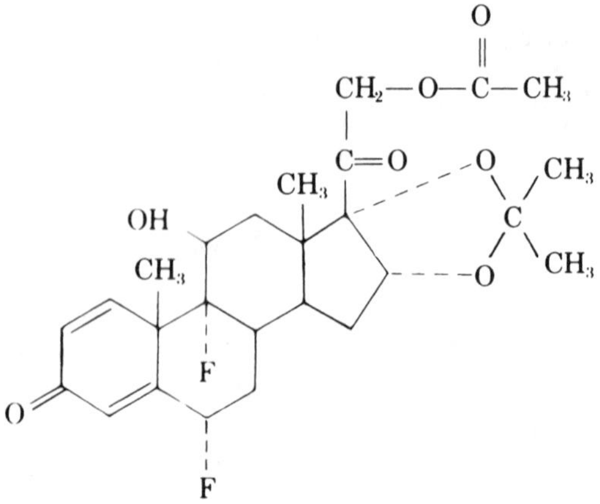

Fluocinonide fluocinolone acetonide acetate

2. **Packaging:**
> Fluocinonide 0.05% gel: 15 g, 30 g, 60 g, 120 g
> Fluocinonide 0.05% cream, ointment: 15 g, 30 g, 60 g, 120 g
> Fluocinonide 0.05% solution: 20 mL, 60 mL

F. Flurandrenolide (Cordran, Cordran SP) is a synthetic fluorinated corticosteroid.

1. **Structure**

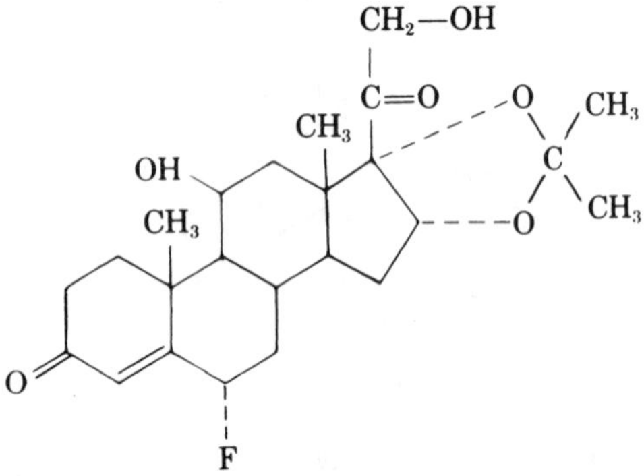

Flurandrenolide

2. **Packaging:**
> Flurandrenolide 0.025% cream, ointment: 30 g, 60 g
> Flurandrenolide 0.05% cream, ointment: 15 g, 30 g, 60 g
> Flurandrenolide lotion 0.05%: 15 mL, 60 mL
> Flurandrenolide tape 4 μg/sq. cm roll: 24 in. × 3 in., 80 in. × 3 in.

G. Halcinonide (Halog, Halog-E) is a synthetic fluorinated corticosteroid.

1. **Structure**

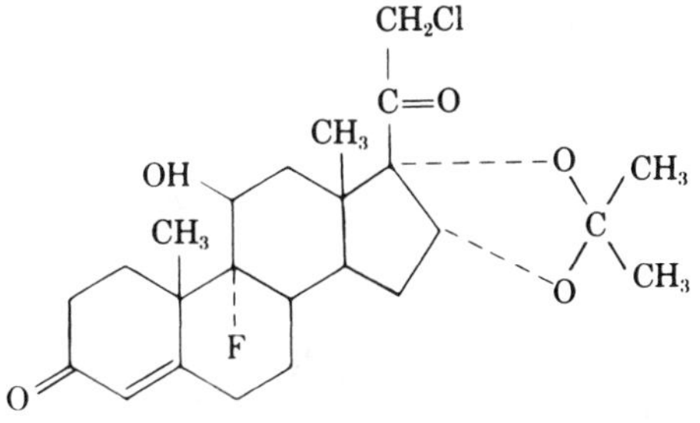

Halcinonide

2. **Packaging:**

Halog 0.025% cream: 15 g, 60 g
Halog 0.1% cream, ointment: 15 g, 30 g, 60 g, 240 g
Halog-E 0.1% cream: 15 g, 30 g, 60 g
Halog 0.1% solution: 20 mL, 60 mL

H. Hydrocortisone (Cortizone, Cortaid, Anusol-HC, Hytone, LactiCare-HC, Sarnol HC, Penecort, Texacort, and many other branded products) may be purchased as a generic drug.

1. **Structure**

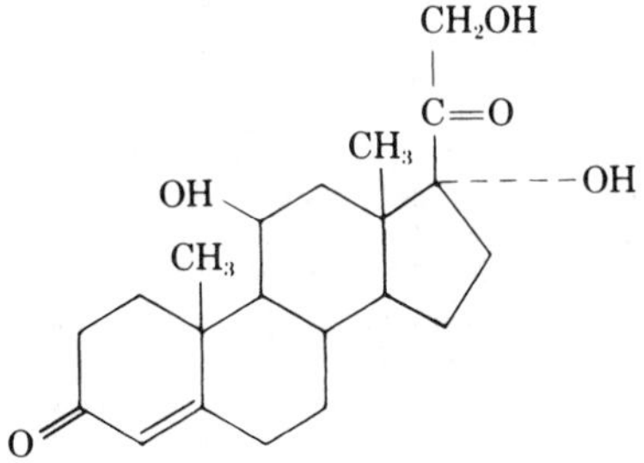

Hydrocortisone

2. **Packaging (OTC):**

Hydrocortisone 0.5% cream, ointment: 15 g, 30 g, 60 g, 120 g, 1 lb
Hydrocortisone 0.5% lotion: 30 mL, 60 mL, 120 mL
Hydrocortisone 1% cream, ointment: 15 g, 20 g, 28 g, 30 g, 56 g, 90 g, 120 g, 240 g, 1 lb
Hydrocortisone 1% gel, solution: 15 g, 30 g
Hydrocortisone 1% liquid, lotion: 45 mL, 60 mL, 75 mL, 118 mL, 120 mL, 600 mL
Hydrocortisone 1% roll-on: 14 g
Hydrocortisone 1% spray: 45 mL
Hydrocortisone 2% lotion: 30 mL
Hydrocortisone 2.5% cream, ointment: 15 g, 20 g, 30 g, 60 g, 120 g, 240 g, 1 lb

I. Prednicarbate (Dermatop E) is a synthetic nonfluorinated topical corticosteroid.

   1. Packaging:

   Prednicarbate 0.1% cream, ointment: 15 g, 60 g

J. Triamcinolone acetonide (Aristocort, Kenalog) is a synthetic fluorinated corticosteroid.

   1. Structure

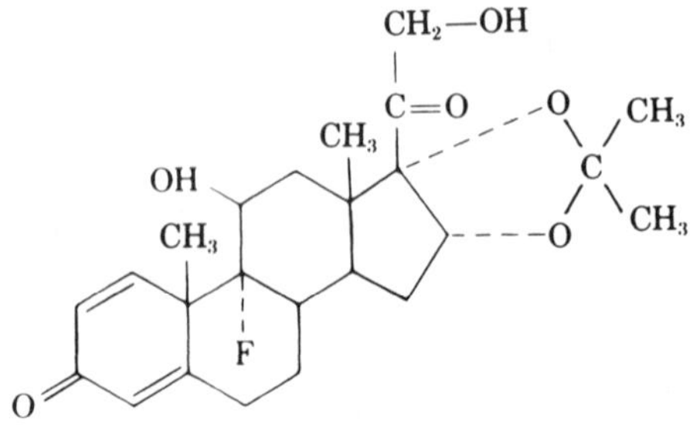

Triamcinolone acetonide

   2. Packaging:

   Triamcinolone acetonide 0.025% cream, ointment: 15 g, 28 g, 30 g, 57 g, 60 g, 80 g, 113 g, 120 g, 240 g, 454 g, 1 lb

   Triamcinolone acetonide 0.1% cream, ointment: 15 g, 20 g, 28 g, 30 g, 57 g, 60 g, 80 g, 90 g, 113 g, 120 g, 240 g, 454 g, 1 lb

   Triamcinolone acetonide 0.5% cream, ointment: 15 g, 20 g, 28 g, 30 g, 57 g, 60 g, 113 g, 120 g, 240 g

   Triamcinolone acetonide 0.1% lotion: 15 mL, 60 mL

   Triamcinolone acetonide 0.025% lotion: 60 mL

   Triamcinolone acetonide aerosol, 2-second spray: 23 g, 63 g

K. Steroid combinations. There are hundreds of topical corticosteroid preparations available in different vehicles and in combination with antibiotics (most frequently neomycin), other antiseptics (iodochlorhydroxyquin), and other agents (tars, keratolytic agents). Some combinations are useful, but there is more flexibility and control over therapy, often at a lower cost to the patient, if separate, identifiable agents are used.

Systemic Corticosteroids

I. DISCUSSION. Systemic corticosteroids are used in the treatment of a number of skin diseases, ranging from pemphigus vulgaris to severe cases of allergic contact dermatitis. Because of their well-known and serious side effects, the decision to use them must be based on careful consideration of the indications, alternatives, contraindications, and risks in each clinical situation. Fortunately, many of the instances for which they are utilized in dermatology are either short-lived or rapidly responsive so that "short courses" of treatment, for which the risks are significantly diminished, may be used.

Virtually every aspect of inflammation and immunologic reactivity is altered—usually diminished—by corticosteroids. For example, neutrophil migration and adherence to endothelium are reduced, capillary permeability and blood flow are diminished, the passage of immune complexes across basement membranes is decreased, and it is thought that lysosomal membranes are stabilized by corticosteroids, among many other effects.

Systemic corticosteroids are either proved or generally acknowledged to be beneficial in the treatment of pemphigus vulgaris, bullous pemphigoid, id (autosensitization) reactions, severe allergic contact dermatitis (such as poison ivy), collagen-vascular diseases, pyoderma gangrenosum, and Sweet's syndrome. Low doses at bedtime may be useful in treating hormonal disorders such as hirsutism or acne. They are also often prescribed for severe erythema multiforme, severe cutaneous drug reactions, toxic epidermal necrolysis, and severe sunburn, although their efficacy in these conditions is based largely on anecdotal clinical experience and has not been demonstrated unequivocally. Experimentally, for example, prednisone was unable to alter the development or course of sunburn erythema induced artificially on small areas of the skin. On the other hand, it is probably true that patients with severe sunburn and toxic symptoms (e.g., fever and chills) may feel better when treated with systemic steroids. Corticosteroids have also been recommended for the prevention of postherpetic neuralgia, particularly when they can be given early enough in the course of herpes zoster in elderly patients.

II. General principles of corticosteroid use in cutaneous disorders

  A. Assess the indications, risks, benefits, alternatives, and possible adjuvant therapies.

  B. Evaluate possible contraindications and side effects, with special attention to any past history of psychiatric illness, osteoporosis, diabetes mellitus, glaucoma, hypertension, and peptic ulcer disease (Tables 40-4 and 40-5).

  C. Corticosteroids are relatively contraindicated in psoriasis, in which their withdrawal may incite a generalized pustular flare, and in atopic dermatitis, in which withdrawal may be extremely difficult and may be accompanied by exacerbation.

  D. Diagnose and treat any secondary infection (such as impetigo, cellulitis, or erysipelas) before starting steroids. Also, a protein-purified derivative (PPD) should be planned at the start of a long course of glucocorticoid therapy. It takes an average of 12 days for a patient to become anergic after starting glucocorticoids, so there is adequate time to discontinue steroid therapy and to start isoniazid if indicated.

  E. While they are on corticosteroid treatment, patients should be monitored, at least monthly, for the presence of any adverse reactions. Development of symptoms such as polyuria, polydipsia, abdominal pain, fever, or joint pain should be assessed. Blood pressure and weight as well as fasting blood sugar, CBC, and lipid and electrolyte levels should also be followed. In addition, a stool hemoccult and eye examination should be checked biannually.

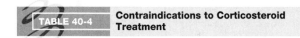

TABLE 40-4   **Contraindications to Corticosteroid Treatment**

Absolute
   Ocular herpes simplex
   Untreated tuberculosis
Relative
   Acute or chronic infections
   Pregnancy
   Diabetes mellitus
   Hypertension
   Peptic ulcer
   Osteoporosis
   Psychotic tendencies
   Renal insufficiency
   CHF (excluding that secondary to active rheumatic carditis)
   Diverticulitis
   Recent intestinal anastomoses

CHF, congestive heart failure.
Modified from Storrs FJ. Use and abuse of systemic corticosteroid therapy. *Man Dermatol Ther* 1979;1:95.

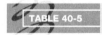

TABLE 40-5	Common Corticosteroid Complications

Central nervous system
  Pseudotumor cerebri
  Psychiatric disorders
Musculoskeletal
  Osteoporosis with spontaneous fractures
  Aseptic necrosis of bone
  Myopathy
Ocular
  Glaucoma
  Cataracts
Gastrointestinal
  Fatty infiltration of the liver
  Nausea, vomiting
  Intestinal perforation
  Pancreatitis
  Peptic ulceration
Cardiovascular and fluid retention
  Hypertension
  Sodium and fluid retention
  Hypokalemic alkalosis
  Atherosclerosis
Suppression of host defenses
  Immunosuppression, anergy
  Effects on phagocyte kinetics and function
  Increased incidence of infections
  Recurrent tuberculosis
Endocrinologic
  Suppression of hypothalamic-pituitary-adrenal axis
  Growth failure
  Secondary amenorrhea
Metabolic
  Hyperglycemia
  Nonketotic hyperosmolar states
  Hyperlipidemia
  Drug interactions
  Fibroblast inhibition
  Inhibition of wound healing
  Subcutaneous atrophy (striae, purpura)
Skin
  Acne
  Alteration of fat distribution (Cushingoid appearance)
  Urticaria

(continued)

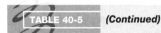

TABLE 40-5	**(Continued)**

Facial erythema
Atrophy
Striae
Lanugo hair
Alopecia

Source: From Fauci AS. Glucocorticosteroid therapy. In: Wyngaarden JB, Smith LH, Bennett JK, eds. *Cecil's textbook of medicine*. Philadelphia, PA: WB Saunders, 1988.

F. If acute infection, trauma, or surgery occurs during treatment, the steroid dose must be increased appropriately. Patients exposed to acute stress are at increased risk of adrenal crisis. Symptoms of adrenal suppression include weakness, lethargy, nausea, anorexia, fever, orthostatic hypotension, hypoglycemia, and weight loss.

G. HPA axis suppression must be considered after short courses. The degree of suppression depends on the patient, dosage (including frequency and amount), duration, and route of treatment. Longer courses and divided doses increase the risk for complications. Pituitary-adrenal reserve in response to stress may be diminished for as long as 5 days after a 5-day course of 25 mg PO b.i.d. A single injection of triamcinolone acetonide may suppress adrenal responsiveness for 2 to 3 weeks or more. Patients should be informed of this potential risk.

H. In most instances, the best route of administration is oral, and the drug of choice is prednisone, which is short acting and inexpensive. To be active, prednisone must be converted to prednisolone in the liver (Table 40-6). Potency and duration of action vary among the multiple drugs available (Table 40-6).

I. Other routes of administration include intralesional, intramuscular, or intravenous. Intralesional corticosteroids allow concentrated delivery directly into the involved area with minimal risk of HPA axis suppression. Intramuscular injection is used less frequently owing to prolonged suppression of the HPA axis and inconsistent absorption. Intravenous corticosteroids may be used in stressful situations in patients already on long-term oral steroids.

J. Although prednisone is not teratogenic, there is some risk of adrenal suppression and growth suppression in infants exposed *in utero* or through breast-feeding.

K. To prevent glucocorticoid-induced osteoporosis, the American College of Rheumatology guidelines recommend bisphosphonate therapy for all patients beginning long-term prednisone at a dose >5 mg/day.

III. DOSAGE CONSIDERATIONS IN ACUTE DERMATOSES. To achieve maximal therapeutic benefit, systemic corticosteroids must be given in adequate dosage for a sufficient length of time. It is also desirable to commence treatment as early as possible in the course of the illness. Alternate-day therapy starting at double the daily dose must be considered when use for >1 month is necessary. The initial dose of prednisone for an adult with conditions such as allergic contact dermatitis should be at least 60 mg daily. The course should be no <2 to 3 weeks. If the dose is too small or duration of treatment too short, a rebound phenomenon with generalized exacerbation of the rash and symptoms can occur.

Prednisone should be given as a single daily dose (before 8:00 a.m.) to minimize suppression of the normal diurnal cortisol secretions. Occasionally, split doses are needed early on in a disease to achieve adequate therapeutic control; once achieved, conversion to an every morning or every other day schedule as soon as possible is recommended. Suggested regimens for acute dermatoses are given in the following text.

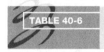

TABLE 40-6	Relative Potencies of Some Glucocorticoids

Drug	Equivalent dose (mg)
Cortisone	25
Cortisol (hydrocortisone)	20
Prednisone, prednisolone	5
Methylprednisolone, triamcinolone	4
Betamethasone	0.60
Dexamethasone	0.75

Prednisone

Prednisolone

A. Preferred methods
  1. Prednisone 60 mg PO each morning for 5 days, 40 mg PO each morning for 5 days, 20 mg PO each morning for 5 days, then discontinue. This is the easiest and least expensive regimen and uses 30 tablets of 20 mg over 15 days.
  2. Prednisone 60 mg PO each morning for 7 days, followed by prednisone 30 mg PO each morning for 7 days, then discontinue (126 tablets of 5 mg or 63 tablets of 10 mg over 14 days).
B. Other schedules
  1. Prednisone 60 mg PO each morning for 3 days, 50 mg PO each morning for 3 days, 40 mg PO each morning for 3 days, and then taper by 5 mg/day to 0 (120 tablets of 5 mg over 16 days).
  2. Prednisone starting with 60 mg PO the first day and decreasing by 5 mg (i.e., 78 tablets of 5 mg over 12 days). The total amount and duration of treatment may be varied

IV. Glucocorticoid adrenocorticotropic hormone (ACTH) suppression by oral corticosteroids
  A. Short acting (24 to 36 hours)
      Cortisone
      Cortisol (hydrocortisone)
  B. Intermediate acting (48 hours)
      Prednisone
      Prednisolone
      Methylprednisolone
    1. Packaging:
        Prednisone oral solution: 5 mg/5 mL: 5 mL, 500 mL
        Prednisone oral solution: 5 mg/mL: 30 mL
        Prednisone syrup, 5 mg/5 mL: 120 mL, 240 mL
        Prednisone tablets: 1 mg, 2.5 mg, 5 mg, 10 mg, 20 mg, 50 mg: 100 mg
      Triamcinolone
    1. Packaging:
        Triamcinolone syrup, 4 mg/5 mL: 120 mL
        Triamcinolone tablets: 4 mg, 8 mg
  C. Long acting (over 48 hours)
      Betamethasone
      Dexamethasone
    1. Packaging:
        Dexamethasone elixir, oral solution 0.5 mg/mL: 5 mL, 20 mL, 100 mL, 120 mL, 240 mL, 500 mL
        Dexamethasone oral solution 0.5 mg/0.5 mL: 30 mL
        Dexamethasone tablets, 0.25 mg, 0.5 mg, 0.75 mg, 1 mg, 1.5 mg, 2 mg, 4 mg, 6 mg
        Dexamethasone therapeutic pack: 6 × 1.5-mg, 8 × 0.75-mg tablets
V. INJECTABLE GLUCOCORTICOIDS. Time noted is the duration of their ability to suppress inflammatory reaction (see sec. II).
  A. Short acting (hours to days)
      Dexamethasone sodium phosphate
  B. Intermediate acting (1 to 2 weeks)
      Betamethasone acetate
      Betamethasone sodium phosphate
      Dexamethasone acetate
      Triamcinolone diacetate
  C. Long acting (3 to 4 weeks)
      Triamcinolone acetonide
      Triamcinolone hexacetonide

 ANTIPERSPIRANTS AND TREATMENT OF HYPERHIDROSIS

I. For hyperhidrosis of palms and soles
  A. Aluminum compounds
    1. For initial treatment of hyperhidrosis, apply 20% aluminum chloride hexahydrate in absolute alcohol (Drysol) to dry palm or sole at bedtime. Discomfort or irritation can be kept to a minimum by avoiding use on moist skin and by using 1% hydrocortisone cream in the morning if necessary. Sweating should decrease to less than 50% of pretreatment levels within 4 weeks. If this treatment process is unsatisfactory, use with occlusion as follows: apply 20% solution of aluminum chloride hexahydrate in 80% absolute anhydrous ethyl alcohol (Drysol; Dab-o-Matic) to affected areas at bedtime and cover with plastic wrap, socks, or gloves. Do not wash the area for close to 2 hours before applying. Wash medication off in the morning. Use for 3 to 5 consecutive nights or more the first week until the desired anhidrosis is achieved and then one to three times weekly thereafter. The number of treatments depends on the individual.

2. The antiperspirant action of aluminum salts is unclear. Physical blockage of the sweat ducts by an aluminum-containing cast is the most widely held opinion, although the possibility that aluminum produces vacuolization and atrophy of the secretory cells has been proposed.

3. The most common adverse effects reported include stinging, burning, pruritus, and irritation. Contact dermatitis is rarely seen.

4. Another metal salt, zirconium, had been used in the past; however, aerosol zirconium–based products were banned by the FDA in 1977 owing to the development of axillary granulomas in patients who used these products. Nonaerosol formulations at concentrations <20% are still allowed.

B. Botulinum A toxin (Botox) has been utilized in the management of hyperhidrosis and is the most effective treatment available. Its mechanism of action is to block the secretion of acetylcholine, resulting in a reversible chemical denervation. Botulinum toxin is delivered to the treatment sites through a series of superficial injections spaced 1 to 2 cm apart in a checkerboard pattern. The toxin is delivered to the superficial dermis to allow for greatest effect. Treatment success depends on the concentration used, depth of injection, and skill in placement. Effects of a single injection session may last between 6 and 9 months.

C. Aldehydes. Aldehydes reduce perspiration by denaturing keratin in the superficial corneocyte, thereby blocking the sweat gland pores. Disadvantages include a short-lasting effect and an increased incidence of contact sensitization. Either formalin (5% to 10%) or nonalkalinized glutaraldehyde applied with a cotton swab is effective. Formalin is a more frequent sensitizer and hence used less often. Unbuffered generic glutaraldehyde is available as a 50% solution through drug supply houses; 2% glutaraldehyde is used most easily as a Cidex solution or Cidex Formula 7 long-life solution (obtained through hospital supply sources).

1. Glutaraldehyde solution is applied three times a week for 2 weeks and then once weekly or as needed. A 10% solution is used for the feet. It will cause a temporary brown discoloration, but this pigmentation will diminish as frequency of application decreases. A 2% solution, which will not stain, may be used on the palms; however, this concentration produces only slight diminution in sweating.

2. Methenamine mandelate is a synthetic antibacterial agent that, when applied to the skin, hydrolyzes to ammonia and formaldehyde. A 5% methenamine stick or a 10% solution is effective in mild to moderate hyperhidrosis and rarely produces allergic reactions.

   a. Structure

Methenamine

   b. Use: Apply three times a week for 2 weeks, then once weekly as needed.
   c. Packaging:
   Methenamine mandelate 10% solution
   Methenamine mandelate 5% stick

D. Iontophoresis with tap water is a simple, safe, and economic treatment for hyperhidrosis; it involves introducing tap water through intact skin by means of an electric current. Although its mechanism of action is still unclear, it is thought to produce a physical blockage in the sweat glands at the level of the stratum corneum. Also, disruption of the electrical gradient of the sweat duct may occur; this gradient is needed for the normal flow of perspiration. Adding anticholinergic drugs such as glycopyrrolate to the water may provide some extra benefit but can also lead to side effects from systemic absorption. A battery-powered iontophoresis unit (Drionic) is available for home use. One study concluded that 80% of hand sites, 33% of sole sites, and 37.5% of axillae sites responded within 14 days, and this increased to 100%, 78%, and 75%, respectively, after 20 days, although patients often report diminished effectiveness over time.

E. Systemic anticholinergic drugs are usually not tolerated in the required doses but may be tried [glycopyrrolate (Robinul) three to five times a day initially, then decreased]. Sedatives or tranquilizing drugs are sometimes helpful.

1. Structure

Glycopyrrolate

F. Relaxation techniques including biofeedback training may decrease excessive palmoplantar and axillary sweating and the symptoms of chronic hyperhidrosis.

G. General measures include careful hygiene of hands and feet, frequent washing with deodorant soap, changing socks daily, and wearing cotton socks and leather shoes without rubber, plastic, or wooden soles.

1. Deodorants function either by masking odor or by decreasing bacteria. Antibacterial agents in deodorants include quaternary ammonium compounds (benzethonium chloride) and cationic compounds (chlorhexidine, triclosan).

II. FOR AXILLARY HYPERHIDROSIS

A. Aluminum compounds. May be used as noted in the preceding text.

B. Injection of botulinum toxin A induces anhidrosis that may last 6 to 9 months.

C. Scopolamine hydrobromide 0.025% applied topically can be an effective antiperspirant. Higher concentrations produce side effects such as diplopia.

D. Systemic anticholinergic and sedative (tranquilizing) drugs, iontophoresis, and relaxation techniques may be of value.

E. Glutaraldehyde is generally not effective in the axillae.

F. Surgical management of the axillary hyperhidrosis includes excision of the sweat gland–containing axillary vault, liposuction of the axillary vault, or upper thoracic sympathectomy. Complications of the surgical approach include Horner syndrome, brachial plexus injuries, pneumothorax, compensatory hyperhidrosis in adjacent regions, and painful scars. Hyperhidrosis may recur following sympathectomy. Plantar hyperhidrosis may be relieved with lumbar sympathectomy. Permanent nonfunction of sweat glands in the palms may result in scaling and fissuring of the palms.

ANTIPRURITIC AND EXTERNAL ANALGESIC AGENTS

I. DISCUSSION. See Chap. 26.

A. Camphor is a ketone which, when applied in 1% to 3% concentration, has mild antipruritic effects through its anesthetic and counterirritant properties. Counterirritants are substances that, by inducing other sensations such as coolness or warmth, "crowd out" the perception of pain or itch. Camphor is used in various OTC topical analgesic products in concentrations as high as 9%.

1. Structure

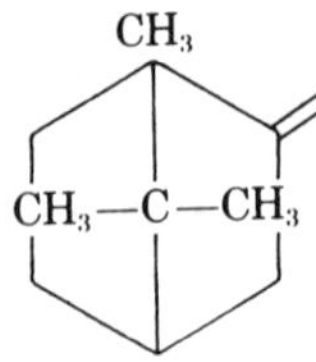

Camphor

B. Menthol, a cyclic alcohol (derived from peppermint, other mint oils, or prepared synthetically), relieves itching by generating a cool sensation. It is usually used in 0.25% to 2% concentrations but is present in concentrations as high as 16% in some OTC products.

1. Structure

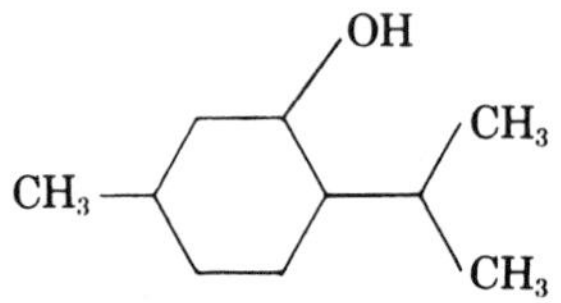

Menthol

C. Phenol in dilute solution (0.5% to 2%) decreases itch by anesthetizing the cutaneous nerve endings. Phenol should never be used on pregnant women or infants younger than 6 months of age.

1. Structure

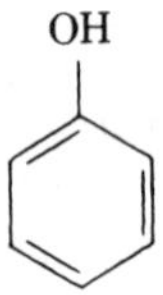

Phenol

D. Pramoxine hydrochloride (Itch-X, PrameGel, Prax, Tronothane, AmLactin AP) is a local anesthetic that is structurally similar to dyclonine and unrelated to the ester- or amide-type compounds.

    1. Structure: (See Anesthetics for Topical Administration, sec. III. B).

    2. Packaging:

        Pramoxine 1% cream: 28.4 g, 30 g, 113.4 g, 140 g, 1 lb

        Pramoxine 1% gel: 35.4 g, 118 g

        Pramoxine 1% lotion: 15 mL, 120 mL, 240 mL

        Pramoxine 1% spray: 60 mL

E. Chlorethane (ethyl chloride) is a highly flammable liquid that acts as a topical vapo-coolant to control pain associated with minor surgical procedures. When applied as a spray, the product produces freezing of superficial tissues to $-20°C$, which results in insensitivity of peripheral nerve endings and local anesthesia that is maintained up to 1 minute. Other coolant sprays can be used with the same effect.

1. Use: Apply immediately before the procedure is initiated.

2. Packaging:

Ethyl chloride spray: 3.5 oz

F. Doxepin is a dibenzoxepin-derivative tricyclic compound that exhibits potent histamine H_1 and H_2 receptor antagonist activity. Although the sedative effect of systemically absorbed doxepin may contribute to the drug's antipruritic activity, the antipruritic efficacy of doxepin does not depend on a sedative effect. It is used topically for the short-term (up to 8 days of therapy) relief of moderately severe pruritus associated with eczematous dermatitis, including lichen simplex chronicus. Patients must be cautioned regarding the potential sedative effects and the risk of contact dermatitis.

1. Use: Apply to affected areas t.i.d.–q.i.d. without occlusion.

2. Packaging:

Zonalon 5% cream: 30 g

G. Salicylic acid (1% to 2%) and tars (coal tar solution, 3% to 10%) are also occasionally useful, although their mode of action is not known.

1. Structure

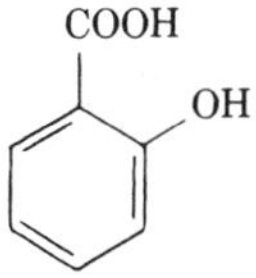

Salicylic acid

H. Crotamiton (Eurax) is not only scabicidal but has also been claimed to have a direct antipruritic effect. This has never been well studied, and the evidence indicates that crotamiton is not a generally effective antipruritic.

I. Local anesthetics are often used to allay pruritus by blocking nerve impulses at sensory nerve endings (see also Anesthetics for Topical Administration).

J. Other ingredients in OTC analgesics include the following:

1. Methyl salicylate, occurring naturally as wintergreen or sweet-birch oil, which, when rubbed on the skin, produces mild irritation and is absorbed to an appreciable extent. Triethanolamine salicylate 10% acts as an analgesic without irritant properties and is readily absorbed.

2. Thymol (see Antiinfective Agents).

3. Turpentine oil is used for its "counterirritant" properties.

4. Allyl isothiocyanate, volatile oil of mustard, acts as a powerful local irritant.

5. Clove oil, which contains eugenol as its main constituent, is used in ointments and is widely used in toothache preparations.

6. Capsaicin oleoresin, an irritant, derived from the plant of Solanaceae family (cayenne pepper), produces a feeling of warmth when applied to intact skin. Capsaicin depletes and prevents reaccumulation of substance P in peripheral neurons and is useful in the treatment of postherpetic neuralgia (see Chap. 16). Substance P is felt to be the principle chemomodulator of pain impulses from the periphery to the CNS. Its use in the therapy of pruritus has not been fully evaluated.

a. Use: Apply t.i.d.–q.i.d.

b. Packaging:

Capsaicin cream, 0.025%, 0.075%, 0.25%: 28 g, 30 g, 45 g, 60 g, 90 g

Capsaicin gel, 0.025%, 0.05%: 15 g, 30 g, 42.5 g

Capsaicin lotion, 0.025%, 0.075%: 59 mL

Capsaicin roll-on, 0.075%: 60 mL

7. Methacholine chloride, histamine dihydrochloride, and methyl nicotinate are used for their local vasodilating properties.

8. Other volatile oils in OTC preparations include wormwood and eucalyptus oils.

K. Dermatologic antipruritic formulations
    1. Lotions, liniments, emulsions
        a. Calamine lotion, USP (drying):
            Calamine (zinc oxide with 0.5% ferric oxide for coloring): 8 g
            Zinc oxide: 8 g
            Glycerin: 2 mL
            Bentonite magma (suspending agent): <25 mL
            Calcium hydroxide solution, to make: 100 mL
        i. Packaging:
            (1) Calamine lotion: 120 mL, 240 mL, 480 mL
            (2) Phenolated calamine, USP: 1% phenol added to calamine formulations: 120 mL, 240 mL
            (3) Alcoholic calamine lotion (more drying):
                Calamine 10 g
                Zinc oxide 10 g
                Bentonite 2 g
                Talc 10 g
                Glycerin 10 g
                Alcohol 40 mL
                Water, to make 100 mL
            (4) Calamine liniment (less drying):
                Calamine 15 g
                Peanut oil 50 mL
                Calcium hydroxide, to make 100 mL
            (5) Menthol lotion with phenol (Schamberg's):
                Menthol 0.5 g
                Phenol 1 g
                Zinc oxide 20 g
                Calcium hydroxide solution <40 mL
                Peanut oil, to make 100 mL
        i. Packaging:
            Schamberg's lotion: 480 mL
    2. Gels and ointments
        a. Menthol 0.5%
            Pramoxine HCl 1.0%
            In gel base
        i. Packaging:
            As PrameGel: 118 g.
        b. Salicylic acid 3%
            Phenol 1%
        i. Packaging:
            As Panscol 3% lotion: 120 mL
            3% ointment: 90 g
    3. Impregnated pads
        a. Glycerin 10%
            Witch hazel (gallic acid, tannin, and volatile oils) 50%
            Water 40%
        i. Use: Apply p.r.n. as replacement for toilet tissue or as cleansing and antipruritic wipe in prevention and therapy of pruritus ani and other perineal pruritic processes.
       ii. Packaging:
            As tucks: box of 12, box of 40, box of 100
            Gel: 19.8 g
    4. Miscellaneous antipruritic preparations (some contain potential allergic sensitizers such as benzocaine and diphenhydramine).
        a. Calamatum contains benzocaine (1.05% in spray, 3% in ointment), calamine, zinc oxide, menthol (in aerosol), camphor, phenol (in ointment), isopropanol (in spray).

　　i. Packaging:
　　　　Aerosol: 85 g
b. Caladryl contains 1% camphor, 8% calamine, 2% alcohol, 1% pramoxine HCl, cetyl alcohol, and parabens.
　　i. Packaging:
　　　　Lotion: 180 mL
c. Caladryl clear contains 1% pramoxine, 0.1% zinc acetate, 2% alcohol, camphor, diazolidinyl urea, and parabens.
　　i. Packaging:
　　　　Lotion: 180 mL
5. Miscellaneous external analgesic products. These multiingredient preparations are used by many patients for muscular aches.
　　a. Ben-Gay ointment contains 18.3% methyl salicylate, 16% menthol; Ultra-Strength cream contains 30% methyl salicylate, 10% menthol.
　　b. Mentholatum ointment contains 9% camphor, 1.35% menthol, and aromatic oils. Mentholatum Deep Heating ointment contains 12.7% methyl salicylate, 5.8% menthol, eucalyptus oil, and turpentine oil.
　　c. Sloan's liniment contains 46.7% turpentine oil, 6.7% pine oil, 3.3% camphor, 2.6% methyl salicylate, 0.6% capsicum, and 40% kerosene.

 CLEANSING AGENTS

I. DISCUSSION. Cleansers are any agents that remove sebum or foreign particles from the skin. A spectrum of cleansers exists, ranging from very drying to very moisturizing. The choice of cleanser depends largely on a particular individual's skin type.

A. Cleaning creams and lotions are useful in patients with very dry or sensitive skin who may react adversely to common soap products. They are generally oil-based, water-based, or water-free oils, the latter being the most moisturizing. Because they may leave an oily residue, they should be avoided in acne-prone patients. Cosmetic companies market most of these products, because they are useful in removing oily cosmetics. Examples of these cleansers include Albolene liquefying cleanser, Oil of Olay daily facial cleansing lotion, Ponds cold cream deep cleanser, and Sea Breeze whipped facial cleanser.

B. Soaps. Surfactants are substances that are able to dissolve both oil and water; soaps and soap-free cleansers (SFCs) are surfactants. Soaps are sodium or potassium salts that are derived from plant and animal oils or fats, whereas SFCs are synthetically derived. The two most common soaps are sodium tallowate and sodium cocoate. Soaps are alkaline (pH 9 to 10), which may irritate intact or damaged skin. Normal skin has a slightly acidic pH of 5.6 to 5.8. Cleansers with a pH closer to normal skin may be less irritating. Modified soaps may be less irritating because they are adjusted to be slightly acidic or neutral. Badly irritated skin should not be exposed to soaps, detergents, or cleansers other than water.

1. Neutral soaps or soap-like preparations contain synthetic detergents and have a pH of 7.5 or less. Preparations include Alpha Keri, Aveeno bar, Dove, Lowila Cake, and Emulave.

2. Superfatted soaps contain increased fat or oil on the assumption that they leave a film of protective oil on the skin. Preparations include Basis, Neutrogena Dry Skin, and Oilatum Soap.

3. Antimicrobial bar soaps contain topical antiseptics such as carbanilide, triclocarban, or the substituted phenol triclosan. They have some deodorant action by inhibiting bacterial growth. Representative soaps include Clearasil Antibacterial (triclosan), Coast (tricloban), Dial (1.5% tricloban), Irish Spring (0.75% tricloban, 0.25% triclosan), Safeguard (1.5% tricloban), Zest (tricloban), Jergens clear complexion (triclocarban), Lever 2000 (triclosan), and Lifebuoy III (triclosan).

　　One study comparing bar and liquid soaps found higher microbial flora in the bar form.

C. SFCs are surfactants that are synthetically produced. They generally have a pH close to that of normal skin and, hence, are less irritating. SFCs that contain oils may be even less irritating. Examples of SFCs include Aquanil lotion, Cetaphil lotion (lipid-free), Basis facial cleanser, Oil of Olay foaming face wash; SFCs containing oils include Aveeno cleansing bar for dry skin (also for normal to oily skin). Eucerin cleansing bar, Lowila cake soap, and pHisoderm skin cleanser for oily skin, regular skin, or for babies.

D. Abrasive cleansers are advertised for acne patients to assist in exfoliating the skin, presumably to "unplug" skin pores or to remove dead sensitive skin. They may contain various amounts and kinds of particulate matter, aluminum oxide, polyethylene, or sodium tetraborate decahydrate or even ground fruit pits or nutshells. The danger of these products is that they may cause some inflammation or damage to the follicles. Preparations include Sastid scrub (20% aluminum oxide), Pernox scrub (1.5% salicylic acid, 2% sulfur, polyethylene, and docusate sodium), Brasivol (aluminum oxide with sodium lauryl sulfate, fine, medium, or rough), and Ionax (polyethylene granules with benzalkonium chloride).

E. Acne cleansers (see Acne Preparations)

F. Shampoos

    1. Coal tar. Coal is a mixture of various tar acids and hydrocarbons. Coal tar is reproduced through the distillation process of coal; it is then further refined by various methods to make it aesthetically more pleasing and pharmaceutically practical.

        The exact method by which coal tars are useful in managing dandruff, seborrheic dermatitis, and psoriasis is not known. It has been suggested that coal tar removes oxygen from the skin, thereby inhibiting mitosis and decreasing the size and number of cells in the stratum germinativum and stratum corneum. It may also have a vasoconstrictive, weak antiseptic, and antipruritic effect. Coal tars have also been used in combination with other drugs (hydrocortisone, salicylic acid, and sulfur) in relieving pruritus, flaking, and irritation of the skin.

        Adverse effects include irritant dermatitis with increased concentrations; folliculitis may be seen after prolonged use. These preparations may stain blonde or gray hair.

    a. Packaging:
            Crude coal tar:
            DHS tar gel (6.5%)
            Doak tar shampoo (3%)
            Zetar (1%)
            MG217 (2%)
            Ionil T Plus (2%)
            Coal tar extract:
            Neutrogena T/Gel (2%)
             Tegrin (5%)
             Pentrax (8.75%)
            Coal tar solution:
            Denorex (9%), with 1.5% menthol
            Duplex T (15%)
             Coal combination:
            T/Sal (2%), with 2% salicylic acid
            MG217 (5%), with colloidal sulfur 1.5% and salicylic acid (2%)

    2. Selenium sulfide suspension (Selsun) is a mixture of selenium monosulfide and a suspension of solid selenium and amorphous sulfur. Selenium acts by inhibiting cellular proliferation, kills yeast organisms, and has high substantivity. Little or no toxicity has been observed when applied directly to normal skin or hair, but these products should not be used on inflamed or exudative skin, where absorption may be increased. They are used in the control of seborrheic dermatitis, dandruff, and tinea versicolor.

a. Packaging:

Selenium sulfide 1% lotion/shampoo: 120 mL, 210 mL, 240 mL, 330 mL

Selenium sulfide 2.5% lotion/shampoo: 120 mL

3. Zinc pyrithione is the active ingredient in several shampoos used to control dandruff and seborrheic dermatitis and is also effective in the therapy of tinea versicolor. It remains unclear whether the beneficial effects are caused by an antiproliferative or antimicrobial effect or both. It is substantive to the hair, allowing continued therapeutic effect after washing.

a. Structure

Zinc pyrithione

b. Packaging:

Shampoos including DHS-Zinc (2%), Head & Shoulders (1%), and Zincon (1%).

4. Ketoconazole (Nizoral) shampoo. See Chap. 29.

COSMETICS AND COVERING AGENTS

I. COSMETICS

A. The FDA defines *cosmetics* as any agent applied to the body for purposes of "cleansing, beautifying, promoting attractiveness, or altering the appearance." As such, the term cosmetics encompasses a broad range of consumer products. Hypoallergenic cosmetics are products intended to cause less allergic reactions, although there is no standard. Companies specifically involved in the manufacture of less allergenic compounds include Almay, Clinique, and Prescriptives.

B. A key reference for cosmetic ingredients is the Cosmetics, Toiletries, and Fragrances Association (CTFA) Cosmetic Ingredient Dictionary. This reference lists >2,500 cosmetic ingredients used to formulate cosmetic products. Also, it contains important information on suppliers of cosmetic ingredients and is recognized as the official labeling compendium by the FDA for generating cosmetic ingredient disclosures under the Fair Packaging and Labeling Act.

C. The best source for cosmetic ingredient patch test concentrations and vehicles is the manufacturer. Many companies in the cosmetic industry provide patch test samples on request. The "Industry on Call" booklet published by the American Academy of Dermatology (AAD) is useful in contacting the appropriate cosmetic company.

II. COSMETIC CAMOUFLAGE. Covering agents are used by patients in a variety of skin diseases, including vitiligo, acne, nevus flammeus, tattoos, other pigmentation abnormalities, and alopecia areata. Dermablend and Covermark are perhaps the most widely used agents. They are available in various skin tones, with a high degree of opacity. They are also effective sunscreens and are waterproof. Cosmeticians can assist patients in learning proper application techniques, which often differ from those of regular cosmetics. Some of these products may require special cleansers for removal. Other brands that specialize in concealing cutaneous defects include Dermage, Chromelin, Vitadye, Recover, and Natural Cover by Linda Seidel.

Product Information

Cover FX, www.coverfx.com

Covermark, www.covermark.com

Dermablend, www.dermablend.com

Dermage, www.dermage.com
MAC/Studio Full Coverage, www.maccosmetics.com
Natural Cover by Linda Seidel, www.lindaseidel.com
Neostrata Coverblend, www.neostrata.com/coverblend/

 DEPILATORIES AND REMOVAL OF EXCESSIVE HAIR

I. HYPERTRICHOSIS

  A. Mild hypertrichosis, most often familial in nature, is a cause of cosmetic concern for many women. It is mandatory that endocrine or local factors be ruled out before dismissing excessive hair as a simple cosmetic problem.

II. HAIR REMOVAL

  A. There are several ways by which the amount or appearance of excessive hair may be decreased.

    1. Bleaching the hair will make it less obvious. A 6% solution of hydrogen peroxide, commonly known as 20-vol peroxide, is most often used. It may be used alone, but the addition of an alkali, usually 10 drops of ammonia per 30 mL of peroxide, immediately before use will activate the hydrogen peroxide and permit more intense bleaching.

    2. Plucking hair is painful but effective. Each pluck will start another growing cycle in the hair root.

    3. Wax epilation is essentially just widespread plucking. A warm wax is placed on the skin, allowed to dry, and then, as it is peeled off, the hairs are pulled out.

    4. Shaving is quick and effective and does not cause the hair to regrow more rapidly or more abundantly.

    5. Rubbing with a pumice stone will remove fine hair.

    6. Depilatories disintegrate and destroy hair on topical application by hydrolyzing disulfide bonds. The hair is left as a gelatinous mass, which is easily wiped off the skin. The following two active ingredients are currently used:

      a. Sulfides of alkali metals and alkaline earths are the most effective, but they also develop a disagreeable hydrogen sulfide odor and are more irritating than thioglycollate products. Strontium sulfide or barium sulfide is the active ingredient. Preparations available include Magic Shaving Powder and Royal Crown Shaving Powder. Both contain barium sulfide and calcium hydroxide.

      b. Thioglycollate-containing agents require increased contact time but are more easily perfumed and are less irritating than other preparations. Preparations available include Nair, Neet, and Nudit.

    7. Vaniqa (eflornithine hydrochloride 13.9%) cream is a unique topical cream that slows anagen hair growth by irreversibly blocking the enzyme ornithine decarboxylase. This enzyme produces polyamines in the hair matrix that are partially responsible for the growth of the anagen hair. The cream was tested only on the upper lip and chin region. The onset of action is usually within 8 weeks of starting the b.i.d. treatment, and the hair growth will return to baseline within 8 weeks of discontinuing the drug. Patients need to be reminded that this product does not remove hair but slows its growth in between whatever they use for hair removal.

      a. Use: Apply a thin layer to the affected area. The most common side effects are stinging, erythema, and acneiform eruptions. It is contraindicated in inflammatory acne, pregnancy, and lactation.

      b. Packaging:
        Vaniqa cream: 30 g; 60 g (2/30 g tubes)

    8. Electrolysis is a permanent method of hair removal by which the hair bulb is destroyed by a high-frequency electric current and the hair will not grow back later. A topical anesthetic cream before treatment may reduce associated discomfort. When performed by a skilled operator, this technique is useful. Pit-like perifollicular scarring and regrowth or incompletely destroyed hairs may follow electrolysis or repeated plucking. Pretreatment with Retin-A cream for 2 weeks may reduce healing time.

9. Laser hair removal is a permanent form of hair removal that requires pigmented hair, with melanin as the target for hair destruction. Utilizing the principle of photothermolysis, a laser wavelength of light is selected and delivered at a specific energy to target the hair follicle, while minimizing surrounding tissue damage. Epidermal melanin decreases the efficacy of the treatment, as it may absorb a portion of the light emitter, with resultant epidermal damage. Numerous lasers and light sources are available at present. Thorough evaluation and patient selection must be performed to determine if the patient is a good candidate for this treatment. In general, patients with Fitzpatrick skin types I–III and dark hair are the best candidates. Longer wavelength lasers such as diode and 1,064 nm Nd:YAG allow for safe and efficacious treatment of patients with Fitzpatrick skin types IV–VI. Treatment should be avoided if the patient is tan. Side effects include localized edema and erythema, postinflammatory hyperpigmentation, blistering, and scarring. Approximately 10% to 20% of treated hairs are reduced with every treatment; therefore, multiple treatments are generally necessary. A topical anesthetic cream before treatment may reduce associated discomfort.

III. STIMULATION OF HAIR GROWTH

A. **Androgenetic alopecia.** Men and women alike may be affected with androgenetic alopecia (pattern hair loss), where terminal hairs are replaced with progressively finer, smaller vellus hairs. Men are generally affected in the bitemporal and vertex regions; women often present with more diffuse alopecia, generally in a frontovertical distribution.

1. Therapy
   a. Minoxidil is a piperidinopyrimadine derivative and potent vasodilator that possesses hair growth stimulant properties. Topical minoxidil solution in 10% propylene glycol has proved effective in approximately 30% of individuals in converting vellus to terminal hairs. It is most effective in younger patients with less chronic hair loss. Hair growth is more likely to be stimulated on the vertex rather than on the bitemporal areas. Its mechanism of action is unknown. Adverse reactions include local irritation and contact dermatitis. If the treatment is discontinued, clinical regression occurs within 3 months to the state of hair thinning that would have occurred had the treatment not been started. Twice-daily treatment is more efficacious than once-daily application. Women who use the 5% concentration may note the development of facial hair, which is reversible on discontinuation of the medication. The 5% concentration can be more irritating than the 2% solution: application of the 5% solution at bedtime and the 2% solution in the morning can leave the hair more manageable and the scalp less irritated. Minoxidil is also used in the treatment of alopecia areata.

      i. **Use:** Apply to scalp b.i.d. and gently massage into scalp.
      ii. **Packaging:**
         Minoxidil 2% solution: 60 mL with dropper
         Minoxidil 5% solution: 60 mL with dropper

2. Finasteride (Propecia) is a synthetic 4-azasteroid compound. It acts as a specific competitive inhibitor of steroid type II 5α-reductase, an intracellular enzyme present in high concentrations in the inner root sheath of the hair follicle and prostate gland. The conversion of testosterone to the active metabolite DHT depends on the presence of this enzyme. In men with androgenetic hair loss, increased amounts of DHT and 5α-reductase lead to miniaturized hair follicles and a shortened hair growth cycle. Inhibition of type II 5α-reductase by finasteride blocks the peripheral conversion of testosterone to DHT, resulting in substantial reductions in serum and tissue DHT concentrations. Oral finasteride has been effective in promoting hair growth in men aged 18 to 41 with mild to moderate androgenetic alopecia. It is most effective for vertex and midscalp loss. Its effectiveness has not been investigated for bitemporal loss. New hair growth is generally detected 6 months after treatment initiation.

Cessation of the medication results in a gradual return to a pretreatment hair loss stage. It is contraindicated in pregnant women and in children, because it inhibits the conversion of testosterone to DHT, which could result in deformities in the external genitalia of a male fetus. Other side effects are rare. Less than 2% men reported sexual dysfunction, including erectile dysfunction, which was only slightly higher than the placebo group and was reversible on discontinuation of the medication. Finasteride has no effect on sperm motility/ejaculate. It slightly lowers the prostate-specific antigen (PSA); therefore, doubling the PSA value before its clinical interpretation should be considered in the evaluation of benign prostatic hypertrophy. A baseline PSA should be obtained in males over 40 or if there is a positive family history of prostate cancer.

a. Use: Take 1 mg/day

b. Packaging (Merck):
Propecia 1 mg tablet: pack of 30 or Pro-Pak (90-day supply)

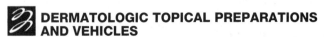

DERMATOLOGIC TOPICAL PREPARATIONS AND VEHICLES

(See also Types of Topical Medications)

Lotions, creams, ointments, and powders can be used alone or may act as vehicles for pharmacologically active substances. Ideally, they are nontoxic, stable, and do not sensitize with repeated use. It should not be assumed that "inert" vehicles or bases have no effect on the skin or epithelial metabolism.

I. CONSTITUENTS OF DERMATOLOGIC PRODUCTS. Dermatologic vehicles are often complex substances that contain many additives. The general classes of vehicle ingredients are emulsifying agents, which are surfactants and improve stability of emulsions; stabilizers, including preservatives and antioxidants, which preserve stability of vehicles both initially and over time; solvents, which increase the solubility of the drug in the vehicle; thickening agents, used to increase viscosity or suspend ingredients in vehicles; emollients; and humectants, agents that are hygroscopic and draw moisture from the skin.

A. Emulsifying or dispersing agents provide stability and homogeneity. Glyceryl monostearate, polyethylene glycol derivatives (polyoxyl 40 stearate, polysorbate 80), and sodium lauryl sulfate are such agents used in preparations containing oily components and water. Sodium lauryl sulfate may act as an irritant.

B. The consistency and appearance of creams are improved by the addition of additives such as ethylenediamines (frequent allergic sensitizers), cetyl palmitate, and related esters.

C. Lubricants, emollients, and/or antifoaming agents include stearic acid, stearyl alcohol, isopropyl myristate, and cetyl alcohol.

D. Methylcellulose and gum tragacanth are used as suspending agents in pastes and ointments.

E. Preservatives include parabens (short alkyl esters of parahydroxybenzoic acid), benzyl alcohol, oxyquinoline sulfate, organic quaternary ammonium compounds, hexachlorophene, parachlorometaxylenol, and chlorobutanol. Methyl and propylparaben may act as allergic sensitizers.

II. LOTIONS, CREAMS, OINTMENTS, AND POWDERS

A. Lotions are usually liquid suspensions or dispersions intended for external application to the body. Solid-in-liquid suspensions are preparations of finely divided, undissolved drugs, or other particulate matter dispersed in liquid vehicles. These suspensions require shaking before application to ensure uniform distribution of solid in the vehicle. Liquid-in-liquid dispersions generally contain higher water content than cream emulsions and can be poured. Lotions provide a protective, drying, and cooling effect and may act as a vehicle for other agents. The addition of alcohol increases the cooling effect. If an astringent, such as aluminum, is present, it will precipitate protein and dry and seal exudating surfaces.

1. Calamine lotion (see Antipruritic and External Analgesic Agents).
2. Alcohol, zinc oxide, and talc lotion (more drying):
   Zinc oxide 15 g
   Talc 15 g
   Glycerin 10 g
   Alcohol 30 mL
   Water, to make 100 mL
3. Burow's emulsion, modified (less drying):
   Zinc oxide 10 g
   Talc 10 g
   Olive oil 45 mL
   Anhydrous lanolin 10 g
   Aluminum acetate solution 2.5 mL
   Water, to make 100 mL

B. Oil-in-water and water-washable cream emulsions are easily washable and will take up water but are not in themselves soluble.

1. Hydrophilic ointment, USP, contains polyoxyl 40 stearate as an emulsifying and wetting agent, stearyl alcohol as a stabilizer, and parabens (parahydroxybenzoic acid) as preservatives. It is a good vehicle for water-soluble medications. If hydrophilic ointment is used under occlusion, an irritant contact dermatitis may result. Sodium lauryl sulfate is the provocative agent.

   a. Contains:
   Methylparaben 0.025 g
   Propylparaben 0.015 g
   Stearyl alcohol 25 g
   White petrolatum 25 g
   Propylene glycol 112 g
   Sodium lauryl sulfate 5 g
   Water, to make 100 mL

2. Glycerin is frequently found in moisturizing creams (such as Complex 15, Curel, DML Forte, Lubriderm, and Jergens). This agent has been termed a **humectant**, which is a substance that is purportedly absorbed into the skin to help replace missing hygroscopic substances or, if absorption does not occur, to attract water from the atmosphere and serve as a reservoir for the stratum corneum. In fact, glycerin appears to be effective in treating dry skin but its mechanism of action is not known.

3. Commercially available oil-in-water emulsion bases include Nivea cream, Purpose Dry Skin cream, and Lubriderm.

C. Ointments. These bland bases may have an antimitotic effect on stripped epidermis, perhaps related to the effects of physical occlusion. The "stickiest" preparations are the most inhibitory.

1. Water-soluble ointments [polyethylene glycols (Carbowax)] are completely water soluble and may also act as lubricants or as water-soluble bases.

2. Emulsifiable ointments

   a. Water-in-oil absorbent ointments are difficult to wash off and are insoluble in water, but will take up water in significant amounts.

   i. Hydrous wool fat, USP (lanolin), although insoluble in water, is capable of absorbing twice its weight in water. It is a yellow-white preparation containing 28% water and is the purified, fat-like substance from the wool of sheep

   Anhydrous lanolin, a brown-yellow absorbent ointment that contains <0.25% water, is more greasy and occlusive.

   (1) Packaging:
   Anhydrous lanolin: 25 g, 500 g

   ii. Cold cream, USP (rose water ointment), is a pleasant-smelling, soft base used chiefly because of its cosmetic appearance and for its lubricating, emollient, and cooling effects (hence its name, cold cream). These preparations are good vehicles for the incorporation of many substances. The official cold cream is a water-in-oil (W/O) emulsion, but there are many variations that approach oil-in-water (O/W) emulsions. These creams are the basis of many cosmetic products such as cleansing, night, moisturizing, and eye creams.

(1) Contains:
Spermaceti 12.5 g
White wax 12.0 g
Mineral oil 56.0 g
Sodium borate 0.5 g
Water, to make 100 g

(2) Packaging:
Pond's Dry Skin Cream: 3.5 oz

b. Similar bases consisting of oils and emulsifying agents but no water are termed **absorbent ointments**. They are difficult to wash off and are insoluble in water, but they will soak up water to become water-in-oil emulsions.

i. Hydrophilic petrolatum, USP, is characterized by its ability to take up large amounts of water. It is less greasy than petrolatum but more greasy than hydrophilic ointment.

(1) Contains:
Cholesterol 3 g
Stearyl alcohol 3 g
White wax 8 g
White petrolatum, to make 100 g

(2) Packaging:
Hydrophilic petrolatum ointment: 1 lb

ii. Commercially available hydrophilic (W/O) bases include Eucerin (which is equal parts of Aquaphor and water), Keri Cream, Nivea oil, Polysorb, and Aquaphor, the latter two when hydrated.

3. Water-repellent ointments consist of inert oils, are insoluble in water, are difficult to wash off, will not dry out, and change little with time.

a. Petrolatum, USP, is a semisolid mixture of hydrocarbons obtained from petrolatum and is the most commonly used base for ointments. White petrolatum (decolorized petrolatum) is more aesthetically appealing and is used most often.

i. Packaging:
Petrolatum: 454 g

b. Liquid petrolatum, USP (mineral oil, liquid paraffin), is a mixture of purified hydrocarbons obtained from petrolatum.

i. Packaging:
Mineral oil: 500 mL

4. Silicone (dimethicone) ointments are excellent water-protective agents because they have an extremely low surface tension and penetrate crevices in the skin to form a plastic-like barrier. Further, they are nontoxic, inert, stable, and water repellent. As such, they are useful as barrier creams in industry or wherever constant or frequent exposure to aqueous compounds is a problem. They will not, however, protect well against solvents, oils, or dusts.

a. Structure

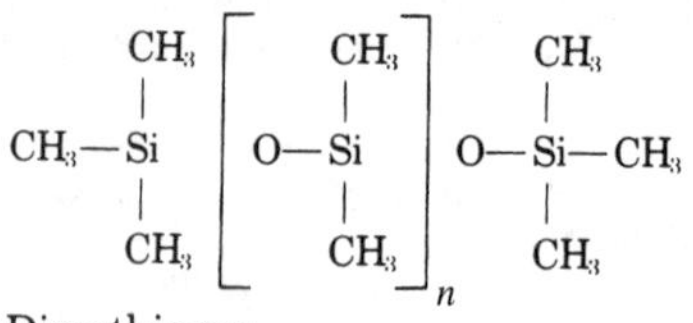

$$CH_3-\underset{\underset{\displaystyle CH_3}{|}}{\overset{\overset{\displaystyle CH_3}{|}}{Si}}\left[O-\underset{\underset{\displaystyle CH_3}{|}}{\overset{\overset{\displaystyle CH_3}{|}}{Si}}\right]_n O-\underset{\underset{\displaystyle CH_3}{|}}{\overset{\overset{\displaystyle CH_3}{|}}{Si}}-CH_3$$

Dimethicone

b. Packaging:
Silicone 10% ointment: 30 g, 480 g

Because there are no all-purpose effective protective agents, it is essential to choose a particular cream for protection against a specific hazard, that is, against dusts and particular matter, aqueous compounds, or solvents.

D. Pastes are made by incorporating a fine powder into an ointment. The base is usually petrolatum, and the powders, which constitute 20% to 50% of the paste, are usually zinc oxide, talc, starch, bentonite, aluminum oxide, or titanium dioxide. Pastes are more absorptive, less greasy, and less effective vehicles than ointments and are less efficient at preventing water evaporation. However, they are excellent protective compounds and may be used in subacute and chronic dermatoses. Pastes should be applied evenly with a tongue blade or finger and may be removed most easily with a cloth soaked in mineral or vegetable oil.

  1. Zinc oxide paste, USP

      Zinc oxide 25 g

      Starch 25 g

      White petrolatum, to make 100 g

    a. Packaging:

        Zinc oxide paste: 28 g, 60 g, 75 g

E. Powders increase evaporation, reduce friction, and provide antipruritic and cooling sensations. Zinc oxide or stearate, magnesium stearate, talc, cornstarch, bentonite, and titanium dioxide may either be used as dusting powders or incorporated into pastes or shake lotions. Talc is the most lubricating, but it does not absorb water; starch is less lubricating and absorbs water; zinc oxide has absorptive properties intermediate between the two. Zeasorb powder, which contains 45% microporous cellulose, has a relative absorbency of water almost twice that of talc-based powders. Talc can cause a granulomatous reaction in wounds, and starch may be metabolized by organisms and cause an increase in *Candida* overgrowth.

  1. Talc, USP (talcum), is a hydrous magnesium silicate that sometimes contains a small amount of aluminum silicate.

    a. Packaging:

        Talc: 500 g

F. Miscellaneous

  1. Collodion is a mixture of pyroxylin (a nitrocellulose derivative), ether, and alcohol that forms an adherent film on the skin after drying. Flexible collodion contains collodion, camphor 0.2%, and castor oil 0.3%. It is used as a vehicle for salicylic and lactic acids in the treatment of warts, as a protective film over herpes zoster lesions, and over fissures as present in chronic hand dermatitis.

  2. N^6-furfuryladenine (Kinerase) is a natural plant growth factor that is purported to retard the aging process and improve fine wrinkles and dyspigmentation with continuous use, with a moisturizing effect. It is nonirritating.

    a. Packaging: (ICN Pharmaceuticals):

        Kinerase 1% cream, lotion

 INSECT REPELLENTS

I. DISCUSSION. See Chap. 5.

II. Effective insect repellents contain diethyltoluamide (DEET), ethyl hexanediol (E-H), or multiple ingredients. The mechanism of action for repellents is not clearly defined. Once applied, they are thought to evaporate a certain distance from the skin, where they are recognized by the insect, irritating their olfactory organs. Agents with faster rates of evaporation are more effective, but these products also lose their effectiveness faster. Because repellents do not kill insects, selection for resistant species does not occur. Most repellents must be reapplied after sweating or bathing.

A. DEET is an organic liquid that is an excellent mosquito repellent; stronger preparations of DEET are also effective against stable flies, although little protection is provided against ticks. Commercial preparations are available in aerosol, cream, or lotion form and vary in concentration from 6% to 100%. Because DEET is absorbed into the bloodstream, it should be applied sparingly. Lesser concentrations of DEET should be used whenever possible, with additional applications to the skin if needed. Reports of a toxic encephalopathy and brief seizures have been documented in children after overzealous use. Less serious neurologic side effects include confusion, irritability, and insomnia. Contact dermatitis has been observed with preparations containing higher concentrations of DEET.

Use preparations with <20% DEET in children. Avoid mucous membranes, broken skin, and hands of children, because they are often in contact with the mouth. Spray clothing instead of skin whenever possible, but avoid contact with rayon, acetate, or spandex, because these materials may be damaged by DEET.

B. Ethyl hexanediol will not irritate human skin but can cause a chemical conjunctivitis. It is a standard repellent for chiggers, mosquitoes, black flies, and other biting flies and is more useful when combined with dimethyl phthalate and indalone. The mixture of these three chemicals will repel ticks and flies when it is applied to clothing.

C. Dimethyl carbate can be applied to clothing to repel ticks.

D. Butopyronoxyl is not water soluble and can be applied to skin and clothing to repel biting stable flies, Lone Star ticks, dog and cat fleas, and chiggers.

E. Butylethylpropandiol is used together with benzyl benzoate as the U.S. Army standard for clothing impregnation to repel ticks and chiggers.

F. Benzyl benzoate can be used in a 5% emulsion to repel many arthropods and can be used as a lotion to treat sarcoptic mange and canine pediculosis.

G. Permethrin 0.5% spray kills ticks and repels mosquitoes and stable flies. It is broken down when applied to skin and, hence, should be applied to clothing, shoes, tents, and so on. Spray only enough to moisten the material. Spray on clothing at least 2 hours before wearing. One treatment should last through a few washings.

III. Systemic allergic reactions to insect stings may include urticaria, bronchospasm, laryngeal edema, hypotension, and death. Approximately 1% to 3% of adults in the United States have had systemic allergic reactions to insect stings. Fifty percent of these adults will have similar reactions if they are stung again as against <5% of such patients who are treated with immunotherapy. Preparations from venom from the honeybee, yellow jacket, yellow hornet, white-faced hornet, and Polistes wasp are available for diagnosis and immunotherapy. Fire ant whole-body extracts are also available. Risks of immunotherapy include large local reactions or systemic reactions in 5% to 15% of patients early in treatment. These reactions are less likely in the maintenance phase of therapy. Generally, venomimmunotherapy may be stopped after 5 years or sooner.

KERATOLYTIC, CYTOTOXIC, AND DESTRUCTIVE AGENTS

I. α-Hydroxy acids represent a group of substances derived from natural products such as fruits (citric acid), milk (lactic acid), sugar cane (glycolic acid), apples (malic acid), and wine (tartaric acid). Variations of these products are effective in treating skin problems such as xerosis, photoaging, and acne. Three prevailing theories postulate how they work, although their exact mechanism is unknown. First, dissolution of the chemical adhesion between cells within the outermost layer of the epidermis may lead to keratolysis or sloughing of excess stratum corneum. Second, alteration in the pH of the skin when the acids contact the epidermis causes irritation, with subsequent increased cell turnover rate and a renewed stratum corneum. Lastly, exposure to the acids may induce slight edema, which plumps the skin, reducing fine lines and wrinkles. In acne, softening of intercellular adhesion may assist in exfoliation, with a comedolytic effect. Overall, tretinoin still seems to be more effective in comedolysis, although the combination of α-hydroxy acids and tretinoin may be synergistic. In treating xerosis, α-hydroxy acids have been shown to thicken the epidermis, as well as thin the stratum corneum. Cracks and fissures in the stratum corneum improve after treatment; histopathologically, a disorganized stratum corneum regains its well-organized, basket-weave appearance. In addition, in a double-blinded trial, Lac-Hydrin (12% ammonium lactate) was shown to increase the glycosaminoglycans in the dermis as well.

Higher concentrations of α-hydroxy acids (30% to 70%) are available for physicians' use in the office for light chemical peels. Rewarding results in reducing fine lines and evening skin tone may be obtained. The patient, however, will not achieve the depth of peeling with these products that can be attained with higher concentrations of trichloroacetic acid or laser resurfacing.

II. Anthralin is a synthetic derivative of a substance that was originally extracted from the araroba tree of Brazil. It is most frequently used in the treatment of psoriasis, although it may also be helpful in alopecia areata. Anthralin reduces epidermal mitotic activity, perhaps through interference with mitochondrial DNA or certain cellular enzyme systems. It may act as an irritant and will stain skin and clothing. Anthralin is most effective when incorporated into a stiff paste or ointment containing salicylic acid. However, because these preparations are messy and difficult to apply, more cosmetically acceptable anthralin creams are preferable to most patients.

A. Structure

Anthralin

B. Use: Apply daily as directed and rinse off. Optimal contact time will vary according to strength used and patient response. Initial contact time is between 15 and 20 minutes. Commence treatment for 1 week at the lowest strength possible and increase the strength as necessary. Continue treatment until clearance is obtained.

C. Packaging:

Anthralin ointments contain anthralin, petrolatum, and mineral oil (0.1%, 0.25%, 0.5%, 1%: 42.5 g).

Anthralin creams (Drithocreme, Micanol) contain anthralin in a vanishing cream base (0.1%, 0.25%, 0.5%, 1%: 50 g).

III. Bleomycin, a cytotoxic antineoplastic agent that inhibits DNA synthesis, is an alternative therapy for recalcitrant warts. It may be administered through a bifurcated needle intralesionally, usually reconstituted in physiologic saline or 1% lidocaine at a concentration of 0.5 to 1 U bleomycin/mL, or by injection. A maximum total dose of 2 U may be administered. The lidocaine suspension reduces the discomfort at the time of injection; however, patients may still experience pain or local tenderness at the treated site for 1 to 7 days following treatment. A hemorrhagic eschar develops that should be pared down 2 to 3 weeks after treatment. Larger warts may require a series of injections every 3 weeks. Caution should be taken when treating distal digits because Raynaud's phenomenon and nail loss have been reported.

A. Structure

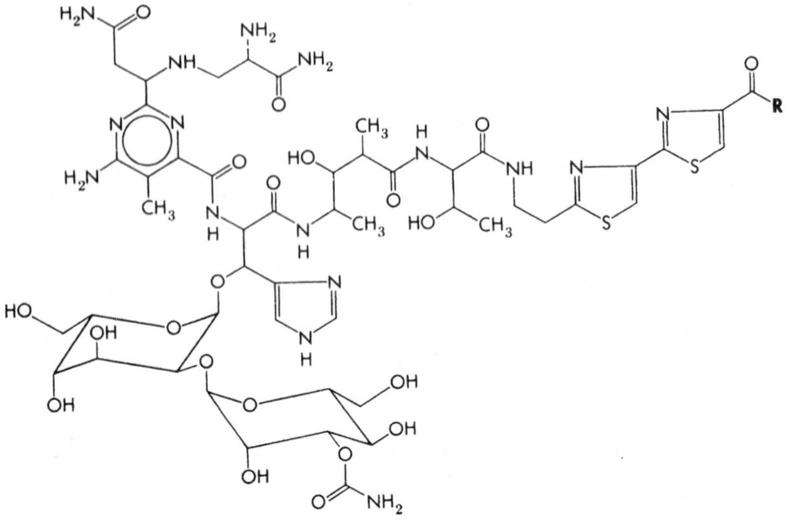

Bleomycinic acid: **R** = OH

Bleomycin A$_2$: **R** = NHCH$_2$CH$_2$CH$_2$—$\overset{+}{S}\overset{CH_3}{\underset{CH_3}{}}$

Bleomycin B$_2$: **R** = NHCH$_2$CH$_2$CH$_2$CH$_2$NHC$\overset{NH}{\underset{NH_2}{}}$

Bleomycin

B. Packaging:

Bleomycin powder: 15 U vials, 30 U vials.

IV. Calcipotriene (calcipotriol) is a synthetic vitamin D$_3$ derivative that is useful for the treatment of patients with moderate plaque psoriasis. Its effects are comparable with those of class II topical steroids, without the associated adverse effects. Its mechanism of action involves both induction of terminal differentiation of keratinocytes and inhibition of keratinocyte production. It should be applied to the face with care, as this region is more susceptible to irritation, burning, and itching, as seen in approximately 10% of patients. Other adverse effects include erythema, peeling, xerosis, dermatitis, or worsening psoriasis in 1% to 10% of patients. Fewer than 1% of patients experience hypercalcemia, atrophy, hyperpigmentation, or folliculitis. Allergic contact dermatitis to calcipotriene has been reported.

Most patients demonstrate improvement after 2 weeks; 70% of patients improve after 8 weeks, with 10% showing complete clearing. It should be avoided in patients with documented impairment in calcium metabolism, hypercalcemia, vitamin D toxicity, or history of renal stones.

Calcipotriene may be used as an adjuvant with psoralens plus ultraviolet A (PUVA) and ultraviolet B (UVB). Pretreatment with or subsequent addition of calcipotriol to PUVA reduces the cumulative doses of UVA needed to achieve >75% reduction in severity and distribution of psoriasis.

A. Structure

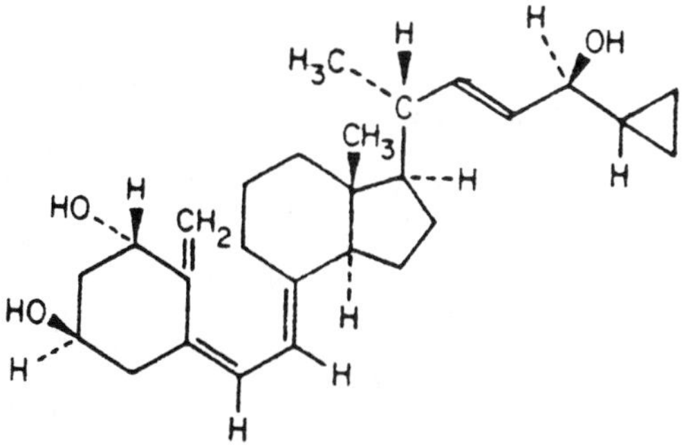

Calciptriene

B. Use: Calcipotriene ointment should be applied thinly to plaques twice daily, with a total dosage not >100 g/week.

C. Packaging:

Dovonex 0.005% cream: 30 g, 60 g, 100 g
Dovonex 0.005% ointment: 30 g, 60 g, 100 g
Dovonex 0.005% solution: 60 mL

V. Cantharidin, from the beetle *Cantharis vesicatoria*, causes intraepidermal vesiculation and is used in the treatment of warts and other benign cutaneous lesions. Cantharidin is extremely toxic if taken internally; it should not be prescribed for at-home use.

A. Structure

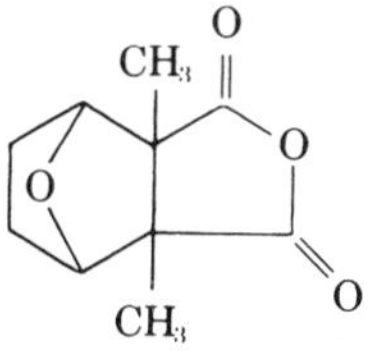

Cantharidin

B. Packaging:

Cantharidin 0.7%, as Cantharone: 7.5 mL

VI. Caustics are used alone in some circumstances and are often used to obtain hemostasis. They are also used in combination with electrosurgery for the superficial treatment of hyperplastic cutaneous lesions (warts, keratoses, xanthelasmas) and are also utilized in cosmetic therapy for aging, wrinkled facial skin.

A. Mono-, di-, and trichloroacetic acids [CCl_3COOH (trichloroacetic acid)] are rapid and effective local cauterizing agents. They are strongly corrosive and act by precipitation and coagulation of skin proteins. The monochloroacetic derivative is more deeply destructive than the trichloroacetic preparation; 35% to 50% trichloroacetic acid is, in general, the most useful preparation.

B. Silver nitrate ($AgNO_3$), in solid form or in solutions stronger than 5%, is used for its caustic action; 5% to 10% solutions may be applied to fissures or excessive granulation tissue. Silver nitrate sticks consist of a head of toughened silver nitrate (>94.5%) prepared by fusing the silver salt with sodium chloride. They are dipped in water and applied as needed.

1. Packaging:

Silver nitrate 100 sticks

VII. FU is a fluorinated pyrimidine antagonist that acts as an antimetabolite by interfering with DNA synthesis by inhibiting thymidylate synthetase activity. It is used topically for the treatment of multiple actinic keratoses, superficial basal cell carcinomas, and Bowen's disease; it also has been found useful in therapy of some types of warts.

The combination of 5-FU and topical tretinoin may be used in treating actinic keratoses resistant to 5-FU alone. Patients may be pretreated with 0.1% tretinoin cream 2 to 3 weeks before starting twice-daily applications of 5% 5-FU cream. The combination is continued until an inflammatory response to the actinic keratosis begins (approximately 2 weeks). The tretinoin is then discontinued, but the 5-FU is continued for an additional 2 to 3 weeks.

The mechanism for the synergy is unclear but may involve enhanced penetration of the 5-FU secondary to the keratolytic effects of the tretinoin. Also, both 5-FU and tretinoin may have complementary dual effects in inhibiting cellular function and better destruction of hyperproliferative cells.

5-FU has also been used topically in treating human papillomavirus (HPV) infections, especially flat facial warts. Erosion and ulceration are not necessary for a therapeutic response. Its use in preventing recurrent disease prophylactically has also been well recognized.

A. Structure

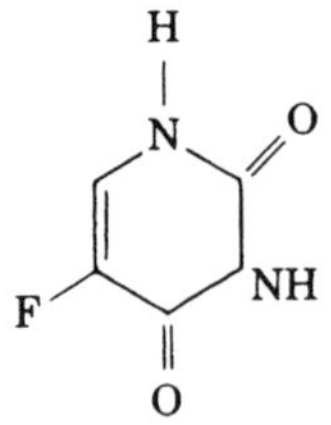

Fluorouracil

B. Packaging:

Fluorouracil 1% cream: 30 g
Fluorouracil 5% cream: 25 g
Fluorouracil 0.5% cream: 30 g
Fluorouracil 1% solution: 30 mL
Fluorouracil 2% solution: 10 mL
Fluorouracil 5% solution: 10 mL

VIII. Imiquimod (Aldara) is an imidazoquinolone amine that is an immune response modifier. Its exact mechanism is unknown in the topical treatment of HPV and molluscum contagiosum but may be related to the immunomodulating effect of the drug. It is also effective in the treatment of actinic keratoses and superficial basal cell carcinoma.

It induces production of a variety of cytokines and can enhance cell-mediated cytolytic antiviral activity. It is a rapid and potent inducer of interferon-α, interleukin-1 α and β, interleukin 6, interleukin 8, tumor necrosis factor-α, granulocyte-macrophage colony-stimulating factor, and granulocyte colony-stimulating factor. Systemic absorption is minimal. It is generally well tolerated. Adverse local reactions include erythema, erosion, excoriation, flaking, and edema of the treatment sites.

A. Use: Apply to affected area three times weekly before normal sleeping hours and leave on the skin for 6 to 10 hours, then rinse off. Treatment is continued until warts have cleared, generally 8 to 12 weeks. Several protocols have been proposed for treatment of actinic keratosis, basal cell carcinomas, and squamous cell carcinomas, including application every other day and application during weekdays only and breaks during weekends for 6 to 16 weeks.

B. Packaging:

Aldara 5% cream: 250 mg single dose packets, box of 12

IX. Podophyllum resin (podophyllin) is a chemically complex extract obtained from the roots of either of the two plants: *Podophyllum peltatum* (American) or *Podophyllum emodi* (Indian) (also called *Mandrake* or *May-apple*). Podofilox is the most cytotoxic ingredient in podophyllum resin (present in concentrations of 15% to 20% in *P. peltatum* and 30% to 40% in *P. emodi* resins) and exerts its effect by binding to intracellular microtubular proteins and thereby preventing the development of the mitotic spindle. *In vitro*, podophyllum also inhibits RNA synthesis. Podophyllum is used in the treatment of condyloma acuminata and other warts. It can induce severe erosive changes in adjacent normal skin and may produce serious systemic effects, including peripheral neuropathy, psychotoxic confusional states, adynamic ileus, renal damage, leukopenia, and thrombocytopenia, if applied too generously, especially on mucosal surfaces. Podophyllum is applied as a 25% suspension in compound tincture of benzoin or in alcohol at weekly intervals. Its use during pregnancy is contraindicated as it is a suspected teratogen.

Podofilox (formerly podophyllotoxin) is the active ingredient in podophyllin resin. It inhibits microtubular function by combining with free dimers of tubulin, the main structural component of microtubules. Application of 0.05 mL of podofilox 0.5% in lactate-buffered ethanol twice daily for 3 consecutive days each week appears safer than conventional podophyllin therapy, even when it is self-administered.

A. Structure

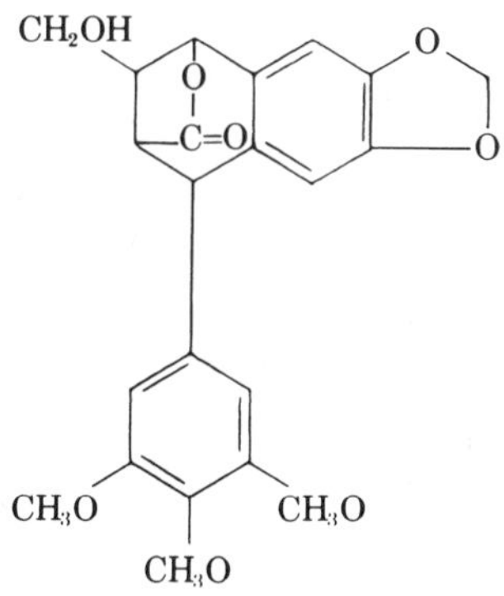

Podofilox

B. Use: Apply to affected areas only. Rinse off after 4 hours. Repeat treatment weekly as necessary.

C. Packaging:

Podofin [25% podophyllum resin (American) in compound tincture of benzoin]: 15 mL

Condylox (0.5% podofilox in lactate-buffered alcohol): 3.5 mL.

Cantharone Plus (podophyllin 5%, cantharidin 1%, salicylic acid 30% in octylphenyl polyethylene glycol 0.5%, cellosolve, ethocel, collodion, castor oil, and acetone): 7.5 mL.

X. Propylene glycol solution (40% to 60%, v/v $CH_2CH[OH]CH_2OH$, propylene glycol) applied to the skin under plastic occlusion hydrates the skin and causes desquamation of scales. Propylene glycol, isotonic in 2% concentration, is a widely used vehicle in dermatologic preparations. Hydroalcoholic gels containing propylene glycol or other substances augment the keratolytic action of salicylic acid. Keralyt gel consists of 6% salicylic acid, 19.4% alcohol, hydroxypropylcellulose, propylene glycol, and water and is an extremely effective keratolytic agent. Overnight occlusion is used nightly until improvement is evident, at which time the frequency of therapy can be decreased to every third night or once weekly. This therapy is well tolerated, is usually nonirritating, and has been most successful in patients with X-linked ichthyosis vulgaris. Burning and stinging may occur when applied to damaged skin. Patients with other abnormalities of keratinization with hyperkeratosis, scaling, and dryness may also benefit.

A. Packaging:
> Keralyt gel: 1 oz
> Epilyt solution (40% propylene glycol): 4 oz

XI. Resorcinol (resorcin), a phenol derivative, is less keratolytic than salicylic acid. This drug is an irritant and sensitizer and reported to be both bactericidal and fungicidal. Solutions containing 1% to 2% have been used in preparations for seborrhea, acne, and psoriasis.

A. Structure

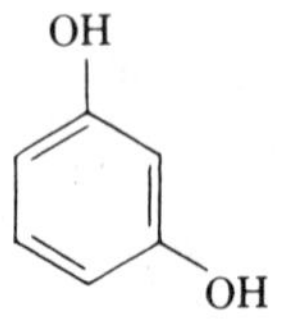

Resorcinol

XII. Retinoids (for information regarding isotretinoin or tretinoin, see Chap. 1). Acitretin (Soriatane) is a synthetic derivative of vitamin A that is particularly effective in treating the pustular and erythrodermic forms of psoriasis. It is the main metabolite of etretinate; ingestion of alcohol with acitretin increases the amount of detectable etretinate. It is accumulated in fatty tissue with a prolonged elimination half-life of approximately 120 days. Most patients show improvement within 2 to 4 weeks, although some patients may need as long as 6 months of therapy before a response is noted. Other disorders of keratinization, which may respond to acitretin, include Darier's disease, pityriasis rubra pilaris, lamellar ichthyosis, and hyperkeratotic palmaris and plantaris. Acitretin is teratogenic and is contraindicated during pregnancy. Pregnancy should be avoided for at least 1 year after discontinuation of treatment. *P. cerebri*, hepatotoxicity, and ocular changes may occur.

A. Structure

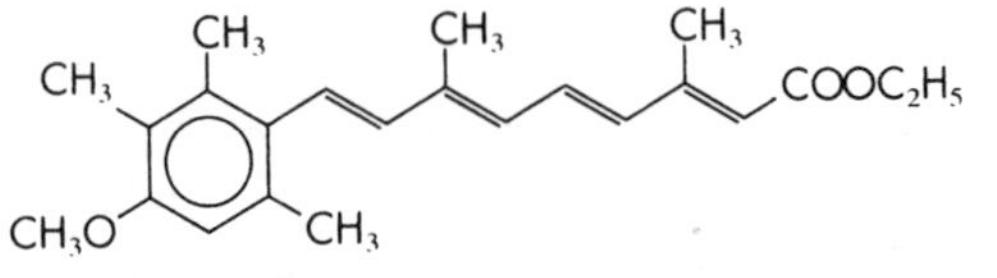

Etretinate

B. Use: Individualization of dosage is required to achieve maximum therapeutic response while minimizing side effects. Initiate treatment at 10 to 25 mg/day with food. Terminate treatment when resolution is achieved. Treat relapses as outlined for initial therapy. Baseline and treatment liver function tests, glucose, and cholesterol/triglyceride panel should be monitored throughout treatment. A baseline and monthly pregnancy test are required.

C. Packaging:
> Soriatane capsules: 10-mg, 25-mg tablets

XIII. Bexarotene (Targretin) is a member of a subclass of retinoids that selectively activate retinoid X receptors. It is used in the management of patch and plaque stages of cutaneous T-cell lymphoma (CTCL). It inhibits growth of tumor cell lines of hematopoietic and squamous cell origin. As it is a teratogen, its use is contraindicated in pregnant women.

A. Use: Apply to affected areas once every other day for the first week, then increase at weekly intervals to a final application of four times daily, depending on patient tolerance. Treatment is continued as long as benefit is appreciated.

B. Packaging:

Targretin 1% gel: 60 g

XIV. Salicylic acid is keratolytic and at concentrations between 3% and 6% causes softening of the horny layers and shedding of scales. It produces this desquamation by solubilizing the intercellular cement and enhances the shedding of corneocytes by decreasing cell-to-cell cohesion. In concentrations >6%, it can be destructive to tissue. Application of large amounts of the higher concentration of salicylic acid can also result in systemic toxicity. Salicylic acid is used in the treatment of superficial fungal infections, acne, psoriasis, seborrheic dermatitis, warts, and other scaling dermatoses. When it is combined with sulfur, some believe that a synergistic keratolytic effect is produced. Common preparations include a 3% and 6% ointment with equal concentration of sulfur; 6% propylene glycol solution (Keralyt); 5% to 20% with equal parts of lactic acid in flexible collodion for warts (Duofilm, Occlusal); in a cream base at any concentration for keratolytic effects; as a 60% ointment for plantar warts; and in a 40% plaster on velvet cloth for the treatment of calluses and warts (40% salicylic acid plaster).

A. Structure

Salicylic acid

B. Packaging:

Gel 17% salicylic acid: 7 g, 14 g, 14.2 g

Liquid 17% salicylic acid: 9 mL, 10 mL, 13.3 mL, 13.5 mL, 15 mL

Plasters 15%, 40%: 40% salicylic acid plasters (Dr Scholls, Mediplast)

XV. SELENIUM SULFIDE (See Cleansing Agents)

XVI. Sulfur is incorporated into many preparations used in the treatment of acne, rosacea, ringworm, psoriasis, scabies, seborrheic dermatitis, and infestations. Sulfur inhibits the growth of microorganisms, particularly fungi and parasites. More effective keratolytic, antifungal, and antibacterial agents are available.

XVII. TAR COMPOUNDS. A tar is a product of destructive distillation of organic substances. Tar is obtained from various sources and, therefore, there are different types. Wood tars include oil of cade, beech, birch, and pine. They do not photosensitize but are more allergenic than coal tars. Bituminous tars include ichthyol and ammonium ichthyosulphonate, a distillation of shale deposits containing fossilized fish. Coal tars are by-products of the destructive distillation of bituminous coals and are ill-defined, aromatic, and complex substances. They contain 2% to 8% light oils (benzene, toluene, xylene), 2% to 10% middle oils (phenols, cresols, naphthaline), 8% to 10% heavy oils (naphthaline and derivatives), 16% to 20% anthracene oils, and approximately 50% pitch. Coal tars are brown black, slightly soluble in water, and partially soluble in many solvents. Only coal tar and coal tar pitch have photosensitizing properties.

In hairless mice, coal tars have been shown to inhibit DNA synthesis. Five-percent crude coal tar ointment applied to normal human skin causes an initial transient hyperplasia followed by a 20% reduction in viable epidermal thickness after 40 days' treatment. These findings indicate that tar by itself can act as a cytostatic agent. Although coal tars are carcinogenic for the skin of experimental animals and are often used along with another oncogenic agent, ultraviolet light (UVL), the risk of developing cancer from therapeutic coal tar products remains unclear. The presence of unidentified mutagenic material(s) in the urine of patients with coal tar has been reported.

Tars have long been found to be useful in patients with eczematous, pruritic, and hyperplastic disease. They are often used in combination with sulfur, salicylic acid, and topical steroids and are used with UVB UVL in the therapy of psoriasis (see Chap. 27).

A. Coal tar products are available OTC or may be compounded to USP, NF, or other formulas.

    1. Estar gel:
        Tar (equivalent to crude coal tar) in hydroalcoholic base 5%

    2. Coal tar creams include Fototar (2%) and Tegrin (5%).

    3. Tar gels include Aquatar (2.5%), Estar (5%), P&S (8%), and PsoriGel (7.5%).

    4. Liquid tar preparations include MG217 lotion (5%), Oxipor (25%), and Doak Tar Distillate (40%)

    5. Tar ointments include Medotar (1%), Taraphilic (1%), and MG217 (10%).

    6. Bath preparations include Balnetar (2.5%), Cutar (7.5%), Polytar (25%)

    7. Examples of shampoos include DHS-T, Ionil T, Pentrax, T/Gel, Tegrin, and Zetar (many other brands are available).

    8. Tar soaps are Packer's Pine Tar, Tegrin, and Polytar.

B. Coal tar solution [liquor carbonis detergens (LCD)] is prepared by extracting coal tar with alcohol and polysorbate (Tween80), an emulsifying agent. Each 100 mL of the solution represents 20 g of coal tar. When mixed with water, a fine dispersion of coal tar results. LCD may be incorporated (at 2% to 5%) in creams or ointments, in tincture of green soap for a shampoo (10%), or added (60 mL) to the bath for antipruritic and other effects.

C. Ichthammol (Ichthyol) is obtained by the destructive distillation of certain bituminous schists (shale rock). It is less irritating than coal or wood tars, is water soluble, stains linens, and is used at 2% to 5% in the treatment of some subacute and chronic dermatoses.

D. Juniper tar, USP (cade oil), is obtained by destructive distillation of the heartwood of *Juniperus oxycedrus*. It contains hydrocarbons, including phenolic and aromatic compounds, and is used in the management of chronic eczema and psoriasis. It is available as an ointment, shampoo, bath solution, and soap.

XVIII. Urea-containing preparations have a softening and moisturizing effect on the stratum corneum and, at times, may provide good therapy for dry skin and the pruritus associated with it. They appear to have an antipruritic effect apart from their hydrating qualities. Urea compounds disrupt the normal hydrogen bonds of epidermal proteins; therefore, their effect in dry hyperkeratotic diseases such as ichthyosis vulgaris and psoriasis is not only to make the skin more pliable but also to help remove adherent scales. Lactic acid also has a softening and moisturizing effect on the stratum corneum.

A. Use: Apply b.i.d. to q.i.d.

B. Packaging:
        Urea 10% cream: 75 g
        Urea 20% cream: 75 g, 90 g, 120 g, 1 lb
        Urea 40% cream: 18.35 g, 30 g, 85 g, 199 g
        Urea 10% lotion: 180 mL, 240 mL
        Urea 25% lotion: 240 mL
        Urea 40% gel: 15 mL

XIX. Zinc pyrithione (see Cleaning Agents).

PIGMENTING AND DEPIGMENTING AGENTS, SUNSCREENS

I. DISCUSSION. See Chap. 17.

II. AGENTS THAT CAUSE HYPOPIGMENTATION

A. Hydroquinone products act to inhibit the enzymatic oxidation of tyrosine and suppress other melanocytic metabolic processes, thereby inhibiting melanin formation. Use of daily sunscreen and sun avoidance is paramount in the prevention of pigment recurrence. Effects are seen between 2 and 6 months.

1. Structure

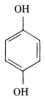

Hydroquinone

2. Use: Apply to hyperpigmented areas b.i.d.

3. Packaging:

Hydroquinone 1.5% cream: 14.2 g, 28.4 g, 85 g, 60 g, 120 g
Hydroquinone 2% cream: 28.4 g
Hydroquinone 2% gel: 14.2 g
Hydroquinone 3% solution: 30 mL
Hydroquinone 3% gel: 30 g
Hydroquinone 4% cream: 14.2 g, 28 g, 28.4 g, 45 g, 56.7 g
Hydroquinone 4% gel: 14.2 g, 28.4 g

B. Monobenzone is the monobenzyl ether of hydroquinone. It acts to increase the excretion of melanin from melanocytes and may prevent melanin production. In some patients, monobenzone causes destruction of melanocytes and permanent depigmentation. This treatment is utilized to irreversibly depigment normal skin surrounding vitiliginous lesions in patients with disseminated idiopathic vitiligo. These products should be used only when permanent depigmentation is desired, only after careful consideration by the patient and physician, and under close supervision. An irritant dermatitis may be seen with ongoing treatment.

1. Structure

Monobenzone

2. Use: Applied to normal skin two to three times a day. Results should be obtained in 1 to 4 months. Discontinue treatment after 4 months.

3. Packaging:

Benoquin 20% cream: 37.4 g

III. AGENTS THAT INDUCE HYPERPIGMENTATION AND REPIGMENTATION

A. Trioxsalen (Trisoralen) followed by UVA exposure is used to repigment vitiliginous areas (see Chap. 17) and in photochemotherapy (see Chaps 27 and 38).

1. Structure

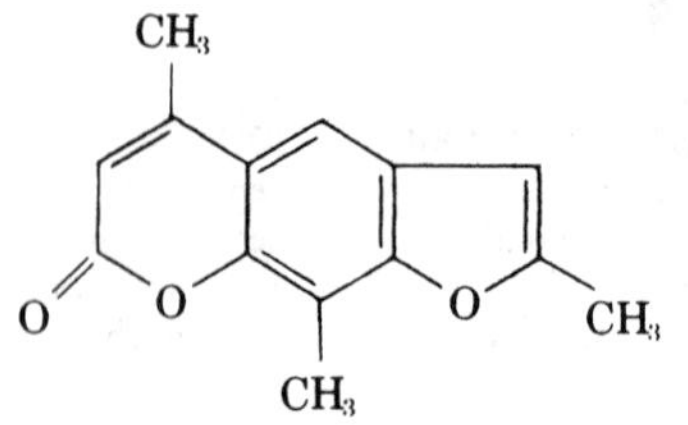

Trioxsalen

2. Packaging:

Trisoralen, 5-mg tablets: 28, 100, 1,000 tablet packs.

B. Methoxsalen has effects similar to those of trioxsalen. Methoxsalen is superior to trioxsalen in producing erythema and tanning and is the drug used in PUVA therapy. Methoxsalen is also available as a 1% lotion.

1. Structure

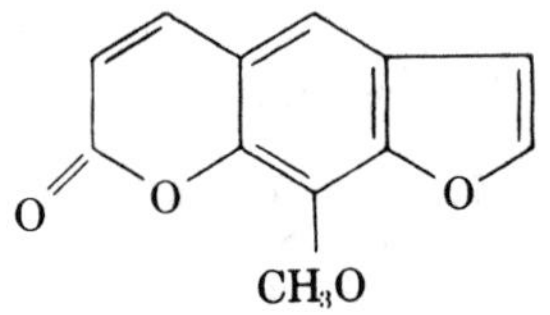

Methoxsalen

2. Packaging:

Oxsoralen-Ultra, 10-mg capsules: 50s
8-MOP 10-mg capsules: 50s
Oxsoralen, 1% lotion: 1 oz

IV. SUNSCREENS (see Chap. 33)

A. Physical blockers reflect and scatter UV rays, infrared radiation, and visible light. Inert compounds are ground into particles and suspended in a variety of bases. Disadvantages include messiness, grittiness, and color. Recently, clothing has also been manufactured to physically block UV rays.

1. Titanium dioxide
Includes Neutrogena Chemical Free, Ti-Screen, Vaseline Intensive Care, Hawaiian Tropic, Durascreen, and Sundown sunblocks

2. Sun Precautions advertises tightly woven lightweight nylon garments that provide SPF 30 protection, wet or dry.

B. Chemical sunscreens absorb various wavelengths of UVL and consequently allow only a limited amount of light to enter the tissue. They can be arbitrarily classified according to their effectiveness in absorbing UVA versus UVB rays.

1. UVA sunscreens

a. Benzophenone compounds absorb UVL well from 250 to 365 nm and somewhat from 365 to 400 nm. They are less effective than PABA compounds in the UVB sunburn spectrum.

i. Structure

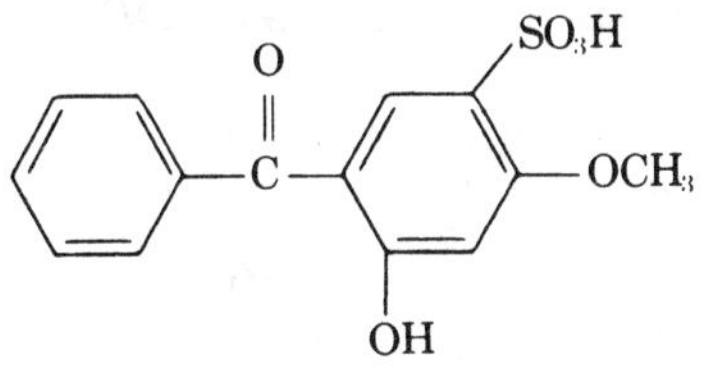

Sulisobenzone

ii. Packaging:

Includes Coppertone, Hawaiian Tropic, Ti-Screen, Tropical Gold, Water Babies, Solbar, Solbar PF, Bullfrog, PreSun, PreSun Ultra, Bain de Soleil, and Shade.

b. Parsol 1789 (Arobenzone) has excellent efficacy throughout the UVA spectrum (305 to 385 nm).

i. Packaging:

Shade UVA guard (octyl methoxycinnamate, arobenzone, oxybenzone): 4 oz

2. UVB sunscreens

a. PABA preparations absorb UVL between 280 and 320 nm. This acid will stain white fabrics, especially cotton. The esters of PABA are slightly less effective and do not stain as much. Cross-sensitization can occur with some sunscreens. In particular, PABA and its derivatives may cross-react with sulfonamides, benzocaine, procaine, paraphenylenediamine, and azo dyes. Padimate-O, the ester form of PABA, is also used for UVB protection. See Chap. 33 for commonly used sunscreens.

i. Structure

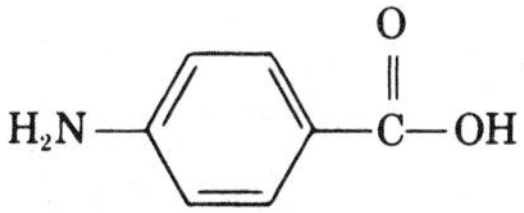

para-Aminobenzoic acid

b. Cinnamates absorb UVL from 390 to 320 nm. Salicylates absorb UVL in the 290- to 320-nm range. These sunscreen agents are often used in combination with benzophenones or PABA esters.

C. Others

1. Red veterinary petrolatum (RVP) has UVL-absorbing qualities to 340 nm and is also a water-protective agent because of its greasy base. It is available as a sunshade with zinc oxide added (RVPaque) and for lip protection with 5% PABA.

a. Packaging: and cost:

RVP (95% RVP): 1.25 oz
RV PABA lipstick (20% RVP, 5% PABA): 3.75 g

2. Sunshades physically block light, usually contain titanium dioxide or zinc oxide powders, and are opaque and usually tinted. They are not very effective unless a thick coat is applied.

WET DRESSINGS, BATHS, ASTRINGENTS

I. WET DRESSINGS
  A. The effects of wet dressings have been previously discussed (see Chap. 39).
  1. Open wet dressings are indicated in acute inflammatory states with exudation, oozing, and crusting. They are applied as follows:
  a. The patient should be in a comfortable position, usually in bed, with an impermeable material under the area to be compressed to prevent wetting the mattress.
  b. The dressings, which need not be sterile, should consist of 2- to 4-in. wide Kerlix, soft gauze, or soft linen such as old sheeting or pillowcases, handkerchiefs, or shirts.
  c. Moisten dressings by immersing them in the solution and then gently wringing them out. They should be sopping wet, but not dripping. Solutions should be warm or tepid. Cover with a soft towel or cloth that will allow evaporation.
  d. Apply or wrap around the skin loosely. Multiple layers, at least six to eight, should be applied to prevent rapid drying and cooling.
  e. Dressings should be removed, remoistened, and reapplied every 10 to 15 minutes, for between 30 minutes and 2 hours t.i.d. It is difficult to completely moisten dressings in place, and resoaking is often needed to remove accumulated and adherent exudate and crusts. If frequent changes are impracticable, an IV bottle with the wet dressing solution may be suspended over the bed and the material slowly fed into the dressing through IV tubing. Alternatively, the dressing should simply be removed every 2 to 3 hours and reapplied. It is usually difficult for patients to care for their own dressings.
  f. After dressings are removed, a lotion, powder, liniment, or paste may be applied to the skin. Occlusion of exudative skin with ointments should be avoided.
  g. Dressing material should be discarded daily, but some, such as Kerlix, may be laundered and reused.
  h. If large areas of skin are compressed at once, chilling and hypothermia may result. In general, no more than one third of the body should be treated at any time.
  2. Closed wet dressings will cause maceration and retain heat and are used in the treatment of conditions such as cellulitis and abscesses. The foregoing instructions should be followed, but warm dressings should be covered with plastic, oilcloth, or other impermeable material.
  B. Solutions for wet dressings are either astringents or antiseptic agents. Astringents precipitate protein and thereby decrease oozing. The principal astringents are salts of aluminum, zinc, lead, iron, bismuth, tannins, or other polyphenolic compounds.
  1. Aluminum acetate [Al(OCOCH$_3$)$_3$, Burow's solution], containing approximately 5% aluminum acetate, is diluted 1:10 to 1:40 for use. Probably the most widely used astringent for wet dressings, it is easy to use, does not stain, and is drying and soothing.

  Domeboro or Bluboro powder packets or tablets quickly dissolve in water to make fresh aluminum diacetate available. One packet or tablet in 1 pt of water yields a 1:40 dilution (two packets at 1:20 dilution); 30 minutes of evaporation, however, will concentrate a 1:40 solution to 1:10, at which point the aluminum salts may become too irritating and drying.
  a. Packaging:
      Domeboro (aluminum sulfate and calcium acetate):
      12 packets
      12 tablets
      Bluboro (aluminum sulfate, calcium acetate, FD&C blue dye):
      12 packets
  2. Potassium permanganate (KMnO$_4$) is an oxidizing agent that is rapidly rendered inactive in the presence of organic material. The oxidizing action of the chemical is purportedly responsible for its germicidal activity. It is also an astringent

and a fungicide. This preparation stains the skin and clothing, and undissolved crystals will cause a chemical burn. It is used less commonly now (primarily as an antifungal agent) and may be little better than water as a wet dressing. A 1:4,000 to 1:16,000 dilution is used on weeping or denuded surfaces (one crushed 65-mg tablet dissolved in 250 to 500 mL; one 330-mg tablet dissolved in 1,500 mL to 3,000 mL). For use as a medicated bath, 8 g (approximately 2 tsp) should be dissolved in 200 L (a full bathtub) of water to produce about a 1:25,000 dilution. Skin stains may be removed with a weak solution of oxalic acid or sodium thiosulfate.

3. Normal saline (0.9% sodium chloride) may be approximated by adding 1 level tsp of salt to 480 mL water.

4. Silver nitrate, 0.1% to 0.5%, is an excellent germicide and astringent. Its germicidal action is due to precipitation of bacterial protein by liberated silver ions. It may cause pain if applied in concentrations >0.5%. A 0.25% solution may be prepared by adding 1 tsp of the stock 50% aqueous solution to 1,000 mL of cool water. Silver nitrate stains skin dark brown after exposure to air and will stain black any metal container (including the teaspoon) and everything else that it touches.

5. Compresses with 5% acetic acid reduce the microbial count in infected wounds and are used primarily for infections involving *P. aeruginosa*.

II. BATHS

A. Baths and soaks are useful in treating widespread eruptions. Evaporation is impeded, and, therefore, there is less drying and cooling. Nevertheless, baths and soaks may be very soothing, antipruritic, and somewhat antiinflammatory. The tub should be half full (approximately 100 L, or 25 gal, of water) and the duration of exposure limited to 30 minutes. Many of the bath oils make the tub very slippery.

1. Soothing and antipruritic colloid additives

a. Oatmeal contains 50% starch with approximately 25% protein and 9% oil. Mix one cup Aveeno oatmeal and two cups of cold tap water, shake, and pour into a tub of lukewarm water. Oilated Aveeno contains an additional 35% mineral oil and lanolin derivative for emollient action.

i. Packaging:
Aveeno, 30-g packets: 454 g
Oilated Aveeno: 240 mL

b. Starch baths are best prepared by mixing two cups of a hydrolyzed starch, such as Linit, with four cups of cold tap water to form a paste, then adding this to a tub of lukewarm water. A mixture of equal parts of sodium bicarbonate (baking soda) and starch is often used as a soothing colloidal bath powder.

2. Bath oils are added to tub water to help prevent drying of the skin. Most contain a mineral or a vegetable oil and also a surfactant. Theoretically, the patient absorbs a portion of the oil around him. There are two types of bath oils: those that are dispersed throughout the bath and those that lie on the surface of the water and coat the surface of the body as the patient leaves the tub. If nothing else, bath oils are pleasant, but patients occasionally note mild pruritus immediately after their use. The following are some pleasing preparations; some patients will prefer one to another: Alpha Keri, Aveeno, Lubriderm, Nutraderm, and RoBathol.

a. Packaging:
Alpha Keri oil bath: 240 mL
Nutraderm oil bath: 240 mL

 WOUND DRESSINGS

I. DISCUSSION. The realization that a moist wound environment facilitates healing can be dated only to the early 1950s. Several types of occlusive dressings have been developed and are currently employed in the treatment of cutaneous ulcers. Each of these dressings has certain advantages and disadvantages, which are summarized in Table 40-7.

TABLE 40-7   Summary of Selected Synthetic Dressings

Type	Advantages	Disadvantages	Brand: packaging/cost: s = sheet(s)
Alginates	1. Absorbent 2. Useful in cavities 3. Hemostatic	1. ± Difficult to remove 2. ± Painful if dries 3. ± Odor	1. Kaltostat: 4 × 4 in. (1s) 2. Sorbsan: 10 × 20 in. (1s) 3. Algosteril: 3-3/4 × 3-3/4 in. (10s)
Films	1. Adherent 2. Transparent 3. Bacterial barrier	1. Nonabsorbent 2. ± Difficult to handle 3. May strip epithelium on removal	1. Bioclusive: 8 × 10 in. (10s) 2. Omniderm: 6 × 8 in. (10s) 3. Opsite: 5 × 4 in. (1s) 4. Tegaderm: 4 × 10 in. (1s)
Foams	1. Absorbent 2. Moist 3. Conforms to contours	1. Can adhere to wound if exudate dries	1. Lyofoam: 11 × 9 in. (30s) 2. Alleryn: 4 × 4 in. (1s)
Hydrocolloids	1. Enhanced wound healing 2. Waterproof 3. Easy to use 4. Adherent	1. Unpleasant odor 2. Yellow drainage 3. Difficult in cavities 4. ± Maceration of surrounding skin 5. Opaque 6. May stimulate excess granulation tissue	1. Comfeel: 8 × 8 in. (5s) 2. Duoderm: 6 × 6 in. (3s) 3. Tegasorb: 4 × 4–3/4 in. (5s)
Hydrogels	1. Comfortable 2. Absorbent 3. Semitransparent	1. Nonadherent 2. Maceration of skin around wound 3. Expensive	1. Nu-Gel: 6 × 8 in. (5s) 2. Vigilon (nonsterile): 4 × 4 in. (10s) 3. Vigilon (sterile): 4 × 4 in. (10s)
Laminates	1. Absorbent 2. Conforms to contours		1. Biobrane: 10 × 10 in. (5s)
Polysaccharides	1. Absorbent 2. Antiseptic 3. Desloughing	1. Odor 2. Difficult to handle/remove 3. Can dry out the wound bed	1. Debrisan: 60 g 2. Duoderm granules: 5 g

Source: Modified from Phillips TJ, Dover JS.JS. Leg ulcers. *J Am Acad Dermatol* 1991;25(6 Pt 1):965–987.

Occlusive dressings alter several aspects of the wound environment that would account for their efficacy. The presence of moisture alone has been shown to enhance the rate of reepithelialization. By trapping wound fluid next to the wound surface, occlusive dressings protect the wound bed from drying and from trauma. There is a transient influx of inflammatory cells into the wound, which may not only aid in the digestion of necrotic debris but also help prevent overt bacterial infection. The wound fluid also contains a variety of growth factors that could affect epidermal migration and connective tissue formation, as well as provide an ideal environment for the survival of epidermal cells. Regardless of whether they are oxygen permeable, occlusive dressings create a low-pH, low-oxygen environment, conditions that apparently facilitate both dermal and epidermal healing. When properly applied, occlusive dressings may act as a physical barrier to outside contaminants. Furthermore, they may ameliorate pain either by a direct cooling effect or, perhaps, by interference with arachidonic acid metabolism.

Occlusive dressings are not without their drawbacks. Improper application with wrinkling and folding may allow the leakage of exudate onto surrounding normal skin with enlargement of the ulcer. A transient increase in bacterial counts is observed after the application of occlusive dressings and does not normally result in clinical signs of infection. Nonetheless, in a study of six commercially available dressings applied to wounds inoculated with bacterial pathogens (*S. aureus, S. pyogenes*, and *P. aeruginosa*), none was able to prevent clinical infection. The fact that overt infection is an uncommon complication of the use of these dressings might simply reflect clinicians' hesitancy to use them on grossly infected wounds. Before choosing an occlusive dressing, it is critical to identify and treat any underlying causes of the wound. For instance, occlusive dressings, often used in treating distal leg ulcers, would be of little benefit in patients with untreated venous insufficiency or malignancy as the cause of the ulcer.

Specifics of the application of these dressings vary depending on the type, particularly whether it is self-adhering. Initially, the dressing should be changed once or twice a day as the amount of accumulating exudate dictates. With time, dressings may need to be changed only once a week. It cannot be overemphasized that occlusive dressings are an adjunct to wound care, and proper assessment and management of any underlying predisposing pathology are imperative.

II. **PACKAGING** (see Table 40-7)
   A. 2-Octyl cyanoacrylate (Dermabond) is a fast-setting topical skin adhesive intended to close easily approximated skin edges of wounds from surgical incisions, including punctures from minimally invasive surgery and simple, thoroughly cleansed, trauma-induced lacerations. It may be used in conjunction with, but not in place of, subcuticular sutures. It is contraindicated for use on any wounds with evidence of active infection, areas under high skin tension, mucocutaneous surfaces, or skin regularly exposed to body fluids. Patients with formaldehyde allergies may react to this topical solution.
      1. Packaging (Ethicon, Inc):
         Dermabond liquid: 0.5-mL single-use crushable glass ampules
   B. Becaplermin (Regranex) is a recombinant platelet-derived growth factor that is used topically as adjunctive therapy in the treatment of lower extremity diabetic neurotropic ulcers that extend into the subcutaneous tissue or deeper.
      1. Use: Apply to ulcer once daily until ulcer is healed.
      2. Packaging (Ortho-McNeil):
         Regranex 100 μg: 2-g, 7.5-g, 15-g multiuse tubes
   C. Apligraf is a bioengineered human skin equivalent used in the treatment of venous ulcers. It is composed of living keratinocytes and dermal fibroblasts derived from neonatal foreskin and propagated in culture. A gel of dermal fibroblasts and type I bovine collagen is formed, allowed to contract, and overlaid with neonatal keratinocytes to form a bilayered construct. It is able to produce its own matrix proteins and growth factors. Melanocytes are absent. It has a 5-day shelf life.
      1. Use: Apply to noninfected ulcer under compression dressing for 2 weeks.
      2. Packaging (Organogenesis, Inc., and Novartis):
         Apligraf: 7.5-cm diameter sheet

Appendix

FOUNDATIONS, INSTITUTES AND SUPPORT GROUPS

AIDS

Foundation for AIDS Research
AMFAR
120 Wall Street, 13th Floor
New York, NY 10005
Phone: 212-806-1600
Fax: 212-806-1601

National HIV/AIDS Hotline
Centers for Disease Control and Prevention
CDC HIV/AIDS Hotline
800-342-AIDS
1600 Clifton Road, Atlanta, GA
30333, U.S.A.
Phone: 404-639-3311/
Public Inquiries:
404-639-3534/800-311–3435
Email: cdcinfo@cdc.gov
Web: www.cdc.gov

Pediatric AIDS Foundation
2950 31st Street
Suite 125
Santa Monica, CA 90405
Phone: 310-395-9051
Fax: 310-314-1469

Albinism

National Organization for Albinism
   & Hypopigmentation
PO Box 959
East Hampstead, NH 03826-0959
Phone: 603-887-2310
Fax: 603-887-6049
E-mail: info@albinsim.org
Web: www.albinism.org

Alopecia Areata

National Alopecia Areata Foundation
PO Box 150760
San Rafael, CA 94915
Phone: 415-472-3780
Fax: 415-472-5343
E-mail: info@naaf.org
Web: www.naaf.org

Behcet's

American Behcet's Disease Association
PO Box 280240
Memphis, TN 38168
Phone: 800-723-4238
Web: www.w2.com/behcets.html

Birthmarks

Vascular Birthmark Foundation
PO Box 106
Latham, NY 12110
Contact: Linda Shannon, Executive
Director
Phone: 877-VBF-LOOK
Phone: 877-VBF-4646 (evenings and
weekends)
Web: www.birthmark.org

Sturge-Weber Foundation
PO Box 418
Mt. Freedom, NJ 07970
Phone: 800-627-5482
Web: www.sturge-weber.com

Cancer

American Cancer Society
100 West Palatine Road
#150 Palatine, IL 60067
Phone: 800-ACS-2345
Web: www.cancer.org

National Cancer Institute
Office of Communications
9000 Rockville Pike
Bldg. 31, Room 10-A-31
Bethesda, MD 20892
Phone: 800-4-CANCER
Fax: 301-402-4945
Web: www.cancer.gov

National Coalition for Cancer Survivorship
1010 Wayne Avenue, Suite 505
Silver Spring, MD 20910-5600
Phone: 888-937-6227
Fax: 301-565-9670
Email: minfo@cansearch.org
Web: www.cansearch.org

Skin Cancer Foundation
245 Fifth Avenue
Suite 1403
New York, NY 10016
Phone: 212-725-5176 or (800) SKIN-490
Fax: 212-725-5751
E-mail: info@skincancer.org
Web: www.skincancer.org

American Melanoma Foundation
3914 Murphy Canyon Road, Suite A132
San Diego, CA 92123
Phone: 858-277-4426
E-mail:
sunsmartz@melanomafoundation.org
Web: www.melanomafoundation.org

Also see:
Skin Cancer Updates on the AAD site
MelanomaNet

Chickenpox
VZV Research Foundation
24 East 64th Street, Floor 2
New York, NY 10021
Phone: 212-371-7280
Fax: 212-371-7277
Web: www.vzvfoundation.org

The National Eczema Association for
Science & Education (N.E.A.S.E.)
4460 Redwood Highway, #16D
San Rafael, CA 94903
Phone: 800-818-7546
Web:www.nationaleczema.org
info@nationaleczema.org

Epidermolysis
National Epidermolysis Bullosa Registry
Jo-David Fine, M.D., Principal Investigator
University of North Carolina—Chapel Hill
National EB Registry
Bolin Heights Building #1
CB #3369
Chapel Hill, NC 27514-3369
Phone: 919-966-2007
Fax: 919-966-7080
Email: EB_registry@med.unc.edu

Epidermodysplasia Verruciformis
Paul E. Keener Registry
Robert Byrd Health Sciences Center
Box 9167
Morgantown, WV 26506
Phone: 304-293-2804
Fax: 304-293-8824

Erythema Multiforme
Stevens-Johnson's Syndrome Foundation
PO Box 350333
Westminster, CO 80035
Phone: 303-635-1241
Fax: 303-469-2528
E-mail: sjsupport@aol.com
Web: www.stevensjohnsonsyndrome.net

General Dermatology
Department of Dermatology
University of Iowa
www.dermatology.uiowa
Infoderm
www.infoderm.com
Dermquest
www.dermquest.com
Matrix
www.matrix.ucdavis.edu
Mayo Clinic
www.mayo.edu

General Information
American Academy of Dermatology
www.aad.org
National Institutes of Health (NIH)
www.nih.gov
National Library of Medicine
www.nlm.nih.gov

Genetic Disease
The Genetic Alliance
4301 Connecticut Avenue, NW
Suite 404
Washington, DE 20008
Phone: 202-966-5557
Fax: 202-966-8553
Helpline 800-336-GENE
E-mail: info@geneticalliance.org
Web: www.geneticalliance.org

Herpes
Herpes Resource Center
American Social Health Association
P.O. Box 13827
Research Triangle Park, NC 27709
Contact: Leigh Jolley, Program
    Coordinator
Phone: 919-361-8488 (National Herpes
    Hotline)
Purchase Herpes Info 800-230-6039
Web: www.ashastd.org

Human Papillomavirus
HPV Support Program
American Social Health Association
P.O. Box 13827
Research Triangle Park, NC 27709
Phone: 919-361-8400
Web: www.ashastd.org

Ichthyosis
Foundation for Ichthyosis & Related
  Skin Types, Inc. (F.I.R.S.T)
1601 Valley Forge Road
Lansdale, PA 19446
Phone: 215-631-1411 or 800-545-3286
Fax: 215-631-1413
Email: info@scalyskin.org
Web: www.scalyskin.org

National Registry for Ichthyosis &
  Related Skin Disorders
University of Washington
PO Box 356524
Seattle, WA 98195
Phone: 800-595-1265 or 206-616-3179
Fax: 206-616-3179
Email: ichreg@u.washington.edu

Lice
See Pediculosis

Lupus
Lupus Foundation of America, Inc.
2000 L St., NW, #710
Washington, DC 20036
Phone: 202-349-1155
Fax: 202-349-1156
Web: info@lupus.org

Melanoma
See Skin Cancer

Nevi
Nevus Network
Congenital Nevus Support Group
PO Box 1981
Woodbridge, VA 22193
Phone: 703-492-0253
Fax: 405-377-3403
Email: nevusnet@bigfoot.com
Web: www.nevusnetwork.org

Nevus Outreach, Inc.
600 S. Delaware, Suite 200
Bartlesville, OK 74003
Phone: 918-331-0595
Fax: 281-417-4020
Nevus Hot Line 877-426-3887
Web: www.nevus.org

Pediculosis
National Pediculosis Association
50 Kearney Road
Needham, MA 02494
Phone: 781- 449-NITS
Fax: 781-449-8129
E-mail: npa@headlice.org
Web: www.headlice.org

Pediatric Dermatology
The Society for Pediatric Dermatology
5422 North Bernard
Chicago, IL 60625
Phone: 773-583-9780
Fax: 773-583-9765
E-mail: Patrici107@aol.com
Web: www.pedsderm.net

Pemphigus
National Pemphigus Foundation
1540 River Park Drive, #208
Sacramento, CA 95815
Phone: 916-922-1298
Fax: 916-922-1458
E-mail: pemphigus@pemphigus.org
Web: www.pemphigus.org

Port Wine Stain
Sturge-Weber Foundation
PO Box 418
Mt. Freedom, NJ 07970
Phone: 800-627-5482
Web: www.sturge-weber.com

Postherpetic Neuralgia
VZV Research Foundation
40 East 72nd Street
New York, NY 10021
Phone: 212-472-3181
Fax: 212-861-7033
E-mail: rtp@vzvfoundation.org
Web: www.vzvfoundation.org

Psoriasis
National Psoriasis Foundation
6600 SW 92nd Avenue, Suite 300
Portland, OR 97223-7195
Phone: 503-244-7404 or 800-723-9166
Fax: 503-245-0626
E-mail: getinfo@psoriasis.org

Rosacea

National Rosacea Society
800 South Northwest Highway
Suite 200
Barrington, IL 60010
Contact: Suzanne Corr
Phone: 847-382-8971 or 888-NO BLUSH
Fax: 847-382-5567
E-mail: rosaceas@aol.com
Web: www.rosacea.org

Shingles (Herpes Zoster)

VZV Research Foundation
40 East 72nd Street
New York, NY 10021
Phone: 800-472-VIRUS or 212-472-3181
Fax: 212-861-7033
E-mail: rtp@vzvfoundation.org
Web: www.vzvfoundation.org

Social Health

American Social Health Association
P.O. Box 13827
Research Triangle Park, NC 27709
Contact: Linda Alexander, PhD, FAAN,
   Executive Director
Phone: 919-361-8400
Fax: 919-361-8425
Web: www.ashastd.org

Surgery

American Society of Dermatologic Surgery
www.asds.net.org

Vitiligo

National Organization for Albinism
   & Hypopigmentation
PO Box 959
East Hampstead, NH 03826-0959
Phone: 603-887-2310
Fax: 603-887-6049
E-mail: info@albinsim.org
Web: www.albinism.org

National Vitiligo Foundation
PO Box 6117
Tyler, TX 75711
Phone: 903-595-3713
Email: info@nvfi.org

Note: Page numbers followed by *f* indicate figures; those followed by *t* indicate tables and those followed by *p* indicate color inserts.